Ototoxic Drugs Exposed

The Shocking Truth About Prescription Drugs, Medications, Chemicals and Herbals That Can (and Do) Damage Our Ears

Ototoxic Drugs Exposed

The Shocking Truth About Prescription Drugs, Medications, Chemicals and Herbals That Can (and Do) Damage Our Ears

Third Edition

Neil G. Bauman, Ph.D.

Integrity First Publications

Lynden, WA

http://IntegrityFirstPublications.com

Ototoxic Drugs Exposed
The Shocking Truth About Prescription Drugs, Medications, Chemicals and Herbals That Can (and Do) Damage Our Ears

Third Edition

Another **Integrity First** book in the series:

Everything You Wanted to Know About Your Hearing Loss But Were Afraid to Ask
(Because You Knew You Wouldn't Hear the Answers Anyway!)

Copyright © 2002, 2003, 2010 by Neil G. Bauman

ISBN 978-1-935939-00-9

Integrity First Publications

1013 Ridgeway Drive,
Lynden, WA 98264-1057
Phone: (360) 778-1266
FAX: (360) 389-5226
Email: info@IntegrityFirstPublications.com
Website: http://IntegrityFirstPublications.com

Printed in the United States of America

Trademarks

Trademarked names appear throughout this book. Rather than list the names and entities that own the trademarks, or insert a trademark symbol with each mention of the trademarked name, the publisher states that it is using the names with no intention of infringing upon that trademark. To this end, all the brand names of drugs and chemicals are printed in italics with the initial letter capitalized. These brand names are the registered trademarks of their respective pharmaceutical and chemical companies.

Warning—Disclaimer

I dedicate this book to

Diane

my wife

helper

encourager

companion

best friend

co-worker

and editor

About the Author

Neil G. Bauman, Ph.D., (Dr. Neil) is the executive director of the Center for Hearing Loss Help in Pennsylvania. He is a hearing loss coping skills specialist, researcher, author and speaker on issues pertaining to hearing loss. No stranger to hearing loss himself, he has lived with a life-long severe hereditary hearing loss.

Dr. Neil did not let his hearing loss stop him from achieving what he wanted to do. He earned several degrees in fields ranging from forestry to ancient astronomy (Ph.D.) and theology (Th.D.) in addition to his extensive studies in fields related to hearing loss.

For the past number of years, Dr. Neil has researched a variety of hearing loss issues, including extensive studies into the effects of ototoxic drugs on our ears. His mission is helping hard of hearing people understand and successfully cope with their hearing losses and other ear conditions. To this end, he provides education, support and counsel to hard of hearing people through personal contact, as well as through his books, articles, presentations and seminars.

Dr. Neil is the author of eleven books and more than 1,000 articles on hearing-loss related topics. (See the back of this book for a list of his books.) He is also a dynamic presenter, and speaks throughout the USA and Canada.

You can contact him at:

Neil Bauman, Ph.D.
Center for Hearing Loss Help
1013 Ridgeway Drive
Lynden, WA 98264-1057
Phone: (360) 778-1266
FAX: (260) 389-5226
Email: neil@hearinglosshelp.com
Web site: http://hearinglosshelp.com

Contents

Preface

Each year more than 1,000,000 people in the United States experience drug-related poisoning.[1] Of these, approximately 100,000 die! According to another source, these figures are much too conservative. They estimate that in 1999, 2,000,000 people were hospitalized and 140,000 died from the side effects of, or reactions to, prescription drugs! Yet another source says that at least a million people are severely injured each year by the medications they take and an additional million people are harmed by drugs given to them during their hospital stays.[2]

Put another way, doctors estimate that between 3 and 7% of adverse drug reactions require hospitalization. While in hospitals, about 20% of the patients experience adverse drug reactions. About 1% of these patients die from these drug reactions.[3]

These are shocking statistics. The cost of this drug-induced carnage is more shocking still. Current estimates tell us that adverse drug events and medical errors cost more than 100 billion dollars a year![4] Not only is this totally ridiculous, it is totally unnecessary.

Of the people who survive this drug assault on their bodies, some soon discover to their shock and sorrow that prescription drugs have also insidiously attacked their ears leaving them condemned to the eerie world of semi-silence.

In the course of talking with and helping thousands of people with hearing losses, I am appalled at the enormous number of people who have lost some (or all) of their hearing or balance from taking drugs prescribed by their doctors. Most of these unfortunate people were never told that taking such drugs could (and often would) damage their ears. In fact, many doctors don't even know that many of the drugs they prescribe do indeed damage ears.

The fancy name for drugs that can damage our ears is ototoxic drugs. (The correct pronunciation is OH-toe-TOX-ik, although some people say AH-toe-TOX-ik).

Ototoxic?

Doctors don't know anywhere near as much as they should about hearing loss and drugs. Shari once asked her doctor if a drug he was prescribing for her was ototoxic. He replied, "Oto *what*?"

One lady told me that when challenged, her doctor couldn't name even one ototoxic drug! Ototoxic drugs are not unknown. In 1999, audiologist Richard Carmen wrote that there were at least 130 drugs and chemicals already identified as ototoxic.[5] (You now hold in your hands a book that lists 1,060 ototoxic substances.) How come no one seems to know about them? There is abysmal ignorance concerning ototoxic drugs by both health care professionals and the public in general. Doctors need to realize that the indiscriminate use of many prescription drugs has been responsible for many people suffering from unnecessary hearing loss, tinnitus and balance problems.

I have attempted to make this book as comprehensive as possible. To this end, I have included all the known (to me) ototoxic drugs used in Canada, the United States, Great Britain and indeed, from any country in the world where I could find reliable information in English.

If you live or travel elsewhere in the world, you should know that there are more than 10,000 prescription drugs that are not available in the USA.[6] No doubt, many of these drugs are also ototoxic. Unfortunately, I can't find much ototoxic information about them, so the information on foreign drugs contained in this book is often incomplete and generally rather sparse. In any case, I have included all the ototoxic information I have come across.

Drugs can be useful in the treatment of various disorders. At the same time, you need to have a realistic understanding of what drugs can and cannot do. Very seldom do drugs miraculously reverse a fatal illness. "Aside from antibiotics for a few infections, drugs that make a disease totally and permanently disappear are almost unknown".[7]

If You Have Further Information

If you have information on ototoxic drugs not listed in this book, or if you have further information on ototoxic side effects not included for a drug in this book, I would be glad to hear from you. I want to continue to make this book as complete as possible.

You can reach me at the Center for Hearing Loss Help (neil@hearinglosshelp.com or www.hearinglosshelp.com) or through the publisher, Integrity First Publications. See either the front or back of this book for contact information.

Drugs usually only relieve the **symptoms** of an illness such as pain, anxiety, angina, etc.,[8] but they do **not** remove or fix the underlying **cause**. At the same time, they cause adverse side effects. This is the reality of drug treatment. You need to decide if you want to risk your precious ears in order to treat a symptom rather than do something to root out the cause of a disorder.

The rule in buying goods and services is *caveat emptor*—let the buyer beware. This is the same warning I leave with you concerning any drugs you may consider taking.

For the record, I am not a medical doctor, audiologist, pharmacist or biochemist, nor do I pretend to be any of these. Rather, my expertise lies in educating people and helping them understand and successfully live with their hearing losses. If this book helps you save even some of your precious hearing or balance, I will have achieved my goal.

Neil Bauman, Ph.D.
Lynden, WA

1   Silverman, 2000. p. xi.
2   Freundlich, 1998. p. 1.
3   DiSogra, 2001. p. 5.
4   Rybacki, 2001. pp. xvii, xxiii.
5   Carmen, 1999. p. 37.
6   *International Retail Prices for Prescription Drugs*, 2001. p. 1.
7   Flieger, 1995. p. 5.
8   Flieger, 1995. p. 2.

Chapter 1

How to Effectively Use This Book

This book contains three types of information. This chapter teaches you how to effectively use this book. The second section (Chapters 2 through 13) explains what ototoxic drugs are, what you need to know about them, and what you can do to help yourself lessen their effects on your ears. The third (and major) section (Chapters 14 through 16) lists specific information on each ototoxic drug, herbal and chemical.

Quick Start

If you want to dive right in and look up a specific drug or chemical and find out what its ototoxic properties are, here's how to do it fast. (However, I strongly urge you to read this entire chapter first, or read along as you are looking up a drug, since this chapter explains what the various headings, authorities and risk assessment classes mean.)

Drugs

If you want to look up a drug, turn to Chapter 14, the main drug section (pages 165 - 627). Drugs are listed in alphabetical order. Brand (trade) names are in *italics*, generic ototoxic drug names in **bold** and alternate generic drug names in regular type.

You will find the details of each drug under the drug's generic name. If you don't know the generic name, look for the brand name and it will "point" you to the correct generic drug where you will find the details about this drug's known ototoxic properties and other information.

Herbals

Chapter 15 contains information on ototoxic herbals (pages 661 – 677). Follow the same procedures used above for looking up drugs. The detailed herbal listings are in alphabetical order by their genus and species (**bold**), while common names are in regular type.

Chemicals

If you want to look up a chemical, go to Chapter 16 (pages 679 - 758). Chemicals are listed in alphabetical order. The most common generic chemical name for each chemical is in **bold**. Alternate names for this chemical are in regular type, while any trade names are in *italics*.

You will find the details of each chemical under its most common generic chemical name. If you don't know the generic chemical name, look for a known brand name or other alternate chemical name, and it will "point" you to the correct generic chemical name where you will find the details about this chemical's known ototoxic properties and other information.

Legend

Throughout this book, I use certain conventions. Drug classes are in SMALLCAPITALLETTERS. The first letter of each generic drug name is capitalized. If the drug is ototoxic, it is printed in **bold**. Trade or brand names of drugs are in *italics* to show they are registered trade names. For example, the AMINO-GLYCOSIDE ANTIBIOTIC **Tobramycin** is sold under such trade names as *Nebcin*, *Tobradex* and *Tobrex* while the LOOP DIURETIC **Furosemide** is sold under such brand names as *Furoside*, *Lasix* and *Uritol* (among others).

If you are unsure whether the substance you want to look up is a drug, herb or chemical, check all three tables.

Now the Details for the Drugs

Each of the individual drug listings follow the same standard format to make it easy for you to find the information you want. This also makes it easy to compare between drugs.

This standard format has the following headings in this order: "Generic drug name," "Pronunciation guide," "Drug classification," "Brand names," "Ototoxic effects," "Risk assessment" and "Notes" (if there are any). The following sections explain the contents under each of these headings.

Generic Drug Name

The drugs in this book are listed in alphabetical order by their common generic names.

Drugs generally have two kinds of names. First, they have an "official" or generic name. Second, each drug generally has a trade or brand name. For example, **Azithromycin** is the "official" or generic drug name of a particular antibiotic. It is sold under the brand name of *Zithromax*. These two names refer to exactly the same drug.

Some drugs have more than one generic name. When this happens, I have chosen the more commonly-used name in North America and put it as the preferred generic name. Any alternate generic names are in brackets beside it, e.g., **Paromomycin (Aminosidine)**. In this case, **Paromomycin** is the more commonly used generic name, and it is under this name that you will find the ototoxic details of this drug. If all you know is the lesser-used name, look up this name in Chapter 14 (e.g., **Aminosidine**), and it will refer you to **Paromomycin**.

Most drugs have two-part generic names. For example, **Acebutolol** is really **Acebutolol hydrochloride**. **Morphine** is really **Morphine sulfate**. The first part of the name is the important one. Therefore, in order to keep things simple and thus easier to understand, I only use the first part of the name as the generic drug name.

Generic Name vs. Generic Drug

Don't confuse the term "generic name" with the terms "generic drug" and "generic product". The generic **name** of a drug is the official chemical name for the active ingredient of a given drug. A generic **drug** or generic **product** is a drug that is not sold under a specific brand or trade name. (They are often called "no name" brands). A few drugs don't have any trade names and are just sold under their generic names.

However, whether a drug is sold by its generic name, a specific brand name or as a generic drug, the active ingredient is the same.

However, to further complicate matters, some drugs have more than one chemical formulation—e.g., **Metoprolol tartrate** and **Metoprolol succinate**. Although these different forms have the same active ototoxic ingredient, they may have slightly different degrees of ototoxicity, but their basic ototoxic properties are there in any case. Likewise, **Erythromycin estolate**, **Erythromycin ethylsuccinate**, **Erythromycin gluceptate** and **Erythromycin stearate** are just slightly different forms of the active ingredient, **Erythromycin**. In such cases, I combine them all under one generic name, in this case, **Erythromycin**.

In a few cases, I include a generic drug with minor ototoxic properties under the listing of another generic drug rather than giving it a separate listing of its own. For example, suppose you want to find the ototoxic properties of the generic drug **Antipyrine**. When you look for it, you will see it listed as "**Antipyrine** (see **Benzocaine**)". This means you will find the details of this drug in the "Notes" section of the drug **Benzocaine**.

Combination Drugs

Combination drugs complicate things. There are many brands of medications that contain two or more drugs combined into one "pill". One or more of these drugs may be ototoxic.

As far as I have been able to determine, just because two or more drugs are combined into one medication does not change the fundamental ototoxic properties of each separate drug. However, depending on the exact combination, the ototoxic properties of one (or more) of these drugs may make the ototoxic side effects of another drug in the combination more severe.

There are many combination drugs that do not list any ototoxic side effects in either of the two main "drug bibles" used in North America; the *Physicians' Desk Reference* (PDR) used in the USA and the *Compendium of Pharmaceuticals and Specialties* (CPS) used in

Canada. However, when you look up each individual drug separately, you often will find their ototoxic properties listed. Since I primarily only list the brand names of those combination drugs that have ototoxic effects listed in the PDR or CPS, the combination drugs I have listed here are the **minimum** number of combination drugs with ototoxic effects—not the actual numbers that are out there.

If your doctor prescribes a medication that contains more than one drug, in order to be safe, look up each of the drugs that are included in the combination and see if any of them are ototoxic. If you don't know what drugs a given medication contains, ask your doctor or pharmacist to give you a list of the generic names in the medication.

I list the brand name for a combination drug under the listing for the main ototoxic ingredient in that drug. In the notes section of that drug, I then list the other drugs in that combination. If any of these drugs are ototoxic, I refer you to the appropriate drug listing for the ototoxic details of those drugs.

Pronunciation Guide

Hard of hearing people have a tough time understanding unusual words so we never quite hear how to pronounce all the "fancy" drug names. Many of these drug names are real tongue twisters if you are not already familiar with them.

To make it easier for you, I have included a pronunciation guide for each drug. Just be aware that in some cases there is more than one "official" way to pronounce a given drug's name. The Canadian (British) way to pronounce drug names may be somewhat different from the American way. Also, different people pronounce these names differently anyway. So use this as a guide only.

Pronounce the name just like it appears. For example, pronounce **Fenofibrate** as "fen-oh-FYE-brate". Put the stress on the syllable in CAPITAL letters.

Drug Classification

I have attempted, whenever possible, to classify drugs by their chemical similarities. The drug classification helps you find other drugs that are in the same class or family of drugs. Thus, if your doctor prescribes a certain drug, you can see if there is another drug with similar medicinal properties that is less ototoxic, and thus might be better for your ears.

Also, since drugs in the same family tend to have similar ototoxic effects, you can see at a glance which drug families you might want to avoid (if possible) in order to protect your ears.

The information under the "Drug classification" heading refers you to the appropriate section in Table 14.1 (the "tabbed" pages—pages 629 through 659). This table shows all the drugs grouped by their chemical (or use) classification. Within each group, the drugs are in alphabetical order by their generic names.

The legend for the various ototoxic abbreviations is found on the last page of Table 14-1. You can find further information on each of these side effects in the Appendix.

Brand Names

Brand names are the registered trade names of specific drug formulations manufactured by specific pharmaceutical companies. In this book I normally only list the more common brand names in use at this time, but these are by no means all, or even most, of the brands that may be used for that drug.

Some drugs only have one brand name. Others can have more than 50 brand names. When a given ototoxic drug has more than about five brand names, I only list a representative sample—normally the more commonly-used ones. (Whether I list a particular brand name or leave it out does not indicate in any way that the brands I list are superior or more highly recommended or less ototoxic than any that I may omit.)

Therefore, if you are taking a certain brand of a drug and it is not listed in this book, don't assume that it is not ototoxic until you check the listing under that drug's generic name.

If you only know the brand name, but you cannot find it listed in Chapter 14, phone your pharmacist and ask him for that brand's generic drug name. Then look under the generic drug name for any ototoxic properties.

Be aware that the same brand name of a combination drug can have different formulations in different countries. When this happens, it can have different ototoxic side effects depending on its formulation, or the one brand (say in the USA) may be ototoxic and the identical brand name in Canada may not be ototoxic. As a result, you need to look up each generic drug name of combination drugs separately to see whether any of them are ototoxic or not.

Note that sometimes there are minor spelling differences between brand names in different countries.

Some Drugs Have Many Brands

Just to show you that some drugs can have enormous numbers of brand names, here is a listing of all the brand names I can find for the drug **Furosemide**. There is quite a pile of them—102 to be exact. However, under the **Furosemide** listing, I only list the one that is currently commonly used—*Lasix*.

Aldic, Aluzine, Anfuramaide, Apo-Frusemide, Apo-Furosemide, Aquarid, Aquamide, Aquasin, Arasemide, Bioretic, Cetasix, Dirine, Discoid, Disemide, Diural, Diuresal, Diurema, Diurin, Diurolasa, Diusil, Dranex, Dryptal, Durafurid, Edenol, Errolon, Eutensin, Fluidrol, Franyl, Frumex, Furmid, Frusedan, Frusema, Frusemid, Frusemide, Frusetic, Frusid, Frusix, Furantril, Furanturil, Furetic, Furex, Furix, Frumide, Furo-Basan, Furocot, Furodiurol, Furomen, Furomex, Furomide M.D., Furo-Puren, Furorese, Furosan, Furoside, Furosix, Furoter, Furovite, Fusid, Golan, Hissuflux, Hydrex, Hydro, Impugan, Kofuzon, Kutrix, Lasemid, Lasiletten, Lasilix, Lasix, Lasix Retard, Laxur, Liside, Marsemide, Naclex, Nadis, Nelsix, Nephron, Nildema, Novosemide, Odemase, Odemex, Oedemex, Promedes, Promide, Radisemide, Radonna, Rasitol, Retep, Rosis, Salinex, Salurid, Seguril, Sigasalur, Trofurit, Uremide, Urenil, Uresix, Urex, Urex-M, Urian, Uridon, Uritol, Yidoli.

For example, *Lopresor* is the Canadian version of **Metoprolol** while *Lopressor* is the United States counterpart.

If a drug only goes by its generic name and has no brand name, I show this simply as "—".

Ototoxic Effects

This is the real "meat" of each listing. This is where you find out how this drug can affect your ears. The ototoxic side effects are broken down into four main areas, then subdivided again by the specific ototoxic effect.

The four main areas are (in this order) "Cochlear," "Vestibular," "Outer/Middle Ear" and "Unspecified/General Ear Conditions". If I have no information available for under a specific heading, I do not use that heading.

"Cochlear" side effects include things to do with hearing, such as hearing loss, hyperacusis and tinnitus.

"Vestibular" side effects include things that affect your balance, such as ataxia, dizziness, nystagmus, oscillopsia and vertigo.

"Outer/Middle Ear" conditions include such things as ear pain, feeling of fullness in ears, increased ear wax, otitis externa and otitis media.

"Unspecified/General Ear Conditions" include such general things as ear disease, ear disorder, inner ear abnormality and ototoxicity.

I describe and explain these terms and a number of others in Chapter 3. There is also a brief description of each of them in the Appendix.

Unfortunately, researchers sometimes use a variety of vague terms that seem to refer to similar conditions. I don't know exactly what they mean by these more general terms. For example, they variously use vague terms such as auditory damage, auditory defects, auditory disorders, auditory disturbances and auditory ototoxicity. I lump all these under the term "auditory disorder". Similarly, I lump other vague terms such as hearing disorder, hearing abnormality, hearing alterations, hearing disturbance, hearing dysfunction and hearing problems under the term "hearing disorder".

In addition, I collect other vague terms under headings such as "ears blocked," "equilibrium disorder," "hearing loss," "labyrinthitis" and "vestibular disorder". See the Appendix for the complete list of synonyms researchers have used for each of these (and other) terms.

For each drug, I list all the ototoxic side effects I have found. I compiled these from numerous sources. Often, the results are somewhat vague. For example, hearing loss could be permanent or temporary. It could be mild or severe or total deafness—but I have no way of knowing, if it is not clearly stated. If a percentage was given for frequency, I give it. If no statistics were given, I am unable to determine whether the side effect is relatively common or extremely rare so could only note that it has been reported.

Keep in mind that drug books such as the CPS and PDR do not necessarily list all the ototoxic side effects for a given generic drug, nor do they necessarily list them all in any one place. For example, both the CPS and PDR list drugs by brand name. I have gathered all the ototoxic side effects from the individual brand-name listings of each generic drug and compiled them under the generic drug. One brand may list several ototoxic side effects while another brand of the identical generic drug may list one (or none). Therefore, if you or your doctor look up the ototoxic side effects of a drug under a particular brand name, you may not find all those side effects there. Consequently, you may think I have padded the results. Rest assured that all the side effects I list have indeed been reported by the authorities cited, maybe just from a different listing in the same book.

Also, be aware that the same side effects are not always reported consistently from year to year. Therefore, if my listing shows "Tinnitus: (PDR)," for example, and you look in the current PDR and do not find it listed—this is **not** a mistake. It just means that this side effect was listed in a previous edition (or perhaps for a different brand) but is not listed in the current edition for whatever reason.

The ototoxic effects of a given drug can vary greatly depending on how it is taken. For example, ototoxic effects may not be apparent if you take a certain drug as a tablet, but if you take the same drug as an intravenous injection, it could be quite ototoxic. Many ototoxic effects also depend on the dose; both how much you take at a time, and for how long you take the drug. The greater the dose and/or the longer the time you take a drug, generally the greater the risk of ototoxic effects showing up.

It is important you realize that ototoxic side effects picked up during the drug trials are generally in people taking the drug at the **recommended** frequency, duration and dosage. A drug may be ototoxic at higher than recommended dosages, but this information may not be known or readily available since the drug trials are conducted at the recommended dose. As a result, if your doctor prescribes a drug at a higher dose, or for longer than recommended, you may experience ototoxic side effects that are not listed in books like the PDR!

After each ototoxic side effect I give one to three pieces of information about that side effect. First, if known, I provide an estimate of frequency of ototoxic occurrence. Second, I show a comparison to placebo results. Third, I provide the source where I got this information.

Here is how to interpret this information.

Frequency of Occurrence

Some drug studies report how many people have experienced a given ototoxic side effect. If I can find the results of such studies, I include the results and convert them to percentages. If there are two or more studies, I combine the results and show the range. This makes things easier to understand. Therefore, if one study reports that hearing loss is 1% and another reports it is less than 3%, I combine these results and show the range as between 1% and 3%. If I do not have any estimate of frequency of occurrence, I leave this blank.

Comparison to Placebo Results

In order to know whether a given ototoxic side effect is really a result of taking a certain drug or not, researchers often conduct special double-blind studies. In double-blind studies, a group of patients or study volunteers are divided into two sub-groups. One group gets the drug under study. The other group gets a "dummy" pill or "placebo" (commonly called a "sugar pill"). Neither the patients taking the drugs/placebo nor the researchers examining the patients and reporting the side effects know which group a patient is in until after the study is completed. This eliminates obvious bias on the part of researchers and "wishful thinking" on the part of the study volunteers.

When reporting on such studies, I show the drug results as compared to the placebo results in square brackets. It might look like this: "Dizziness: 6.8% [1% above placebo results]". This means that in the drug study 6.8% of the patients who received the drug had resulting dizziness but only 5.8% of the test (placebo) group had dizziness.

Symbols

The symbol "<" before a number means "less than". Likewise, the symbol ">" means "greater than". Therefore, you would read "<4%" as "less than 4%" and ">0.1%" as "greater than 0.1%".

I want to emphasize that these results only apply to the studies reported. They are not necessarily indicative of how another group of people might respond, or how the population in general would respond, but are the best information we have at the moment.

Authorities Cited

The third piece of information beside any ototoxic side effect is the authoritative source from which I got that information. It is usually in the form of two three-character abbreviations in round brackets like this: "(CPS, PDR)".

I use these same abbreviations throughout this book. Table 1-1 lists all the abbreviations and acronyms used.

In order to keep this list of abbreviations manageable, I use footnote references instead of abbreviations if a source is only quoted a few times.

The two main references I quote are the CPS and the PDR. In addition, I compiled information from a number of other drug books, and from various other sources (see Table 1-1).

I cite a maximum of two sources if they are available and place them in alphabetical order. This keeps things from getting too cumbersome. My first choices are always the PDR and the CPS. If one or both of these two sources do not list that ototoxic side effect, I cite any other sources I have. If I only cite one source, that is the only source I have for that side effect.

Table 1-1. Authorities Cited (Abbreviations & Acronyms)

AHF   *AHFS Drug Information.* 2002, 2009.

ATS   Agency for Toxic Substances and Disease Registry. 2001.

BNF   *British National Formulary.* 2002, 2009.

CP2   *Clinical Pharmacology 2000.* 2001.

CPS   *Compendium of Pharmaceuticals and Specialties.* 1998, 2000, 2003, 2010.

DFC   *Drug Facts and Comparisons.* 2009.

DIO   Drug Information Online. www.drugs.com. 2010.

Eps   Epstein. 2002. *Drugs That Can Cause Hearing Loss/Drugs That Can Cause Tinnitus.*

Ka7   Kaufman. 1997. *Ototoxic Medications: Drugs That Can Cause Hearing Loss and Tinnitus.*

Ka8   Kaufman. 1998. *Ototoxic Drugs.*

Med   *Medscape DrugInfo.* 1998-2010.

Med+   *Medline Plus.* 2001.

NDH   *Nursing 2010 Drug Handbook.* 2010.

Nia   Niall, Paul. 1998. *The Effects of Industrial Ototoxic Agents and Noise on Hearing.*

NTP   *National Toxicology Program.* 2001.

PDR   *Physicians' Desk Reference* (PDR). 1997, 2000, 2002, 2003, 2007, 2008, 2009, 2010 (and PDR.COM on-line 2001).

PDR-H   *Physicians' Desk Reference for Herbal Medicines.* 2000, 2007.

PDR-N   *Physicians' Desk Reference for Nonprescription Drugs and Dietary Supplements* and *PDR for Nonprescription Drugs, Dietary Supplements, and Herbs.* 2002, 2008, 2009.

RXL   *RxList Monographs.* 1997-2010 RxList.com.

Ryb   Rybak, Leonard. 1992. *Hearing: The Effects of Chemicals.*

San   Sanders, Melodie. 1997. *Drugs Which Can Cause Ototoxicity and/or Tinnitus.*

She   Shemesh, Zecharya. 2001. *List of Drugs Which May Cause Tinnitus.*

Str   Strain, George. 1996. *Aetiologies of Deafness.*

USP   *United States Pharmacopeia.* 1997, 2001. Complete Drug Reference.

WIK   Wikipedia. 2010.

See the "Literature Cited" section at the back of this book for complete citations for these authorities.

Risk Assessment

Before you take a drug that might be ototoxic, you probably want to know two things. First, you want to know what your chances are of experiencing one or more of its ototoxic side effects. Second, you want to know how bad those side effects could be if you do experience any. You want to know, for example, if you will just experience a bit of temporary dizziness, or if your world will be flipped upside down as a result of permanently losing all your hearing or balance.

Unfortunately for us, not much is known about the risks of many ototoxic drugs. Therefore, I have come up with a rough guide to assessing that risk. Note that this is my own personal subjective assessment of a drug's risk. You do not have to agree with me at all. You and/or your doctor may come to an entirely different conclusion. That is quite all right.

I have placed each of the ototoxic drugs into one of five risk classes. Class 1 is the lowest risk and Class 5 is the highest. I base the largest share of this risk assessment on how frequently people have these side effects. For example, if it only affects 1 person in 1,000, I may put it in Class 1. However, if it affects 20% of the people that take it, I may put it in Class 4 or 5.

I then modify this basic risk assessment with three other factors. The first one is how many different ototoxic side effects this drug can cause. If it only can cause tinnitus and dizziness I would rate the risk lower than if this drug produced hearing loss, tinnitus, hyperacusis, dizziness and vertigo, for example. If a drug has more than four ototoxic side effects, or if it can cause hearing loss, this drug automatically gets a minimum of a Class 2 rating. The second factor is how severe the resulting side effects may be. Constant, loud, debilitating tinnitus would be in a higher class than mild temporary tinnitus. Finally, I factor in how these side effects could affect a person's lifestyle. For example, mild temporary hearing loss is one thing and would be in a lower risk class than total permanent deafness.

Fortunately for our ears, most drugs are in the lower risk classes. Few of them are Class 5 drugs. Table 1-2 shows the five risk classes, together with the number of drugs in this book in each risk class.

If I don't feel I have enough reliable information to make a reasonable assessment for a given drug, I show it as "Not enough information to rate". This indicates a considerable degree of uncertainty as to the completeness (or accuracy) of the specific ototoxic properties of this drug.

Table 1-2. Number of Drugs by Risk Class

Risk Class	Number	Percent
1 (low)	380	43%
2	350	40%
3 (moderate)	68	8%
4	39	5%
5 (high)	13	1%
Not rated	27	3%

This is because there are several lists of ototoxic drugs and chemicals, both published and on the Internet, where the authors simply give a list of drugs and/or chemicals that are ototoxic but do not cite the source, or cite a source to which I do not have access. In other cases, a drug may be part of a list of drugs labeled as causing tinnitus or part of a list simply labeled "ototoxic drugs". Do these drugs have other ototoxic side effects that are not listed? Are they even ototoxic? I don't know.

I have no particular reason to doubt the accuracy of the sources I quote. I believe they had good reasons for listing each drug or chemical where they did (although I cannot vouch for their accuracy/completeness).

Some drugs may be new, foreign, experimental, restricted or withdrawn. Thus there is little information on their ototoxic side effects readily available. This is especially true if these drugs are foreign and there is not much information available on them in English.

Since these drugs are either not included in, or are not listed as being ototoxic in recent editions of the *Physicians' Desk Reference* (PDR), the *Compendium of Pharmaceuticals and Specialties* (CPS) or other sources I trust, I show their risk assessment as "Not enough information to rate". In these cases, you'll have to make up your own mind as to what risk assessment you think might be appropriate.

This risk assessment is a measure of what I might do if I were prescribed this drug. The higher the risk class, the more I'd need to be convinced that this drug was absolutely necessary. Never forget that even a Class 1 drug has a very real risk, and some people do experience the side effects listed or I would not have included it in this book. As a result, I'd always ask my doctor to prescribe non-ototoxic drugs, if any are available that will do the job.

At the same time, you need to remember that this risk assessment only applies to ototoxic side effects—not to all the other adverse side effects these drugs may have. Since all drugs have adverse side effects, you always want to weigh **all** adverse side effects when considering taking any medication.

With Class 4 and 5 drugs, you have a much greater chance of getting one or more of the ototoxic side effects. Therefore, you need to carefully weigh the benefits of not taking such drugs against the proposed benefits of taking them and be satisfied in your own mind that the resulting trade-off will be worth it. Consider the risk factors that may apply to you when making this decision. (See Chapter 4 for these risk factors and how you can help put the odds in your favor.)

Notes

The notes section gives additional information about a given drug. Many drugs do not have any notes.

There are four basic kinds of information I list here. First, for combination drugs, I list all the drugs contained in this compound. I indicate which of them are ototoxic and which listings to go to for further information on their ototoxic properties. Second, I give further information on this drug's ototoxicity and use, if available. Third, I give personal (anecdotal) stories of real people and their experiences with the ototoxic side effects of this drug. Fourth, I refer you to other chapters in this book for further information on this drug or things related to this drug.

Ototoxic Drugs by Drug Class (Table 14-1 Explained)

Table 14-1 (pages 629 – 659) follows the drug listings. It is easy to find as it is "tabbed" on the front edge of the pages in this table.

Drugs in Table 14-1 are arranged in alphabetical order by drug class, then subclass and finally alphabetically by generic name within each drug class/subclass. Note that many drugs fall into two or more classes. I show each drug under only one class. Where possible, I've tried to arrange the classes so that they contain chemically-similar drugs, since they will be more inclined to have similar ototoxic properties. If their chemical class is unknown, I tried to group them in classes by their most common use.

You can use this table to quickly see the ototoxic properties of a given class of drugs. You can also see how many of the drugs in a given class have the same ototoxic side effects. Even more importantly, you can use this table to easily determine which drug is likely to be the least ototoxic of the drugs listed in a given class of drugs.

The column on the right lets you quickly see the ototoxic effects of each drug. The abbreviations of the ototoxic side effects are fairly intuitive. For example, "HL" stands for hearing loss, "T" for tinnitus and "V" for vertigo, etc. The complete list of abbreviations is on the last page of this table.

Here is an example of how you could benefit by using this table. Let's assume your doctor prescribed the ACE INHIBITOR **Moexipril** for your high blood pressure. You could turn to section 20.8.8 in Table 14-1 and see all the ACE INHIBITORS and their ototoxic side effects at a glance. Upon inspection, you can see that **Moexipril** has the greatest number of ototoxic side effects in this class of drugs. You can also see that **Benazepril**, **Captopril** and **Imidapril** have the fewest. Therefore, you might suggest to your doctor that if any of these drugs would do the job, you would rather he prescribe one of them for you, as you want to save your ears from further damage as much as possible.

What To Do If You Can't Find a Particular Drug/ Chemical

There are five reasons why a drug or chemical for which you are looking might not be listed in this book.

1.   The most obvious reason is that the drug or chemical is not known to be ototoxic. This book only contains drugs known to be ototoxic. However, don't assume that if a drug/chemical is not listed in this book, it is not ototoxic. It may be. Read on.

2.   It is a new drug put on the market after I did the research for this book, or its ototoxic properties have been newly discovered/reported. Some existing drugs once thought to have no effect on our ears, later prove to be ototoxic months, years or even decades after they are released. A good recent example is the drug **Acetaminophen**. It wasn't

listed at all in the Second Edition as it wasn't then known to be ototoxic, but it has now been found to be quite ototoxic.

3.   It is a foreign drug. There are a number of ototoxic drugs used in foreign countries that are not listed in this book. This is because I have a difficult time getting reliable information on many foreign drugs. However, I have listed all the foreign ototoxic drugs I have come across.

4.   It is an "old" drug or chemical that is no longer used. There are a number of drugs that have been used in the past and are not used any more, or are no longer used in Canada and the USA. When this happens, current drug publications such as the CPS, PDR or on-line databases cease listing these drugs. However, just because they are no longer being used does not mean that they were not ototoxic. In fact, some of these were highly ototoxic. The problem is that since they are no longer listed, it is hard to dig up the specific ototoxic properties of these drugs. Therefore, reliable information on some of these discontinued drugs may be meager or non-existent.

5.   I missed it somehow. I'm certainly not infallible. Furthermore, I don't have access to all the ototoxic drug information that is squirreled away in various places all over the planet. Thus, I have no idea how many ototoxic drugs I may have missed while compiling this book.

If you are suspicious that a drug may be ototoxic yet it is not listed in this book, there are a couple of things you can do. First, realize that this book will be obsolete before it is even published since there are two or three new ototoxic drugs coming on the market every month!

Therefore, always look up any drug not listed here in the latest version of the PDR if you are in the USA or the CPS if you are in Canada. You can often find these books in your public library, or ask your doctor or pharmacist if you can look at theirs.

Second, you can often make an educated guess as to a drug's ototoxic properties. Here's how to do it.

Begin by determining what class of drug you have or ask your pharmacist. Then turn to Table 14-1 at the end of the drug listings (tabbed pages). Find that class of drugs and see what their various ototoxic properties are. You could

Similar Drugs Often Have Similar Ototoxic Side Effects

You should know that **all** drugs in a given class of drugs likely have the same (or similar) ototoxic effects to some degree or other. Therefore, even if a certain drug in a given class is not listed in this book, that does not mean it is not ototoxic. It may just mean that its ototoxic side effects have not yet been reported.

make a reasonable assumption that any new drugs in that class might have similar ototoxic properties—although this is not always true. Some of the newer drugs are more ototoxic and some of them are not so ototoxic.

Let's say you are wondering about the drug *Terramycin*. You don't find it listed in the drug listings. You know that *Terramycin* is the brand name of the generic drug Oxytetracycline. You have discovered that it is a member of the **Tetracycline** class of drugs. You turn to the TETRACYCLINES (section 7.4.60) in Table 14-1. There you see seven drugs listed. Five of them have either hearing loss (HL) or ototoxicity (OX) listed as a side effect and two don't. You could then assume that *Terramycin* has a good chance of causing hearing loss although that has not yet been reported.

Next, look up the various drugs in this class and see what the individual drug listings say about the degree of ototoxicity of each of these drugs. At this point, decide if you want to risk taking that drug. All you are really doing is making an educated guess, but by doing so, you are putting the odds in your favor.

Herbals

Herbals follow the same general format as do the drugs. They are in alphabetical order by their scientific names. Herbs do not have headings for "Drug classification," "Pronunciation guide," "Brand names" and "Risk assessment".

Two new headings they do have are: "Common name" and "Main active ingredient".

Common Name

This is the common English name(s) by which most people know this herb.

Main Active Ingredients

These are the active chemical constituents that can cause ototoxic side effects.

Chemicals

The chemical section also follows the same general format as does the drug section, but with a few differences. There are no headings for "Drug classification" and "Risk assessment," but I have added two others.

Other Names

The "Brand names" heading used for ototoxic drugs is now the more general heading, "Other names". This is because it includes not only trade names, but alternate chemical names for this substance. Trade (brand) names (at least what I think are trade names) are in *italics*. Other chemical names are in normal type.

Sometimes it is hard to tell which is the most commonly used name for a chemical. In these cases, I have chosen one and placed the synonyms listed under "Other names".

Uses

Unlike drugs, which you basically take when you are sick, chemicals are used all the time and can be found everywhere. As a result, knowing where a given chemical is used gives you a clue as to whether you may have been exposed to it or not.

Glossary

If you come across unfamiliar words, see the Appendix for a brief definition.

Chapter 2

Ototoxic Drugs—What Are They?

Ototoxic Drugs Defined

Drugs whose side effects can damage your ears, particularly your inner ears, go by the name of ototoxic drugs. "Oto" refers to ears, and "toxic" means something that is poisonous. Therefore, ototoxic really means "ear poisoning".

Generally, ototoxic drugs damage either your cochlear (hearing) system or your vestibular (balance) system. Since your inner ear processes both hearing and balance information, ototoxicity can "mess up" either or both of these senses. Thus, the side effects of ototoxic drugs can have far-reaching consequences, ranging from not being able to hear on a phone to not being able to drive a vehicle because of non-existent balance.

There seems to be some confusion as to exactly what constitutes an ototoxic drug. In an on-line chat room for hard of hearing people, one lady asked me if a certain drug was ototoxic. I replied, "It can cause hyperacusis, tinnitus, ataxia, dizziness, vertigo and ear pain". She typed back, "But is it ototoxic?" To her, ototoxicity was hearing loss and nothing else. Other people consider tinnitus also to be an ototoxic side effect. To me, all of the above are symptoms of ototoxicity.

Many doctors consider ototoxicity to be only those non-medical conditions that affect the inner ear and associated nerves (auditory nerve and vestibular nerve). To them, those structures of your ear subject to ototoxicity include your cochlea, vestibule, semicircular canals and related structures.[1] Thus, according to their concept of ototoxicity, ear pain, for example, is not ototoxic, even though it is caused by taking a given drug.

The *American Heritage Dictionary* currently defines "ototoxic" as "having a toxic effect on the structures of the ear, especially on its nerve supply".[2] Consequently, in a restricted sense, ototoxic refers to drugs and chemicals that damage the inner ear and/or the hearing and balance nerves going from the inner ear to the brain (vestibulocochlear nerve).

However, the authoritative source, *Stedman's Medical Dictionary*, simply defines ototoxicity as "the property of being injurious to the ear".[3]

Thus, ototoxicity refers to toxic damage to any parts of the ear, including damage to the outer and middle ear. Therefore, a drug that causes hearing loss by producing excessive ear wax so it blocks the ear canal is ototoxic. So too are drugs that cause ear pain and middle ear inflammation. Furthermore, drugs that damage the auditory circuits in the base of the brain are also ototoxic since they result in our inability to understand what we hear.

For the purposes of this book, I follow Stedman's definition when considering whether a drug is ototoxic or not. Simply put, if a side effect of a drug can adversely affect our ears, that drug is ototoxic.

> ## Ototoxic Drugs Aren't New
>
> Ototoxic medications have been around for a long time. In fact, ototoxic substances have been recognized since the 15th or 16th century B.C.![4] However, it was only in the past 130 years that doctors recognized the ototoxic potential of certain drugs.
>
> For example, **Quinine**, found in the bark of the cinchona tree, has been used by the natives in South America for centuries to treat malaria. About 1630, Europeans also began using this drug for treating malaria. Even so, it wasn't until the late 1800s that doctors began to realize the ototoxic effects of **Quinine**.
>
> Here is another example. In 1829, researchers discovered salicin, the active ingredient of SALICYLATES (of which *Aspirin* is one), but it took another 48 years (until 1877) before they first noticed its ototoxic properties.[5]

How Common Are Ototoxic Drugs?

Until now, ototoxic drugs have been largely ignored. Few doctors can name more than a handful of ototoxic drugs.

However, ototoxic substances are much more common than people realize. For example, researchers estimate that between 1.5% and 16% of the more than 1,000,000 different chemical compounds (which includes drugs, industrial chemicals and metals) may be sensory toxicants. This means that between 15,000 and 160,000 chemical compounds likely affect our senses.[6]

Those chemical compounds that specifically damage our ears are a subset of this number. We have five senses, with our eyes and ears being the major ones. I am going to take a guess (this is just my own personal unsupported opinion here, and it may be totally wrong) and say that our eyes and ears respectively each account for 35% of this total and that our other three senses (taste, touch and smell) account for approximately 10% each.

If my 35% figure is in the ballpark, there may be between 5,200 and 56,000 ototoxic chemical agents out there. (Even if we assume that each of the 5 senses has an equal share at 20%, these figures would still range between 3,000 and 32,000 ototoxic agents.)

This book contains information on the 1,060 ototoxic agents known to me at the time of writing, but obviously this is a small fraction of the ototoxic agents that exist—a miniscule 2% to 20% (or 3% to 35% if you take the 20% figure) of the ototoxic substances thought to be out there. No matter which way you figure it, there are still an enormous number of ototoxic agents of which we know nothing at this time!

The 1,060 ototoxic substances in this book break down into three categories: 877 drugs, 35 herbs and 148 chemicals.

As I mentioned previously, some drugs have only one brand name; others have more than 50! (I've included the more common brands—a total of about 1,660 brand names.) In the "Ototoxic Chemicals" section I list a total of 697 brand names and alternate chemical names.

Drug manufacturers release a number of new drugs each year. Unfortunately, many of these new drugs are ototoxic. I was looking at the 1998 edition of the *Complete Drug Reference*. They include a number of "Introductory Version Patient Education Leaflets" in their Appendix I. These are leaflets for the new drugs that have not gone through the formal review process yet. This is a great idea since it provides consumers with relevant information on medications as soon as possible after these new drugs hit the market.

In their Appendix I, they list 53 new drugs. I was shocked to see that fully 28% already had known ototoxic side effects.[7] Remember, these are all new drugs. Field testing of new drugs (meaning we are the guinea pigs) often reveals a host of further ototoxic side effects.

In fact, we knew by 2001 that at least 62% of these drugs had ototoxic side effects. This means almost two-thirds of the new drugs that come on the market each year are found to be ototoxic within 3 years of their release! This is scary and something we all need to know. I would have hoped that new drugs would be safer for our ears, not the other way around. However, this does not seem to be the case.

As further corroboration, *Supplement A*, the semi-annual supplement to the *Physicians' Desk Reference*, listed 15 new ototoxic drugs in the 2000 edition.[8] Therefore, it is likely that about 30 new drugs with ototoxic properties are coming on the market each and every year in America alone!

Ototoxic Side Effects

Ototoxic drugs typically damage the sensitive hair cells in your cochlea and/or in your vestibular (balance) system. This can result in a whole bunch of side effects, depending on the exact site of the damage. Some ototoxic drugs cause permanent damage, and others only have a temporary effect on your ears. A few of the ototoxic side effects you may experience include temporary or permanent hearing loss in both ears, generally, but not always, at the higher frequencies; ringing or other noises in your ears; dizziness or vertigo; eye problems; and balance problems. (Chapter 3 gives a comprehensive list and explanation of many ototoxic side effects.)

Often the first warning you get of impending damage to your ears is when your ears begin to ring (tinnitus) or, if you already have tinnitus, your tinnitus gets worse.[9] Tinnitus usually appears first as a continuous high-pitched sound. The reason for this is that ototoxic drugs generally damage the hair cells at the base of the cochlea—which is where the high-frequency sounds are detected and passed on to the brain. If your ears begin to ring, you should immediately report this to your doctor, then together you and your doctor should decide what to do—whether to reduce the dose, change the medication or stop taking that medication altogether.

One of the treacherous things about tinnitus is that, if it is not very loud to begin with, or if you are quite sick, you may not even be aware of this warning signal until after it is too late.

The same holds true for some of the warning symptoms of vestibular damage. If you are bedridden, or in the hospital, you may not notice that your balance is affected until later when you are feeling better and try to get up. By then, it may be much too late. Doctors often attribute this unsteadiness to the results of your sickness, or to being bedridden, not to drug-induced damage to your vestibular system. As a result, doctors may overlook such ototoxic damage, or fail to diagnose it right away.[10]

Therefore, if you find that you have balance problems after you get out of the hospital, both you and your doctor need to carefully review your hospital records for any ototoxic drugs you may have taken. Be aware that symptoms may not appear until several days after you get home.[11]

Another warning you may have is a feeling of fullness or pressure in your ears. Your ears may feel "blocked" or "full". Rarely will your first warning be a noticeable hearing loss.

If you complete a course of drug therapy with apparently no ill side effects to your ears, don't assume that the drug did not harm your ears in any way. The time for ototoxic damage to show up varies tremendously. For example, intravenous LOOP DIURETICS or high-dose SALICYLATE therapy can bring on hearing loss in a matter of minutes. The ototoxic effects of **Erythromycin** and **Cisplatin** normally show up in the first 4 days of therapy.

Unfortunately, the ototoxic side effects of some drugs don't show up for several days, weeks or months after you stop taking them. By then, it is much too late for your doctor to do anything about it. The ototoxic effects of AMINOGLYCOSIDE ANTIBIOTICS can take from a few days to 6 months[12] or more to reveal themselves.[13] Also, be aware that when you take various drugs from time to time over many years, each different drug may have a minor effect on your ears, but taken together, they may result in noticeable hearing loss or other ear damage.

However, don't blame drugs for all of your ear problems. You do not want to automatically assume that there must be a cause and effect relationship between any drug you are taking and any symptoms of ear damage you are experiencing. For example, just because tinnitus develops while you are taking a certain drug does not necessarily mean that the drug caused the tinnitus. It might have. Then again, your tinnitus might have come from an entirely different source—for example, being overtired, or stressed out, or from exposing your ears to loud sounds.

If you are in doubt as to whether a drug is causing ototoxic damage to your ears or not, stop taking the medication (with your doctor's permission, of course) and see if the symptoms go away. You need to allow your body time to get rid of the drug, so give it at least two weeks or so. If the symptoms go away, begin taking the drug again and watch if the symptoms come back. If they return, that is a strong indication that this drug is indeed ototoxic to your ears.

The Main Ototoxic Drug Classes

There are five main classes of ototoxic drugs that doctors commonly recognize today (although there are many more drugs in various classes that they should recognize). These five main classes include the AMINOGLYCOSIDE antibiotics (**Amikacin**, **Gentamicin**, **Neomycin**, etc.), SALICYLATES (**Aspirin**, etc.), QUININES (**Chloroquine**, **Quinine**, etc.), LOOP DIURETICS (**Ethacrynic acid**, **Furosemide**, etc.), and some ANTI-NEOPLASTICS (anti-cancer drugs such as **Buserelin**, **Cisplatin**, **Vinblastine**, **Vincristine**, etc.).

In addition, many NSAIDs (NON-STEROIDAL ANTI-INFLAMMATORY DRUGS), ANTIBIOTICS, ANTIHISTAMINES, CARDIOVASCULAR drugs, ANTI-CONVULSANT drugs, ANTI-DEPRESSANT drugs and ANTI-PHYSCHOTIC drugs (tranquilizers) are also ototoxic.

Furthermore, there are a bunch of drugs in other classes that are ototoxic to some degree or other. For more information on the ototoxic drugs in this book by their classes, see Table 14-1 (tabbed pages).

Ototoxicity Often Minimized

Most people, many doctors included, do not think about ototoxic drugs. In fact, ototoxic drugs are so far removed from the stream of human consciousness that until very recently the word "ototoxic" was not even listed in regular dictionaries!

How is the average person supposed to find out about ototoxic drugs when the word isn't even mentioned? It should be no surprise then, that drug books downplay the seriousness of ototoxic side effects. For example, in the 2006 edition of *The Essential Guide to Prescription Drugs* the author compiled 12 tables of drugs that cause "important" side effects for various conditions.

Does this book have a special table for ototoxicity? Definitely not! There are tables for such important things as drugs that may cause damage to your blood, nerves, heart, lungs, liver and kidneys. There are tables for drugs that might increase your sensitivity to sunlight; drugs that can adversely affect your sexuality; and drugs that may interact with alcohol. There is even a table for drugs that may adversely affect your vision. Yes! Good vision is vital to people with poor hearing. Hard of hearing people use their eyes as their ears. However, there is no table specifically for drugs that adversely affect ears. This needs to change!

Because the incidence of ototoxicity is minimized, it is easy to fall into the trap of believing that because ototoxic side effects have not been reported for a given drug, it must be safe for your ears. A good quote to remember is, "absence of evidence does not equal evidence of absence". In other words, just because an ototoxic side effect has not been reported for a specific drug does not mean that that drug never causes ototoxic damage. In fact, as you will see in Chapter 5, **most** occurrences of ototoxic side effects are **never** reported.

Ototoxic Drugs and You

Be careful about taking any drugs, especially ototoxic drugs, if you are hard of hearing. Most drugs coming on the market have not been thoroughly studied for potential side effects. As a result, if you take them, you end up as the guinea pig. Is this what you want? Never forget that all drugs have side effects. Some of these side effects may be much worse for the rest of your body than are the effects of certain ototoxic ones on your ears.

For example, did you know that an estimated one and a half million people in the United States end up in the hospital each year as a result of adverse side effects from taking drugs? Another 100,000 people die each year from these adverse side effects![14] You do not want to be a part of these statistics.

There are many drugs that are ototoxic to some degree. For example, taking 6 to 8 **Aspirin** a day can cause ringing in your ears (tinnitus) and temporary hearing loss.[15] Other drugs will quickly and permanently damage your ears. You may be left with little or no hearing. This happened to Elizabeth after she took an antibiotic to fight a life-threatening infection. Now she cannot hear any high-frequency sounds.

Other drugs can have both temporary and permanent effects. While taking chemotherapy, Ruby temporarily lost most of her hearing. After her treatments were over, most of her hearing returned, but she was left with permanent and annoying tinnitus.

When looking at side effects, always compare **all** the side effects you may experience against the good the drug is supposed to do you, then make your choice based upon how much risk you are willing to accept. Only you, yourself, know how much "pain" you are willing to endure to avoid the risk of losing any more of your hearing or causing other ear damage from taking drugs.

Carefully weigh the benefits you hope to receive from taking ototoxic drugs against their potential for causing permanent damage to your ears. Sometimes, the side effects of the drugs are much less severe than the result of not taking them, namely certain death. It's a no-brainer when

We All React Differently

Just because a drug is listed here doesn't necessarily mean you will damage your ears if you take it. Ototoxic drugs do not always (or even mostly) cause ototoxicity—but be warned, they may. Each person's body is slightly different and reacts differently. For example, Marcia has been taking **Diclofenac** for 15 years and does not have any noticeable hearing damage, although the drug she is taking can cause hearing loss, balance problems and tinnitus. She is one of the fortunate ones.

On the other hand, Flo took **Fluoxetine** for 5 years and had never been told it could cause hearing loss. Within 3 weeks after she finally stopped taking it, she noticed a significant improvement in her hearing.

the choice is either deaf or death. If it's not a matter of life and death, do your research, then make an informed decision.

In order to make an informed decision, before beginning drug therapy, you need to know what drugs you are going to be taking. You need to know **all** the side effects of these drugs. You need to know the interactions that may occur between these drugs. Finally, and this is most important, you need to carefully consider the role that hearing and balance play in maintaining the quality of your life and how your quality of life could change when the drug treatment is over. Too often, people neglect this important aspect until they lose their hearing or balance. At that point it is too late to say, "Oops, we should have thought of that before!"

It is not easy to determine what effects any ototoxic drug may have on your life. This is because there is enormous variation in how ototoxic side effects affect different people. The side effects you experience may be temporary or permanent; the symptoms may be mild or severe; the ototoxic damage may be the same in both ears or totally different in each ear; and the damage may affect both ears (bilateral) or just appear in one ear.

After you have carefully considered all these factors, you need to sit down with your doctor and decide whether you are prepared to accept the risk of those side effects if you take the proposed course of drugs.

You need to be aware that damage to your ears can result in serious vocational, educational and social problems. You can minimize or prevent these effects if you can detect any ototoxic side effects early enough in the treatment process. Therefore, you and your doctor have to work together to closely monitor the effects of any drugs on your body. Unfortunately, monitoring for the effects of ototoxic drugs is not a common practice. This is another thing that needs to change!

Don't let your doctor railroad you into taking his recommended course of drugs. Your body may react differently than he expects. For example, certain drugs may build up to toxic levels in your blood if your body does not metabolize them as expected. Each person's reaction to any given drug or medication is unique.[16] In fact, studies show that people vary widely in how much of a drug they need to take before it begins to adversely affect their ears.[17]

You may not have a single noticeable side effect from a given drug while the next person has several severe side effects. Betty found this out to her sorrow. Her doctor told her that a certain antibiotic he prescribed would only damage her hearing if taken in large doses for a prolonged time. What happened to her? The very first (relatively low) dose permanently damaged her hearing. For the past twenty-five years she has had to wear two hearing aids just to be able to get most of what people say.

Always ask your doctor or pharmacist about the possible side effects of any medications (or combinations of medications) you are taking. Have them look it up in their "drug bibles" (the PDR in the USA, the CPS in Canada and the BNF in Great Britain) and show you. Remember, it's your hearing that is at risk. You are the one who will have to live with the results day after day, month after month, year after year, not your doctor or pharmacist. I know that I, for one, always want to err on the side of caution. I avoid all ototoxic (and other) drugs if that is possible.

You also need to be aware that sometimes you do not find the ototoxic information where you would expect to find it. For example, I looked up the drugs *Ecotrin* (**Acetylsalicylic acid**) and *Demadex* (**Torsemide**) in the PDR. To my surprise, it did not list any ototoxic side effects for these drugs where you would normally look to find such information—under the section headed "Adverse Reactions". Yet these drugs are indeed ototoxic. I found this out when I looked under "Warnings" on a different page. There I read "If ringing in the ears or a loss of hearing occurs…" and "Tinnitus and hearing loss…have been observed…". There was not even a "See WARNINGS" as is customary if side effects are listed elsewhere. If you want to be sure you have found all the ototoxic side effects, you need to read all the fine print on any drug, no matter what the heading says.[19]

> ### Top Prescription Drugs for 2008
>
> Here's a shocking statistic. Of the top 200 prescriptions written in America in the year 2008 (representing more than 2 billion prescriptions), 83% of them have ototoxic side effects listed for them! Now that's scary.
>
> The number one prescription drug of 2008 was *Lipitor* (**Atorvastatin**). This drug is known to both cause hearing loss and tinnitus.
>
> The number two drug was *Lortab* (**Hydrocodone** and **Acetaminophen**). This drug is addictive and is subject to abuse. Recently, researchers have discovered that it can cause sudden severe hearing loss when it is taken for too long or in large doses.[18]

Here is something else you should know. If you read the "Patient Product Information" sheets that come with your drugs or if you read the "Patient Product Information" area on the manufacturer's web site, you likely are not getting much if any of the information you are wanting on ototoxic side effects. These information sheets are "dummied down" for the layperson, and also greatly shortened. Thus a lot of information is left out. For example, one manufacturer's "Patient Product Information" sheet on their web site only listed one ototoxic side effect—dizziness—yet this drug has a number of other ototoxic side effects.

True, the manufacturer listed a bunch of "serious" side effects, but not the ototoxic ones we want to know. At the bottom of the page they gave this warning. **Be sure to heed it!** It said:

> The side effects described above do **not** include **all** the side effects reported with this drug. **Do not rely on this leaflet alone** for information about side effects. Your doctor or pharmacist can discuss with you a more complete list of side effects.

When you see something like this, you need to look elsewhere for a more complete list of the side effects. In this case, if you go to the "Physician Prescribing Information" page on this same web site, you will find the missing ototoxic side effects. These are the same side effects as those you find in the PDR. There you will discover that, in addition to dizziness, this drug could cause vertigo, tinnitus, otitis media and earache. Now you know you are getting nearer to the truth.

Deaf People and Ototoxicity

Just because you may be deaf already doesn't mean that you are immune to the side effects of ototoxic drugs. True, you will not experience any further hearing loss since your hearing is gone. However, ototoxic drugs can still damage your vestibular (balance) system. Most of the drugs in this book are known to affect the vestibular system in some way. Therefore, whether you are deaf or not, you still want to be very careful when taking any ototoxic drugs.

If you are almost deaf (severe or profound hearing loss), you certainly don't want to lose the remaining precious bit of your hearing. Some health care professionals might wonder what difference a little hearing makes. To them it may be insignificant. To us, it is extremely important.

Take Responsibility for Yourself

You, and you alone, are responsible for the body God gave you. Therefore, although you may go to doctors for help, the final decision on any treatment, including any drugs your doctor may want you to take, is up to you.

As a result, you need good information so you can make good decisions. Since doctors seldom are reliable sources of ototoxic drug information, you need to check things out for yourself. If you don't, it is your ears that will suffer—not the ears of your doctor, nor the ears of your pharmacist. You alone are ultimately responsible for everything that goes into your body.

Therefore, before you take a drug, check out the side effects listed on the box/bottle or the insert that comes with it. Do this with over the counter medications too. Better yet, check out the side effects in the CPS or PDR (or this book).

Some people take the time to check things out and thus save themselves a lot of grief later. One lady I know went to her local drug store to pick up some *Excedrin* (**Acetylsalicylic acid**) at her doctor's suggestion. Being diligent, she read the fine print on the box and was surprised to see that it could cause tinnitus and hearing loss. This is great, a bit of "ototoxic truth" on the boxes now! But you have to watch out. She told me that these side effects were listed on the larger box, but not on a smaller box of the same drug.

She was further surprised when she asked the pharmacist about these ototoxic side effects and he immediately told her that *Extra Strength Tylenol* would be much less ototoxic for her.

This was so unusual (truth in labeling and a pharmacist that knew about ototoxicity) that she emailed me to see if both were telling the truth! (At the time this incident happened, both were telling the truth as far as anyone knew. However, since then researchers have discovered that *Tylenol* [**Acetaminophen**] is actually quite ototoxic—but they didn't know that back then.)

The unfortunate thing about this whole incident is that her doctor either didn't know or didn't care about the fact that he was recommending an ototoxic drug to a hard of hearing person. He should have known better! Therefore, I re-emphasize, check every drug out for yourself. You may be extremely glad you did!

---

1   *Guidelines for the Audiologic Management of Individuals Receiving Cochleotoxic Drug Therapy*, 1994. p. 1.
2   *American Heritage Dictionary*, 2000.
3   *Stedman's Medical Dictionary*, 2000. p. 1288.
4   Haybach, 1998. p. 6.
5   Haybach, 1999. pp. 16-17.
6   *Environmental Impact on Hearing: Is Anyone Listening*, 1994. p. 5.
7   *United States Pharmacopeia*, 1998. pp. 1672-1725.
8   *Physicians' Desk Reference. 54th Edition. Supplement A*, 2000.
9   *Compendium of Pharmaceuticals and Specialties*, 2000. pp. 1589, 1669.
10 Troost, 1998b. p. 1.
11 Troost, 1998b. p. 2.
12 Haybach, 1999. p. 62.
13 Haybach, 1998. p. 3.
14 Waltermire, 1998. p. 1.
15 Stanten, 1996. p. 16.
16 *Medroxyprogesterone acetate*, 2001. p. 2.
17 Fausti, 1993a. p. 664.
18 *Top 200 Prescriptions*, 2008. p. 1.
19 *Physicians' Desk Reference*, 1997. pp. 2625-2626.; PDR, 2000. pp. 2629-2630.

Chapter 3

Ototoxic Side Effects and Your Ears

The Effects of Drugs

All drugs potentially have four kinds of effects on your body. First, there is the intended therapeutic effect. This is why you are taking this drug in the first place. Second are the side effects. These are mild reactions other than the intended effect. Third are the allergic effects. Fourth are the toxic effects. These are severe effects up to, and including, death.

According to Dr. Harold McPheeters, "It has become fashionable in recent years to refer in drug advertisements and promotions to the latter three kinds of effects as 'side effects.' In reality, some of the toxic effects (such as damage to the liver, kidneys and nervous system) are becoming more dangerous as medications themselves become more powerful". [1]

The effects of drugs on our ears mostly fall in group 4, toxic effects rather than into group 2, side effects. However, in keeping with current usage, I'll refer to groups 2-4 simply as "ototoxic side effects," "adverse side effects" or just plain "side effects".

Ototoxic Side Effects

When you think of ototoxic side effects you likely think of things such as hearing loss and tinnitus, and you would be right. However, this is just barely scratching the surface. There are a whole host of other ototoxic side effects. Some of these give rise to problems that you might never suspect were related to your ears.

Drugs can damage or cause problems in various parts of our ears. I have broken these side effects down into four basic groups. First, I discuss those side effects arising from damage to the cochlear (hearing) system. Second, I deal with those side effects arising from damage to the vestibular (balance) system. Third, I comment on those side effects arising from damage to the central nervous system (nerve and brain). Finally, I touch on those side effects arising from the outer and middle ear.

Cochlear Side Effects

The cochlea is the part of your inner ear that converts mechanical sound vibrations into electrical signals. It contains thousands of tiny hair cells that relay hearing information to the auditory nerve and from there up to your brain.

Cochlear damage from ototoxic drugs can result in such side effects as tinnitus, hearing loss, distorted hearing, hyperacusis, a feeling of fullness in your ears and auditory hallucinations.

Tinnitus

Tinnitus is a phantom sound. You "hear" it in your brain when there is no external sound present. Sometimes people refer to it as a ringing in their ears or ear noises.

Tinnitus can manifest itself as a wide variety of sounds. It may be a ringing, roaring, beating, clicking, banging, buzzing, hissing, humming, blowing, chirping, clanging, sizzling, whooshing, rumbling, whistling or dreadful shrieking noise in your head. It may also sound like rushing water, radio static, breaking glass, bells ringing, owls hooting or chainsaws running.[2] Some people hear several of these sounds at the same time.

Often tinnitus precedes or accompanies hearing loss from ototoxic drugs. In fact, tinnitus is the **number one** indicator that you may be doing further damage to your ears. It also may be the **only** warning you'll ever get. Pay attention to it!

Table 3-1. The More Common Ototoxic Side Effects

Side Effect	No. of Drugs*	% of Ototoxic Drugs**
Dizziness	728	83
Vertigo	560	64
Tinnitus	529	60
Ataxia	350	40
Hearing loss	294	34
Earache	218	25
Otitis media	132	15
Nystagmus	117	13
Ototoxicity	75	9
Ear disorder, unspecified	69	8
Labyrinthitis/vestibular disturbances	64	7
Hyperacusis	53	6
Auditory/Hearing disturbances	40	5
Otitis externa	40	5
Loss of balance/equilibrium disorder	38	4
Otitis	37	4
Auditory hallucinations	30	3
Ears blocked/pressure	28	3

*This is the number of drugs in this book with this side effect.
**These percentages are based on the 877 ototoxic drugs in this book. A lot of these drugs have more than one ototoxic side effect. The average is 3.9 ototoxic side effects per drug.

Although tinnitus from ototoxic drugs is generally high-pitched, continuous and occurs in both ears, certain ototoxic drugs produce distinctive tinnitus sounds. For example, tinnitus caused by SALICYLATES is generally high-pitched and sounds like a continuous musical note. It usually stops when you stop taking the drug. Tinnitus from **Quinine** and related drugs produces similar sounds. In contrast, taking **Erythromycin** can produce what sounds like "blowing" while LOOP DIURETICS may produce a middle-frequency sound.[3]

Tinnitus arising from taking ototoxic drugs may or may not be permanent.[4] If you are taking an AMINOGLYCOSIDE antibiotic, you are one of the lucky ones if it stops within a couple of weeks after you finish the drug therapy. For some people, it never goes away.

Tinnitus may show up very quickly after you begin taking an ototoxic medication or it may take several days to months to years to become apparent. For example, tinnitus from LOOP DIURETICS may start just minutes after you begin receiving it as an I.V. In contrast, tinnitus may not show up until 2 or 3 days after taking an AMINOGLYCOSIDE antibiotic. With the BENZODIAZEPINES, tinnitus may only show up **after** you stop taking the drug.

For Further Information

To learn more about tinnitus and how you can bring it under control, order the book *When Your Ears Ring!—Cope With Your Tinnitus— Here's How*. (See the back of this book for ordering information.)

Hearing Loss

Hearing loss may be the first thing you associate with ototoxic drugs. Although it is not the most common ototoxic side effect, the results of hearing loss certainly can have an enormous effect on your life.

Hearing loss may occur as the only ototoxic side effect, but many times tinnitus or a feeling of fullness in your ears (or both) precede or accompany it. This makes these side effects important indicators of an impending hearing loss and should never be ignored.

Typically, ototoxic drugs first damage the hair cells (cilia) at the base of the cochlea. The cilia at the base of the cochlea are sensitive to high-frequency sounds. The damage then progresses towards the tip where the cilia are sensitive to low-frequency sounds. This is why hearing loss typically begins in the very high frequencies and steadily moves down the frequency spectrum to the speech frequencies.

Hearing Loss Synonyms

The PDR and CPS list this side effect variously as hearing loss, decreased hearing, diminished hearing or even disturbed hearing (whatever that really means). Other times they call it deafness. However, I think they generally mean hearing loss to some degree or other—not total deafness.

You may have a hearing loss from taking an ototoxic drug and never know it unless you have special high-frequency audiograms done. As your hearing loss progresses to the lower frequencies, a regular audiogram will begin to reveal your hearing loss. It is not unusual to be unaware of any hearing loss until it has reached mild to moderate status. By that time, your hearing loss will be more than 30 dB in the speech frequencies,[5] and it may be much too late to do anything to restore your hearing.

Ototoxic drugs almost always cause sensorineural hearing losses (SNHL) (the old term was nerve deafness). This is opposed to conductive losses, which stem from damage to the middle ear. However, taking certain drugs may result in clogged middle ears with a resultant conductive hearing loss. Hearing loss can range from mild high-frequency loss to total deafness. Also, drug-induced hearing loss is generally, but not always, the same in both ears (bilaterally symmetrical), although sometimes it can be different in each ear (asymmetrical)[6], or only affect one ear. Sensorineural hearing loss may be permanent or temporary depending on the drug and a number of other factors.

Distorted Hearing

Even though an ototoxic drug may not cause a hearing loss, it can still damage your hearing. Sometimes it will cause you to experience distorted hearing—everything may sound "tinny" or "funny".

The typical "ski slope" hearing loss means you hear the lower frequency sounds close to normal, but you don't hear high frequency sounds at all. (Your audiogram looks like a ski slope that slopes down to the right.) This, by itself, will make speech sound distorted or different.

Furthermore, auditory system damage caused by ototoxicity may impair your ability to discriminate between spoken words. You may be able to hear speech, but don't understand some/most/all of the words you hear, even when they are loud enough for you.[7]

If you have a sensorineural hearing loss, generally the worse the loss, the worse your discrimination will be.

Hyperacusis

Hyperacusis is a fairly rare condition where you perceive normal sounds as abnormally loud. In fact, many sounds may seem painfully loud. Yet these same sounds are at a comfortable level for those with normal hearing. It's as though your internal volume control is stuck on high.

At least 53 drugs can cause hyperacusis.

Do not confuse hyperacusis with recruitment. Recruitment is an abnormal rate of **increase**

For Further Information

To learn more about hyperacusis and how you can help bring it under control, order the book *Supersensitive To Sound? You May Have Hyperacusis.* (See the back of this book for ordering information.)

Recruitment is clearly explained in the book *When Hearing Loss Ambushes Your Ears—Here's What Happens When Your Hearing Goes On the Fritz.* (Again, see the back of this book for ordering information.)

in sound due to hearing loss. When you double a sound in volume, a person with normal hearing perceives it as twice as loud. A person with recruitment may perceive it as **seven times** as loud, for example.

Hyperacusis more often occurs if you have normal or near normal hearing. Recruitment is **always** a function of a sensorineural hearing loss. Generally, the worse your hearing, the worse your recruitment.

Feeling of Fullness in Your Ears

Another ototoxic side effect of some drugs is a feeling of fullness in your ears or head. This may feel like pressure in your ears, your ears may feel "plugged up", stuffed up, clogged or blocked, or you may have a general feeling of pressure in your head.[8] This feeling of fullness in your ears often precedes or appears at the same time you first notice a hearing loss.

The professional health care people seem baffled by this symptom. As one health care professional explained, "Not only is the reason for this sensation unknown, but no nerve able to sense a pressure change in the inner-ear areas has been identified".[9]

I think they are looking in the wrong place. They are expecting to find the Eustachian tube or the middle ear itself clogged due to an infection. This can certainly give a clogged up feeling.

However, there is another reason of this feeling of fullness that few seem to understand, and that is a **psychological** feeling of pressure in response to hearing loss. When you suddenly lose some hearing, your brain tells you that your ears **must** be blocked (or else sounds would keep coming through, wouldn't they?). Hence, the stuffed up feeling.

I get this same sensation when I take my hearing aids off—all of a sudden it is too quiet and my ears feel "blocked". This feeling eventually goes away as my brain gets used to not hearing much of anything again.

Therefore, if your ears feel "blocked" after taking an ototoxic drug, you may be losing your hearing and your ears are warning you in this manner. It's a good idea at this point to have your hearing checked by an audiologist.

Auditory Hallucinations

A good number of drugs cause hallucinations—auditory or otherwise. There are two basic classes of auditory hallucinations. For lack of a better term, I'll call them "psychiatric" auditory hallucinations and "psychological" auditory hallucinations.

Psychiatric auditory hallucinations are where a person clearly hears and understands voices speaking to him when no one is there. Often the person knows exactly who or what is talking to him—for example, a departed loved one, a chair or a tree, etc. Sometimes the person carries on a conversation or responds to these voices. These kind of hallucinations are an indication of mental illness (schizophrenia, for example). If you hear these kinds of voices, you should seek treatment by a competent psychiatrist.

At the same time, be aware that certain drugs can cause this effect. Therefore, if your medication is causing these voices, just stopping the drug (in consultation with your doctor) may be the best solution.

Much more common in my opinion, but far less talked about for fear of being labeled mentally ill, are the psychological variety of auditory hallucinations, previously referred to as musical hallucinations or musical tinnitus, but now known as Musical Ear Syndrome (MES).

Musical Ear Syndrome is not a sign of mental illness, but rather is a by-product of something not working quite right in the auditory system. From time to time, numerous hard of hearing people hear such sounds. This is generally nothing to worry about. Many people hear tinnitus—one class of phantom sounds—but they are not thought to be "crazy". MES is somewhat related to tinnitus, but consists of complex phantom sounds such as music and voices whereas tinnitus is comprised of simple (unmodulated) sounds. A person who hears these MES sounds is no more suffering from mental illness than a person who hears tinnitus.

If you have MES, you may hear what sounds vaguely like voices or singing or music. For example, you may hear what sounds like a radio program, but you cannot quite distinguish the words although it sounds like someone talking. Similarly, you might hear music. The tune is vaguely familiar, but you cannot quite place it.

At other times, you may clearly hear the phantom music. Generally this music is pleasant to neutral. Two common tunes in America are "The Star Spangled Banner" and "Amazing Grace". Sometimes you may hear classical music. Often, older hard of hearing people seem especially prone to hearing these phantom sounds.

No doubt, some drugs cause psychiatric auditory hallucinations and others result in Musical Ear Syndrome. Since the drug reference books such as the PDR and CPS do not define what they mean by auditory hallucinations, they may be referring to either of the above classes. Furthermore, the professionals recording the side effects may not be aware of the difference between the two classes of hallucinations in the first place so just lump them together as "auditory hallucinations".

I have found at least 369 drugs and herbals that can cause hallucinations. Of this number, only 30 specifically state that the resulting hallucinations are the auditory variety. It is these 30 drugs that I have included in this book. (Incidentally, probably most of these 369 drugs do cause auditory hallucinations of one kind or another since auditory hallucinations are the most common kind of hallucinations.)

For Further Information

If you hear these strange phantom sounds, learn more about your Musical Ear Syndrome and how you can help bring it under your control in the book *Phantom Voices, Ethereal Music & Other Spooky Sounds*. (See the back of this book for ordering information.)

Vestibular Side Effects (tabulated in the drug listings)

The vestibular (balance) system is that part of your inner ear that consists of the three semicircular canals (anterior, posterior and lateral), the saccule, the utricle and the vestibular nerve. Like the cochlea, these structures contain thousands of tiny hair cells that generate and relay balance signals to your brain.

As long as your vestibular system is working properly, you seldom give your ability to keep your balance a thought. However, if your vestibular system ever fails, it can impose enormous changes on your lifestyle.

Perhaps you weren't aware of this, but your vestibular system does not work alone to maintain your balance. Actually, there are three separate systems that help you maintain your balance. The other two systems are your visual and your proprioceptive (proh-pree-oh-SEP-tiv) systems.

The vestibular portion of your inner ear continuously senses gravity and both straight and curved movement. Your eyes see both your position in space and movement. Your proprioceptive system uses special pressure sensors in your muscles, tendons and joints to sense gravity and joint position. Most of your proprioceptive sensors are in your feet and leg joints.

Your vestibular system works together with your eyes in what doctors call the vestibulo-ocular reflex. This reflex instantly adjusts the position of your eyes to prevent blurred vision and to prevent your vision from bouncing when you move your head, walk or even breathe.

Your vestibular system also works together with the muscles of your body via your spinal cord in what doctors call the vestibulo-spinal reflex. This instantaneous reflex allows for continual, coordinated muscle adjustments so you can maintain your balance as you change position. It involves the vestibular system, vestibulocochlear nerve, brain, spinal cord and the muscles you use for standing and walking.[10]

In addition, your vestibular system works together with your vestibulo-sympathetic reflex to keep your blood pressure and respirations normal while you are moving.[11]

Your brain uses the separate signals from your vestibular, visual and proprioceptive systems to instantly and subconsciously maintain clear vision and to make rapid muscle adjustments to prevent you from falling. You need at least two of these three systems working properly in order to effectively maintain your balance.[12]

When all three systems are working properly, you have no trouble keeping your balance. However, when you lose your vestibular system, your brain has to rely on the other two systems, but without the critical vestibular information, problems can arise.

One of the insidious things about taking ototoxic drugs is that vestibular damage does not usually show up right away. As a result, you may not stop taking an ototoxic drug soon enough to prevent severe vestibular damage. Vestibular ototoxicity may follow the signs and symptoms of cochlear ototoxicity. However, be aware that sometimes its onset can be both sudden and severe.[13]

Ototoxic drugs can cause a number of vestibular side effects. Some of the more common ones include the inability to tolerate head movement, dizziness, lightheadedness, nausea, vomiting, vertigo, oscillopsia, visual problems, loss of balance, difficulty walking in the dark, nystagmus,[14] ataxia[15] and severe fatigue.[16] Note that many of these symptoms are not specific to ototoxic drug damage alone, but can result from several other causes as well.

Vestibular side effects generally are worse in the first few weeks after vestibular damage occurs. As time goes by, your brain gets less confused by the loss of vestibular information because it learns to rely more on your visual and proprioceptive systems. Walking becomes easier. Your ataxia will slowly resolve to some extent as your brain puts this alternative information to use. However, if you had severe vestibular damage, you will be left with permanent side effects that can alter your lifestyle dramatically.[17]

There are numerous ototoxic side effects that affect the balance system. The drug listings in this book only tabulate the effects of those ototoxic side effects more directly associated with the inner ear, namely: dizziness, vertigo, ataxia, nystagmus, labyrinthitis, loss of balance/equilibrium and oscillopsia.

Dizziness

Dizziness is a very common side effect of taking drugs. In fact, the majority of the drugs available today can cause dizziness.[18] Many of these drugs are ototoxic, so it should be no surprise that dizziness is also the most common ototoxic symptom. According to a pamphlet put out by Audiologic Consultants, fully 85% of dizziness symptoms can be attributed to inner ear disturbance (ototoxicity).[19] Of the 877 ototoxic drugs in this book, 728 (83%) are known to cause dizziness.

Because dizziness may or may not be an ototoxic side effect, and since I have no way of knowing for sure what the case is for any particular drug, I have not listed a drug in this book if its sole ototoxic side effect is dizziness. As a result, I will have left out a number of drugs that do indeed cause dizziness as an ototoxic side effect and thus should have been included.

Not only is dizziness a common ototoxic side effect, I also believe dizziness is one of the early symptoms of ear damage. Whether your dizziness is actually caused by ototoxic damage to your balance system or whether the vestibular damage results from the same cause as the dizziness—namely a lack of oxygen getting to your inner ears—doesn't really matter. The end result is the same, very real damage to the delicate hair cells in the vestibular portion of your inner ears.

Dizziness comes in two basic types. With near-syncope dizziness, not enough blood gets to your brain. Symptoms usually appear over a few seconds. Typically, if you have this type of dizziness your vision dims, you are uncoordinated, confused, pale and perspiring. If these symptoms improve rapidly when you either sit down, squat down or lay down, you likely had this kind of dizziness.[20] You may describe it by such terms as feeling woozy, feeling you are going to faint, feeling light-headed, feeling that you are going to black out or feeling you have tunnel vision. For example, you could get this kind of dizziness from standing up too quickly (orthostatic dizziness). Also, some medications can lead to hypovolemia (which basically results in low blood pressure) or autonomic reflex loss with the resulting dizziness.[21]

The second type, non-syncope dizziness manifests itself as a feeling of vague disequilibrium. You can get this of dizziness from hyperventilating (breathing too fast or too deeply),[22] hypoglycemia, anxiety or migraine headaches, among other things.[23]

Unfortunately, sometimes people use the term "dizzy" when they really mean "vertigo" and vice versa. Unlike dizziness, if you have vertigo, you have a false sensation of moving or spinning.

Vertigo

Vertigo (VER-tih-goe) is a medical term reserved for the perception of movement when the body is really at rest. You most often experience vertigo as a spinning sensation much like what you experience after getting off of a merry-go-round. You have the sensation that your surroundings are continuing to spin even though they aren't.[24] If you have vertigo, you may feel that the room you are in is spinning around you, or that you are spinning around and the room is still. Sometimes, you just have the sensation that the ceiling of the room is slowly spinning around. Vertigo can also appear as linear motion or even a rocking motion.[25]

A person with vestibular ototoxicity may also complain of transient positional vertigo (a sensation of movement that is not occurring stimulated by certain head positions or by rapid head movements).[26]

Vertigo results from a mismatch of vestibular, visual, and proprioceptive inputs. When all three are telling your brain the same thing, all is well. However, when your ears tell your brain one thing and your eyes and proprioceptive system tell it another thing, your brain doesn't know who to believe. In this case, your brain's confusion manifests itself as vertigo.

Benign Paroxysmal Positional Vertigo

If your vertigo is brought on by certain particular head positions, then you likely have benign paroxysmal positional vertigo.[27] This kind of vertigo occurs when the "rocks in your head" (the technical name is otoconia)—tiny crystals of calcium carbonate—get into the wrong places. They normally are in a tiny structure in your inner ear called the utricle. If they get jiggled out of the utricle and get into one of your semi-circular canals, you get benign paroxysmal positional vertigo. This kind of vertigo has nothing whatsoever to do with ototoxicity. It is typically treated with the Epley maneuver.

Symptoms of vertigo may start instantly, or they may develop over a few seconds. If you are experiencing vertigo, you typically become pale and may have some of the symptoms of motion sickness such as nausea, vomiting, headache and fatigue. The typical vertigo attack gradually goes away, often leaving you feeling queasy and tired for some time afterwards.[28]

Ataxia

Ataxia (ah-TAKS-see-ah) is the loss of your ability to coordinate your muscles properly such that it affects your gait. As a result, when you walk you may stagger as if you were drunk.

Ataxia is one of the results of a damaged vestibular system. Normally, your vestibular system sends balance information to those areas of your brain and nervous system involved in the motor control of your muscles. This balance information allows your brain to continuously make little adjustments in muscle activity and body position to allow you to stand upright and maintain your balance.[29]

If your vestibular system doesn't pass this information to your brain or if it passes faulty information, your brain does not order these tiny adjustments. As a result, you will lurch and stagger (staggering gait) as the other two parts of your balance system try to compensate. You will likely have an unsteady gait and stumble a lot.

You may try to compensate by standing and walking with your legs farther apart than normal in order to give you better control of your balance (wide-based gait), and you may keep looking down while you are walking.[30] Even so, you may lose your balance or stagger when turning quickly (whole body or head only), and need to hold on to walls or furniture when you are walking.

In addition, you may have difficulty walking on slippery, soft or slanted surfaces or on uneven ground. You may have difficulty standing or walking in dim or dark places or when you have your eyes closed. Even under good lighting conditions, you will still tend to stagger. You may also feel unsteady, have problems standing with your feet together, be uncoordinated and clumsy and overreach when grabbing for objects.[31]

Nystagmus

Nystagmus (nye-STAG-muss) is another side effect that at first glance doesn't seem to have anything to do with your ears. Nystagmus is technically not a "ear" problem. However, it shows the powerful influence the vestibular (balance) system has on the motor neurons of the III (oculomotor), IV (trochlear) and VI (abducens) cranial nerves. These nerves control various eye movements.

Nystagmus refers to abnormal rapid rhythmic back-and-forth involuntary eye movements (eye jerking),[32] usually side to side, rarely in the vertical plane.[33] With nystagmus, both of your eyes drift slowly in one direction and then suddenly jerk in the opposite direction. When nystagmus is caused by vestibular problems, your eyes jerk horizontally (sideways).

You get nystagmus if only one side of your vestibular system is damaged, or if one side is damaged worse than the other side. Your eyes will jerk toward the undamaged (less damaged) side and will drift back towards the (more) damaged side. This abnormal eye movement can cause vertigo, nausea, vomiting and a host of other visual complaints.[34]

Labyrinthitis

Labyrinthitis (lah-brin-THY-tis) is simply an inflammation of the labyrinth. The labyrinth includes all the structures in your inner ear (cochlear and vestibular systems).

Labyrinthitis may show up as many different symptoms some of which include vertigo, nystagmus, sensorineural hearing loss, nausea and vomiting.[35]

Loss of Balance/Equilibrium Disorder

When you damage your vestibular system, one result is that you have difficulty keeping your balance. When your finely-tuned sense of equilibrium is damaged, you may suddenly lose your balance or stagger like you are drunk. You may feel unsteady. You may bump into things and have difficulty walking straight. In extreme cases you may not be able to stand erect without support.

Oscillopsia

You get oscillopsia (ah-sih-LOP-see-ah) when you are unable to sense minute head movements and thus make compensatory eye adjustments to keep the "picture" you are seeing stable. When your eyes can't maintain a stable horizon, you see a "jumbling of the panorama"[36] and have "bouncing vision". [37]

Oscillopsia is common if your vestibular system is severely damaged in both ears. Here is what happens. When you walk, your head moves up and down with your body movement. Your vestibulo-ocular reflex (involving your vestibular system, vestibulocochlear nerve, brain and the muscles of your eyes) normally keeps your eyes clearly focused on your surroundings by instantly and continuously changing your eye position as you move.[38] You think nothing of this. It is totally subconscious and automatic. However, if your eyes and your ears lose this coordination due to vestibular damage,[39] your eye muscles do not receive the proper signals to automatically adjust to movement. As a result, your surroundings will appear to move, bounce, jiggle and jump about as you move, and your vision may be blurry.[40]

When your surroundings "bounce" it can make walking extremely difficult or even impossible. This is because under these conditions it is difficult to see and respond to obstacles in your path and to sense the exact location of the floor or ground.[41]

Vestibular Side Effects (not tabulated in the drug listings)

The following ototoxic side effects of vestibular damage are not tabulated in the drug listings, but they are just as much the product of ototoxic drug damage to the balance system as those mentioned previously. You may experience some, all or none of the following side effects when an ototoxic drug damages your vestibular system.

If you experience any of the following side effects after taking an ototoxic drug, very likely they were also caused by the same ototoxic drug that produced any listed side effects.

Emotional Problems

Damage to your vestibular system can result in emotional problems, especially if your lack of balance causes major changes in your life. For example, emotional problems may surface if you go from self-sufficiency to near total incapacitation. Your emotions can also take a beating if others don't understand your situation, or if your mental abilities change. You may experience anxiety, frustration, anger and depression.[42] You may mourn your loss of self-reliance. Your feelings of self-confidence and self-esteem may plummet.

You may also experience similar emotional problems as a result of hearing loss since hearing loss can cut you off socially from those around you.

Fatigue

A seemingly unlikely result of vestibular ototoxicity is fatigue. If your balance system is severely damaged, you may be exhausted all the time. This is because keeping your balance is now no longer a subconscious event, but something that you must consciously work hard to maintain. In addition, your eyes and proprioceptive system must work overtime too. The result may be that everyday tasks are now exhausting.

Fatigue may also result from hearing loss. When you lose some hearing, you strain to hear and intently watch people's faces in order to speechread them. This, just by itself, is also exhausting.

Memory Problems

Strange as it may seem, vestibular ototoxicity can cause memory problems. Here is why. When you damage your vestibular system, keeping your balance is now largely a conscious effort, not the automatic effortless procedure it once was. Consequently, those areas of your brain that you once just used for thought and memory, now must constantly work on keeping you balanced. As a result, your memory may suffer. You may grope for words when talking. You may easily forget what is being spoken about during a conversation. You may be easily distracted. You may have difficulty comprehending directions or instructions. You may have trouble concentrating and may feel disoriented at times.

Older people may have similar problems as they age. However, you can't blame everything on aging if you are taking ototoxic drugs. Ototoxic side effects may be partly/largely responsible for these symptoms.

Muscular Aches and Pains

Another seemingly unlikely result of vestibular ototoxicity is muscular aches and pains and headaches. Your muscles may become sore and tense when your automatic vestibulo-spinal reflex (the reflex dictating automatic muscle changes in response to changing movement situations) no longer works automatically and you have to consciously control it. You may do this by making your muscles rigid and less relaxed as you strain to keep your balance. In addition, you may get headaches and a stiff/sore neck from trying to hold your head absolutely still so you won't feel dizzy or nauseous.

Nausea

You might not associate nausea with damage to your inner ears, but it is actually a relatively common side effect of vestibular damage.[43] When you damage your vestibular (balance) system, the confusion of sensory inputs your brain experiences can result in nausea. The nausea may be continual or intermittent. You may feel like you have a hangover all the time or you may feel "seasick".

Visual Problems

Whether you realize it or not, your eyes are inextricably tied to your ears. You need your eyes to help maintain your balance. At the same time, you need your ears (vestibular system) to maintain clear vision. Thus, when you damage your vestibular system, you will almost certainly have visual difficulties as well. In fact, visual complaints may be one of the first clues you have that you have damaged your vestibular system. These resulting visual problems may even cause you more trouble than the "normal" vestibular side effects.

Earlier in this chapter, you learned that one of the functions of the vestibular system is to send certain information to your brain and nervous system in order to control your eye movements (vestibulo-ocular reflex). This information helps stabilize your eyes in space when you move your head. It also reduces the movement of the image of a fixed object on your retinas thus giving you clear vision.[44]

You might not think just how important your balance system is to your eyes. Every time your heart beats or you breathe, your head moves a tiny bit. Your vestibular system senses these tiny changes in position and tiny movements (as well as all the major movements too) and your brain sends messages to your eye muscles to correct for it, all unknown to you.

Anything that disrupts your vestibulo-ocular reflex directly affects your vision.[45] Therefore, if your vestibular system is damaged, you will likely have fuzzy or blurred vision. Furthermore, you will likely have difficulty focusing on objects, or holding your eyes on a printed page since your hands can't hold a book completely steady.[46] This makes it very difficult to read.[47] It can also make it difficult to write. Also, you probably will have difficulty with depth perception, and focusing on, or watching, moving objects.

In addition, you may feel dizzy, experience nausea or have a sense of moving, particularly at the onset, if you move your eyes, move your head and eyes simultaneously, or watch moving objects. This can make being around traffic, riding in a vehicle, watching TV or watching a movie in a movie theater very unpleasant. You may find moving or flickering lights bother you.

You may find that you no longer can tolerate head movement, that you no longer can determine when movement has stopped, and that you no longer can determine your bodily position in space, especially with your eyes closed.[48]

Just the act of focusing your eyes may be difficult and can lead to dizziness and nausea. You may have a tendency to look down because it is harder to focus on more distant objects. In addition, a visually "busy" scene may make you feel sick. Looking at the floor with its (generally) simple patterns makes it much easier to "take in". Your ability to accurately determine distances may also be disrupted. This can lead to even more difficulty when you are walking. Poor depth perception may result in your bumping into things. People may think you are clumsy.

Never underestimate how experiencing both eye and balance problems at the same time can have an enormous impact on your life and lifestyle.[49]

Vomiting

When you see a person vomiting, your first reaction is not, "Aha, that person has a damaged balance system!" You think stomach flu, food poisoning, sickness and anything else but ear damage, don't you? Yet vomiting may be the result of a damaged vestibular system—especially at the beginning.[50] As time goes by, your brain attempts to compensate for the vestibular damage and generally the vomiting ceases. Quite often vomiting and vertigo occur together. When the room is spinning around, you feel so sick you often "toss your cookies".

Vague Feelings of Unease

Sometimes you can't put your finger on exactly what is wrong. You may feel vaguely uneasy. You may feel that things seem wrong or unreal. You may feel tired and listless without knowing why. You may feel lightheaded or faint.[51] As unlikely as it may seem, all these symptoms may be the result of a damaged vestibular system.

By now you should have developed a sense of awe at the marvelous balance system God designed for you. At the same time, you now also realize the tremendous upsets that may come into your life and lifestyle if you allow ototoxic drugs to damage this wonderful system.

Central Nervous System (CNS) Side Effects

Ototoxic drugs can also mess up our brains and/or scramble the message as it passes along our auditory nerves. The PDR and CPS sometimes refer to this by the ambiguous term "CNS toxicity". Unfortunately, this may or may not have anything to do with our auditory systems. Be aware that anything that affects our brains can just as easily affect our auditory networks. However, since there is no way of telling whether "CNS toxicity" specifically includes ototoxic side effects, I have not included it as one of the ototoxic side effects for the purposes of this book.

Central Processing Disorder

Sounds may enter our ears and be processed correctly, but these sound signals may be delayed or scrambled after they leave our inner ears. This scrambling can occur as the sound signals are processed by the neuronal networks that make up our auditory nerves, or in auditory parts of our brains. When this processed sound reaches the conscious levels in our brains where we "hear", we may hear a bunch of gibberish. The proper name for this is a central processing disorder.

Several ototoxic chemicals have this effect. These chemicals do not necessarily cause a hearing loss as such, but they prevent our brains from processing sounds normally. As a result, we may not understand speech well (or at all).

Outer/Middle Ear Side Effects

Outer or middle ear side effects include such things as excessive ear wax production, swelling or redness in your ear canals, middle ear infections and ear pain or earaches. Occasionally you will see terms such as otorrhagia (bleeding from the ear), otorrhea (purulent discharge or puss from the ear), ruptured or perforated tympanic membrane (hole in the ear drum) and cholesteatoma (tumor of the middle ear).

Ceruminosis

This is the medical way of saying excessive ear wax production and build-up. A few drugs have this side effect.

Ear Pain

The fancy word for ear pain is otalgia. Typically, ear pain is a result of ear infections, particularly in the middle ear. Ear pain and otitis (see below) often go together. However, ear pain (and earache and ear discomfort) can be the result of taking an ototoxic drug apart from any ear infection. A lot of drugs (218) have ear pain associated with them.

Otitis

Otitis is an inflammation of the ear. Normally doctors define where this inflammation occurs by adding a modifier to the word "otitis". Thus, **"otitis externa"** refers to conditions of the outer ear and ear canal. Typically they include infections that have symptoms such as redness, swelling and itching.

"Otitis media" typically refers to infections of the middle ear. Terms used to describe this condition include fluid in ear, ear pressure, pressure/throbbing in ears and ear disorder.

Some of the drugs listed in this book as having otitis, otitis externa or otitis media as an ototoxic side effect do not directly cause these conditions. Rather, these infections come in and take over when an opportunity presents itself. Thus these infections are sometimes called "opportunistic infections". For example, this could happen as the result of an ototoxic antibiotic killing off the "good bacteria" in the ear canal, leaving it wide open to an opportunistic invasion of "bad bacteria".

Another scenario is where an ototoxic drug suppresses the immune system to some degree, thus letting a "bad guy" get a foothold where it otherwise would not be able to do so. Sometimes these are classified under the heading of "resistance mechanism".

---

1   McPheeters, 2000-2001. p. 1.
2   Bauman, 2002. p. 7.
3   Haybach, 1999. pp. 33-34.
4   Haybach, 1998. p. 3.
5   Kalkanis, 2001. p. 2.
6   Kalkanis, 2001. p. 1.
7   Kalkanis, 2001. p. 8.
8   Haybach, 1998. p. 3.
9   Haybach, 1999. p. 34.
10   Haybach, 1998. p. 2.
11   Haybach, 1998. p. 2.
12   Haybach, 1999. pp. 6-7.
13   Troost, 1998b. p. 1.
14   *Disorders of the Inner Ear*, 2000. p. 8.
15   *Compendium of Pharmaceuticals and Specialties*, 2000. p. 1499; *Physicians' Desk Reference*, 2000. p. 2803.
16   Haybach, 1996. pp. 3-4.
17   Haybach, 1999. p. 36.
18   Haybach, 1999. p. 33.
19   *Are You Dizzy*, 2001. p. 1.
20   Bowen, 1998. pp. 2-3.
21   Bowen, 1998. p. 4.
22   *Vestibular Frequently Asked Questions*, 1995. p. 1.
23   Bowen, 1998. p. 9.
24   Haybach, 1998. p. 6.
25   *Vestibular Frequently Asked Questions*, 1995. p. 1.
26   Haybach, 1998. p, 6.
27   Bowen, 1998. p. 5.
28   Bowen, 1998. p. 3.
29   *Vestibular Apparatus*, 2000. p. 1.
30   Haybach, 1998. p. 6.
31   Haybach, 1998. p. 6.
32   Haybach, 1998. p. 6.
33   Hull, 2000. p. 1.
34   Haybach, 1999. pp. 7-8.
35   *Disorders of the Inner Ear*, 2000. p. 11.
36   Kalkanis, 2001. p. 2.
37   Haybach, 1998. p. 6.
38   Haybach, 1998. p. 2.
39   Troost, 1998b. p. 1.
40   Haybach, 1999. p. 7.
41   Haybach, 1999. pp. 36-37.
42   Haybach, 1999. p. 38.
43   *Compendium of Pharmaceuticals & Specialties*, 2003. p. 1612.
44   Vestibular Apparatus, 2000. p. 1.

45   Haybach, 1998. p. 4.
46   Haybach, 1998. p. 6.
47   Haybach, 1998. p. 6.
48   Haybach, 1998. p. 6.
49   Haybach, 1999. pp. 37-38.
50   *Compendium of Pharmaceuticals & Specialties*, 2003. p. 1612.
51   Haybach, 1999. p. 36.

Chapter 4

Are You at Risk?

Some people take ototoxic drugs with seeming impunity. Others take one dose of an ototoxic drug and wham—there goes their hearing. Why? The short answer is, "We are all different". Therefore, it should be no surprise that we also vary in our sensitivity to ototoxic drugs.

Risk Factors

Researchers have identified a number of factors that increase the risk of our having an ototoxic reaction when taking certain drugs. This chapter explains 20 of these risk factors (in no particular order of importance).

You are more at risk of an ototoxic reaction to a given drug than the general population if any of these risk factors apply to you. The more that apply, the higher your risk.

1. You are very young. This includes as yet unborn children. If you are pregnant when you take an ototoxic drug, it can have devastating effects on your unborn child including damaging both the auditory and vestibular systems resulting in permanent deafness and/or balance problems. Your unborn baby is particularly vulnerable during the first trimester, especially between weeks 6 and 8. **Quinine**, the SALICYLATE family, **Streptomycin** and **Dihydrostreptomycin** are among the dastardly drugs that do this.[1]

2. You are a senior (over 60). You very likely already have minor hearing problems. The effects of taking ototoxic drugs are additive and can compound your hearing loss.

3. You have certain hereditary (genetic) factors that make you more susceptible than the general population. This seems particularly true if you take AMINOGLYCOSIDE antibiotics. (For further information, see the section "Genetics and Aminoglycoside Ototoxicity" in Chapter 9.)

4.   You already have a sensorineural hearing loss, balance problems or some other form of pre-existing ear damage.[2] People with a pre-existing hearing loss may actually be at greater risk of incurring further hearing loss than people with normal hearing. This is the case with **Cisplatin**, and there is no reason to believe the situation is any different with other ototoxic drugs. One study found that people with pre-existing hearing loss on their baseline audiogram (taken before **Cisplatin** treatment) had greater subsequent hearing loss than those with normal hearing.[3]

Since ototoxic damage is probably cumulative, pre-existing ear damage, whatever the cause, can result in measurable or observable damage more quickly. This could include ear problems such as Meniere's Disease (syndrome of fluctuating hearing loss, tinnitus and vertigo), Cogan's disease (a syndrome of visual, hearing and balance problems), Lermoyez syndrome (increasing deafness, interrupted by a sudden attack of dizziness, after which hearing improves), endolymphatic hydrops (similar to Meniere's Disease), autoimmune inner-ear disease (AIED) and perilymphatic fistula (inner ear fluid leaking into the middle ear).[4]

5.   You have had previous ear damage (hearing loss) from excessive noise.[5] The amount of noise predisposing you to ototoxicity is not well defined. You could assume you are at greater risk if you have been around artillery fire, jet aircraft, rock concerts (as either a performer or a fan), or use jackhammers, fire guns, work at construction sites, or work or play in noisy environments.

6.   You have problems with either your liver or kidneys (whether pre-existing or developing during drug treatment). For some unknown reason, people with kidney problems have an unusually high incidence of hearing loss, even without drug use.[6] Chinese herbalists have known this for hundreds of years. They still teach that your ears and your kidneys are "connected". Therefore, if you are taking any medications that affect your kidneys, or if your kidneys are not working properly (possibly from taking nephrotoxic [kidney-damaging] drugs such as the AMINOGLYCOSIDE antibiotics), watch out for any ototoxic changes to your ears.

Your body eliminates many drugs through your kidneys. If your kidneys aren't working properly, ototoxic drugs can spend more time in your body, thereby increasing your chances of ototoxic side effects.[7]

7.   You are extremely sensitive to drugs or have a low tolerance for drugs.

8.   You have previously had ototoxic reactions to drugs. This proves your ears are particularly sensitive to ototoxic drugs. Your risk of ototoxic reactions to current or future drug therapy is much higher. Not only does the risk increase, but the resulting ototoxic damage has a tendency to be more severe and is more likely to be permanent.[8]

9.   You have previously used ototoxic drugs, or you have taken repeated courses of the same ototoxic drug. This is especially true if you have previously used AMINOGLYCOSIDE antibiotics.

10.   You have taken certain drugs for a long time (especially if you have taken a drug for longer than the manufacturer recommended). You have to watch this as doctors often prescribe drugs for longer periods than the manufacturer recommends.

11.   You can be at higher risk if an ototoxic drug is not administered properly. Proper administration is critically important if you want to avoid permanent, severe ototoxic damage.[9] For example, you increase the risk if you have taken ototoxic drugs in large doses than recommended; if you have been given a larger single dose of an ototoxic drug than recommended; if you have been given a higher than recommended cumulative (total) dose; or you have been given a rapid or faster than recommended dose (injection or intravenous). This could show up as higher than recommended peak serum levels and/or higher than recommended trough serum levels.[10]

12.   You have been given an inappropriate dose (children, elderly people, obese people)— e.g., a child given an adult's dose. If you are overweight, it is important that your doctor calculates any AMINOGLYCOSIDE antibiotic doses based on your lean muscle mass, not on your total body weight including fat or you could have an overdose resulting in more severe ototoxic side effects.[11]

13.   You are dehydrated. This can occur if you are taking DIURETICS. Dehydration can lead to higher than normal blood/serum levels of ototoxic drugs.[12] (Incidentally, if you have a fever it is very easy to become dehydrated.)

14.   You have taken ototoxic DIURETICS at the same time as other ototoxic drugs or if you have used or are using two or more ototoxic and/or nephrotoxic (toxic to the kidneys) drugs at the same time. Since various drug interactions increase the risk of ototoxicity, taking two or more ototoxic drugs sharply increases your chances of ototoxic reactions. You also increase your risk if you take drugs that cause nephrotoxicity (kidney toxicity) because this, in turn, increases the likelihood of ototoxicity.

Taking two or more ototoxic drugs at the same time or consecutively may cause severe permanent ototoxicity. The damage may occur at lower cumulative doses and much more rapidly, even when the doses of both drugs are within acceptable, published therapeutic ranges[13] as a result of potentiation.

Some drug combinations that will increase your risk of having ototoxic reactions include: AMINOGLYCOSIDE antibiotics and **Indomethacin** (in newly-born babies); AMINOGLYCOSIDE antibiotics and LOOP DIURETICS; AMINOGLYCOSIDE antibiotics and **Vancomycin**; **Ampicillin** and **Amphotericin B**; **Bumetanide** and **Cisplatin**; **Capreomycin** and **Kanamycin**; and **Ethacrynic acid** and some CEPHALOSPORIN antibiotics.[14][15]

LOOP DIURETICS and AMINOGLYCOSIDE antibiotics are one particularly bad combination. Not only are they both ototoxic, but the LOOP DIURETICS may change the antibiotic concentration in serum and tissue, increasing the possibility of ototoxic damage. These DIURETICS also increase the chance that dehydration will develop, another risk factor for ototoxicity.[16]

15. You have had previous ear infections.

16. You are generally in poor health in the first place. This also includes poor nutrition at the time you are taking any ototoxic drug.[17]

17. You have abnormal laboratory values such as reductions in serum albumin, serum red blood cells, hematocrit, hemoglobin or you have rising serum creatinine levels.[18]

18. You have had radiation treatments on your head or ear.[19]

19. You have bacteremia (bacteria in the bloodstream) (AMINOGLYCOSIDE antibiotics).[20]

20. You have either eye or proprioceptive (balance) problems. This increases the chances that vestibular ototoxicity will have a more serious impact on your life if it does occur. If ototoxic drugs destroy your vestibular system and you already have a visual or proprioceptive problem, you will not be able to maintain your balance. Therefore, if you have visual or proprioceptive problems, you should take potentially vestibular ototoxic drugs with great care, and only if you have a life-threatening condition.[21]

Here's How You Can Reduce Your Risk

You cannot do anything about certain ototoxic risk factors such as your age or your genetic makeup. However, there are still some things you (and your doctor) can do to lessen your risk of having an ototoxic reaction from taking certain drugs.

It is very important that you discuss any hearing and balance conditions you have with your doctor so both of you can work together to protect your ears.

Here is a list of some things you and your doctor can do.

1. Be aware of the early warning signs of ototoxicity. They are (in order of frequency): you feel dizzy; your ears begin ringing (tinnitus); your existing tinnitus gets worse or you hear a new kind of tinnitus; you feel pressure in your ears (unless you have a head cold); your hearing gets worse or begins fluctuating; you develop vertigo (spinning sensation). Should any of these symptoms develop while taking any medication, stop the medication immediately and call your doctor.[22]

2. Tell your doctor that you are hard of hearing, especially if you have a sensorineural hearing loss and/or suffer from balance problems. Also, tell your doctor if you currently have any ringing in your ears (tinnitus). This is very important, as you may be much more susceptible to drugs than the general population. Dr. Epstein cautions, "If you have an existing sensorineural hearing loss, regardless of the cause, when using ototoxic medications, you are more vulnerable to aggravation of that hearing loss".[23]

3. Always discuss possible side effects (including ototoxic side effects) with your doctor before you begin taking a new medication.

4.   Follow your doctor's dosage instructions exactly. Make sure your doctor writes dosage information down clearly for you. Don't trust your (faulty) hearing or your (equally faulty) memory. Overdosing could certainly adversely affect your hearing.

Also, make sure your doctor does not exceed the manufacturer's dosage instructions when he prescribes drugs for you. During the drug approval process, researchers determine the safe dose of each drug. These dosage instructions are listed in drug books such as the PDR along with warnings that drugs are not to be taken for longer than a certain number of days and/or that the dose is not to exceed a certain amount. This information is vitally important if you want to avoid adverse ototoxic side effects.

Do doctors heed these guidelines? Not on your life! For example, a 1996 report by the FDA found that for a certain drug they had specifically warned doctors about, 85% of the prescriptions were still for longer periods than was safe![24]

Did you know that your doctor does not have to follow these recommended guidelines when prescribing drugs? He can prescribe as much as he wants, as often as he wants—but it is you (and your ears) that will suffer the consequences. Therefore, make sure your doctor adheres to the manufacturer's guidelines.

5.   Use the same pharmacy for all your prescriptions so they know all the drugs you are taking. That way they can quickly advise you of any known dangerous drug combinations.[25]

6.   Always read the labels on over-the-counter (OTC) medications and particularly watch for ototoxic side effects. You can also ask your pharmacist about potential ototoxic effects of OTC medications. Just because they are OTC drugs doesn't mean they can't damage your ears.

> **Medic Alert**
>
> If you have read this far, you likely know the ototoxic risk factors that pertain to you. Perhaps you even know your body is particularly susceptible to the ototoxic effects of certain drugs.
>
> One way to help protect yourself is to wear a Medic Alert tag. This tag can do two important things. First, it can warn health care professionals that you have a hearing loss and/ or balance problems. Second, it can warn them about specific ototoxic drugs that you know will further damage your hearing or balance.
>
> For further information, contact Medic Alert, phone 1-888-633-4298 or visit their web site at http://www.medicalert.org.

7.   Make sure you drink plenty of fluids so you don't get dehydrated. This is especially important if you have a fever or are taking LOOP DIURETICS.

8.   If you have kidney problems, have your health care professionals carefully monitor your kidney function and report abnormalities immediately. It is most important

that your doctor determine how well your kidneys are working before he prescribes various medications. This is because your body excretes many drugs through your kidneys. If they are not working properly, some drugs can quickly rise to dangerous levels of ototoxicity in your bloodstream and may result in permanent hearing loss and other ear damage.

9. Avoid using multiple ototoxic drugs at the same time (particularly AMINOGLYCOSIDE antibiotics, **Cisplatin** and LOOP DIURETICS). Also do not take nephrotoxic (kidney damaging) and ototoxic drugs at the same time.[26]

10. Avoid noisy environments for at least 6 months after you have completed a course of an AMINOGLYCOSIDE antibiotic or a platinum compound such as **Cisplatin**. This is because your ears can still be supersensitive to noise-induced hearing loss.[27] The residual drug in your inner ears can team up with noise in a synergistic relationship to cause even more hearing damage. If you wear or obtain hearing aids during this time, you need to keep the volume down as well.[28] Tell you audiologist about this so she can program them correctly for you. (See Chapter 8 for more information on this important subject.)

11. It is most important, if you are beginning treatment with an ototoxic drug such as any of the AMINOGLYCOSIDE antibiotics, LOOP DIURETICS or platinum compounds such as **Cisplatin**, that you have a baseline high-frequency audiogram done before you begin treatment and then serial high-frequency audiograms (testing those frequencies between 8,000 Hz and the highest frequency you can hear [or up to 20,000 Hz]) during and after drug therapy. This is essential as conventional audiograms cannot catch the first indications of high-frequency hearing loss.[29] If this is done, your doctor likely can either modify or stop treatment before significant hearing loss occurs.

12. If you have had vestibular (balance) problems from taking any drug, for example, **Gentamicin**, you want to be very careful not to damage your vestibular system further—unless it is so extensively damaged that you have nothing further to lose. To protect the remaining function of your vestibular system, according to Dr. Hain, you should stay away from any of the AMINOGLYCOSIDE antibiotics, ANTIHISTAMINES like **Meclizine** and **Promethazine**, TRICYCLIC ANTIDEPRESSANTS such as **Amitriptyline**, **Aspirin (ASA)** and other NON-STEROIDAL ANTI-INFLAMMATORY DRUGS such as **Ibuprofen** and **Naproxen** (in large doses), **Cisplatin** and related anti-cancer drugs, **Erythromycin**, LOOP DIURETICS like **Furosemide** and **Ethacrynic acid**, BENZODIAZEPINES such as **Alprazolam**, **Clonazepam**, **Diazepam**, **Lorazepam** and related drugs, and **Quinine** and related drugs.[30]

---

1   Troost, 1998b. p. 2.

2   Troost, 1998b. p. 3.

3   Fausti, 1993a. p. 664.

4   Haybach, 1999. p. 45.

5   Shearer, 1994.

6   Staab, 1991. p. 38.

7   Haybach, 1999. p. 45.
8   Haybach, 1999. p. 45.
9   Haybach, 1999. pp. 48-49.
10   Haybach, 1999. p. 44.
11   Haybach, 1999. p. 50.
12   Haybach, 1998. p. 3.
13   Haybach, 1999. p. 47.
14   Haybach, 1998. p. 3.
15   Haybach, 1999. p. 47.
16   Haybach, 1999. p. 47.
17   Priuska, 1997. p. 3.
18   Haybach, 1999. p. 44.
19   Haybach, 1998. p. 3.
20   Haybach, 1999. p. 44.
21   Haybach, 1999. p. 45.
22   Epstein, 1995. pp. 1-2.
23   Epstein, 1995. p. 1.
24   Freundlich, 1998. p. 2.
25   Shearer, 1994.
26   Haybach, 1998. p. 5.
27   Kalkanis, 2001. p. 3.
28   Kalkanis, 2001. pp. 8-9.
29   Kalkanis, 2001. p. 8.
30   Hain, 1999. p. 3.

Chapter 5

Here's How the System Works

Drugs are damaging our ears at an alarming rate. This disturbs me. The system that should be protecting us and our ears is letting us fall through the cracks. Thus, what appears to be a "minor" problem on the surface, is in reality the tip of an immense iceberg. The real problem (and it is enormous) is hidden below the surface where few see it or do anything about it. For better or worse, that is the way the system "works".

The Tip of the Iceberg

All drugs have side effects. This is no secret. The United States Food and Drug Administration (FDA) is the government's watchdog on the drug industry. The FDA warns, "When it comes to using medicine, there is no such thing as a completely safe drug. **All** medicines have risks".[1] Notice this, "**No** drug is perfectly safe. **Every single drug** that affects our bodies will have some **side effects**".[2]

In order to keep track of how common and severe these side effects are, this information needs to be reported to a central clearinghouse. In the USA, that organization is the FDA. Here is how the system should work in an ideal world.

When people experience side effects, they report those side effects to their doctors. Their doctors, in turn, report them to the FDA. The FDA compiles this information and passes it on to the pharmaceutical manufacturers. The drug companies update the "Adverse Reactions" section on their product information sheets and pass this information along to the publishers of drug books such as the *Physicians' Desk Reference* (PDR). This updated information is printed in the next edition of the PDR. As a result, the PDR always contains the latest and most reliable information on the risk of side effects for each drug.

Our world is far from ideal, so it should be no surprise that this process breaks down all along the line. We need to change this. The first step in working to bring about change is to have a clear understanding of how the system currently "works". As we investigate, we begin to see where the system breaks down and where things can be improved.

Why Side Effects Get Overlooked

The frequency of occurrence of the ototoxic side effects of drugs is grossly under-reported. Indeed, I think this is true for all side effects. Many ototoxic (and other) side effects never get reported. The few adverse side effects that doctors report are the absolute **minimum** that exist. We only know the best case scenario. We certainly don't have a grasp on the most likely scenario, and I don't think anyone knows just how bad the situation really is.

Ototoxic side effects often go unrecognized and unreported for a variety of reasons. Here are some of them.

First, many people do not recognize the ototoxic side effects of the drugs they are taking. Few people are told what ototoxic side effects they should watch for. Therefore, they may not even recognize ototoxic side effects when they do occur. For example, a bit of hearing loss may easily go unnoticed. People may not connect dizzy spells or ringing in their ears to the medications they are taking. What it boils down to is, if you aren't aware you have a given side effect, you certainly won't report it.

Second, when researchers and doctors are doing their studies, they may not be looking for those specific side effects. Unless those side effects reach out and grab them somehow, it's almost certain they will miss them. There's an old adage that says, "You won't find it unless you are looking for it". How true this is in the case of the side effects of ototoxic drugs. Therefore, when drug studies are done, researchers must carefully and deliberately investigate whether any kind of damage is being done to our ears.

Hearing testing is not done often enough to catch many cases of drug-induced hearing loss. One doctor wrote that ototoxicity from taking Loop DIURETICS is probably under-reported because audiometric testing, which could detect early hearing loss, is seldom, if ever, done.[3]

Recording hearing loss by subjective means is not accurate. You likely aren't even aware of having a slight hearing loss. Without the proper testing equipment, you'll never know if an ototoxic drug has given you a mild hearing loss or not. A study revealed that only one person in 250 reported subjective hearing loss from a certain drug. However, conventional audiometric testing revealed that the true number was **ten times** higher![4] The results would have likely been much higher still if the researchers had tested for sub-clinical hearing loss by testing the high frequencies.

Sub-clinical hearing loss is hearing loss that only occurs in the high frequencies. It is not readily detected in an audiological clinic because few audiologists currently have the equipment to test hearing above 8 kHz. Chapter 6 reveals that many drugs cause hearing loss starting at the top end of the high frequencies. Since almost no one tests these high frequencies, a lot of drug-induced hearing loss goes undetected and thus unreported.

Third, another reason ototoxic side effects are often under-reported is because drugs are released to the public before they are thoroughly tested. Did you know that 51% of the approved drugs released in the past few years are now known to have had serious side effects that had not been detected at the time of their release to the public?[5] Some side effects only become evident after long-term drug use, yet drug trials are normally short-term affairs.

It can take years, and even decades after a drug is released, before its ototoxic properties are discovered. For example, **Erythromycin** was introduced in 1952, yet it was not until the mid 1970s that **Erythromycin** was recognized as ototoxic—a period of more than 20 years![6]

Fourth, some people who are being given ototoxic drugs may be unconscious, lethargic, confused, disoriented, sick or otherwise not mentally alert enough to adequately describe the side effects they feel. In these cases, they are not able to report ototoxic effects to their doctors. Then, too, some drugs are sedative in nature. Consequently, the people taking them may be less aware of some of the milder side effects. Thus, the incidence of such side effects is likely much higher than officially reported.[7]

Fifth, it is not easy to monitor a person for vestibular ototoxicity. It is both time-consuming and expensive. Drugs such as antiemetics and motion sickness drugs (**Dimenhydrinate—Dramamine**) may mask the nausea that frequently accompanies vestibular ototoxicity. In addition, if you are sick and confined to bed (perhaps in a hospital) you are not the most reliable person for describing side effects such as balance problems since you do not have to stand up or walk around.[8]

Finally, language can be a major barrier. If your first language is different from that of the medical staff, you may have great difficulty communicating any ototoxic side effects you experience.

Both Patients and Doctors Grossly Under-report Ototoxic Side Effects

The first link in reporting ototoxic side effects is you. Before you take a drug, you need to learn about all its known side effects. Then, if you experience any side effects, you need to report them to your doctor.

Often the system breaks down right here. Many people don't bother to learn which side effects they may experience. According to one FDA survey, 7 out of 10 patients never were told about the side effects of the drugs their doctors prescribed.[9] If your doctor or pharmacist doesn't tell you about the side effects of the drugs you are taking, you need to ask. This is **your** responsibility.

A further breakdown occurs, because even if you do notice a side effect, you may fail to attribute it to the drug you are taking. Thus you may never report it to your doctor. As a result, this side effect may never be written up in the PDR, and people will continue to damage their ears because they don't know the truth.

Even more important, if you don't report all side effects to your doctor, how will he know to adjust your medication so it won't do further damage your body?

A few months ago I was talking to a lady on the phone. She told me she had been taking **Erythromycin** for an infection. I knew it was ototoxic, so I asked her if it had bothered her ears. She didn't think so. I asked her if she had had any of the ototoxic effects you can see listed under **Erythromycin**. Right away she exclaimed, "Yes, I got that, and I had that". The upshot was that she had experienced fairly severe ototoxic side effects from taking this drug and hadn't realized it was caused by this drug at all! She thought it was just some of the effects of the illness she had.

I then asked her if she had reported these side effects to her doctor. No, she hadn't. There she was, damaging her ears, and her doctor was in the dark about the whole episode. I'm afraid this happens far too often.

Not only do you have a responsibility to report side effects to your doctor, he also has a responsibility. Doctors are supposed to report side effects to the FDA. Do you know whether your doctor reports to the FDA any the side effects you tell him about? I'll bet he doesn't! According to former FDA Commissioner, David Kessler, only about 1% ever get reported.[10]

Notice that! Doctors report to the FDA less that 1% of the **serious** side effects they come across. What happens to less serious side effects? Are they ever reported?

In one study of Rhode Island doctors, researchers found that the doctors in the study had recorded 26,000 adverse reactions in their patient's files. According to FDA guidelines, these doctors should have reported these side effects to the FDA. Now, here's the question. How many of these 26,000 side effects do you think these doctors actually reported to the FDA? You are going to be shocked by the answer. Did these doctors report all these 26,000 adverse reactions to the FDA, or even most of them? No sir, they did not! They only reported 11![11] Shocking isn't it?

If this study is representative of the whole country (and there is no compelling reason to believe otherwise), only 1 out of every 2,364 reports of serious adverse reactions ever reaches the FDA. Add to this total, the number of serious side effects that people do not report to their doctors in the first place. The result is that only a miniscule fraction of 1% of adverse side effects ever reach the FDA. Obviously, less serious and "minor" side effects such as hearing loss and tinnitus are rarely, if ever, reported.

The truth is, hearing loss is **not** a minor side effect at all, even though many doctors seem to treat it as such. Here is an example. Peggy lost all the hearing in one ear and some in her other ear from an ototoxic reaction to **Atenolol**. She hurried to her doctor. Did her doctor say, "Wow, I need to get you off this medication and report this side effect now!"? Absolutely not. He downplayed the seriousness of the situation, and treated her as a neurotic woman instead. He actually wrote on her chart that she was "just a little scared" because she had a little "reduced hearing" like it was no big deal and she was being emotional about nothing. Doctors need to realize that sudden hearing loss is a medical emergency! It **is** a big deal, not a minor annoyance that doesn't have to be reported.

Because her doctor (and others like him) do not report these kinds of ototoxic side effects, the current PDR still does not list hearing loss as a side effect for **Atenolol**. Interestingly enough, in other parts of the world, hearing loss is indeed linked to **Atenolol**. We need to get on the ball over here!

What Does Rare Really Mean?

Pharmacists fill billions of prescriptions each year in the USA. This translates into vast amounts of drugs consumed. For example, people consume *Aspirin* (**Acetylsalicylic acid**) by the truckload. As hard as it is to believe, Americans alone consume 40 million pounds of *Aspirin* each year![12] According to Bayer, people take more than 50 billion *Aspirin* tablets worldwide each year. These figures refer to only one drug. Add to this number the thousands of other drugs used worldwide. The total is truly monumental. As a result, "rare" ototoxic side effects can translate into enormous numbers of ears damaged.

The PDR uses the words "frequent," "infrequent" and "rare" to describe how often a given side effect occurs. In the PDR "frequent" generally means occurring in at least 1 person out of 100 (>1%). "Infrequent" side effects occur in fewer than 1 out of 100 people, but in more than 1 out of 1,000 people (0.1-1%) and "rare" side effects occur in fewer than 1 out of 1,000 (<0.1%) people taking a given drug.[13]

You will find some side effects listed as occurring only in 1 out of every 10,000 (0.01%) people taking that drug (very rare). You might consider this to be such a rare occurrence that it is not worth bothering about. Let me put these figures into perspective for you.

Consider a drug that supposedly only causes hearing loss in 1 person out of every 10,000 people taking it. This would be considered very rare. Even so, this "very rare" side effect is still going to affect a lot of people. For example, the population of the United States is approximately 280,000,000. At a chance of only 1 in 10,000 (0.01%), if all the people in the USA took a certain drug that caused hearing loss, 28,000 people would end up with a hearing loss. Would you take solace in the fact that 28,000 other people now can't hear either? That is small comfort!

If the occurrence of hearing loss was rare—only 1 out of 1,000—you would be part of over a quarter of a million people in the USA who would now be hard of hearing from taking that drug. This is certainly not a trivial number. We are talking about a **lot** of people! The comparable figures for China would be 1,200,000 people. Worldwide, the resulting hearing loss would affect over 5,000,000 people each and every year! They may call this "rare," but in reality, it is catastrophic—yet this is how many people would be affected if only one-tenth of 1% of the people taking a given drug had this side effect! Don't be fooled by the word "rare". The suffering caused by a "rare" side effect can be enormous.

The above figures are based on the assumption that the incidence statistics are correct, but are they? As we have seen, only a small fraction of 1% of side effects are ever reported to the FDA. Thus the true incidence of a given side effect is likely much, much higher than the figures you see reported in the PDR.

Put another way, the published figures for a given side effect are grossly low. For example, a side effect that is said to occur in less than 0.01% (1 in 10,000) of the people taking it, may in actual fact, be occurring 2,364 times more often than reported (based on the results of the Rhode Island study). Therefore, instead of only occurring once in every 10,000 people and thus being truly a very rare side effect, this side effect theoretically might be occurring once in every four people (23.6%)! That is not rare at all!

The risk incidence figures in this book all come from reputable sources. If you see "PDR" after an incidence figure, you know that these are the figures that were reported to the FDA during the drug approval process. You can take them at face value if you want. However, now that you know how seldom side effects are really reported, you might want to factor in some constant to allow for a large margin of error in the reported figures. I think these published incidence figures warrant a healthy dose of skepticism.

Furthermore, until widespread studies have been done, no one knows if the results of the specific controlled studies that are reported in the PDR and other similar drug books are reliable indicators of the true incidence of those side effects in the population at large. This is because the population at large may have different characteristics and other factors from those that prevailed during the clinical trials.

Similarly, you cannot accurately compare the cited frequencies with figures obtained from other clinical investigations involving different treatments, uses, and investigators. The cited figures just provide you with a basis for estimating the frequency of occurrence of side effects in the populations studied.[14]

In real life, the figures may vary all over the place. For this reason, you need to know the specific risk factors for your own body. (See Chapter 4 for information on risk factors.) You don't really care what the risk is to the general population. You really want to know how a certain drug is going to affect your own body. You need to interpret any risk statistics in this book in light of the specific risk factors you know you have. Thus a drug with a rare risk of occurrence in the general population, may really be a high risk drug to you. Don't just assume that because the published risk figures are "rare" that the side effect won't happen to you. You may be right, but if you read your risk factors wrongly, you may end up very sorry!

How Serious Are "Serious" Side Effects?

What ototoxic side effects should you be reporting? FDA guidelines say to report **serious** adverse events. They define serious side effects [from drugs] as those that cause death; are life-threatening; cause hospitalization; result in a significant, persistent or permanent disability; and those that require [medical] intervention to prevent permanent impairment or damage.

They further explain their definition of a disability—"a significant, persistent, or permanent change, impairment, damage or disruption in the patient's body function/structure, physical activities or quality of life".[15]

This description fits conditions such as hearing loss, hyperacusis, tinnitus, ataxia, dizziness, nystagmus, oscillopsia, vertigo and various balance problems. These are significant conditions. Many times they are permanent. Furthermore, they all can cause a very definite change in our physical activities, and they most definitely affect the quality of our lives. Therefore, whether doctors and other medical professionals think of ear damage as serious or not, ototoxic damage to our ears **is** a serious adverse event and thus they need to report it!

The FDA requests you (or your doctor) report such events even if you are not absolutely certain a given drug caused the side effect you are reporting. If you are suspicious that it did, report it.

Increasing the Percentage of Side Effects Reported

The FDA largely relies on doctors to **voluntarily** report any side effects they come across in order to catch unreported and under-reported side effects. This is a serious weakness in the system. Doctors can report side effects if they wish but, except for certain serious side effects, they are not bound by law to do this. Thus, as we have seen, they only report a small fraction of 1% of all side effects.

One solution would be for the government to step in and make it mandatory for doctors and pharmacists to report adverse side effects. At least that way, we would have a better grasp of the true frequency and severity of ototoxic side effects.

There are at least three reasons why doctors do not currently report all the side effects they come across.

The first reason is "just because they don't have to". It is human nature not to do more than you have to. Thus, they don't bother.

Second, doctors do not think this is important enough when looking at the whole scheme of things. Since they are pressed for time, they do only those things **they** feel are important. To them, serious heart problems may be important—ears apparently aren't.

Third, doctors have no economic incentive to do so. In fact, they have a big incentive **not** to do so. It takes time to fill out reports. The time spent filling out and filing such reports actually takes money out of their pockets! The FDA suggests it will take 30 minutes for the average person to fill out the necessary form for reporting an ototoxic side effect. Doctors may be able to shorten this time considerably. However, even if it only takes a doctor 5 to 7 minutes to fill out the form and submit it, that is the equivalent of the time many doctors take to examine a patient. This means a doctor can't see as many patients as he would otherwise. Consequently, he will not make as much money. As a result, it is the rare doctor that will take the time to report to the FDA the side effects he comes across.

Assuming the government does not change the current system any time soon, we need to encourage/urge our doctors to file ototoxic drug side-effect reports on our behalf. The FDA has made it relatively easy to file these reports.

If your doctor won't file an ototoxic side-effect report, all is not lost. According to FDA guidelines, these forms do not have to be submitted by doctors. Anybody can file such a report, including you.

How to Report Side Effects

Doctors (and anyone else) can use one of three methods to report ototoxic side effects. The important thing is that someone reports the occurrence of ototoxic side effects.

Phone It In

Anyone can pick up the phone and report side effects verbally to the FDA's MedWatch hotline. The number to call is 1-800-332-1088.

Report It On-line

If you want to fill out the form on-line, go to the FDA web site, fill it in and submit it instantly—all from your keyboard. You can do this from:

https://www.accessdata.fda.gov/scripts/medwatch/

Click the "Begin" button on the right side. If you need instructions, you can access the instructions on how to fill out this form by clicking on the "instructions page" link.

Print It Out and Mail It In

You can download the appropriate form, print it out, fill it out manually and mail it in, or you can fill it in online, then print it out and mail it in. Download this form from:

http://www.fda.gov/medwatch/getforms.htm

When you are at this web site, click on "Form 3500 Voluntary Reporting". (Note this form is in PDF format, so you will need to have Adobe's free Acrobat Reader program already installed on your computer in order to read it.)

A neat feature is that when you print out this form you also print out a prepaid mailer so you don't even have to pay any postage.

To further encourage your doctor to report any ototoxic side effects, print a copy of this form from the FDA's web site and take it with you to your next doctor's appointment. If you do this, your doctor can't say he doesn't have a form handy!

The Way the System "Works"

We like to think that researchers, doctors, drug companies, the FDA and other government agencies all are looking out for our best interests. This is the way it should be. However, in actual fact, this is not exactly the way the system works. Each of these entities are really looking out for themselves, not specifically for you. As a result, you need to watch out for "you".

The Drug Approval Process

Very briefly, here is how drug testing is done. When a new drug is being developed, the drug manufacturer has to follow specific steps. Initially, they accumulate tissue cultures and animal safety data. The proposed new drug (called the Investigational New Drug or IND) is tested on animals to determine how toxic it is, to see if it does what it is supposed to do and to watch for any side effects. Obviously, not all side effects are caught because animals cannot tell you if they are experiencing tinnitus or the feeling their ears are blocked.

If the initial testing is favorable, the FDA approves the results of the animal studies. The drug manufacturer then moves on to the first of four phases of human testing.

Phase 1. In Phase 1, approximately 20 to 80 healthy male volunteers between the age of 18 and 45 take the test drug in small doses until the first signs of toxicity appear. Researchers also watch to see how the drug is metabolized, how quickly it is eliminated from the body and if there are any side effects.

Phase 2. In Phase 2 researchers evaluate approximately 80 to 100 people who have the same disorder this drug is intended to treat. During this phase, researchers look for the optimal dose that has the fewest side effects. They closely monitor adverse drug reactions.

Phase 3. Phase 3 is a full clinical trial where many physicians test the drug on hundreds or even thousands of patients. They compare the test drug results with the results of other drugs to see how "good" it is. If there are no other drugs to use as controls, they do a double-blind study where neither the researchers nor the patients know which patients are given the drug and which patients are given a placebo until after the study is over. The analysis of these data shows whether those getting the drug do better than those that get the placebo. During this phase, the patients are closely monitored to detect any side effects that were not identified in the earlier phases.

Unfortunately, it appears that some drug manufacturers select only the lowest-risk or "best-case" patients on whom to conduct trials. These are the people with little or no history of adverse side effects and/or those with the less severe illnesses.[16]

Phase 4. During Phase 4, the test drug is evaluated on specific groups of people such as children, pregnant women, and seniors. Side effects are reported to the FDA at prescribed intervals throughout this process.[17]

Records are kept of the benefits and the adverse side effects observed over the course of the trials. When the study is over, the drug company compiles these adverse side effects and sends this information together with other descriptive, warning and prescribing information to the FDA for approval. The FDA reviews this information, and if all is to its liking, approves the drug for use by doctors. This approved product information then becomes the official data sheet that is released by the drug company for that product.

The drug approval process, like anything else involved with statistics, has some inherent weaknesses. It is very easy to manipulate statistics whether intentionally or not. "Hard" data such as is reported by the drug companies are really only "estimates of reality". For most drugs, only a comparatively small number of doses have been given in the pre-marketing phase. Many (most) of these data are derived from administering a given drug under carefully controlled conditions. Unfortunately, the same conditions do not prevail in real life.

> ## New is Not Always Better!
>
> Dr. Harold McPheeters has spent a lifetime practicing medicine. He writes:
>
> "Be cautious of the newer medications that have recently been introduced and are being heavily marketed by the drug companies. Most drugs are systematically tested only for life threatening conditions such as heart damage, liver and kidney damage and **not** for other toxic effects such as ototoxicity, neurotoxicity, etc.
>
> Conditions such as ototoxicity will be reported **if they are noticed** as side effects on the initial life-safety tests, but otherwise drugs go to market without systematic investigation for other forms of toxicity. Those conditions are then supposed to be reported as they are observed by physicians and pharmacists in the course of using the drugs on their patients.
>
> Many of the newer medications are very powerful and are inclined to have more serious toxic effects than some of the older medications that were previously used for the same conditions. This seems to be especially true in the field of psychiatry in which the newer psychotropic medications may have many serious side effects—especially on the nervous system".[18]

Once a drug is approved and is in the hands of doctors, the process of reporting side effects becomes unreliable. Many ototoxic side effects just don't get reported—even if they are detected as we have already seen! The problem is compounded because many people take more than one drug at a time. Furthermore, they may have more than one medical condition that predisposes them to developing an ototoxic side effect. Finally, they may be taking higher doses than what is recommended. All of these factors may render supposedly "hard" data soft.[19]

Each drug company is solely responsible for any information they include on the product information sheets they release about the drugs they manufacture, although the FDA may insist that they include certain specific information.

This begs the question, "What happens when more information is discovered about a drug months or years after it has been released?" If it is good—new benefits and such—the drug company will naturally approach the FDA with a revised product information sheet for approval. However, if the new information is negative, for example, if more adverse side effects are discovered, the drug companies have no incentive to make this information public. Why should we even expect a company to "bad mouth" its own products?

Therefore, unless the FDA receives enough information on adverse side effects from other sources (meaning you, me and our doctors), and insists that it be included in the next product information sheet for that drug, these new side effects may never see the light of day. Who knows how many adverse side effects never appear in the PDR and CPS because of this?

If the PDR and CPS do not list all adverse side effects, neither we, as consumers, nor our doctors have any easy way of knowing the truth about any given drug. This is a very serious flaw in the current system that needs fixing.

Unless all side effects are required to be included on product information sheets (and subsequently added to the PDR), more people are needlessly going to lose their hearing as the following story attests.

The Story of Vicodin

Vicodin, a narcotic painkiller, is a brand name for the combination drug **Hydrocodone** and **Acetaminophen**. (There are also other brands by other manufacturers containing these same two drugs such as *Lortab*, *Norco* and *Zydone*.) Originally, during the pre-approval trials, apparently no sign of hearing loss was found. As far as anyone knew, it was not ototoxic. Since its release, neither the PDR nor the CPS have mentioned any ototoxic side effects (until the 2002 PDR finally contained a warning). For 17 years everything went well. By the year 2000, *Vicodin* had climbed to become the most prescribed drug in America.[20] Then it happened.

On April 26, 1999, House Ear Institute physicians reported a previously unknown and devastating side effect of *Vicodin*—rapid, profound, bilateral, irreversible hearing loss after overuse of this drug.[21]

According to Dr. John W. House, "Some patients have retained some hearing if they stop using the painkillers immediately, but for most, the damage is already done. Once the process starts, it seems irreversible".[22]

Although *Vicodin* had been on the market since 1982, hearing loss attributed to *Vicodin* did not begin showing up until 11 years later, in 1993.[23] This was likely because no one was looking for a link between sudden hearing loss and *Vicodin*.

In one report, a man was taking 20 to 30 *Vicodin* pills a day for pain. One day he noticed his ears were ringing. From the time he first noticed his ears ringing until he was completely deaf was only 4 weeks.[24]

After the House report was published, two audiologists called the journal that published this study to report that each of them had had a patient who experienced sudden and significant hearing loss after taking *Vicodin*.

Soon other stories began to surface. Since the House Ear Institute report came out, and while I was writing the first edition of this book, several people wrote to me telling how they too had lost their hearing from taking *Vicodin*. In my files I have anecdotal reports of two women who took *Vicodin* for several months. During that time both noticed a definite drop in their hearing.

Furthermore, I have correspondence in my files with a woman who totally lost her hearing from taking *Vicodin*. Here is her story. Jodi had back surgery so her doctor put her on *Vicodin* for the pain. She built up a tolerance to it and had to take more and more. The pain persisted, and she ended up taking high doses of *Vicodin* for several years. Then one day she noticed her ears were ringing and she couldn't hear things she used to hear. In a matter of months her hearing dropped from normal to so bad that even hearing aids couldn't help her. Now she has a cochlear implant to help her hear.

Vicodin is typically prescribed for short-term use of 2 to 3 weeks at most. A typical dose is one pill every 6 hours. Hearing loss has not been reported when taking *Vicodin* at recommended dosages. Trouble to your ears develops when you take much higher doses such as 20 or more pills a day for 2 months or longer.[25]

You should be aware that *Vicodin* is addictive and thus subject to abuse. As a result, it has a staggering potential for severe hearing loss when used wrongly.

Because the potential for severe hearing loss is enormous, you would have thought that both the FDA and the drug companies would scramble to amend their product information sheets on drugs using the **Acetaminophen/Hydrocodone** combination and get that information widely distributed. Apparently this was not the case. Neither the 2000 PDR nor the 2001 PDR gave any indication that such drugs can cause hearing loss.

According to a news report, the doctors at the House Ear Institute reported hearing loss incidents to the FDA in 1999 (and again in August 2001). To their credit, in 2000 the firm that manufactures *Vicodin* added a warning about the potential for hearing loss to the drug's label. However, it seems that the label change has gone largely unnoticed, even among top hearing specialists.[26]

In September 2001, another article blowing the whistle on *Vicodin* appeared in the papers.[27] Finally, in the 2002 edition of the PDR things begin to change. Under the brands containing the **Hydrocodone/Acetaminophen** combination such as *Lortab*, *Norco* and *Vicodin*, it warns, "Very rare cases of hearing loss have been reported in patients predominantly receiving very high doses of **Hydrocodone/Acetaminophen** for long periods of time".[28]

What I want to know is why in this same PDR the other drugs that contain both **Acetaminophen** and **Hydrocodone** do not have this same warning? For example, in the 2003 edition of the PDR, there are three different brands of drugs containing **Acetaminophen** and **Hydrocodone** that do not have any warning about hearing loss whatsoever.[29]

Is this side effect all that rare? Officially, there were only 48 cases of hearing loss reported as of September 2001, although there have been millions of prescriptions written for *Vicodin*. Since many of these prescriptions were for refills, not for new patients, the incidence is not really as rare as it first appears.

On top of that, hearing loss may be "much more prevalent than we think" according to Dr. Akira Ishiyama, an assistant professor of otolaryngology at UCLA Medical School. According to him, some doctors have not drawn a connection between *Vicodin* use and sudden hearing loss in their patients because they haven't been looking for it.[30]

Apparently the FDA isn't ordering the drug companies to include this new information in future editions of the PDR. As a result, unless doctors know of this information from some other source, they will continue to prescribe *Vicodin* to their patients and will not warn them that they could lose much of their hearing because of it.

This is the way the present system "works". How many more people have to lose their hearing before an effective warning is distributed to doctors and consumers alike?

It's about time things changed. Instead of worrying about politics and the almighty dollar, governments and companies need to concern themselves with people and their well-being. At the same time, people have to take responsibility for their own health and carefully follow the dosage guidelines for taking drugs and not insist their doctors prescribe them drugs for longer than the guidelines recommend.

Pharmaceutical Companies

Drug companies do the research needed to get a new drug approved by the FDA. Then they get it on the market and begin making money. As we have seen, many side effects only show up later when the general population begins taking that drug. Apparently the FDA seems more concerned about claims of how good a drug is (you can't say a drug will cure a certain condition without proper proof) than it is with listing all the side effects that could result. Therefore, the drug companies do not have to list every side effect they have found or know about.

Drug companies spend billions of dollars each year advertising their products in order to get you to take their drugs. The drug industry aggressively promotes drugs to consumers

Drug Advertising—A Disturbing Trend

A disturbing trend today is the numerous drug ads you see on TV. Even more disturbing, these ads are not primarily intended to benefit your health. They are intended to make more money for the drug companies. They are a tool to sell a product. After all, drug companies are in business like any other company and want to boost their bottom lines.

According to Nancy Chockley, President of the National Institute for Health Care Management Research and Education Foundation, you need to be wary because these ads are "presented to influence decisions rather than truly inform". They are "neither substantive nor objective". She cautions, "Drug ads downplay the limitations or side effects of a drug".

What this means is that these drug ads do not give you the whole story. As a result, you cannot make well-informed decisions. She warns, "Consumers need better, more balanced information in order to engage in a genuinely informed discussion with their doctors".[31]

A lot of the drugs you see regularly advertised on TV have ototoxic side effects. (You'll find these drugs and ototoxic side effects described in this book.) However, you seldom, if ever, see these ototoxic side effects listed in the TV ads, although ads for *Viagra* do mention hearing loss, but not its other ototoxic side effects.

and doctors to the tune of $16 billion a year. This advertising pays off handsomely for them. Business is good for the newer and most expensive drugs. In its first year on the market, *Celebrex* racked up sales of $1 billion. *Vioxx* had sales of $1.5 billion in 2000.[32]

Sales increases of the 50 most advertised drugs made up almost half of the increase in drug spending leaving the other 9,850 drugs on the market to make up the other half.[33]

Consumers are going to their doctors and asking/demanding the drugs they see advertised. Research reveals that if 100 million Americans saw a specific drug ad, as a result, 30 million would ask their doctor about it, and doctors would prescribe it to 13.2 million of them.

Television ads by the pharmaceutical companies downplay the many potential side effects of the various drugs they advertise. How often have you ever seen an advertisement for a drug list hearing loss, balance problems and tinnitus as side effects that you need to watch out for? None? Nada? Zero? Zilch? Same here. If people understood all the potential side effects of a given drug, they might think twice before taking it.[34]

Drug companies are in the business of making money—lots of money! They only make money when they are selling drugs to you. Therefore, it should be no surprise that they are aggressive in their quest to get drugs approved so they can sell them and make even more money.

Unfortunately, sometimes they may push too hard. One researcher, Dr. Richard Deyo, wrote about "problems usually discussed only in whispers: powerful constituencies with vested financial interests are routinely intimidating investigators who point out the health risks of drugs". "This is business as usual," he says. "Intimidation and attacks are the way business is conducted".[35]

As wise consumers, we need to know what is going on so we can make informed decisions on the drugs we take. For example, did you know that researcher Dr. Bruce Psaty found that CALCIUM-CHANNEL BLOCKERS were "associated with 60 per cent more heart attacks than other older and cheaper forms of blood pressure medication". Another researcher, Dr. Detsky, took this one step further and published his findings on these new CALCIUM-CHANNEL BLOCKERS and the glowing reports other researchers had reported. He writes, "90 per cent of researchers who had reached positive conclusions about the drugs had economic links to their manufacturers".[36]

You can draw your own conclusions what this could mean to your health and to your ears. If you look at section 20.8.16 in Table 14-1, you can see at a glance the many ototoxic side effects you may experience as a result of taking CALCIUM-CHANNEL BLOCKERS. These are things of which you should be aware.

Here is another example. There are lots of men (and their wives) who are excited about the drug **Sildenafil** (*Viagra* is the most popular brand) and what it can do to enrich their sex lives. However, I think few of them ever really consider the host of side effects that can result—including death! For those of us concerned about our ears, **Sildenafil** can cause hearing loss, tinnitus, vertigo and other bad things. We need to be aware of these things and **then** make an **informed** decision whether or not we are prepared to accept these risks.

Doctors' Ties to Drug Manufacturers Result in Biased Drug Reviews

When you go to your doctor, you expect him to do what is best for you. You want his unbiased advice. You want the best (and cheapest) prescriptions with the fewest side effects to restore your health.

Is this what you get? Or is your doctor's advice skewed by drug company influence? You may never know. Here's why. The experts who write about drugs all seem to have financial ties to the drug companies. As a result, how could you expect them to give the plain, unvarnished truth? Their reports, whether consciously or otherwise, are biased because of these financial ties.

Even the last bastion of unbiased drug reporting, *The New England Journal of Medicine* "recently loosened its guidelines regarding financial ties of experts who write for it".

Why? According to Dr. Jeffrey Drazen, the journal's editor, he couldn't find unbiased experts to write for him. "Everyone he found had financial ties to the firm that made the drugs they would be writing about!"

According to Dr. Ivan Oransky in his article *Ties to drug manufacturers deform medical reviews* says, "Researchers can slant reviews in many ways: by not offering their results for publication if the data undermine a desired outcome; by writing conclusions that are contradicted by their own data; or by emphasizing certain studies while ignoring others".

He warns: "Doctors should know what's influencing the articles they read—and you should know what's influencing your doctor's decisions".[37]

It should be even more obvious now why you have to do your own research if you want to protect your ears (and the rest of your body) from the side effects of ototoxic (and other) drugs. You cannot depend on receiving unbiased professional advice.

Until doctors are required to report **all** side effects, and the FDA requires the drug companies to **compile and report all these side effects** and see that they are included in books such as the PDR and CPS, how will we ever be able to make truly informed decisions?

The Role of the PDR and Other Drug Books

Many people are not clear exactly how the PDR (and CPS and other drug books) fit into the present "system". There are several misconceptions I'd like to address.

First, the PDR is not a complete listing of all the drugs that are available in the USA. (The same is true for the CPS in Canada.) It only contains the drugs that the drug companies want listed there in that particular year. Thus, if a drug company wants a new (or existing) drug included in the next edition of the PDR, it forwards the official product information sheets to the PDR Network, LLC, the publisher of the PDR. (In Canada, these product information sheets go to the Canadian Pharmacists Association for inclusion in the Canadian counterpart to the PDR, the *Compendium of Pharmaceuticals and Specialties*, commonly called the CPS.)

The decision whether a drug is included in the PDR or not appears to be entirely up to the company that manufactures the drugs. For whatever reason, a pharmaceutical company can choose **not** to send this information to be included in the next edition of the PDR. Thus a given drug can be listed there one year and not the next. You can be sure that some older, less profitable, but equally effective drugs are dropped in favor of new, high-profit medications. This is just how it is.

Second, the PDR only lists the information about each drug that the drug companies send it. After the FDA approves the wording on the product information sheets, it is basically set in stone. This—and only this—information is printed in the PDR. The PDR Network, LLC (the publisher of the PDR) publishes the product information sheets in the PDR exactly as they come from the drug manufacturers. They do not edit or change in any way the official product information sheets they receive. They are not a clearinghouse for such information, nor do they compile drug information from various sources. They do not verify the accuracy or completeness of the information contained on the product information sheets. They act solely as a compiler and publisher of this information whether it is right or wrong, complete or incomplete. If new information comes to light on a given drug, unless the drug company includes this new information in a revised product information sheet and sends it to the publisher, that information will never be printed in the PDR. Also, be aware that recalled, discontinued, experimental or foreign drugs are not included in the PDR. Again, this is just how it is.

Third, not all the drugs in the PDR have complete drug listings. Some are quite abbreviated and others basically only give the names of the drug. Again, it seems to be up to the drug companies as to how complete each listing will be that is included in the PDR. Abbreviated drug listings obviously cannot contain as much information as full listings. Thus, the adverse side effects section is greatly abbreviated too, so ototoxic side effects may not even be listed.

Fourth, the drug companies only need to list the side effects the FDA requires. As a result, the PDR listings are not necessarily complete records of all known side effects of any listed drugs.Obviously, not everything that is known about a drug and its side effects is included in the PDR.

Fifth, when independent labs, researchers or doctors find other adverse side effects, and even after these side effects are documented in one of the respected medical journals, this information is not updated in the PDR, **unless** the drug company sends updated product information sheets to the PDR. Since there is no incentive for drug companies to bad-mouth their own drugs, they often leave well enough alone unless the FDA directs them to include this new information. Otherwise, these new side effects stay safely buried and we, the hard-of-hearing consumers, are the ones that lose out.

Sometimes the information for a given drug is identical in both the CPS and PDR. Other times this information is quite different. You should be aware of this. For example, the CPS lists hearing loss as a side effect of **Itraconazole**, but the PDR doesn't. With **Lorazepam**, the situation is reversed, and hearing loss is listed in the PDR but not in the CPS.

At times, the ototoxic side effects listed can be very different. For example, the CPS lists hearing loss, tinnitus, dizziness and vertigo as side effects of **Cephalexin**, yet the PDR only lists dizziness. For **Quetiapine** the PDR lists hearing loss, tinnitus, ataxia, dizziness, vertigo and earache, yet the CPS only lists dizziness and earache for the identical brand of this same drug.

These discrepancies exist because the drug companies and drug regulatory bodies in each country decide which side effects are to be included and which may be left off the official product information sheets. What this means is that you cannot get the whole truth from any given drug source. Some sources list some side effects while other sources may list different side effects.

Therefore, do not be surprised if your doctor or pharmacist doesn't know that a given drug can damage your ears. Your doctor might prescribe **Itraconazole** for you. You ask him to see if it can cause hearing loss. He looks it up in his PDR and assures you it does not cause hearing loss. He is telling you the truth as he knows it since the PDR doesn't list hearing loss as a side effect. However, he will still be wrong, and your ears may suffer for it!

You can't expect to come close to finding all the published information about the ototoxic side effects of drugs unless you take the time to research **all** the drug lists, books and databases in the world. That is why this book is so valuable. I have scoured the literature searching for all reported ototoxic side effects. This book contains the information I have gleaned, not only from the PDR, CPS and BNF, but also from other reliable drug books and drug sources from around the world as well.

This book is as complete as I can make it, but you need to remember that it does not include every ototoxic drug and ototoxic side effect because I do not have access to all the repositories of ototoxic drug information on the planet.

Of the 877 ototoxic drugs listed in this book, the PDR lists at least one ototoxic side effect for only 558 (64%) of them. The CPS lists at least one ototoxic side effect for 544 (62%) ototoxic drugs. However, there are 178 (20%) ototoxic drugs that either are not listed in either the PDR or the CPS or they are listed there, but do not have any ototoxic side effects listed. (To be fair, some of these are foreign drugs and are not used here.)

Now you can see why you need to be extremely careful so you don't inadvertently damage your ears by taking a drug that you and your doctor did not know was ototoxic.

Table 5-1. Ototoxic Drugs in This Book

	Number	Percent
In PDR but not CPS	155	18%
In CPS but not PDR	141	16%
In both PDR and CPS	403	46%
Not in PDR or CPS	178	20%
TOTAL	877	100%

The FDA's Role

The FDA plays a critical role in the present drug system. You may be surprised to learn exactly what they do and do not do.

The FDA is the government body that approves and regulates drug use in the USA. Here is a shocking statistic. "The FDA regulates fewer than 1% of the drugs [chemicals] brought into the market-place".[38] These unregulated drugs are used in all sorts of things like cosmetics and cleaners and on and on.

When the FDA approves a drug, it doesn't mean that drug is "safe". It just means that the supposed benefits outweigh the known risks that are outlined on the drug's label. Note the words "known risks". If hearing wasn't checked during the drug trials, then hearing loss is not considered as one of the "known risks". Likewise, if a study wasn't continued long enough to bring to light certain side effects, then those side effects are not part of the "known risks". You need to understand that the risks listed in any FDA-approved materials are the **minimum** risks you will encounter. The real-life risks may be much, much higher.

The FDA may approve a drug following clinical trials of a few months, involving controlled populations of several hundred people. But later, surprises can occur. To detect these problems, the FDA relies on doctors submitting **voluntary** reports. This is a big mistake. Unfortunately, as we saw previously, once a drug is released for public consumption, the data about side effects does not pour into the FDA from the doctors like it is supposed to. Thus the incidence of side effects of drugs continue to be grossly under-reported.

Although the FDA regulates drugs, you should know that the FDA neither develops or tests drugs. That is left up to the drug manufacturers. They do the studies and submit them to the FDA. The FDA then evaluates the data and assesses the benefit-to-risk relationship based solely on the data submitted. Then they either approve or reject that drug without doing any independent testing to verify the accuracy and efficacy of the drug they are approving![39] The FDA only evaluates the information given to them. If the studies they receive are flawed, less than thorough, or biased, how would they ever know? The system breaks down here too. There needs to be independent corroboration.

You also should be aware that the FDA has extremely limited resources to monitor the safety of all the thousands of drugs on the market today. Around the year 2000 only 52 employees were dedicated to monitoring drug safety. Their Department of Pharmacovigilance and Epidemiology (DPE) comprised only 8 physicians and 1 Ph.D. The DPE has the task of "protecting the American public from the health risks of marketed drugs". How can we expect this miniscule staff to do an effective job for us?[40]

The FDA needs to allocate more resources to monitoring drug safety. They are already stretched much too thinly to effectively monitor all these new drugs coming on the market each year.

In fact, things are going from bad to worse. In order to keep up with the volume of new drugs, the FDA even created a new "fast-track" system where the drug manufacturers can pay a fee to accelerate the release of their new drugs. This translates into a system that approves more drugs with even less information documenting their safety![41]

Is this what we want? Do we like being the guinea pigs and risking our health and our precious ears? If not, we have to speak up and do something to change this inadequate system.

The FDA Sits on an Enormous Database of Drug Side Effects

Here's another thing that needs to change. The FDA sits on an enormous database of largely-inaccessible, yet vitally-important information on drug side effects that have surfaced since the drugs were approved and put on the market. If the FDA has our best interests at heart, why don't they make this information readily available to the public as fast as it comes in?

This information could be invaluable to people wondering about the side effects of any given drug—information that is not otherwise available—that is, the millions of reports of side effects collected by the FDA that are not included in drug books such as the PDR like you think they would be.

Let me give you one small example that I happened to run across serendipitously. This report by the FDA concerns the drug **Omeprazole**.[42] Between September 14, 1989, when **Omeprazole** was approved to be released to the public, and March 31, 2000, when this report was compiled (a period of about 10½ years), the FDA had accumulated 10,005 reports of side effects of **Omeprazole** (and they consider this pile of reports to be "**low**" compared to other drugs). As I read this report, I realized that some of the ototoxic side effects contained in this report had not been listed in the PDR when this drug first came out, and they **still** are **not** mentioned in the latest edition of the PDR. This leads the public to believe that this drug is safer that it really is.

In spite of all its shortcomings, the FDA could help right things if it would make available to the public the enormous amount of information on drug side effects it has buried in its humongous database. As a minimum, they could list all the side effects reported to it for each drug in this database, together with the number of reports of each side effect.

Let's look at this information on **Omeprazole** since it's the only report I've come across on a specific drug. First, here's what's readily available. The PDR (after 10 years of reporting on **Omeprazole**) lists tinnitus, dizziness and vertigo as the only ototoxic side effects of this drug. However, in this FDA report we find that in addition to these side effects, the FDA also had reports on hearing loss, ear pain and ototoxicity.

If you had been prescribed **Omeprazole**, wouldn't you have liked to know **before** you started taking it that taking it could cause hearing loss? Wouldn't you have liked to know how many people had lost their hearing due to taking this drug, so you could estimate your chances of having the same side effect?

You won't find those pieces of information in the PDR. And if you were one of the unfortunate people to lose their hearing from taking **Omeprazole**, wouldn't you wish to know what the chances are of your hearing loss being permanent or temporary? All of the above information is contained in the FDA's database.

For example, this report explains that 35% of the 17 people who experienced hearing loss from taking **Omeprazole** had permanent loss. In the remaining 65% of the cases, the hearing loss was either temporary, or at least some degree of hearing returned. This report also contains the kind of anecdotal reports I have included in this book. As an example, it mentions the case of a 42-year-old man who was prescribed **Omeprazole**. Seven days later he experienced hearing loss in one ear and stopped taking this drug. Since that time his hearing has only improved slightly.[43]

This is the kind of information that could be extracted from this database for every drug it contains. I'd love to include all of the ototoxic information it contains for every drug in this book, but I can't. I don't have access to this information. Neither do you. This too needs to change.

Here's something else that needs to change. The FDA needs to give timely reports of the information it has in its database—not sit on it and hide this information from the public while people die from the side effects of taking various drugs.

For example, think of **Rofecoxib** (*Vioxx*). This popular drug was only on the market for about 5 years. It was withdrawn on September 30, 2004 because of concerns that it was causing heart attacks. Yet this information had been available (but hidden from the public) for some years at that point. The prestigious medical journal, *The Lancet*, published an article on November 5, 2004 where the authors concluded that "owing to the known cardiovascular risk, **Rofecoxib** should have been withdrawn several years earlier". If this had been done thousands of people would still be alive that died due to heart attacks from taking **Rofecoxib**.

How bad was it? In the 5 years **Rofecoxib** was on the market, the FDA estimated that between 88,000 and 139,000 people had experienced heart attacks from taking **Rofecoxib**, and of this number an estimated 26,400 to 55,600 people died.[44] That's scary!

If you had been prescribed **Rofecoxib**, wouldn't you have wanted this information regarding heart problems, as well as its ototoxic properties, as this information was being reported to the FDA? Wouldn't you want to learn this information promptly, rather than waiting for 5 years until tens of thousands of people had died from taking this drug? I know I would have.

This is one reason that Dr. Wolfe of *Worst Pills, Best Pills* typically recommends waiting for 7 years after a new drug comes out before you begin taking it. In that time, many of the "missed" side effects come to light, and the worst drug offenders are often removed from the market in that time frame—as was the case with **Rofecoxib**.[45]

Your Role

You, as the consumer, are the final link in this drug-system chain. You are now aware of how the system works. Since you are the consumer and have the most to lose, you need to be constantly alert to the unexpected damage drugs can do to your body.

Here are some words of warning from a medical doctor. "The most highly promoted and advertised drugs are the very ones that have not yet been fully tested for all kinds of toxic reactions. They are the newer drugs that are still under patent, but the main safety testing has been on the heart and vital functions—not 'minor' effects such as ototoxicity, neurotoxicity or toxic effects on the skin, digestion, muscles, etc. These effects are reported as they are discovered in various patients, in part, during the original drug evaluations, but primarily after the drug is already on the market".[46]

According to Dr. McPheeters, if you already have a hearing loss, it is important that you know which drugs most likely have ototoxic effects. If your doctor prescribes one of these for you, you need to ask him to choose another medication with less risk if possible. You should also avoid neurotoxic drugs whenever possible since the hair cells in the cochlea are basically part of your nervous system and are likely to be similarly affected. Also, avoid taking combinations of medications.

Furthermore, Dr. McPheeters warns that if you are hard of hearing, you should choose well-established medications that are known to be relatively free from ototoxic effects over newly-introduced medications that have not been fully evaluated for possible ototoxic effects.[49] Since new drugs are more powerful and have far greater potential for serious toxic side effects, if you have sensorineural hearing loss or Meniere's disease, you should be very cautious about using them. Only use drugs if there is a very definite need. Take them only as

Warning! Drugs Are Not a Panacea.

Dr. Harold McPheeters, MD, who is himself hard of hearing, is concerned about the indiscriminate use of drugs today. Listen to him as we warns:

"I get concerned at how many folks, influenced by all the drug advertising and promotions, are seeking medications for the most inconsequential and trivial ailments".

"I continue to be dismayed at how frequently folks with hearing losses seem to be searching for some new medications that will solve some relatively minor problem they have. They would be much better advised to avoid medications whenever possible because of the very good chance that such medicines and combinations of medications will cause further assaults to their hearing.

The risks of toxic and allergic reactions are just too great to take unnecessary chances, especially when medications are combined.

The pharmaceutical industry has been remarkably successful in convincing Americans that they should never suffer any discomfort—that there is a medication that will solve or relieve any distress. Too often, those medications have serious side effects that are likely to include ototoxicity".[47]

Doctors need to help their patients understand that often they really need to change their lifestyles, rather than putting their faith in yet another prescription for the latest "miracle" drug.[48]

prescribed, for as long as prescribed and then stop. Do not take additional medications that will only compound the possibility of trouble.[50]

Always tell your doctor about your hearing loss. Emphasize that you want to avoid ototoxic medications if at all possible. At the same time, be on your guard. Some doctors really don't have a clue about hearing loss and how ototoxic drugs can affect our ears.

Once when Malisa had a case of viral flu, she went to her doctor. He prescribed a medication for her condition. When she asked him if it was ototoxic both he and his nurse said, "Oh, no problem with this drug". To be sure, Malisa took out the list of ototoxic drugs she carried with her and said, "Look!" Right there at the top of her list was the drug he was prescribing for her!

Malisa severely admonished them, "I take this very seriously. One physician has already cost me the majority of my hearing and I won't give up what tiny bit of hearing I still have because a physician and nurse won't look things up!"[51]

You have to learn to speak up for yourself. If Malisa's physician—bright and knowledgeable in other areas—will try that stunt with her (and she is **very** assertive when it comes to her health), imagine what happens to all the shy and timid folk who are afraid to confront their physicians. They lose more of their precious hearing without so much as a whimper.

Malisa isn't alone in losing her hearing because a doctor was too busy/lazy to check whether a drug was ototoxic before prescribing it to a patient. One man wrote me, "I was deafened by a doctor who didn't have time to

> ### Medication Error
>
> "Medication error is **not** just giving the wrong pill or the wrong dosage—it is also giving the **wrong medication** to a person who cannot tolerate ototoxic drugs"—Malisa Janes, Rh.D.

look up the potential side effects of an antibiotic he prescribed for me. I trusted this doctor implicitly, so I never looked it up myself". This is a mistake so many people make. Don't trust your doctor. Check things out for yourself! It's your ears—not your doctor's ears—that will be damaged.

This man continues, "I resent apologists for doctors who invalidate the 'do no harm' aspect of the Hippocratic Oath and the system that protects them. If more doctors were made accountable and responsible for their medical 'mistakes' in courts of law, they would not take the cavalier attitude that they do. In my state, a doctor is not required by law to inform patients of adverse events of any medications they prescribe".[52]

You need to take responsibility for yourself. The FDA urges you to put together a health care team consisting of your doctor/physician, nurse, pharmacist and yourself. You have to play an active role on this team if you want to reduce your risk to drug-related side effects while, at the same time, getting the maximum benefit from taking those drugs.

The FDA has an excellent web page called "Be an Active Member of Your Health Care Team" at:

http://www.fda.gov/Drugs/ResourcesForYou/ucm079487.htm

Before you fill a prescription or purchase an over-the-counter (OTC) medicine, learn as much about it as you can, including any adverse side effects that could harm your ears.

After you have learned all you can about the proposed drug treatment and have discussed it thoroughly with your health care team, then weigh your options. You and your health care team need to decide if the supposed benefit from taking any drug outweighs the risk of damage to **you**. However, the final choice is always **yours**.

If you choose to go ahead, but later experience an adverse side effect, let your health care team know immediately! If the side effect is ototoxic, you do not want to wait and risk permanent damage to your ears.

For better or for worse, this is how the system works. Now it is up to you. You are free to believe what you wish from whatever sources you choose to trust. You are free to take the drugs you choose to take and avoid those you choose not to take. Use the information in this book however you want. Most importantly, whatever you do, consult with your doctor. Never take more than the recommended dose, at the recommended times/intervals. Never, never fall into the trap of thinking that "if one 'pill' is good, more is even better". The health of your ears is **your** responsibility. If you won't watch out for them, who will?

---

1   *Be an Active Member of Your Health Care Team*, 2001. p. 1.
2   *Questions about CDER*, 2001. p. 3.
3   Shlafer, 2000. p. 10.
4   *Physicians' Desk Reference*, 2000. p. 2822.
5   Waltermire, 1998. p. 1.
6   Troost, 1998d. p. 3.
7   *Physicians' Desk Reference*, 2000. p. 2748.
8   Troost, 1998b. p. 3.
9   Freundlich, 1998. p. 2.
10 Freundlich, 1998. p. 2.
11 Freundlich, 1998. p. 2.
12 Haybach, 1999. p. v.
13 *Physicians' Desk Reference*, 2000. p. 2111.
14 *Physicians' Desk Reference*, 1997. p. 822.
15 *What is a Serious Adverse Event*, 2001. p. 1.
16 Waltermire, 1998. p. 2.
17 DiSogra, 2001. pp. 4-5.
18 McPheeters, 2001. p. 1.
19 Shlafer, 2000. p. 3.
20 *Top 200 Prescriptions*, 2001. p. 1.
21 PRNewswire, April 26, 1999.
22 Jaeger, 2001. p. 5.

23   Jaeger, 2001. p. 4.
24   Jaeger, 2001. p. 4.
25   Jaeger, 2001. p. 3.
26   Jaeger, 2001. p. 3.
27   Jaeger, 2001. p. 1.
28   *Physicians' Desk Reference*, 2002. p. 518.
29   *Physicians' Desk Reference*, 2003. pp. 1308-9. 3302 and 3327-8.
30   Jaeger, 2001. p. 3.
31   Chockley, 2001. p. 29.
32   Goodman, 2002. p. 17.
33   Barry, 2002. pp. 3, 17-18.
34   Waltermire, 1998. p. 1.
35   O'Hara, 1998. p. 67.
36   O'Hara, 1998. p. 67.
37   Oransky, 2002. p11A.
38   Carmen, 1999. p. 37.
39   *Questions About CDER*, 2001. p. 3.
40   Waltermire, 1998. p. 2.
41   Waltermire, 1998. p. 4.
42   *Omeprazole (Prilosec) OPDA Post-marketing Safety Review*, 2000. pp. 24-25.
43   *Omeprazole (Prilosec) OPDA Post-marketing Safety Review*, 2000. pp. 24-25.
44   *Rofecoxib*, 2010. "Withdrawal".
45   Wolfe, 2010.
46   McPheeters, 2000-2001. p. 1.
47   McPheeters, 2001. p. 1.
48   Waltermire, 1998. p. 4.
49   McPheeters, 2000-2001. p. 1.
50   McPheeters, 1999. p. 1.
51   Janes, 2000. p. 1.
52   Personal communication, 2000.

Chapter 6

The Shocking Truth About Hearing Testing and Ototoxic Drugs

How Bad Is It?

In one of my Hearing Loss Coping Skills classes, I was shocked to find that about one-quarter of the people in that class had ear damage from taking ototoxic drugs. Unlike what doctors would have you believe, this is not an isolated case. One hard of hearing doctor wrote to me concerning the members of his HLAA[1] group. "It seems to me that nearly half of our members with severe hearing loss developed their loss from ototoxic drugs". Another doctor asserts that we know some drugs cause hearing/balance problems in up to 92% of the people taking them.[2]

Cisplatin is very likely the most ototoxic drug used in medicine today. According to one study, **Cisplatin** caused hearing loss in 86% of those studied.[3] Another study revealed that approximately 40% ended up with hearing loss from taking it.[4] The PDR reports an incidence of 31%.

In actual fact, the results reported in the literature range all over the place. Some researchers report that this drug only produces ototoxic side effects in 3% of the people taking it,[5] that it "occasionally causes ototoxicity"[6] and that this ototoxicity is "seldom permanent". Other researchers just as authoritatively assert that not a single person escapes its ravages—that 100% of the people taking **Cisplatin** damage their ears[7]—and that the resulting hearing loss "is usually irreversible (permanent)".[8]

Why the enormous difference in opinion? Who is right? What are we to believe? If the former researchers are right, then ototoxic drugs are probably few and the damage they cause is minimal—nothing to worry about at all. However, if the latter researchers are correct, then there are likely lots of ototoxic drugs out there that can seriously damage our ears.

As I see it, there are two main factors for this enormous variation. First, in real life, people only report a small fraction of 1% of all ototoxic side effects as we saw in Chapter

5. Therefore, if a researcher is really looking for ototoxic side effects, he will likely find far more of them than another researcher who only reports ototoxic side effects if he happens to stumble over them. This alone could account for much of the difference between the 3% and the 100% results.

Second, there are no set standards for determining ototoxicity. There are several definitions of ototoxicity and several different ways of monitoring for ototoxicity. As a result, one researcher decides whether a drug is ototoxic by using one set of rules and another uses completely different criteria.

The Need for Standards

There is a real need for standardized guidelines so research results will be consistent.[9] Some researchers consider there must be a resulting 10 dB hearing loss at any frequency in both ears (or 15 dB in one ear) before they will classify the drug as being ototoxic. Others use 15 dB or 20 dB at any given frequency.[10] Still others use a decrease of hearing of at least 15 dB over two or more adjacent frequencies. Some researchers say that for the purposes of determining ototoxicity, the results have to be repeated for a minimum of two consecutive test sessions,[11] and on it goes.[12]

This means that while some researchers will say a given drug is ototoxic, other researchers—using different criteria—will give it a clean bill of health. Some researchers base their conclusions on objective test results. Others reach more nebulous, subjective conclusions. Still others are so sloppy that they don't even report the basis for their findings.

Back in 1994, the American Speech-Language-Hearing Association (ASHA) proposed some guidelines to clear up this confusion. Let's hope doctors and researchers finally adopt these (or similar) guidelines and bring some semblance of order to this mess.

Here is ASHA's six-step program.

1. Specific criteria for identifying ototoxicity. For example, they suggest that a drug be considered ototoxic if hearing loss drops 20 dB or more at any one test frequency, or if it drops 10 dB or more at two or more consecutive (adjacent) test frequencies, or if there is no response at three consecutive test frequencies where there was a response before.[13]

2. Timely identification of at-risk patients. Generally people are at greater risk if they are either very young or old; if they have a pre-existing hearing loss; if they have kidney problems; or if they have had previous ototoxic reactions to drugs. (See Chapter 4 for further information on numerous ototoxic risk factors.)

3. Pre-treatment counseling regarding potential ototoxic side effects. Prior to ototoxic drug treatment, doctors should counsel their patients regarding the potential ototoxic side effects of the drugs they will be taking. Doctors should carefully and completely explain the risks and benefits of such drug therapy. Counseling should include the ototoxic signs and symptoms to watch for (such as hearing loss, tinnitus, loss of balance, etc.) and what to do if such signs or symptoms occur. (Chapter 3 describes in detail many of the ototoxic side effects that may occur.) Furthermore, counseling needs to cover how the potential side effects can affect a person's ability to communicate effectively. In addition, people need to know how noise and certain drugs can team up to cause even more ear damage than would normally be expected. (Chapter 8 explains this very important topic in detail.)

4. Have valid baseline measures. This means that a person needs to have a full hearing assessment **before** starting drug treatment. The purpose of baseline testing is to document the status of hearing prior to drug treatment. This testing needs to include word discrimination scores in addition to pure-tone hearing testing.

5. Monitor hearing at sufficient intervals to document the progression of hearing loss (or fluctuations in hearing sensitivity). The monitoring intervals need to be such that they will detect the first signs of ototoxic effects. For people receiving AMINOGLYCOSIDE antibiotics, this monitoring interval may be as short as every 2 or 3 days.

6. Follow-up evaluations to determine and document the permanent ototoxic effects of this drug treatment. Such follow-up evaluations should be done immediately after the end of the drug treatment and 3 and 6 months later.[14]

This six-step program is an excellent start to consistent care for people receiving ototoxic drugs. However, it has one serious flaw. It fails to mention the range of frequencies that must be tested during audiometric evaluation—specifically those frequencies above the conventional testing range where most drug-induced hearing loss first occurs.

High-frequency Hearing Testing Needed

One of the reasons doctors and researchers do not know the true incidence of hearing loss in the ototoxic drugs they prescribe is because the initial damage to the hearing system occurs in those frequencies of sound well outside the speech range. The way it stands today, these frequencies are seldom tested for hearing loss. Incidentally, this same problem also occurs in the vestibular (balance) system. Initial ototoxic damage in the vestibular system occurs well outside the normal active and passive head movement range.[15] This means that a lot of damage can be done to both our cochlear and vestibular systems **before** ear specialists can detect it using the methods in common use today.

Research on how ototoxic drugs affect high-frequency hearing began back in the early 1980s and was reported in the mid-1980s.

Researchers are now beginning to realize just how important it is to detect high-frequency hearing loss as early as possible. For example, did you know that high-frequency audiometry can reveal the early effects of an ototoxic drug long before tinnitus appears or actual damage is visible on a conventional audiogram?

Here are some things you should know. People with normal hearing can typically hear up to 18,000 or 20,000 Hz or even higher. The frequencies you use for speech generally lie between 500 and 6000 Hz. Therefore, when you take a hearing test, your audiologist will test your hearing between 250 and 8000 Hz. This is the normal or "conventional" testing range (Fig. 6-1).

Conventional Audiogram

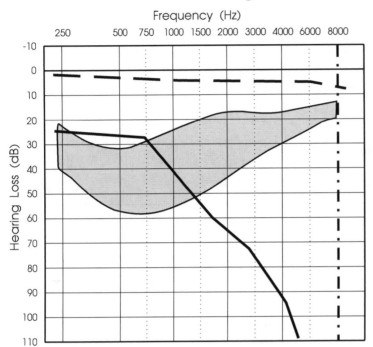

Fig. 6-1. An audiogram in the conventional frequencies. The shaded area is the "speech banana". It shows the frequencies and loudness covered by normal speech sounds. The horizontal dashed line represents normal hearing. The solid sloping line indicates a ski-slope-shaped hearing loss in the conventional frequencies.

Now comes the insidious part. Many ototoxic drugs begin their nefarious work way up in the highest frequencies you can hear where you do not notice it (and where audiologists do not test), and then work their way down. This high-frequency hearing loss is undetectable using modern audiometers since most audiometers only test between 250 and 8,000 Hz.

In studies done on **Cisplatin**, the first indications of hearing loss always showed up between 10,000 and 16,000 Hz. All of these frequencies are well above those shown on conventional audiograms.[16]

This means that even with complete standard audiometric testing, your ears could test at normal—indicating that a certain drug is not ototoxic—yet you could have lost your hearing from 20,000 Hz down to 8,000 Hz and no one would know. You could actually have lost 60% of your hearing spectrum, yet the drug gets a clean bill of health as far as ototoxicity goes (Fig 6-2)!

Ototoxic chemicals have this same characteristic. For example, high-frequency hearing testing revealed that workers exposed to low concentrations of **Styrene** fumes for 5 years had hearing losses in the high frequencies even though their hearing tests in the conventional frequencies were normal. If high-frequency hearing testing hadn't been done, **Styrene** could have been given a clean bill of health even though it is ototoxic.

Breathing **Styrene** fumes is now known to cause a reduction in the upper limit of hearing. (The upper limit of hearing is the highest frequency that you can hear.) Researchers have concluded that the upper limit of hearing is a sensitive indicator for early detection of ototoxicity in workers exposed to **Styrene**[17] and indeed, probably for most drugs and chemicals.

Therefore, if you want to know the truth about your hearing and whether drugs or chemicals are insidiously stealing your hearing from you without your being aware of it, your audiologist needs to **test your hearing right up to the highest frequency you can hear**.

High-frequency Audiogram

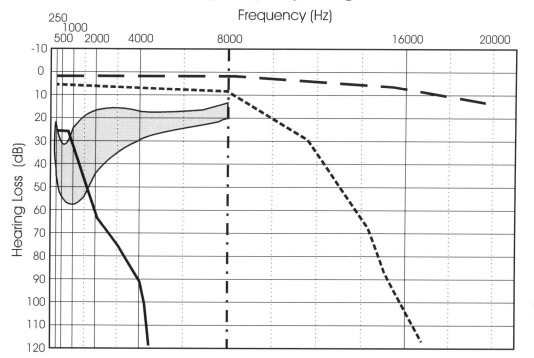

Fig. 6-2. An audiogram showing both the conventional frequencies (below 8,000 Hz) and the high frequencies. The horizontal dashed line represents normal hearing. The dotted line shows a ski-slope hearing loss only noticeable when testing in the high frequencies. Note: hearing is completely normal in the conventional frequencies yet ranges to a profound loss in the high frequencies. The solid line indicates a ski-slope hearing loss in the conventional frequencies. (This line is identical to the solid line in Fig. 6.1 but looks different because of differences in the horizontal scale. Likewise, the speech banana is really identical, but looks different in the two graphs.)

As we have already seen, when researchers document hearing loss, they typically limit their testing to the conventional frequencies between 250 Hz and 8,000 Hz.[18] When they do this, they miss all the hearing loss that shows up in the high frequencies, even though one study demonstrated that testing only the conventional hearing range is the **least effective** method to determine initial hearing loss.[19] Because of this, the real incidence of hearing loss is much higher than is commonly reported.

It's not that doctors and audiologists can't readily test these high-frequency sounds. They can—if they had the desire to do so. All it takes is an audiometer designed and calibrated to test hearing loss at higher frequencies. Such audiometers are available. It's just that most doctors and audiologists don't think such extended testing is necessary. How wrong can they be?

Since hearing loss typically begins at the highest frequencies and progresses to the lower ones, it is essential that doctors monitor the highest measurable frequencies in people with pre-existing hearing loss in order to provide the earliest possible warning of any incipient hearing loss.

Early detection does not, by itself, prevent further damage to your ears. However, it does give doctors time to adjust the dose or stop the medication altogether before hearing loss spreads into the conventional frequencies.[20] If monitoring is restricted to frequencies below 8000 Hz, by the time doctors detect any hearing loss, it is already too late. Hearing loss will have already affected those frequencies necessary for speech.[21]

High-frequency testing is even more important in young people because they likely still have more residual high-frequency hearing than older people, therefore they could suffer a greater loss before it is detected.

How good is high-frequency testing? When researchers compared testing the high frequencies with testing the conventional frequencies only, here is what one study revealed. In the high frequencies only, 45% had initial hearing loss. However, just 29% showed initial hearing loss in the conventional frequencies only, while 26% showed initial hearing loss in both frequency ranges at the same time. Thus, if only the high frequencies had been tested, 71% of the ears tested would have revealed the initial hearing loss.[22]

In a study on the ototoxic effects of AMINOGLYCOSIDES and **Cisplatin**, 70% of the ears tested showed hearing loss due to ototoxicity. (Note that 70% is a far cry from the 3% some researchers have reported when testing these drugs.) Of the ears with drug-induced hearing loss, 52% were first detected in the high-frequency range only. This study again shows that more than half of the people with drug-induced hearing loss have hearing loss that was **not** detected by conventional means. In this case, if only high-frequency hearing testing had been done, 67% of all the ears demonstrating initial hearing loss due to ototoxicity would have been found.[23]

Another study revealed that only 13.5% of the people (ears) studied had initial drug-related hearing loss in the conventional frequencies. An additional 24% had initial detectable hearing loss in the conventional frequencies as well as the high frequencies. This means that if you suspect you have drug-induced hearing loss, your audiologist only has a 37.5% chance of catching it. Thus, a whopping 62.5% of drug-induced hearing loss likely goes undetected because it initially **only** occurs in the high frequencies![24] However, if only the high frequencies had been tested, audiologists would have detected 86% of all cases of drug-induced hearing loss.

The Five-frequency Hearing Testing Process

It is now clear that doctors and audiologists need to test the entire hearing spectrum if they want accurate results. However, there are a couple of problems to overcome.

First, testing all the frequencies between 125 Hz and 20,000 Hz is both time consuming and tiring, especially to the person being tested. Furthermore, if the people being tested are already sick, they may not have the stamina to get through a complete audiometric test.

Second, as people age, their hearing deteriorates especially at the high frequencies. Thus, researchers need to factor this in when testing the higher frequencies of older people. Some people may not have any hearing at all above 10,000 Hz, for example.

In one study, although the average age of the subjects was 55 years, 93% of the ears tested had measurable baseline hearing up to 12,500 Hz, while 48% had responses up to 16,000 Hz. This means that even if older people cannot hear anything at 20,000 Hz, there is still plenty of usable high-frequency spectrum to test.

Fortunately for us, a few researchers have been concerned about drug-induced high-frequency hearing loss. They have been searching for the most effective and accurate way to test for the ototoxic effects of drugs in any given person without the draining and time-consuming process of testing all sound frequencies below 20,000 Hz.

One of their goals was to determine where drugs first affect our hearing. They have recently discovered that there is a five-frequency slope that is very sensitive to the ravages of ototoxic drugs. This is the frequency range they recommend be tested.

The beauty of the five-frequency slope testing is that it is highly sensitive to **initial** ototoxic hearing loss. This range varies depending on each person's pre-existing hearing loss and thus is unique to each person. These five frequencies are generally separated by 1/6 octave. For example, a person with pre-existing hearing loss might have a five-frequency slope consisting of 8, 9, 10, 11.2 and 12.5 kHz.[25]

Since each person's hearing loss is unique, audiologists can't just test for five specific frequencies. They have to tailor the testing process for each individual person. Here is how they can do this easily and accurately.

First, using an audiometer calibrated to accurately test up to 20,000 Hz, the audiologist determines the highest frequency a person can hear. (Note: the hearing loss at this frequency must be 100 dB or less. The reason for the 100 dB cut-off is because researchers noticed that at hearing losses greater than 100 dB, they saw fewer changes in ototoxic activity. After all, at that point, there isn't much hearing left to lose!)

Audiometric Test Frequencies

Audiologists test your hearing at selected intervals. For the conventional frequencies, they normally test in whole "octaves". An octave is exactly double the frequency of the preceding frequency tested. Therefore, they test at 125, 250, 500, 1000, 2000, 4000 and 8000 Hz.

Notice that as the frequency goes up, the interval between adjacent octaves increases. Therefore, they may test fractional octaves like half-octaves between 1000 and 8,000 Hz. These intermediate test frequencies would be close to 1600, 3150, and 6300 Hz.

For the purposes of high-frequency testing, Dr. Fausti recommends that testing should be at one-sixth octave spacing.[26] Above 8,000 Hz, the one-sixth octave testing frequencies are 9000, 10,000, 11,200, 12,500, 14,000, 16,000, 18,000 and 20,000 Hz.

Second, they test both this frequency and the next four lower consecutive audiometric test frequencies. They call this the five-frequency slope range.[27]

Depending on your particular hearing loss, this five-frequency slope may all lie within the extended high-frequency range, it may straddle the 8,000 Hz boundary between the conventional and high frequencies, or it may only reside in the conventional frequencies (Fig. 6-3). It doesn't matter where this slope is, as long as your audiologist finds it and carefully tests you in that range.

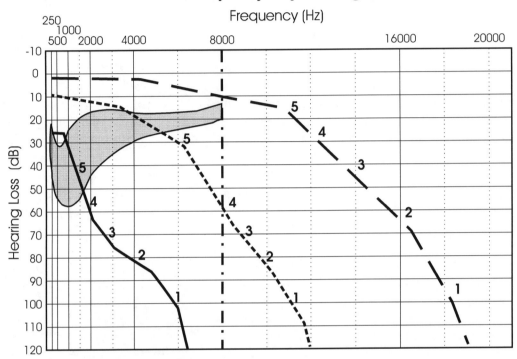

Five-frequency Slope Audiogram

Fig. 6-3. An audiogram showing the five-frequency slope testing profile. Hearing loss from oto-toxic drugs will normally be the most noticeable and be the most sensitive in this five-frequency slope range. The dashed line shows hearing loss only in the high frequencies. The dotted line indicates hearing loss straddling the 8,000 Hz boundary between the conventional frequencies normally tested and the high frequencies. The solid line reveals hearing exclusively in the conventional frequencies (no high-frequency hearing remaining). It is here that any change in hearing loss becomes obvious to conventional testing. The numbers on the lines indicate the location of each of the five frequencies of the five-frequency test protocol.

The worse your high-frequency hearing is, the greater the chance that conventional testing will reveal any ototoxic drug damage. Therefore, when testing older people or people with severe losses, there may be no need for high-frequency testing. In contrast, if children or people with normal hearing are being tested, almost all of them will likely fall into the high-frequency only range. However, a good number of adults will fall into the range that straddles the 8,000 Hz line. Therefore, apart from people with obvious ski-slope losses entirely in the conventional frequencies, everyone else needs high-frequency testing.

Just how effective is this five-frequency slope in detecting hearing loss from ototoxic drugs? The results may surprise you!

In one study on the ototoxic effects of **Cisplatin**, if only the five frequencies in the five-frequency slope had been tested, 93% of the people with ototoxic drug-induced hearing loss would have been detected.[28] This is in sharp contrast to the 39% detected in this same study using only the conventional frequencies. If they had tested **both** the five-frequency slope frequencies and the conventional frequencies, they would have detected 100% of the cases of ototoxic drug induced hearing loss.

This study reveals that conventional audiometric testing would miss five people with drug-induced hearing loss for every two people it detects. This is just not acceptable!

Other studies have yielded similar results. For example, in one case, researchers found that if only the five-frequency slope frequencies had been tested, initial hearing loss would have been detected in 82%, instead of just 42% using only the conventional frequencies.[29]

Another study reported that if only the five-frequency slope values were tested, hearing loss due to AMINOGLYCOSIDE antibiotics would be detected 84% of the time, and for **Cisplatin**, the results would be even higher at 94%.[30]

Yet, another study revealed that initial hearing loss would have been detected in 89% of the people with hearing loss if only the five-frequency slope had been tested. Testing only the conventional frequencies caught just 37%. This would be missing five people with drug-induced hearing loss for every two people detected![31]

In all these cases, if the conventional frequencies and any portion of the five-frequency slope values above the conventional frequencies had been tested, 100% of all drug-induced hearing loss would have been detected.

I think it is about time we insist that our ears get tested at those frequencies that will best detect the initial effects of ototoxic drugs. The routine use of high-frequency audiometry is not just "nice," it is essential.[32]

Many doctors reject high-frequency monitoring of hearing loss for two reasons. First, they think that many of the patients being given massive doses of ototoxic drugs will die (of cancer) anyway, so there is no need to worry about their hearing. Second, they think that middle-aged and older people with pre-existing hearing losses have no useful high-frequency hearing left to monitor.

Both of these assumptions are wrong. Many people are now surviving drug therapy (for cancer) and need their hearing to facilitate their recovery and for their emotional and mental well-being. Also, as studies have shown, doctors can obtain high-frequency thresholds in people with pre-existing hearing loss.[33] True, they may not hear up to 20,000 Hz like they used to, but many can still hear up to 10,000 or 12,000 Hz.

There are several advantages to using the five-frequency protocol. First, of course, is that it is much more accurate in detecting initial hearing loss. Second, the testing procedure is significantly shorter.

However, for those in hospitals that have to undergo drug therapy with ototoxic drugs, having audiograms can be a problem, especially if they are unconscious, semi-conscious or very sick. In that case, instead of doing the hearing testing using a conventional audiometer, it can be done reliably using auditory brainstem response (ABR) techniques modified to work in the higher frequencies. In one such study, high-frequency tone-burst-evoked ABRs alone identified 93% of the initial changes in hearing loss.[34]

The five-frequency slope protocol is fast. It has been proven effective in providing early warning of hearing loss. The final step is to get our doctors and audiologists to use this five-frequency slope audiometric testing procedure in their everyday practice and help us save our precious hearing.

1   HLAA—Hearing Loss Association of America—a national organization for hard of hearing people headquartered in Bethesda, MD, USA.
2   Tange, 1985. p. 77.
3   Fausti, 1993a. p. 663.
4   Tange, 1985. p. 77.
5   *Guidelines for the Audiologic Management of Individuals Receiving Cochleotoxic Drug Therapy*, 1994. p. 4.
6   Shlafer, 2000. p. 12.
7   *Guidelines for the Audiologic Management of Individuals Receiving Cochleotoxic Drug Therapy*, 1994. p. 4.
8   Kalkanis, 2001. p. 1.
9   Fausti, 1993a. p. 662.
10   Troost, 1998a. p. 1.
11   Fausti, 1993a. p. 662.
12   *Guidelines for the Audiologic Management of Individuals Receiving Cochleotoxic Drug Therapy*, 1994. p. 4.
13   *Guidelines for the Audiologic Management of Individuals Receiving Cochleotoxic Drug Therapy*, 1994. p. 5.
14   *Guidelines for the Audiologic Management of Individuals Receiving Cochleotoxic Drug Therapy*, 1994. pp. 5-7.
15   Troost, 1998b. p. 1.
16   Tange, 1985. pp. 77-80.
17   Morioka, 1999. pp. 1-5.
18   *Guidelines for the Audiologic Management of Individuals Receiving Cochleotoxic Drug Therapy*, 1994. p. 4.
19   Fausti, 1992, p. 1031.
20   Fausti, 1993a. p. 661.
21   Fausti, 1993a. p. 664.
22   Fausti, 1993a. p. 663.
23   Fausti, 1993b. p. 4.
24   Fausti, 1994. pp. 232-9.
25   Fausti, 1999. p. 1.
26   Fausti, 1999. p. 1.
27   Fausti, 1993a. p. 663.
28   Fausti, 1993a. pp. 663-664.
29   Fausti, 1993b. p. 5.
30   Fausti, 1999. p. 1.
31   Fausti, 1994. p. 1.
32   Kalkanis, 2001. p. 8.
33   Fausti, 1993b. p. 6.
34   Fausti, 1993b. p. 1.

Chapter 7

We "Hear" with Our Eyes

Ototoxic drugs aren't the only drugs for which we hard of hearing people have to be wary. We also need to watch out for drugs that can damage our eyes. This is critical because so often our eyes have to take over to help out our damaged ears.

Vision Is Vitally Important

Your eyes fill in for your ears in several capacities. For example, if you have a severe hearing loss, your eyes become the primary means of warning you of impending danger. Furthermore, your eyes help you to communicate, whether it be by speechreading, thus supplementing what your faulty ears hear, or by reading the written word. Thus in a very real sense, hard of hearing people "hear" with their eyes.

Your eyes have another critical function. Along with your proprioceptive system, they help you maintain your balance. (See Chapter 3 for information about how your eyes and your proprioceptive system work together to maintain your balance.) If you already have poor vestibular function, possibly from taking ototoxic drugs, then you **need** your eyes. Thus you must protect your vision at all costs.

Very few people, doctors included, realize the immense importance of this. You need to emphasize to your doctor that you don't want any drugs that will damage either your ears **or** your eyes.

Sharon knows what it is like to have both her eyes and her ears damaged by drugs. She writes, "One thing that bugs me is doctors that seem to think because I already have a hearing loss, it doesn't matter if they give me more ototoxic drugs. They load me up with ototoxic antibiotics at the slightest sign of an infection".

Another of Sharon's pet peeves is, "doctors that disregard the concerns of a hard of hearing or deaf patient about being given a drug that has a high risk of both cataracts and glaucoma". She specifically singles out **Prednisone** "which frequently results in people developing both cataracts and glaucoma with the resultant blindness". She laments, "Doctors don't understand that my eyes are my ears".

This is a most serious concern. Imagine for a moment that you are now both deaf and blind. Think of the enormous changes that will bring to your lifestyle. This is nothing to take lightly. The psychological impact will be enormous! Would you want to live under such conditions?

Sharon has already lost much of her hearing. and some of her vision. She explains, "If I become blind, I'm afraid I would lose my will to live because my eyes are my connection to the world around me. I already have severe visual difficulties due to the **Prednisone**. I have cataracts in both eyes and the pain in my eyes from glaucoma is really bad. I tapered myself off the **Prednisone** on my own. My doctor just did not understand my concerns about blindness and what my eyes mean to me. This kind of attitude towards the drugs given to us really bothers me".[1]

You have been warned folks. Sharon has been there—is still there—and tells it like it is.

You Need to Watch Out for Yourself

Since this book only deals with ototoxic drugs and their side effects, it is up to you to check out the visual side effects of any drugs you take. While you are busy protecting your remaining hearing, you also need to be protecting your precious vision.

Here's another thing. Don't let your guard down—even when visiting your eye doctor. The truth is that your eye doctor may be unwittingly prescribing drugs that could damage your ears because the "drug bible" he uses, the *Physicians' Desk Reference for Ophthalmic Medicines* does a poor job (in my opinion) of listing ototoxic side effects for the drugs it describes.

The 2002 edition of the *Physicians' Desk Reference for Ophthalmic Medicines* lists about 108 different generic drugs used in treating eye problems. As you would expect, it has a reasonably comprehensive list of side effects reflecting various eye conditions. However, when it comes to listing the side effects affecting the rest of the body, particularly the ears, that's a different story.

For example, of the 108 drugs mentioned above, 42 can be ototoxic, yet only 11 of these drugs had even one ototoxic side effect listed.[2] Three of these eleven only report dizziness although the *Physicians' Desk Reference* lists several other ototoxic side effects in addition to dizziness. Now comes the scary part. Thirty-one of these forty-two ototoxic drugs (including extremely ototoxic drugs such as **Gentamicin**, **Neomycin** and **Tobramycin**) didn't have even one ototoxic side effect listed!

The 2010 edition of the *Physicians' Desk Reference for Ophthalmic Medicines* is no better. It lists about 71 different generic drugs of which 34 (48%) can be ototoxic, yet it only lists side effects for 2 of these drugs! This is why you have to do your homework before it is too late.

Drugs That Can Damage Our Eyes

In the back of the book, *Essential Guide to Prescription Drugs 2001,* Table 4 lists many of the drugs that can adversely affect our vision. The opening preamble to this table states, "A significant percentage of all adverse drug effects involve visual changes or eye damage". This is something we hard of hearing people need to know!

This table lists 117 specific drugs that can damage our eyes.[3] The really scary thing is that of these 117 drugs, 80 (68%) of them not only can damage our eyes, but at the same time, they can damage our ears, and thus seriously compromise our balance!

Table 7-1 lists drugs that can damage our eyes, but are not known to be ototoxic. I sincerely doubt that this list is anywhere near complete. However, at least you can watch out for these drugs. The drugs in this table are not otherwise listed in this book.

Table 7-2 lists drugs that can damage **both** our eyes and our ears. All the drugs in this table are included in this book, but I only list their ototoxic side effects. I do not mention any of their visual side effects. These drugs can zap us with a "double whammy".

Knowing what I know now, I think if I made a thorough search, I would find this list grossly incomplete. However, it serves as a warning. Check things out for yourself if you want to protect **both** your eyes and your ears.

Table 7-1. Drugs That Can Have Adverse Side Effects on Our Eyes (But Not Our Ears)

Amodiaquine	Fluphenazine
Amyl nitrite	Guanethidine
Atacurium	Hydrochloroquine
Belladonna	Latanoprost
Carbachol	Mephenesin
Carbinoxamine	Mephenytoin
Cephaloglycin	Methotrimeprazine
Chlorpromazine	Nialamide
Chlorpropamide	Oxyphenbutazone
Chlorprothixene	Paramethadione
Cimetidine	Pargyline
Colchicine	Pentylenetetrazol
Dexbrompheniramine	Phenacetin
Dicloxacillin	Phenmetrazine
Diethylstibestrol	Phensuximide
Digitalis	Prochlorperazine
Digitoxin	Promazine
Dimethindene	Terfenadine
Epinephrine	Trifluoperazine
Ethambutol	Triflupromazine
Ethchlorvynol	Trimethadione[4]
Fenfluramine	

Table 7-2. Drugs That Can Have Adverse Side Effects on Both Our Eyes and Our Ears

Acetaminophen
Acetazolamide
Allopurinol
Amantadine
Amiodarone
Aspirin
Atropine
Botulinum Toxin Type A
Bromopheniramine
Bupivacaine
Busulfan
Carbamazepine
Carisoprodol
Cephalexin
Chloramphenicol
Chlordiazepoxide
Chloroquine
Chlorpheniramine
Chlortetracycline
Chlorthalidone
Ciprofloxacin
Cisplatin
Clomiphene
Clonidine
Codeine
Colistin
Cyclizine
Cycloserine
Cyproheptadine
Dapsone
Dexchlorpheniramine
Digoxin
Diphenhydramine
Disulfiram
Doxepin
Ephedrine
Ergotamine
Erythromycin
Ethionamide
Ethosuximide
Etretinate
Fenoprofen
Furosemide
Gabapentin

Griseofulvin
Haloperidol
Hydroxychloroquine
Ibuprofen
Imatinib
Indomethacin
Interferon alpha-n3
Isocarboxazid
Isoniazid
Isosorbide
Levodopa
Lisinopril
Lithium
Mefenamic acid
Memantine
Mesoridazine
Methocarbamol
Methsuximide
Methysergide
Morphine
Nalidixic acid
Nicotine
Nitrofurantoin
Nitroglycerin
Norfloxacin
Orphenadrine
Penicillamine
Pentazocine
Perphenazine
Phenelzine
Phentermine
Phenylbutazone
Phenytoin
Pilocarpine
Pregabalin
Primidone
Promethazine
Propranolol
Quinacrine
Quinidine
Quinine
Rabies vaccine
Reserpine
Sildenafil

Table 7-2. Drugs That Can Have Adverse Side Effects on Both Our Eyes and Our Ears (Cont'd.)

Sodium salicylate	**Tolbutamide**
Spironolactone	**Tranylcypromine**
Streptomycin	**Travoprost**
Tacrolimus	**Trimeprazine**
Tadalafil	**Tripelennamine**
Tetracycline	**Vardenafil**
Thioridazine	**Ziconotide**[5, 6]
Thiothixene	

In addition to the above individual drugs, there are a number of drug classes where all the drugs in that class can affect both your eyes and your ears. Some of these clearly-defined drug classes include:

Barbiturates	(see section 60.12.4 in Table 14-1)
Benzodiazepines	(see section 60.12.8 in Table 14-1)
Cortisone-like drugs	(see section 40.1.4 in Table 14-1)
Monoamine oxidase inhibitors	(see section 60.1.1 in Table 14-1)
Oral contraceptives	(see section 40.12 in Table 14-1)
Phenothiazines	(see section 60.8.1 in Table 14-1)
Sulfonamides	(see section 7.4.56 in Table 14-1)
Tetracyclines	(see section 7.4.60 in Table 14-1)
Thiazide diuretics	(see section 30.5.12 in Table 14-1)
Tricyclic antidepressants[7]	(see section 60.1.8 in Table 14-1)

---

1 Cohen, 2000. p. 1.
2 *Physicians' Desk Reference for Ophthalmic Medicines*, 2002. pp. VIII-XII.
3 Rybacki, 2001. pp. 1099-1202.
4 Rybacki, 2001. pp. 1200-1202.
5 Rybacki, 2001. pp. 1200-1202.
6 Rybacki, 2006. pp. 1219-1221.
7 Rybacki, 2006. pp. 1219-1221.

Chapter 8

The Sinister Partnership Between Ototoxic Agents and Noise

It is no secret that noise damages our ears. Since you are reading this book, you know that many drugs and chemicals also can damage our ears. Studies are now revealing there is often a sinister partnership between ototoxic agents and noise. In a review of some studies, researchers observed that the incidence of sensorineural hearing loss was higher than expected in those workers who were exposed to both noise and organic solvents at the same time.

This had puzzled researchers. Why could some people working in noisy places not seem to suffer any hearing loss, while others working in quieter places end up with severe hearing loss and other ear damage? What factor was increasing the risk of ototoxic damage? They know now. Being exposed to ototoxic agents and noise at the same time can make all the difference.

Unfortunately, two of the more common ototoxic hazards that occur in many work environments are noise and organic solvents. Researchers have found that taking an ototoxic drug, or being exposed to an ototoxic industrial solvent, might not cause noticeable damage to your ears if you are in a relatively quiet place. However, if you take the same dose, and at the same time are exposed to loud noise for any length of time (say at work on a construction site or in a factory), the result could be significant ear damage. In fact, the combination of noise and drugs/chemicals can increase the risk of hearing damage many times over!

In a 20-year study of hearing sensitivity in 319 employees, a remarkably large proportion (23%) of the workers in the chemical sector showed pronounced hearing loss as compared with employees in non-chemical environments (5-8%). These results were found in spite of the fact that the noise levels in the chemical sector (80-90 dB) were less than those in other divisions (95-100 dB).[1]

Not only can hearing loss be worse in the presence of both noise and chemicals, but so can be our ability to understand speech. By comparing pure tone audiometry results to speech audiometry results, researchers determined that the chemical solvents not only caused hearing loss in the cochlea, but also damaged the auditory circuits in the brain so that speech was not processed as clearly as before. This gives rise to lower than expected discrimination scores.[2]

Researchers are just beginning to understand how noise and ototoxic chemicals team up to damage our ears. In some cases, it appears that the noise changes the rate of blood flow and thus allows the ototoxic agent to reach a higher level of penetration than otherwise. In other cases, the noise apparently increases hair cell activity to such an extent that it leads to their injury. Also, researchers think that both noise and ototoxic chemicals can upset intracellular energy production, which could compound the effects of each.[3]

Additive vs. Synergistic Effects

When noise and ototoxic drugs or chemicals get together in our ears, the resulting damage can either be "additive" or "synergistic".

If you were exposed to an ototoxic chemical (or drug) that caused you to lose 20 dB of hearing and at the same time you were exposed to noise that caused you to also lose 20 dB of hearing, the total effect would be a 20 + 20 dB = 23 dB of hearing loss. This is the additive effect—the total is **equal to** the sum of its parts.

However, let's say you were exposed to exactly the same situation above and your resulting hearing loss was 33 dB instead of the expected 23 dB. This loss would be 10 **times** worse than expected. This extra loss above the expected additive effect is called the synergistic effect—where the result is **greater** than the sum of the individual parts.

Adding Decibels Looks Weird

Adding decibels together looks weird since decibels are a logarithmic scale. 23 dB really is twice as loud as 20 dB. If sound levels were measured in linear units rather than in logarithmic units then the result would have been the familiar 20 units plus 20 units = 40 units.

Think of it this way. To get the additive effect, you **add** the two separate effects together. However, you "**multiply**" the two effects together to get the synergistic effect.

Just how pronounced is this synergistic effect? Sometimes the results can be dramatic! In one study, workers were grouped into one of four groups—those exposed to both noise and **Toluene**, those exposed to **Toluene** alone, those exposed to noise alone, and those not exposed to either **Toluene** or noise (the control group). The hearing loss of those exposed to noise alone was 4 times greater than the control group; the hearing loss of those exposed to **Toluene** alone was 5 times greater; and the hearing loss of those exposed to both noise and **Toluene** was 11 times greater![4]

Decibels and Powers of Ten

Since decibels are logarithmic units, if one number is 10 dB greater than another, it is one order of magnitude greater (10 times greater). If one sound level is 20 dB greater than another, then the second sound is 2 orders of magnitude greater (100 times greater) and so forth.

In a study of Brazilian workers, those exposed to both noise and **Toluene** had a 53% incidence of hearing loss. In contrast, those exposed to noise alone had a 26% incidence rate while the control group had an incidence rate of only 8%. When these results were adjusted for age, they showed that noise exposure increased the risk of hearing loss by 4.6 times. When the noise was combined with exposure to **Toluene**, the risk jumped a whopping 27.5 times![5]

One very interesting thing that has come out of animal studies is that the order of exposure seems to determine how bad the resulting hearing loss will be. If the noise exposure comes **before** the drug/chemical exposure, the effect is **additive** at best. However, if the noise exposure comes **after** exposure to the drug/chemical, the effect is **synergistic**.[6]

For example, in a **Toluene** study using rats, **Toluene** alone and noise alone each caused considerable hearing loss, particularly in the high frequencies. However, the hearing loss of rats exposed to **Toluene** followed by noise was greater than the sum of the effects of **Toluene** and noise alone.

Who Are the Guilty Parties?

Not all drugs and chemicals work together to smash your ears, but certain classes of drugs and chemicals are definitely part of this unholy alliance. Unfortunately, not much is known about many of the ototoxic agents and the damage they cause to your ears in the presence of noise. Here are the ones we know to be guilty at the present time.

Drugs

Noise is often a co-factor in medication type ototoxicity, especially when combined with antibiotics. For example, if you get a hearing loss from taking an ototoxic antibiotic, you may, at the same time, also be at much greater risk of additional hearing loss from exposure to noise.[7]

The AMINOGLYCOSIDE class of antibiotics appears to exacerbate the damaging effects of noise exposure on your hearing. This means that if you are taking any of these antibiotics and are exposed to loud noise at the same time, the effects on your hearing may be considerably worse than either one by itself (the synergistic effect).[8]

For example, exposing your ears to loud noise while you are taking **Gentamicin** can make the ototoxic effects worse than if you are not around loud noise when taking this drug.[9] Numerous studies of people taking **Kanamycin** plus being exposed to noise at the same time have revealed both additive and synergistic effects.[10]

In addition to the AMINOGLYCOSIDE antibiotics, **Nicotine** and the anti-cancer drug **Cisplatin** can act together with noise to cause even greater damage to your hearing.[11] This is also true of over-the-counter drugs such as **Aspirin**. Studies have shown that taking higher doses of SALICYLATES like **Aspirin** in the presence of noise causes a greater temporary hearing loss. Furthermore, it takes longer for hearing to return to normal than when taking **Aspirin** without the noise component.[12]

When **Chloramphenicol**, a common microbial antibiotic, is taken alone, it supposedly is not very ototoxic. However, in the presence of noise, the synergistic effect of this drug and noise shoots the risk way up![13]

Chemicals

Until recently, not much was known or done about identifying the high-risk chemicals, especially those that have synergistic effects in relation to hearing loss.

So far, the high-risk chemicals seem to be the organic solvents. Ototoxic organic solvents known to cause even greater damage to our ears in the presence of noise include **Carbon disulfide**, **Dinitrobenzene**, **Styrene**, **Trichloroethylene**, **Toluene** and **Xylene**. In addition, both **Carbon monoxide** (an asphyxiant) and **Lead** (a heavy metal) have this same nefarious characteristic.[14,15,16,17]

Another researcher adds to this list chemicals such as **Arsenic**, **Butyl alcohol**, **Butyl nitrite**, **Heptane**, **Hexane**, **Manganese**, **Mercury** and **Trimethyltin**.[18]

This is just the tip of the iceberg it seems. Suspicion is already cast on **Carbon tetrachloride**, various other metals and other asphyxiants.[19,20] Strange as it may seem, there is even some evidence that heavy salt eaters are more susceptible to damage from noise.[21] Who knows what other chemicals will be implicated in the future?

A review of studies suggested that organic solvents such as those present in oil-based paints interact synergistically with noise to cause increased hearing loss in humans.[22]

In one study almost half of the workers exposed to synthetic varnishes and noise were found to have permanent hearing losses ranging from 10 dB to 60 dB. These varnishes contained organic solvents such as **Benzene**, Butyl acetate, **Styrene**, **Toluene** and **Xylene.**[23]

A **Carbon disulfide** study revealed that the incidence of hearing loss was higher than expected among workers exposed to both noise and **Carbon disulfide** at the same time. In addition, researchers also found that the hearing losses were more severe and began sooner than in those workers only exposed to noise and not to **Carbon disulfide**.[24]

In a 1989 study of 258 workers in a viscose rayon factory, the incidence of hearing loss increased with the duration of exposure from 47% for the group exposed up to 2 years to 71% for the group exposed for 3 years or longer. Not only did the incidence of hearing loss increase with time, but also so did the severity of the resulting hearing losses. These findings help show the synergistic relationship that exists between **Carbon disulfide** exposure and noise.[25]

Carbon monoxide in the presence of noise also has a synergistic effect and makes threshold shifts worse and causes more hair cell damage, particularly in the outer hair cells.[26]

Manganese is a heavy metal that interacts synergistically with noise exposure to cause increased hearing loss. Workers exposed to both noise and **Manganese** had accelerated hearing loss compared to those exposed to **Manganese** alone.[27]

New Standards Needed

Researchers were surprised to discover that when noise and ototoxic agents team up to damage our ears, this damage can occur even though exposure to both noise and chemicals are within currently acceptable limits![28] For example, you may work in an environment where exposure to ototoxic chemicals is kept in what is generally considered the "safe" range for those chemicals. At the same time, you may also work in an environment where the noise level is kept below the level considered at risk for noise. Your ears are thus safe, right? Wrong! You may still be damaging your ears. Therefore, the government needs to set more stringent standards. That way, people exposed to both ototoxic chemicals **and** noise will not inadvertently lose their hearing while their companies are complying with all current government standards.

Much more work needs to be done in this field. Unfortunately, even now, the association between occupational exposure to solvents and hearing loss is rarely evaluated. Since noise is often present in most occupational settings where solvent exposures occur, the hearing losses observed in these situations are often attributed to noise alone. Even studying audiograms is of little help. This is because the pure tone audiogram can look identical whether the hearing loss was caused by noise or by ototoxic chemicals or drugs.[29]

Watch the Noise for a Long Time

One of the treacherous effects of ototoxic drugs teaming up with noise is something you'd probably never suspect. This is the length of time your ears are susceptible to damage after taking certain ototoxic drugs.

When you are warned not to take certain drugs at the same time as you are exposed to noise, you might think this is referring to just the days you are actually taking the drug therapy. Surprise! Not true! You have to avoid noise for much, much longer.

When you take AMINOGLYCOSIDE antibiotics and platinum anti-cancer drugs, such as **Cisplatin**, they are quickly transported to your inner ears. The problem is that, once there, they persist in your inner-ear fluids, not just for a few days, but for several weeks to several months, and up to a year!

During this time, your ears are still very susceptible to the synergistic effects of loud noise.[30] This means that if you have taken an AMINOGLYCOSIDE antibiotic or **Cisplatin** and are now finished with this drug therapy, your ears are still in danger of even more hearing loss if you expose them to loud noise any time in the next few months or more, depending on your specific body chemistry. Heed this warning if you want to protect your ears from additional hearing loss!

Here is something else you should know, as I don't think many audiologists are aware of this yet. If you are getting a hearing aid, instruct your audiologist to set the gain and maximum power output as low as possible in order to protect your ears during this critical time when your ears are still very sensitive to the effects of noise. If you already wear hearing aids, keep the volume down during this time.[31]

Avoiding noise is important, but even here the story is complicated. Research indicates that moderate amounts of noise may protect your ears from extreme amounts of noise so you don't need to try to live in silence. Your ears need sound!

Now the Good News

Here's some good news. Research now shows that anti-oxidants help protect your ears from noise.[32]

Some other exciting news is that the glutamate receptor antagonist MK-801 appears to block the ototoxic effects of **Trimethyltin** in rats. The aim is for researchers to develop new drugs that can prevent or reverse ototoxicity caused by exposure to chemicals and drugs.

In the past, researchers have been working more or less randomly identifying those chemicals that are ototoxic. Now, however, they are beginning to understand the fundamental mechanisms of how these chemicals damage our ears. This should allow them to more effectively predict new ototoxic chemicals and drugs in the future and to develop ways to protect our ears from ototoxic damage.[33]

Researchers have recently discovered that antioxidants can help prevent noise-induced hearing loss. This may also work for drugs that cause hearing loss.

Here's how this works. When hair cells are overstressed by loud noise, free radicals—unstable oxygen atoms that are short an electron—are produced. The free radicals steal electrons from nearby molecules, like the hair cell's fatty walls. Enough of this thievery will kill the hair cell and with it more of our hearing.

Think of these free radicals as tiny enemy bullets. If they "zap" and fatally damage a cell, the cell goes into a process called **apotosis**—in which it systematically shuts itself down and dies. If those cells are the hair cells in your inner ears, then you lose hearing when those hair cells die. Thus, it is important to zap the free radicals before they do their dastardly deeds.

The anti-oxidants are the "good guys". They act as tiny missiles that shoot down the free radicals before they can cause any damage.

Researchers have discovered that if enough powerful antioxidants are supplied before and/or shortly after noise exposure, these antioxidants in our inner ears can largely prevent much of the resulting noise damage that usually occurs.[34]

Glutathione is considered the most powerful natural antioxidant there is. Your body makes this antioxidant naturally from compounds such as N-acetyl-cysteine and D-methionine which in turn are made from three amino acids–cysteine, glycine and glutamic acid.

When your ears need extra help, taking N-acetyl-cysteine and D-methionine helps your body quickly make more glutathione. You can buy both glutathione and N-acetyl-cysteine in health food stores or on-line.

Note: you don't want to overdose on N-acetyl-cysteine, as it can actually work against you and cause even more ear damage. I've seen figures that if you take more than 2,800 mg. of N-acetyl-cysteine a day it can reverse its activity and become a pro-oxidant rather than the beneficial antioxidant. Your ears need some N-acetyl-cysteine, but too much can be dangerous.

In addition, researchers now know that the mineral **magnesium** plays an important part in hearing. Scientists have found that a magnesium deficiency increases susceptibility to noise damage. One of the things that happens is the lack of magnesium causes the tiny blood vessels in your ears to constrict, thus depriving them of an adequate supply of oxygen. At the same time, loud noise depletes your ears of magnesium—so loud noise actually causes a double-whammy. There is evidence that high doses of magnesium taken soon after a sudden hearing loss from loud noise can sometimes help restore hearing.[35]

There are other mechanisms by which we can also help protect our ears from the side effects of ototoxic drugs.

A person once asked me: "I was wondering if you had an opinion on a drug called STS (Sodium thiosulfate). It's being developed to protect chemotherapy patients taking platinum-based anti-cancer drugs from hearing loss. Is this (STS) something that could be more broadly applied to the numerous drugs that can cause ototoxicity?"

I explained: "The research looks promising so far. It's certainly possible that STS will help protect against hearing loss from **some** ototoxic drugs. Because different ototoxic drugs have different mechanisms of damage, the trick is to find an "antidote" that interacts specifically with each ototoxic drug.

I think more likely, that there will be different drugs found to protect hearing against specific classes of ototoxic drugs. For example, Sodium thiosulfate may work best for the platinum-based drugs such as **Cisplatin**, **Carboplatin** and **Oxaliplatin**.

For the AMINOGLYCOSIDE antibiotics, maybe iron chelators such as **Deferoxamine** will prove to be the ticket. Unlike how **Cisplatin** affects our ears, preliminary research indicates that AMINOGLYCOSIDES such as **Gentamicin** only are ototoxic when they react with iron found in the bloodstream. Thus, in this case, iron chelators that "soak up" excess iron in the bloodstream may prove to be the route to go. Another possibility is **Aspirin** taken with **Gentamicin** to do the same job.

Unfortunately, few drugs are specifically studied to determine their ototoxic mechanisms. The notable exceptions are the platinum drugs and the AMINOGLYCOSIDE antibiotics. The rest mostly get the short end of the stick, so it may be a long time before anyone finds a specific antidote for them. However, in general, powerful antioxidants look like the most promising line of protection against ototoxicity available at this time".[36]

---

1   Morata, 1994. pp. 359-366.
2   Morata, 1994. pp. 359-366.

3   Niall, 1998. p. 3.
4   Morata, 1994. pp. 359-366.
5   Rybak, 1992. p. 679.
6   Rybak, 1992. pp. 679-680.
7   Hain, 2001b. p. 6.
8   *Noise And Hearing Loss*, 1990. p. 8.
9   Hain, 2001a. p. 3.
10   Suter, 1991. p. 17.
11   Soh, 1999. p. 2.
12   Rosen, 2001. p. 5.
13   Carmen, 1999. p. 37.
14   Cary, 1997. pp. 455-465.
15   WorkPro, 1999. p. 1.
16   Forge, 1999. p. 1250.
17   Morata, 1994. pp. 359-366.
18   Niall, 1998. p. 3.
19   Morata, 1994. pp. 359-366.
20   Rosen, 2001. p. 6.
21   Hain, 2001b. p. 6.
22   Bisesi, 1994. p. 4.
23   Rybak, 1992. p. 677.
24   Morata, 1994. pp. 359-366.
25   Rybak, 1992. p. 678.
26   Rybak, 1992. p. 680.
27   Rybak, 1992. p. 684.
28   Forge, 1999. p. 1250.
29   Morata, 1994. pp. 359-366.
30   Kalkanis, 2001. p. 2.
31   Kalkanis, 2001. pp. 8-9.
32   Hain, 2001b. p. 6.
33   *Environmental Impact on Hearing: Is Anyone Listening*, 1994. p. 4.
34   Shachtman, 2003. pp. 1-3.
35   Bauman, 2005. p. 1.
36   Bauman, 2009. p. 1.

Chapter 9

Aminoglycoside Antibiotics Are the Ototoxic "Bad Boys"

What Are Aminoglycosides?

The AMINOGLYCOSIDE antibiotics are probably the most ototoxic of all the classes of drugs. Taken as a whole, these drugs are the "bad boys" as far as your ears are concerned. Every doctor, nurse and pharmacist should know this well. Unfortunately, some either never learned this, don't believe it, or have forgotten it. As a result, our ears often have to pay the penalty.

Be wary of the AMINOGLYCOSIDES. They are "high-powered" antibiotics and are normally reserved for life and death situations, or for bacteria that just won't respond to other antibiotics.

There are a bunch of AMINOGLYCOSIDE antibiotics in existence and new ones are being produced all the time. Here in North America, some of the more common ones include **Amikacin**, **Gentamicin**, **Kanamycin**, **Neomycin**, **Netilmicin**, **Streptomycin** and **Tobramycin**.

In Europe, Japan and the Far East, they use a number of others including **Arbekacin**, **Astromicin**, **Betanamycin** (**Aminodeoxy-kanamycin**), **Dibekacin**, **Isepamicin**, **Lividomycin**, **Micronomicin**, **Paromomycin** (**Aminosidine**), **Ribostamycin**, **Sisomicin** and **Spectinomycin**.[1]

Some AMINOGLYCOSIDES like **Hygromycin** are just too dangerous and are not used on people.

I have not included all the foreign AMINOGLYCOSIDES in this book simply because I do not have any ototoxic information on them. However, you can assume that they are all ototoxic, just like the other members of their class.

Before you take any AMINOGLYCOSIDES, both you and your doctor should carefully weigh the potential risks to your ears (and to other parts of your body) against the expected benefits you hope to obtain from taking one of these drugs. Depending on your situation, the risk of hearing loss may be largely insignificant compared to the situation you face. For example, if you have a life-threatening infection from a particularly virulent bacteria, an AMINOGLYCOSIDE may be your only option. Your choice may be simple—be deaf or be dead!

However, there are often alternatives that would allow you to continue with effective treatment while minimizing the risk to your ears. For example, you might ask your doctor to substitute another drug that is just as effective, yet is not as ototoxic. You could ask him to try a less effective drug that has fewer ototoxic risks. You could also have your doctor adjust the dose to minimize the side effects to your ears. Finally, you could suggest he combine the AMINOGLYCOSIDE with another antibiotic that would reduce the overall dose of the AMINOGLYCOSIDE.[2] If you fail to consider these alternatives, or if you fail to optimize treatment based on them, you can greatly increase your risk of hearing loss and other damage to your ears.

AMINOGLYCOSIDE ANTIBIOTICS

Here are all the AMINOGLYCOSIDE antibiotics mentioned in this book.

Amikacin
Arbekacin [++]
Astromicin
Betanamycin (Aminodeoxy-kanamycin) [++]
Capreomycin
Dibekacin
Dihydrostreptomycin
Framycetin
Gentamicin
Hygromycin B
Isepamicin
Kanamycin
Lividomycin [++]
Micronomicin
Neomycin (Fradiomycin)
Netilmicin
Paromomycin (Aminosidine)
Ribostamycin
Sisomicin
Spectinomycin [++]
Streptomycin
Tobramycin
Viomycin

[++] Drugs marked with a [++] do not have separate listings in this book since I do not have information on their ototoxicity at this time.

In the past, some AMINOGLYCOSIDES such as **Streptomycin** had largely been replaced by less ototoxic drugs. Unfortunately, in recent years, AMINOGLYCOSIDE use has been increasing again. This is due to the increasing number of tuberculosis infections and because organisms resistant to other drugs are becoming more prevalent.[3]

What's the Damage?

One of the interesting things about AMINOGLYCOSIDE antibiotics is how some of them mainly damage the cochlear (hearing) system while others mainly attack the vestibular (balance) system. Of course, a few of them attack both systems equally. However, make no mistake about it, **all** the AMINOGLYCOSIDE antibiotics can damage **both** systems to a greater or lesser degree.

Those AMINOGLYCOSIDES that have a decided preference for attacking the cochlear (hearing) system include **Amikacin, Dihydrostreptomycin, Kanamycin** and **Neomycin**.[4] Those that tend to mainly cause damage to the vestibular (balance) system include **Netilmicin** and **Streptomycin**. In contrast, **Gentamicin** and **Tobramycin** attack both systems equally, although **Gentamicin** tends more towards vestibular damage.[5, 6]

Here is something important that few people know about the AMINOGLYCOSIDE antibiotics. When you take them, they head straight for your inner ear fluids—the endolymph and perilymph. They dive in there quickly and easily. The problem is that they persist in your inner ear fluids for a long time after they disappear from your bloodstream[7]—from several weeks to several months[8] and even up to a year. During all the time that AMINOGLYCOSIDES are present in your inner ear fluids, they can be damaging your ears. Also, during this time, your ears are especially susceptible to noise-induced hearing loss. (See Chapter 8 for more information on this.)

Since AMINOGLYCOSIDES persist in your ears for such a long time, hearing loss (and other ear damage) may occur any time up to 6 months after you stop taking them. Even after you have detected a hearing loss, your hearing can continue to deteriorate for up to 12 months.[9] In extreme cases, AMINOGLYCOSIDE ototoxicity may not show up for many months or not until years later.[10]

However, don't get the idea that you always have to wait a long time for AMINOGLYCOSIDE damage to show up. There is a lot of variation. The first symptoms you experience may be sudden; or they may appear slowly during the time you are taking the AMINOGLYCOSIDE; or they may not even appear until sometime after you have stopped the treatment. Watch for any early symptoms of ototoxicity. One problem is that any early symptoms may go unrecognized or may not even be looked for until it is too late. By then, irreversible damage may have already occurred.

AMINOGLYCOSIDE damage begins at the base of the cochlea and progresses to the tip. Since the high-frequency hair cells are at the base of the cochlea and the low frequency ones are at the tip, hearing loss begins at the very high frequencies and progresses to the lower frequencies as the damage increases.

Damage also begins with the outer rows of hair cells and progresses to the row of inner hair cells. Apparently the inner row of the outer rows of hair cells is affected first, followed by the other two rows of outer hair cells. Finally, it affects the inner hair cells.[11]

One of the more insidious things about hearing loss due to AMINOGLYCOSIDE antibiotics is that hearing loss begins in the very high frequencies where we don't notice it and slowly works its way down to the speech frequencies where it eventually becomes apparent. The problem is, testing high-frequency hearing loss needs specially calibrated audiometers to detect it as we saw in Chapter 6. Since audiologists currently only measure the speech frequencies, hearing loss can go totally unnoticed for a considerable period of time.[12] In fact, because of the insidious nature of these ototoxic effects and the minimal symptoms at first, significant hearing loss and vestibular dysfunction may occur before ototoxicity is even detected.

Therefore, if you have any warning symptoms, you need to immediately contact your doctor and stop taking the drug, if possible, before it is too late. Typically, ototoxic damage first manifests itself as high-pitched tinnitus. It then progresses to high-frequency hearing loss and vestibular problems. Early detection of these ototoxic side effects provides critical information that allows your doctor to implement alternate treatment strategies in order to minimize the risk of further damage to your ears.[13]

If you are taking an AMINOGLYCOSIDE antibiotic, you should receive a complete baseline audiometric evaluation consisting of the frequencies between 250 Hz and the highest frequency you can hear (or up to 20,000 Hz). Ideally, you should have your hearing tested at these same frequencies every 2 to 3 days during treatment in order to detect the first indications of hearing loss.[14]

After you stop taking an AMINOGLYCOSIDE, you may continue to notice progressive hearing loss over the next several weeks and months. That is why audiometric testing, particularly in the high-frequency range, is so important. You need audiograms done before, during and for several months after taking any AMINOGLYCOSIDE antibiotic.[15]

If you stop audiometric testing at the same time you stop taking an AMINOGLYCOSIDE, you will miss any hearing loss that shows up later. In one study, 61% of the people tested showed initial hearing loss during or immediately after treatment. However 78% showed change one month after treatment stopped.[16] Thus, if follow-up testing had not been done, doctors would have missed all this delayed hearing loss.[17]

If you lose your hearing or balance from taking an AMINOGLYCOSIDE, you are anxious to know what chance you have of getting your hearing (and/or balance) back. If you recognized the early warning symptoms in time and stopped the drug treatment, your chances are much better. In these cases, the damage is not total. Therefore, your chances for improvement are about 10 to 15% depending on the drugs involved and your particular risk factors. The tinnitus normally goes away in a week or two.

However, if you are unlucky or the resulting damage is severe, there is little chance of recovery. Any damage is likely permanent.[18] However, rarely, recovery does occur, so don't completely give up hope.

How you take an AMINOGLYCOSIDE is also important. Studies are now showing that giving the total daily dose at one time, rather than spreading it throughout the day, does not result in higher rates of ototoxicity. In fact, it may actually decrease the incidence.[20]

Furthermore, if you are taking another ototoxic drug and an

Overweight?

Note: if you are overweight and are taking an AMINOGLYCOSIDE antibiotic, it is most important that your doctor calculates your dose based on your lean muscle mass, not on your total body weight including fat. Otherwise, you may receive an overdose that can cause severe permanent ototoxic damage.[19]

AMINOGLYCOSIDE at the same time, the **order** you take them is most important. Animal studies have shown that giving a LOOP DIURETIC followed by an AMINOGLYCOSIDE does not affect cochlear toxicity (hearing loss) any more than these drugs taken singly. However, reverse the order and wham—the two drugs act synergistically to really damage your ears.[21] So the secret is, never take an AMINOGLYCOSIDE antibiotic at the same time as other ototoxic drugs if you can avoid it. However, if you must take another ototoxic drug and an AMINOGLYCOSIDE, if possible, **take the other drug first**. Then, when you have completed that prescription, begin the AMINOGLYCOSIDE antibiotic. Your ears will thank you for doing this.

Genetics and Aminoglycoside Ototoxicity

Researchers have puzzled over why some people can take an AMINOGLYCOSIDE with seeming impunity, and other people taking the same dose end up with severe hearing loss and/or no balance. There is extreme variability in the resulting hearing loss.[22] Recent studies reveal that some families have a higher incidence than others.[23] This implicates genetics in AMINOGLYCOSIDE ototoxicity.

Researchers now know that you can inherit a genetic susceptibility to hearing loss. Here is an example of the way medications and genes interact.[24] You are more likely to have a resulting hearing loss from taking an AMINOGLYCOSIDE if you have a particular variant of the 12S rRNA gene present.[25]

The relationship between the 12S rRNA gene and hearing loss caused by AMINOGLYCOSIDE antibiotics is very interesting. Here is how it works. AMINOGLYCOSIDE antibiotics kill bacteria by interfering with the normal operation of certain proteins in the bacteria. Fortunately for us, these proteins are either unimportant or not present in humans. This is why AMINOGLYCOSIDES do not kill us.

However, the 1555A>G variant of the 12S rRNA gene changes this balance. The 1555A>G variant "looks" similar to a protein in the bacteria the AMINOGLYCOSIDE is targeting. When this variant is present in humans, an AMINOGLYCOSIDE can interfere with the function of this variant protein. For reasons still unknown, this leads to loss of hearing.[26]

Incidentally, people carrying the 1555A>G mutation are also more likely to develop hearing loss over time even if they never take AMINOGLYCOSIDE antibiotics.[27]

How Ototoxic Are the Aminoglycosides?

All the AMINOGLYCOSIDE antibiotics can cause auditory (hearing loss) and vestibular (balance) toxicity. These symptoms occur more frequently in people with a present or past history of kidney impairment, in people treated with other ototoxic or nephrotoxic (kidney-damaging) drugs, and in people treated for longer periods and/or with higher doses than recommended.

Exactly how common is AMINOGLYCOSIDE ototoxicity? According to one study, you have a 25% chance of incurring a hearing loss from taking any of the AMINOGLYCOSIDE antibiotics.[28]

In fact, these figures may be too low. This is because many people receiving AMINOGLYCOSIDES are not tested for high-frequency hearing loss as we saw in Chapter 6.

Researchers estimate that between one and four million Americans receive AMINOGLYCOSIDE antibiotics each year.[29] Thus up to four million people each year are potentially at risk for hearing loss associated with taking AMINOGLYCOSIDES.[30] Based on the above 25% incidence figure, between 250,000 and 1,000,000 people a year in the United States end up with hearing losses from taking these drugs. That is a staggering number of people with hearing loss! Many more millions are at potential risk to get tinnitus and a whole host of balance problems related to taking AMINOGLYCOSIDE antibiotics.

Other studies show that even this figure is much too low and is really only the tip of the iceberg. One researcher reports that, depending on the specific AMINOGLYCOSIDE and the dose, one-third of the people taking an AMINOGLYCOSIDE antibiotic have a resulting hearing loss as confirmed by (conventional) audiometric testing.[31]

Another researcher reveals that a staggering percentage of the people taking AMINOGLYCOSIDE antibiotics experience ototoxic side effects.[32] For example, of 53 people treated with AMINOGLYCOSIDE antibiotics (4 with **Amikacin**, 47 with **Gentamicin** and 2 with **Tobramycin**), 63% had resulting ototoxic hearing loss.

Of those with hearing loss, 62% revealed initial hearing loss in the high-frequency range, 29% showed initial hearing loss in the conventional frequencies, while 9% showed initial hearing loss in both frequency ranges at the same time.[33] This is why it is critical to have your hearing checked at the highest frequencies you can hear. When only the conventional frequencies are tested, most hearing loss (62%) is missed! (See Chapter 6 for more information on this important subject.)

Here are some more shocking statistics from around the world. "Up to two-thirds of all cases of hearing loss in many parts of the developing world are caused by the indiscriminate use of AMINOGLYCOSIDE antibiotics such as **Streptomycin** and **Gentamicin**".[34] It is bad in Canada and the United States, but it is horrible in many third world countries.

Part of the problem is that in certain countries, antibiotics are prescribed freely, or are available without a prescription. In these areas, AMINOGLYCOSIDE antibiotics account for up to 66% of the deaf people found there.[35] According to Dr. Dinesh Kumar, deafness from ototoxic drugs is "becoming quite common in India" since many of the people there believe in self-medication. The drugs causing much of the hearing losses there include the AMINOGLYCOSIDE **Gentamicin**, and other ototoxic drugs such as **Erythromycin**, **Chloroquine** and **Furosemide**.[36]

In China, up to two-thirds of the cases of deafness may be caused by AMINOGLYCOSIDE antibiotics, which are frequently given to children for upper respiratory tract infections.[37] One study of hard of hearing children in China revealed that 123 of the 154 studied had lost their hearing from taking antibiotics. Of these 123 children, 60 of them had hearing problems due to taking **Gentamicin**.[38]

There are three prime reasons for this needless carnage. First, AMINOGLYCOSIDE antibiotics are relatively cheap. Second, people are ignorant of the devastating effects on these drugs on their ears. Third, far too many people have as their philosophy "a pill for every ill" and even worse, "for each infection, an injection".[39] Thus, sadly, millions of people around the world continue to needlessly lose their hearing from these drugs and few seem to care.

No matter what doctors may say to the contrary, using AMINOGLYCOSIDE eardrops to fight middle-ear infections is not without risk. Many doctors will tell you that there is no risk unless you have a hole in your eardrum. Even then, they don't seem to take the risk of hearing loss and other ototoxic effects seriously. This needs to change.

Bad things do indeed happen to our ears from taking eardrops. It must be much more common than the doctors think. For example, in one study, seven people with middle ear infections and eardrum "defects" were given AMINOGLYCOSIDE eardrops. Guess what? Surprise! **Every single one** ended up with ototoxic effects like hearing loss, tinnitus, vertigo, ataxia, and oscillopsia. In fact **all** were **severely** affected and some incapacitated![40] Does this sound harmless to you?

> ### Wobble, Wobble, Wobble
>
> When an AMINOGLYCOSIDE antibiotic attacks your balance system, it can turn your life upside down. Such occurrences are not as rare as you might be led to believe. You can read a number of the tragic stories of people who now wobble instead of walk in the notes section under the generic drug **Gentamicin**.

Furthermore, these people were carefully monitored. What happens to the masses of people who are given eardrops and never closely monitored? Do the doctors just assume that there is no ototoxic damage? Bet they do—if they give it any thought at all—but they are wrong.

According to one researcher, the incidence and prevalence of ototoxicity may be higher than reported because of the difficulty in distinguishing between the natural course of the inner ear infections and the ototoxic drugs. Since the hearing loss first occurs far above the speech frequencies, people don't notice this loss right away. At the same time, doctors often miss the vestibular toxicity or blame it on labyrinthitis. Since hearing loss and vestibular damage are generally permanent, both you and your doctor need to carefully monitor what is happening to your ears whenever you are taking ear drops.[41]

Neomycin, besides being used in ear drops, has proven to be ototoxic whether injected, taken orally or used externally on a wound. Yes, when just used for cleaning and sterilizing wounds, it has caused deafness in a number of people.[42]

When you are around AMINOGLYCOSIDES remember, they are the ototoxic "bad boys" and you always need to treat them with respect.

Preventing Aminoglycoside Ototoxicity

There is some exciting news coming out concerning Aminoglycoside antibiotics. Researchers are studying iron chelators, antioxidants and gene therapy as possible ways of preventing hearing loss as a result of taking Aminoglycosides.[43]

Current research indicates that it is not the Aminoglycoside antibiotics themselves that destroy the hair cells in our hearing and balance systems. Rather, the by-products of these drugs cause free radicals to be formed. It is these free radicals that cause the ototoxicity. Here is how it works.

In 1995, Dr. Jochen Schacht and his colleagues discovered a surprising fact. **Gentamicin** is not ototoxic until it combines with iron in the bloodstream and becomes "activated". As **Gentamicin**-iron molecules form, they trigger production of free radicals—unstable molecules that rip apart and damage cells. Unfortunately, the thousands of tiny hair cells in the cochlea are particularly vulnerable to free radical attacks. When these hair cells are damaged or die, we don't hear. It's that simple.

To prevent the iron binding with the **Gentamicin**, Schacht decided to try iron chelators to "soak up" the excess iron in the bloodstream. The iron chelators he used were **Deferoxamine** (DFO) and 2,3-Dihydroxybenzoate (DHB). He also tried the antioxidant **Mannitol**.

In low doses, **Deferoxamine** helps to protect against this type of Aminoglycoside ototoxicity.[44] In addition, laboratory test animals injected with **Gentamicin** as well as Dihydroxybenzoate and **Mannitol** had complete protection at all measured hearing frequencies. Equally important, this treatment did not affect the antibiotic properties of **Gentamicin**. This is the good news. Now this needs to be tested on people to see if it will prevent hearing loss in humans like it did in the animal studies.[45]

The bad news is that this medical advance may never see the light of day. More research needs to be done to confirm preliminary studies, but funds are not forthcoming. Apparently, the big pharmaceutical companies do not want to invest their research dollars in "old" drugs whose patents have expired.[46]

Other researchers have recently discovered that **Acetylsalicylic acid (ASA** or **Aspirin)** is also a good chelator and thus may also help protect our ears from the damaging effects of taking Aminoglycoside antibiotics. **ASA** quickly breaks down in our bodies to produce Salicylate, a compound that soaks up any extra iron and thereby prevents the Aminoglycosides from forming free radicals.

Again, the results in animal studies are impressive. Guinea pigs receiving **Gentamicin** alone had severe hearing loss of up to 70 dB and almost complete destruction of the outer hair cells in the cochlea. In contrast, guinea pigs given both **Gentamicin** and **Aspirin** only had minor hearing loss of less than 20 dB and minimal hair cell damage.[47] Current research is now determining if **Aspirin** affords the same protection in humans. Let's hope it does!

Still other researchers have discovered that when glial cell line-derived neurotrophic factor (GDNF) is present, it helps protect inner-ear hair cell degeneration from the effects of both loud noise and ototoxic drugs. This is good news for our ears. Now researchers are looking into whether GDNF can still provide this protection if given shortly after a person has taken an AMINOGLYCOSIDE antibiotic. Preliminary results suggest that this is the case and hair cell destruction is not as great when GDNF is given following an ototoxic antibiotic.[48]

Perhaps the day will come when doctors will give an AMINOGLYCOSIDE antidote at the same time they give the AMINOGLYCOSIDE antibiotic. If that ever happens, one of the biggest ototoxic threats to our ears will have been eliminated!

1   *Antibiotics Index*, 2001. p. 4.
2   Fausti, 1992. p. 1026.
3   Kalkanis, 2001. p. 2.
4   Kalkanis, 2001. p. 2.
5   Shlafer, 2000. p. 6.
6   *Guidelines for the Audiologic Management of Individuals Receiving Cochleotoxic Drug Therapy*, 1994. pp. 2-3.
7   *Guidelines for the Audiologic Management of Individuals Receiving Cochleotoxic Drug Therapy*, 1994. p. 3.
8   Kalkanis, 2001. p. 2.
9   Haybach, 1999. p. 35.
10   Oghalai, 1996. p. 1.
11   Lyos, 1992. p. 1.
12   Troost, 1998d. p. 3.
13   Fausti, 1992. p. 1026.
14   Fausti, 1992. p. 1030.
15   Shlafer, 2000. p. 7.
16   Fausti, 1992. p. 1030.
17   Shlafer, 2000. p. 7.
18   Troost, 1998b. p. 3.
19   Haybach, 1999. p. 50.
20   Haybach, 1999. p. 50.
21   Troost, 1998a. p. 1.
22   Fausti, 1992. p. 1029.
23   Haybach, 1999. p. 44.
24   WebMDHealth, 2001. p.3.
25   WebMDHealth, 2001. p.2.
26   WebMDHealth, 2001. p.5.
27   Snow & Wackym, 2008. p.276
28   Shlafer, 2000. p. 7.
29   Haybach, 1999. p. 19.
30   *Guidelines for the Audiologic Management of Individuals Receiving Cochleotoxic Drug Therapy*, 1994. p. 2.
31   Kalkanis, 2001. p. 2.
32   *Guidelines for the Audiologic Management of Individuals Receiving Cochleotoxic Drug Therapy*, 1994. p. 4.
33   Fausti, 1992. p. 1028.
34   Abdulla, 1996. p. 648.
35   Kalkanis, 2001. p. 2.
36   Kumar, 1998. p. 1.

37   Priuska, 1997. p. 2.

38   Shearer, 1991. pp. 74-75.

39   Abdulla, 1996. p. 648.

40   Helal, 1997. pp. 1056-59.

41   Helal, 1997. pp. 1056-59.

42   Suss, 1993. p. 183.

43   Kalkanis, 2001. p. 3.

44   Priuska, 1997. p. 5.

45   Schacht, 1997. pp. 1-2.

46   Abdulla, 1996. p. 648.

47   *Aspirin Component Prevents Antibiotic-induced Deafness*, 1999. pp. 1-2.

48   Yagi, 1999. p. 1.

Chapter 10

Beware of Benzodiazepines—Don't Let This Nasty Time-Bomb Ambush You and Your Ears

Another "nasty" class of ototoxic drugs is the BENZODIAZEPINES (pronounced ben-zoe-die-AZ-eh-peens). Unlike the AMINOGLYCOSIDES, the BENZODIAZEPINES are not extremely ototoxic, but what they lack in their degree of ototoxicity, they make up for in their "nastiness". You see, the BENZODIAZEPINES are dependence-forming drugs, so any ototoxic side effects they may cause—including tinnitus, hyperacusis and balance problems—are very difficult to bring under control once they get started.

What Are Benzodiazepines?

The BENZODIAZEPINES are a class of drugs commonly known as tranquilizers and sleeping pills. They are predominantly prescribed for anything associated with anxiety or sleeping problems.

Some of the more common BENZODIAZEPINES include **Alprazolam** (*Xanax*), **Diazepam** (*Valium*), **Lorazepam** (*Ativan*), **Clonazepam** (*Rivotril & Klonopin*) and **Triazolam** (*Halcion*). There are at least 20 different BENZODIAZEPINES (see Section 60.12.8 in Table 14-1). The generic names (with three exceptions) either end in "lam" or "pam".

In addition to the BENZODIAZEPINES, there are three other drugs that, although not BENZODIAZEPINES, have similar effects including the same horrible dependence and withdrawal problems. They are **Zaleplon** (*Sonata*), **Zolpidem** (*Ambien*) and **Zopiclone** (*Imovane*). What I say about the BENZODIAZEPINES largely applies to these drugs too.

How It All Begins

When people go to their doctors with problems sleeping or feeling anxious, and are prescribed one of the BENZODIAZEPINES, the last thing on their minds is that years later they will be "hooked" on a horror drug. That's how it all begins.

BENZODIAZEPINES are only meant to be taken for short periods of time. They are **temporary** solutions to problems such as anxiety and sleeplessness. In fact, safe and appropriate use of BENZODIAZEPINES is for **no longer** that 2 to 3 weeks if taken daily.[1] They were **never** meant to be the long-term solution to these problems. Unfortunately, doctors allow multitudes of people to stay on these drugs for months, and in many cases, years.

When you stay on a BENZODIAZEPINE for too long, bad things begin to happen. First, the longer you take a BENZODIAZEPINE, the less effective it becomes. For example, for problems sleeping, BENZODIAZEPINES are only effective for about 1 to 2 weeks. When your symptoms begin to get worse, doctors typically increase your dose. This works for a few more weeks, then you begin to feel even worse.[2]

This is because if you take BENZODIAZEPINES for inappropriately long periods of time, not only does the drug become ineffective, it also induces drug dependency. When this happens, your body comes to depend on the drug to function. Thus you are "hooked" much as a person becomes addicted to certain drugs. (Note: technically, BENZODIAZEPINES cause dependency, not addiction, but the end result is similar.)

Here is some shocking information about BENZODIAZEPINE dependence. You would do well to heed it before you ever begin taking one of these drugs (see sidebar).

Benzodiazepine "Addiction" Warning

"The biggest drug-addiction problem in the world doesn't involve heroin, cocaine or marijuana. In fact, it doesn't involve an illegal drug at all. The world's biggest drug-addiction problem is posed by a group of drugs, the BENZODIAZEPINES, which are widely prescribed by doctors and taken by countless millions of perfectly ordinary people around the world".

"Drug-addiction experts claim that getting people off the BENZODIAZEPINES is more difficult than getting addicts off heroin. The only genuine long-term solution is to be aware of these drugs and to avoid them like the plague".

"It seems that the dependency is so ingrained, and the withdrawal symptoms you get are so intolerable, that people have a great deal of problem coming off BENZODIAZEPINES. The other aspect is that with heroin, usually the withdrawal is over within a week or so. With BENZODIAZEPINES, a proportion of patients go on to long term withdrawal, and they have very unpleasant symptoms for month after month, and this can go on for two years or more. Some of the tranquilizer groups document people who still have symptoms ten years after stopping".[3]

Used responsibly and taken in the short term to tide you over a rough spot, BENZODIAZEPINES can do some good. However, so often these drugs are abused. For example, according to one estimate, 1 person in every 50 people has been taking a BENZODIAZEPINE **for longer than 6 months!**[4]

Furthermore, research indicates that 30% to 50% of regular BENZODIAZEPINE users will develop a dependency to these drugs. In addition, the longer you take a BENZODIAZEPINE, the greater your risk of becoming dependent on that drug.[5]

This makes it very difficult to get off BENZODIAZEPINES. In fact, researchers estimate that between 50% and 80% of people who have taken BENZODIAZEPINES continually for 6 months or longer will experience withdrawal symptoms when reducing the dose or stopping completely.[6]

Here's What It's Like When the Benzos Grip You

Some people seem to be able to take BENZODIAZEPINES with seeming impunity, however many people have such bad experiences they sincerely wish they had never taken the first pill. Here is one such example.

A lady explained: "About 15 years ago I started having panic attacks and began taking **Alprazolam** (*Xanax*) at 1.5 mg/day and have been on it ever since. Two years ago I had some really bad panic attacks so my doctor doubled my *Xanax* medication to 3 mg/day.

Now everything is out of control for some reason. In the past year or two, in spite of the increased dose, things have been getting much worse to the point I don't feel normal any more.

My hearing is a lot worse, I have vertigo and balance problems. I feel unsteady on my feet. My ears are ringing. They are also supersensitive to sounds. As a result, I can't wear a hearing aid in one ear any more.

I feel like I am only 50% here—kind of like a bad head cold feeling, or living in a dream state. I feel shaky and out of sorts and panicky. I feel weird and feel like I am going to pass out. I can be fine one minute, then bam—all of a sudden I feel this odd feeling coming on as if my hearing gets very quiet. I feel as if I am chilled. I get a tingly feeling in my head, and then I feel a sort of darkness and closed-in feeling about to happen. I start to shake and sweat, and I just feel as if I am drifting away.

I have always thought that my medications could be hurting me more than helping me. Why did the doctor do this to me? My neurologist feels I won't be able to stop taking the *Xanax* as my body is now dependent on it. If I would go off this drug, he feels I would spin out of control—but I'm already out of control!

For some time I have wanted to try to taper down, or get off the *Xanax*, but I am scared I will feel worse. How am I going to live my life without the *Xanax*? I want to be able to get through the day, but not like this! I would love to be **free** and be **me** again!"

Unfortunately, this lady is not alone. I have heard a number of similar stories from people who have been taking BENZODIAZEPINES for a number of months or years. Eventually, like this lady, they realize the drugs are not helping them, yet when they try to go off them, the nasty time-bomb hidden in these drugs not only ambushes their ears, but also flips their lives upside down and leaves them worried about their ability to function in the future.

Getting Off Benzodiazepines

Getting on BENZODIAZEPINES is easy, but getting off them once you have built up a dependence to them is very hard, and for some people almost impossible. You see, dependence on the BENZODIAZEPINES is insidious and sneaks up on you without your even being aware of it—often until it is too late.

This drug dependency actually makes your original symptoms worse. For example, BENZODIAZEPINES eventually make your sleep problems even **worse** than they were before you began taking these drugs.

The same thing happens with anxiety. Initially, the BENZODIAZEPINES help, but if you continue to take them for extended periods of time, the resulting physical dependency can actually cause an **increase** in anxiety—even while taking the same low dose![7]

Myriads of side effects begin to emerge. Taking BENZODIAZEPINES can have several negative side effects on your ears. For example, those side effects that act on your cochlea include hearing loss, auditory hallucinations, hyperacusis and tinnitus.

Those side effects that act on your vestibular system and affect your balance in one way or another include dizziness, ataxia, loss of balance, vertigo and nystagmus.

In addition to messing up your ears, taking BENZODIAZEPINES can cause a number of other scary side effects such as anxiety, fears, feelings of unreality, hypersensitivity to light, insomnia, lack of concentration, loss of memory, nightmares, panic attacks, rapid mood changes, shaking, sweating, depersonalization (a feeling of not knowing who you are), outbursts of rage or aggression, paranoia, persistent unpleasant memories, feeling of pins and needles, rapid changes in body temperature, blackouts and a host of other symptoms.

When I mentioned to the lady in the above story that she likely would be shocked to learn that almost all of her symptoms, both ear-related and otherwise, were known side effects of taking BENZODIAZEPINES, she replied, "I'm scared. Everything you have said about the drugs I take really hit home".

Since the side effects of BENZODIAZEPINES can be so insidious, your first line of defense is knowledge. You now know that BENZODIAZEPINES are only supposed to be used for short periods of time—2 to 3 weeks at the most! Any doctor who prescribes these drugs for longer periods than that is doing you a disservice, and may be harming you. Thus, refuse to take any BENZODIAZEPINE for longer than 3 weeks. By doing so, you will avoid these withdrawal problems.

When you finally decide the BENZODIAZEPINES aren't doing you any good, and indeed are causing you much more harm than good, you try to go off them. The range and severity of the resulting BENZODIAZEPINE withdrawal symptoms will likely take you by surprise. This is when you discover to your horror that when you try to go off them, your existing symptoms intensify and still other side effects appear. For many people, the intensity of BENZODIAZEPINE withdrawal is overwhelming. Unfortunately, there are no predictors for who will likely suffer severe withdrawal, and who will likely have a mild withdrawal experience.[8]

Some people, for example, get hyperacusis when they try to go off BENZODIAZEPINES. In one study of 22 people, 4 (18%) had hyperacusis. Fortunately, by 3 months, only 1 person of the 4 still had hyperacusis.[9]

Other people end up with protracted tinnitus when they try to go off a BENZODIAZEPINE. For example, one man who had taken **Diazepam** for 8 years for anxiety, got obnoxious tinnitus just 4 days after discontinuing **Diazepam**. His tinnitus persisted for 3 months. Fortunately, after 6 months, his tinnitus was only occasional and of short duration, and by 1 year it had completely disappeared.[10]

Another man began to hear high-pitched ringing tinnitus in both his ears for the first time in his life as he reduced his **Diazepam** dose to a low level. Unfortunately, in his case, he still had tinnitus 1 year later, but was learning to cope with it.

The withdrawal side effects can be so incapacitating that some people choose to stay on these drugs because they cannot cope with these horrible side effects when they try to stop taking BENZODIAZEPINES. By doing so, they condemn themselves to a miserable existence for the rest of their lives.

For example, one man, after taking **Diazepam** for 12 years for anxiety had severe tinnitus upon discontinuing **Diazepam**. In his case, he discovered he couldn't stop taking the **Diazepam** because of his incapacitating high-pitched intense tinnitus in both his ears which began each time he reduced his dose of **Diazepam**.[11]

Make Haste Slowly

In order to go off any BENZODIAZEPINE, you will have to taper off extremely slowly—and under your doctor's guidance, of course. Reducing the dose of the drug very slowly minimizes the severity of the withdrawal symptoms.

One lady that that had built up a drug dependence explained: "The secret to getting off these drugs is to do it **very** slowly. You may or may not know this, but the medical community is in the dark ages about tapering off anti-psychotic medications. There is a significant minority, including me, who have trouble big time, if we were to taper by their protocol which is very fast. (Actually, I suspect we are far more than a minority.)

One psychiatrist told me that anti-psychotic medicine should not be tapered any faster than 10% of the current dose every 4 weeks. Yes, it is a slow process, but here is the proof. I have had minimal side effects and can hold down a full-time job. The people who taper off too quickly have a totally different experience, and it is not pleasant!"

Another tip from this lady is that you slowly taper off only **one** drug at a time. Since she was on several drugs, at her safe taper rate it was going to still take her another **six years** to be drug free. This is the way to do it if you don't want unpleasant side effects cropping up because of tapering off too fast. It also gives your brain a chance to get its brain chemistry working properly again without the help of drugs.

As you can see, overcoming the withdrawal side effects of Benzodiazepines can take many weeks, months or years. Usually the length of time someone has been taking a Benzodiazepine, and the amount they have been taking, will have the most impact on how long it takes for their withdrawal symptoms to pass.

If you want to stop taking Benzodiazepines, read the excellent manual *Benzodiazepines: How They Work and How To Withdraw* by Dr. Heather Ashton, one of the foremost authorities on the planet on how to break free from these drugs. Not only is it free, it's easy to read and packed with the information you need to help you.[12]

The goal is to become healthy and drug free. Then you won't have to worry about ototoxic (or other) adverse side effects. The good news is that if you persist through the agonies of the withdrawal stage—no matter how long it takes—in the end, as the lady in the lead story expressed it, you will be free and be "me" again!

---

1   *About Benzodiazepines*, 2005. p. 5.

2   *About Benzodiazepines*, 2005. p. 4.

3   *Benzodiazepine Addiction, Withdrawal & Recovery*, 2006.

4   *About Benzodiazepines*, 2005. p. 3.

5   *About Benzodiazepines*, 2005. p. 6.

6   *About Benzodiazepines*, 2005. p. 7.

7   *About Benzodiazepines*, 2005. p. 4.

8   *About Benzodiazepines*, 2005. p. 8.

9   Busto, 1988. p. 4.

10   Busto, 1988. p. 3.

11   Busto, 1988. p. 3.

12   Ashton, 2002.

Chapter 11

Grapefruit Juice and Ototoxic Drugs

Drinking grapefruit juice could be hazardous to your ears. Surprised? Here's the scoop. It's not that grapefruit juice isn't good for you—it is. The problem is that grapefruit juice also contains a substance that can greatly increase the potency of some drugs.[1]

You probably know that mixing medications can be dangerous to your health. This is because certain drugs can enhance the effects of other drugs leaving you with a dangerously high level of a given drug in your body. Your doctor and your pharmacist normally watch out for such interactions and prescribe accordingly.

What is not very well known yet is that downing certain drugs with a drink of grapefruit juice can be just as harmful. Researchers stumbled on to this effect in 1991.[2]

None of the other citrus fruits contain these chemicals called furanocoumarins. However, they are abundant in grapefruit.

Mary Anne Hochadel, a pharmacist, warns that while many doctors know that grapefruit juice can be a problem, they might not understand that all parts of the grapefruit, whether fresh, juiced or concentrated in any quantity has the same effect. Earlier studies implicated the concentrated forms, but newer studies have shown that all parts of the grapefruit have an effect.[3]

Here is how it all works. When you drink a glass of grapefruit juice, these furanocoumarins chemically bond to the Cytochrome P-450 3A4 (CYP 3A4 for short) enzymes located in the lining of your intestines. This prevents these enzymes from doing their work.[4]

One of the things these enzymes do is to break down certain compounds before they are absorbed into your bloodstream. This is what God designed them to do.

The trick is to get your body to absorb the medication compounds before the CYP 3A4 enzymes break them down and render them useless. If the medication doesn't break down at the "normal" rate, a problem arises because this changes the effective dose.

What normally happens is that, for instance, maybe 10% of a given drug is absorbed into your bloodstream before the enzymes break it down. As a result, doctors prescribe pills that in this hypothetical example would contain ten times the amount they want to be absorbed—knowing that 90% will be destroyed by these enzymes.

However, if you drink grapefruit juice, these enzymes can no longer do their normal work of breaking down such drugs. When that happens your body absorbs all (or almost all) of the drug into your bloodstream possibly giving you a horrendous overdose that your doctor never intended. This overdose could wreak havoc in your body or even kill you. If those drugs were ototoxic, this dose could result in various kinds of damage to your ears.

Your Body Does Not Absorb All the Medications You Take

Surprising as it may seem, your body does **not** normally absorb much of the medications you take. According to Dr. Paul Watkins, "For many medications that are taken orally in pill form, the majority of the drug is not absorbed from the digestive tract but instead passes out of the body and is, in effect, wasted".[5]

This grapefruit juice effect may last only a few hours. However, taking some drugs as much as 24 hours after drinking some grapefruit juice will result in higher drug levels in your blood than would normally occur.

Furthermore, the effects of drinking grapefruit juice are cumulative. This means that if you drink a glass of grapefruit juice daily for a week, the drug interaction would be stronger than if you only occasionally drink some grapefruit juice.[6] Mixing grapefruit juice with certain medications causes the body to react as if up to 15 **times** the recommended drug dose had been taken. As you can imagine, that could be pretty dangerous!

Studies Show Significant Blood Drug Level Increases

Studies report that **Felodipine** concentrations increased an average of 300% (with peak concentrations as high as 600%) when taken with grapefruit juice. Similarly, **Nisoldipine** levels increased 500% with peak concentrations increasing to 900%.[7]

Other studies report levels of **Lovastatin** increasing by a whopping 1,500% and **Simvastatin** increasing by 1,513%! These are the largest effects of grapefruit juice reported so far.[8]

For older people, the difference in drug levels in the blood can be higher than for younger people. One study reported that older people had a given drug blood level 3.5 times higher than normal after taking grapefruit juice. Other studies have shown that younger people had drug blood levels between 2 and 2.5 times higher than did those who took their medications with water instead of grapefruit juice.[9]

At the present time, I am not aware of the literature reporting anyone having specific ototoxic side effects from drinking grapefruit juice while taking certain drugs, but it may have already happened since such things seldom are reported anyway. Doctors are currently more worried about "serious" side effects like severe heart problems and death than they are with damage to our ears.

There are a number of drugs that "interact" with grapefruit juice. The following list is not exhaustive but gives you a good idea of the kinds of drugs for which you have to watch. If you are in doubt, have your pharmacist look up the specific information on grapefruit juice/drug interactions for that drug.

This list only includes drugs that have known ototoxic properties **and** were known to interact with grapefruit juice in 2002. (There may be other drugs with this property discovered since then.) They include:

ANGIOTENSIN-2-RECEPTOR ANTAGONISTS such as **Losartan** (*Cozaar, Hyzaar*).[10]

> ### Increases in Blood Drug Levels
>
> The percentages in square brackets are the increase over normal in drug blood levels for that drug after taking grapefruit juice according to a specific study.

ANTI-ARRHYTHMICS such as **Propafenone** (*Rythmol*).[11]

ANTI-CONVULSANT DRUGS such as **Carbamazepine** (*Tegretol*) [40%].[12, 13]

ANTIFUNGAL ANTIBIOTICS like **Itraconazole** (*Sporanox*)[14, 15] and **Ketoconazole** (*Nizoral*).[16]

ANTIHISTAMINES (H$_1$ RECEPTOR ANTAGONISTS) such as **Diphenhydramine** (*Benadyl, Tylenol*),[17] **Fexofenadine** (*Allegra*)[18] and **Loratadine** (*Claritin*).[19]

ANTI-NEOPLASTICS such as **Vinblastine** (*Velban*).[20]

ANTI-RETROVIRAL PROTEASE INHIBITORS such as **Indinavir** (*Crixivan*)[21] and **Saquinavir** (*Fortovase, Invirase*) [200%].[22, 23, 24]

BENZODIAZEPINES such as **Alprazolam** (*Xanax*),[25] **Diazepam** (*Valium*) [320%],[26] **Midazolam** (*Versed*) [240%],[27, 28, 29] and **Triazolam** (*Halcion*) [48%].[30, 31]

BETA BLOCKERS such as **Carvedilol** (*Coreg*) [16%].[32]

CALCIUM-CHANNEL BLOCKERS such as **Amlodipine** (*Lotrel, Norvasc*)[16%],[33] **Felodipine** (*Plendil*) [600%],[34, 35, 36] **Nifedipine** (*Adalat, Procardia*)[200%],[37] **Nimodipine** (*Nimotop*),[38] **Nisoldipine** (*Sular*) [900%][39, 40] and **Verapamil** (*Calan, Isoptin*)[43%].[41, 42]

CARDIAC GLYCOSIDES such as **Digoxin** (*Lanoxin*).[43]

Cholesterol lowering drugs (HMG-CoA REDUCTASE INHIBITORS) such as **Atorvastatin** (*Lipitor*)[250%],[44] **Cerivastatin** (*Baycol*),[45] **Lovastatin** (*Mevacor*)[1500%],[46, 47] **Pravastatin** (*Pravachol*)[48] and **Simvastatin** (*Zocor*)[1513%].[49, 50]

GASTRO-INTESTINAL DRUGS such as **Cisapride** (*Prepulsid*) [39%].[51]

IMMUNOSUPPRESSANT DRUGS such as **Cyclosporine** (*Sandimune, Neoral*)[300%][52, 53, 54] and **Tacrolimus** (*Prograf*)[400%].[55, 56]

MACROLIDE ANTIBIOTICS such as **Erythromycin** (*Ery-Tab*).[57, 58]

TRICYCLIC ANTI-DEPRESSANTS such as **Clomipramine** (*Anafranil*) [300%][59] and **Imipramine**.[60]

There were several reports that **Caffeine** was affected by grapefruit juice. This is not true. Further research shows that **Caffeine** is metabolized by the 1A2 isoenzyme not the 3A4 isoenzyme found in grapefruit juice.[61]

There are several potentially ototoxic drugs that are metabolized by the Cytochrome P450 3A4 enzyme according to available data. Many of these have not yet been specifically studied for their grapefruit juice interactions. Therefore, it would be prudent to avoid taking grapefruit juice if you are taking any of the following medications: **Amiodarone** (*Cordarone*), **Cilostazol** (*Pletal*), **Donepezil** (*Aricept*), **Montelukast** (*Singulair*), **Pimozide** (*Orap*), **Quetiapine** (*Seroquel*), **Sildenafil** (*Viagra*), **Tadalafil** (*Cialis*), **Tamoxifen** (*Nolvadex*), **Tamsulosin** (*Flomax*)[62] and **Vardenafil** (*Levitra*).

It is important for you to know that people differ greatly in their ability to absorb varying amounts of many medications. Thus it is very difficult for researchers to predict exactly how much grapefruit juice is going to affect blood drug levels in any given person. Some people might absorb only one-tenth of a pill and others might absorb five times more.[63] Thus, a dose that does not hurt one person's ears could cause hearing loss in another.

This is because people have widely varying levels of the CYP 3A4 enzymes in their intestinal tract.[64] Dr. Paul Watkins, a professor of medicine, explains, "The amount of the enzyme in the intestinal wall varies greatly among people, which explains why the grapefruit juice effect may be serious for some people and unimportant for others".[65]

He adds, "It probably makes very little difference if people with relatively low levels of the intestinal enzyme take their medicine with grapefruit juice or with water. But for others with a great deal of the enzyme, an unaccustomed glass of juice in the morning may send enzyme levels plummeting and drug levels soaring as much as nine-fold".[66]

Dean Elbe, a pharmacist, suggests that a reasonable guideline is simply this. If you are not currently taking your medications with grapefruit juice regularly, don't start. If you are

---

CYP 3A4 Stabilizes Drug Absorption

One most interesting finding in the studies Dr. Watkins was associated with, is that after taking grapefruit juice, CYP 3A4 levels were virtually the same for everyone in the study instead of the large differences normally found between people.[67]

This means that adding the active ingredient in grapefruit juice to given medications could ensure that much more of the drug would be absorbed and less wasted. At the same time, it would produce nearly the same effect in each person. Research is continuing on this.

already taking your medications with grapefruit juice regularly and are not experiencing any adverse side effects, don't stop.[68]

If you are unsure about your medications and how grapefruit juice will affect their absorption in your body, you can prevent any negative reactions by simply bypassing grapefruit altogether and drink orange juice instead. It's that simple!

Not only does grapefruit juice inhibit the action of CYP 3A4 enzymes, so do some drugs. Drugs known to be CYP 3A4 inhibitors include **Ketoconazole**, **Ritonavir**, **Indinavir**[69] and **Telithromycin**[70].

Taking any of these above drugs with the drugs listed in this chapter could give the same effect as taking grapefruit with them.

There is obviously a problem with two of these drugs as both **Ketoconazole** and **Indinavir** are listed as being **affected** by grapefruit juice, and now these two drugs are supposed to be CYP 3A4 **inhibitors**. They can't be on both sides of the fence at the same time.

---

1   *Grapefruit Juice Can Interact with Medications*, 1999. p. 1.
2   *Grapefruit Juice Can Interact with Medications*, 1999. p. 1.
3   *Grapefruit Interferes with Select Medications*, 2000. p. 1.
4   *Grapefruit Juice Can Interact with Medications*, 1999. p. 1.
5   *It's Not Pulp Fiction: Taking Medications with Grapefruit Juice May Increase Their Potency*, 1996. p. 1.
6   *Grapefruit and Serious Drug Interactions*, 2000. p. 1.
7   *The Grapefruit Juice Effect*, 1997. p. 3.
8   Elbe, 1999c. pp. 1-2.
9   *New Grapefruit Juice—Drug Interactions Found*, 1998. p. 1.
10 *Be Careful When Mixing Grapefruit Juice with Your RX*, 1999. p.1.
11 *The Grapefruit Juice Effect*, 1997. p.3.
12 Elbe, 1999e. p. 2.
13 *New Grapefruit Juice—Drug Interactions Found*, 1998. p. 1.
14 *Grapefruit Juice and Medications*, 1997. p. 1.
15 *The Grapefruit Juice Effect*, 1997. p.2.
16 *Grapefruit Juice and Medications*, 1997. p. 1.
17 *Food and Medication Interactions Can Be Very Harmful*, 1999. p. 1.
18 *Be Careful When Mixing Grapefruit Juice with Your RX*, 1999. p.1.
19 *Food and Medication Interactions Can Be Very Harmful*, 1999. p. 1.
20 *Be Careful When Mixing Grapefruit Juice with Your RX*, 1999. p.1.
21 *Food and Medication Interactions Can Be Very Harmful*, 1999. p. 1.
22 Elbe, 1999e. p. 3.
23 Zuger, 1997. p. 1.
24 *Be Careful When Mixing Grapefruit Juice with Your RX*, 1999. p.1.
25 *Grapefruit Juice and Drugs*, 2000. p. 2.
26 Elbe, 1999a. p. 1.
27 Elbe, 1999a. p. 1.
28 *Grapefruit Juice and Drugs*, 2000. p. 2.
29 *Grapefruit Juice and Medications*, 1997. p. 1.

30 Elbe, 1999a. p. 1.
31 *Grapefruit Juice Can Interact with Medications*, 1999. p. 1.
32 Elbe, 1999e. p. 3.
33 Elbe, 1999b. p. 1.
34 Zuger, 1997. p. 1.
35 *Be Careful When Mixing Grapefruit Juice with Your RX*, 1999. p.1.
36 *The Grapefruit Juice Effect*, 1997. p.3.
37 *Procardia (Nifedipine) Capsules*, 2002. p. 1.
38 *Grapefruit Juice Can Interact with Medications*, 1999. p. 1.
39 *The Grapefruit Juice Effect*, 1997. p.1.
40 Elbe, 1999b. p. 1.
41 Elbe, 1999b. p. 1.
42 *Grapefruit Juice and Drugs*, 2000. p. 2.
43 *Be Careful When Mixing Grapefruit Juice with Your RX*, 1999. p.1.
44 Elbe, 1999c. p. 2.
45 Elbe, 1999c. p. 1.
46 Elbe, 1999c. p. 1.
47 *Grapefruit Juice and Medications*, 1997. p. 1.
48 *Grapefruit Juice and Medications*, 1997. p. 1.
49 Elbe, 1999c. p. 2.
50 *Grapefruit Juice and Drugs*, 2000. p. 3.
51 Elbe, 1999e. p. 1.
52 Elbe, 1999d. p. 1.
53 *Be Careful When Mixing Grapefruit Juice with Your RX*, 1999. p. 1.
54 *Grapefruit Juice and Medications*, 1997. p. 1.
55 Elbe, 1999d. p. 1.
56 *Grapefruit Juice and Drugs*, 2000. p. 3.
57 *Grapefruit Juice and Medications*, 1997. p. 1.
58 *The Grapefruit Juice Effect*, 1997. p.2.
59 Elbe, 1999e. p. 1.
60 *Grapefruit and Serious Drug Interactions*, 2000. p. 1.
61 Elbe, 1999f. p. 1.
62 Elbe, 1999g. p. 1.
63 *It's Not Pulp Fiction: Taking Medications with Grapefruit Juice May Increase Their Potency*, 1996. p. 1.
64 *Grapefruit Juice Can Interact with Medications*, 1999. p. 2.
65 Zuger, 1997. p. 2.
66 Zuger, 1997. p. 2.
67 *The Grapefruit Juice Effect*, 1997. p. 5.
68 Elbe, 1999b. p. 1.
69 *Desyrel*, 2004. p. 3.
70 Ketek, 2004. p. 11.

Chapter 12

Potpourri

When Ototoxic Drugs Team Up, They Can Smash Your Ears

Not only do ototoxic drugs team up with noise to destroy your ears, they also team up with other ototoxic drugs to continue their assault on your ears. The sad fact is that there are thousands of drugs on the market, yet very little hard data exists on what taking these drugs in various combinations can do to your ears.

When you take two or more drugs at the same time, there can (and will) be interactions between these drugs. These interactions can produce one of the following results.

1.   The effect on the drug is unchanged. It would be wonderful if this was always the case.

2.   The drug will be less effective. In other words, it is not doing what your doctor intended.

3.   The drug may be more effective. This means you are essentially receiving an overdose. If the drug is ototoxic, the enhanced effects may damage your ears more than you would have expected this drug to do.

4.   There may be unexpected side effects. If these side effects are ototoxic, you could damage your ears whereas taking each drug separately would not have done so.

If you are only taking one drug at a time, there won't be interactions with other drugs, but you still have to be careful as any given drug may interact with the food you eat or the beverages you drink. The result of this could be to increase the ototoxicity of the drug you are taking. For example, one such interaction is taking certain drugs with grapefruit juice. This could result in your body receiving an overdose of that drug. If that drug is ototoxic, you could inadvertently damage your ears. (See the Chapter 11 for more information about this interaction.)

The United States Food and Drug Administration (FDA), has a lot of good information on their web site for you to study. Check out their web page called "Drug Interactions: What You Should Know" at:

http://www.fda.gov/Drugs/ResourcesForYou/ucm163354.htm

Which drug combinations are particularly dangerous to your ears? One of the worst combinations is taking LOOP DIURETICS (**Ethacrynic acid**, **Furosemide** or **Torsemide**) and AMINOGLYCOSIDE antibiotics (**Gentamicin**, **Kanamycin**, **Neomycin**, **Streptomycin**, **Tobramycin**) at the same time. In fact, taking drugs of these two classes together greatly increases your chance of having permanent ototoxic results[1] as the ototoxic effects are synergistic.

Another nasty combination is **Cisplatin** when used in combination with an AMINOGLYCOSIDE antibiotic and a LOOP DIURETIC like **Furosemide**—a typical combination used to treat cancer.[2]

LOOP DIURETICS can also team up with other antibiotics such as **Polymyxin B**,[3] which can greatly increase the risk of ototoxicity.

This is just scratching the surface of drug combinations. When taking several different drugs at the same time, you need to practice your ABCs—Always Be Careful!

Non-steroidal Anti-inflammatory Drugs (NSAIDs) Can Cause Meningitis and Hearing Loss!

One little-known side effect of taking NON-STEROIDAL ANTI-INFLAMMATORY DRUGS (NSAIDs) is aseptic meningitis. Aseptic meningitis can, in turn, cause hearing loss and tinnitus. The signs and symptoms of NSAID-induced meningitis are similar to those of viral or bacterial meningitis.

One of the symptoms of aseptic meningitis can be a bilateral sudden sensorineural hearing loss while a person is on NSAIDs.

Doctors are not sure why NSAIDs can cause aseptic meningitis. Some think it is a hypersensitivity reaction to the drug. They are also unclear how it causes the hearing loss—whether in the cochlea or

> ### Types of Meningitis
>
> Meningitis may be caused by a virus (viral meningitis), or by bacteria (bacterial meningitis). If it is not caused by either of these pathogens, doctors call it aseptic meningitis. Drug-induced meningitis is a type of aseptic meningitis.

in the brain. One theory is that the endolymphatic sac is irritated, which may account for the predominantly low-tone pattern of the resulting hearing loss.

The NSAIDs most frequently associated with this disorder include **Ibuprofen**, **Sulindac**, **Naproxen** and **Tolmetin**. Other ototoxic drugs that may cause aseptic meningitis are the ANTIBIOTIC drugs **Trimethoprim** and **Sulfamethoxazole**,[4] the ACETIC ACIDS **Diclofenac**[5] and **Ketorolac**,[6] the PROPIONIC ACID **Ketoprofen**,[7] the COX-2 INHIBITOR **Rofecoxib**,[8] the ANTICONVULSANT drug **Carbamazepine**,[9] and the **Mumps vaccine**.[10]

The risk factors discovered so far that appear to be associated with NSAID-induced aseptic meningitis include heavy use of drugs, systemic lupus erythematosus and mixed connective tissue disease.

Fortunately, with the cases studied so far, when NSAID use is stopped, hearing returns to normal within a few months and tinnitus subsides.[11]

Watch Out for Your Pet's Ears Too

If you are hard of hearing, you probably rely to a certain extent on your dog to be your ears like I do with our dog, Riley. Dogs make excellent "furry ears" to help us hear. In fact, many deaf and hard of hearing people have specially-trained service dogs (called "hearing ear dogs" in Canada and "hearing dogs" in the USA) to alert them to all kinds of things they can't hear. This is wonderful!

However, all may not be well in doggy-land. Your faithful Fido can get sick. Perhaps you notice he is scratching at his ear. You take him to the veterinarian. The vet looks into his ears and prescribes an antibiotic to clear up an ear infection.

After a few days of faithfully applying the eardrops, the infection clears up. Both of you are now happy—until a few days later you discover to your horror that Fido is now deaf! He can't hear you yelling right by his head. Whatever happened to his hearing?

Surprise! Dog's ears are very susceptible to the ototoxic effects of drugs just like your own ears are. I know. It happened to our Riley too.

One lady wrote to me about her pet going deaf from taking ototoxic drugs, "It is an eye opening experience to realize that drugs specifically prescribed for treatment of the ear could damage it!"

Make no mistake. This stuff happens. Even though our vet said this was the only case he had seen in his 25 years of practice as a veterinarian, it must occur much more frequently than is commonly thought. Just 4 or 5 weeks later, I was talking to the phone repairman. I happened to mention that our dog was still pretty deaf from taking a course of eardrops to clear up an ear infection so the dog might not let me know if anyone was knocking on my door.

Imagine my surprise when the repairman exclaimed, "That happened to my dog too! He had an ear infection so the vet gave me some drops for him. Within a week he was totally deaf. Fortunately, most of his hearing came back about 3 weeks later".

I further questioned him about whether his dog's hearing all returned, and he said it was not back to what it was before. This is the same experience with Riley. He cannot hear as well as he used to—but at least he can hear some sounds! I think he now has a moderate hearing loss.

Certainly not every pet taking an ototoxic medication loses his hearing any more than that happens to people. Just as in humans, some are more susceptible than others. There are a lot of factors that put your pet at higher risk of ototoxic damage. These include such things as age, concurrent infections, anesthesia, pre-existing cochlear damage and repeated courses of antibiotics.[12]

Unfortunately, by the time you notice that your pet is losing his hearing, it is already too late and the ototoxic effects may be permanent. The AMINOGLYCOSIDE antibiotics are very ototoxic to dogs, just as they are to humans. The two most commonly used AMINOGLYCOSIDES in veterinary practice are **Gentamicin** and **Neomycin**. They often come in the form of ear drops or topical creams.[13]

For example, the drug compound we used on Riley's ears is sold under the trade name of *Otomax*. *Otomax* is an ointment used for ear infections. Notice that it is a combination of three drugs: **Gentamicin**, **Betamethasone** and Clotrimazole. The first two are known to be ototoxic.

You may be staggered to discover that many of the drugs your veterinarian prescribes are ototoxic! I wonder how many vets know this. One article I read stated that there are more than 180 ototoxic compounds. The author then listed 57 of the more common ones likely to be seen in veterinary practice.[14] In my research, I came across a reasonably comprehensive data base of veterinary drugs used in the United States, Britain, France, Germany and Holland that listed 687 different drugs.[15] Other lists yield additional veterinary drugs.[16] In one list, I recognized well over 220 veterinary drugs that are ototoxic to humans. In addition, I'm positive there must be drugs only used in veterinary medicine that are also ototoxic. If pets are affected by the same drugs as humans, it would appear that at least 30% of veterinary medicines have the potential to damage your pet's ears.

Table 12-1 lists the enormous number of drugs (271 to be exact) that veterinarians use that are known to be ototoxic to humans. Your pet may have the same ototoxic reactions to these drugs as you do.

The next time your veterinarian prescribes a drug for your dog, check it out. If it is ototoxic to humans, there is a good chance it will also be ototoxic to your pooch. Watch him closely for any signs of ototoxic side effects since he can't tell you if his ears are ringing or that he is going deaf. He looks out for you. The least you can do is watch out for him!

Table 12-1. Drugs Used in Veterinary Practice That Are Known to be Ototoxic to Humans and Thus May Damage Your Pets Ears Too

Acebutolol	Centrimide
Acetazolamide	Cephalexin
Acetylsalicylic acid	Chloral hydrate
Albendazole	Chlorambucil
Albuterol	Chloramphenicol
Alclofenac	Chlordiazepoxide
Allopurinol	Chlorhexidine
Alprazolam	Chloroquine
Amikacin	Chlorothiazide
Amiloride	Chlorpheniramine
Aminosalicylic acid	Chlortetracycline
Amiodarone	Chlorthalidone
Amitriptyline	Cholecalciferol
Amlodipine	Cholestyramine
Amobarbital	Ciprofloxacin
Amphotericin B	Cisapride
Ampicillin	Cisplatin
Arsenic trioxide	Clemastine
Atenolol	Clindamycin
Atropine	Clomiphene
Auranofin	Clomipramine
Bacitracin	Clonazepam
Baclofen	Clonidine
Benazepril	Codeine
Benzalkonium	Colistin
Benzethonium	Cortisone
Benzocaine	Cyclizine
Betamethasone	Cyclophosphamide
Bismuth subsalicylate	Cyclosporine
Bretylium	Cyproheptadine
Bromocriptine	Cyproterone
Bumetanide	Cytarabine
Bupivacaine	Dactinomycin
Buprenorphine	Danazol
Buspirone	Dapsone
Butorphanol	Deferoxamine
Cabergoline	Dexamethasone
Caffeine	Diazepam
Calcitonin	Diazoxide
Calcitriol	Dibekacin
Captopril	Dichlorphenamide
Carbamazepine	Diclofenac
Carprofen	Digoxin

Table 12-1. Drugs Used in Veterinary Practice That Are Known to be Ototoxic to Humans and Thus May Damage Your Pets Ears Too (Cont'd.)

Dihydrochysterol	Hydrocodone
Diltiazem	Hydrocortisone
Diphenhydramine	Hygromycin B
Diphenylhydantoin	Hyoscyamine
Diphenylhydrazine	Ibuprofen
Dipyridamole	Imipenem
Disopyramide	Imipramine
Doxepin	Indomethacin
Doxorubicin	Ipratropium
Doxycycline	Isoniazid
Doxylamine	Isosorbide
Enalapril	Isotretinoin
Ephedrine	Itraconazole
Ergonovine	Ivermectin
Erythromycin	Kanamycin
Estradiol	Ketoconazole
Ethacrynic acid	Ketoprofen
Ethosuximide	Ketorolac
Etodolac	Levamisole
Etretinate	Lidocaine
Famotidine	Lincomycin
Fenoprofen	Lisinopril
Fentanyl	Lithium
Flavoxate	Lorazepam
Flecainide	Magnesium salicylate
Fluconazole	Mannitol
Flucytosine	Meclizine
Fludrocortisone	Medroxyprogesterone
Flumazenil	Mefenamic acid
Fluorouracil	Megestrol
Fluoxetine	Meloxicam
Flurazepam	Mepacrine
Framycetin	Meperidine
Frusemide	Meprobamate
Furosemide	Mesalazine
Gemfibrozil	Methazolamide
Gentamicin	Methenamine
Glibenclamide	Methimazole
Glipizide	Methocarbamol
Glyburide	Methotrexate
Griseofulvin	Methylprednisolone
Haloperidol	Metoprolol
Hydrochlorothiazide	Metronidazole

Table 12-1. Drugs Used in Veterinary Practice That Are Known to be Ototoxic to Humans and Thus May Damage Your Pets Ears Too (Cont'd.)

Mexiletine	Primidone
Midazolam	Procainamide
Minocycline	Procarbazine
Misoprostol	Progesterone
Mitotane	Promethazine
Morphine	Propafenone
Nadolol	Propofol
Nalbuphine	Propranolol
Nalidixic acid	Propylene glycol
Naltrexone	Propylthiouracil
Naproxen	Protriptyline
Neomycin	Pseudoephedrine
Netilmicin	Pyridostigmine
Nifedipine	Quinidine
Nitrogen mustard	Quinine
Nitroglycerin	Ranitidine
Norethindrone	Ribavirin
Nortriptyline	Rifampin
Octreotide	Scopolamine
Olsalazine	Secobarbital
Omeprazole	Sertraline
Oxazepam	Sisomicin
Papaverine	Sodium salicylate
Paroxetine	Sotalol
Penicillamine	Spironolactone
Penicillin	Streptomycin
Pentazocine	Sucralfate
Pentobarbital	Sulfamethazine
Perphenazine	Suramin
Phenobarbital	Tamoxifen
Phenylbutazone	Tenoxicam
Phenylephrine	Terbutaline
Phenytoin	Testosterone
Pilocarpine	Tetracycline
Pimozide	Theophylline
Pindolol	Thiabendazole
Piperazine	Thioridazine
Piroxicam	Timolol
Polymyxin B	Tobramycin
Praziquantel	Tocainide
Prazosin	Tolbutamide
Prednisolone	Tranylcypromine
Prednisone	Triamcinolone

Table 12-1. Drugs Used in Veterinary Practice That Are Known to be Ototoxic to Humans and Thus May Damage Your Pets Ears Too (Cont'd.)

Triamterene	**Vasopressin**
Triazolam	**Verapamil**
Trimeprazine	**Vinblastine**
Trimethoprim	**Vincristine**
Tripelennamine	**Vitamin B$_{12}$**
Valproic acid	**Zidovudine** [17] [18] [19]
Vancomycin	

1   Haybach, 1998. p. 6.

2   *Audiological Aspects of Ototoxicity*, 1996. p. 1.

3   *Guidelines for the Audiologic Management of Individuals Receiving Cochleotoxic Drug Therapy*, 1994. p. 3.

4   *Physicians' Desk Reference*, 2003. p. 2184.

5   *Physicians' Desk Reference*, 2003. p. 2236.

6   *Physicians' Desk Reference*, 2003. p. 2945.

7   *Physicians' Desk Reference*, 2002. p. 3550.

8   *Physicians' Desk Reference*, 2003. p. 2124.

9   *Physicians' Desk Reference*, 2003. p. 3145.

10   *Physicians' Desk Reference*, 2003. p. 2046.

11   Davison, 1998. p. 820.

12   Strain, 1996. p. 2.

13   Strain, 1996. p. 2.

14   Strain, 1996. pp. 2-4.

15   *VetBase: List of Drugs*, 2000. pp. 1-7.

16   *Veterinary Formulary*, 2001. pp. 2-3.

17   *VetBase: List of Drugs*, 2000. pp. 1-7.

18   Strain, 1996. pp. 2-4.

19   *Veterinary Formulary*, 2001. pp. 2-3.

Chapter 13: Keep Yourself Healthy While Taking Few or No Drugs

Chapter 13

Keep Yourself Healthy While Taking Few or No Drugs

People often ask me how they can protect their ears from the ravages of ototoxic drugs. They want to know about safer alternatives. In fact, one man took me to task. He wrote, "You keep saying what drugs are ototoxic and should not be used if we want to protect our ears and hearing. However, you don't tell us what we should be taking. It would enlighten us all if you explained some of the safer treatments we can use".

With this in mind, I have added this chapter. The information in this chapter is not intended to be comprehensive, as that would be a major book in itself, but I'm giving examples of some things you can do in order to help protect yourself from the side effects of ototoxic drugs. Here are a number of things you should consider.

Educational, Not Medical Advice

Do not take the information in this book as medical advice. I am not a medical doctor, and therefore I do not diagnose conditions and prescribe treatments. However, I do provide educational information that you and your doctor can use to help prevent drugs from damaging your ears.

Take Responsibility for Your Own Health

"If it's to be, it's up to me". This was one of the slogans I heard repeatedly in one multi-level company I was once a part of. The meaning is clear. If you want something to happen, you have to make it happen yourself. Don't expect someone else to do it.

What does this have to do with ototoxic drugs? Simply this. If you want to protect your ears from the ravages of ototoxic drugs, you have to be eternally vigilant. This means you have to become **informed** on the side effects of drugs **before** you take them.

If you don't know anything else about ototoxic drugs, this book is a good place to obtain this information. Take the time to look up any drugs your doctor wants to prescribe for you. This way you will know the risks to your ears from taking that drug before you take it. Then you and your doctor can mutually decide what drugs may work for you while still protecting your ears. If your doctor brushes you off, maybe it's time to find another doctor—one that is willing to work with you to save your ears.

Part of taking responsibility for your own health is that you need to learn how to become and stay healthy. Therefore, you need to research any proposed treatments in light of good health before you begin them.

For example, my experience reveals that many prescription drugs cause unnecessary damage to our bodies. Thus, I use other means in order to stay healthy. There are many alternative ways of achieving health without taking drugs. Talk to various alternative medicine practitioners—for example, naturopathic doctors, herbalists, chiropractors, acupuncturists, massage therapists and so on. These practitioners have a wealth of knowledge about good health, and the wisdom to help you become, and stay, healthy.

When you do this, not only will you save the money that you now spend on drugs, but you will also likely feel ever so much better. Furthermore, you'll never have to worry about drugs damaging your ears either!

It takes time and effort to maintain good health. It doesn't just happen by itself. You have to be involved. Remember, "If it's to be, it's up to me!"

Choose a Health Care Professional Who Knows About Health, Not Just About Sickness

If you want to stay healthy, you need to choose your health care professionals wisely. If you are sick, who would you rather go to—a doctor who is an expert in health and can teach you how to become and stay healthy, or a doctor who is an expert in sickness and treats the symptoms of your condition with drugs and/or surgery, but never treats the fundamental cause, so you are never really cured?

You might be shocked to know that in medical school the typical MD gets extremely limited training in good health. He spends the bulk of his time learning about sickness. In contrast the typical ND (naturopathic doctor) spends much of his time learning about health and how to keep the body healthy.

Check out the various health care professionals that practice alternative medicine and therapies. For example, some medical doctors have learned a lot about good health and practice some alternative therapies. Naturopathic doctors are trained in how to restore you to health, and use natural means to accomplish that. Sometimes what your body needs is not a medical doctor, but the skills of a chiropractor. Other conditions respond best to an acupuncturist. Other times, a herbalist may be the person to see, or a massage therapist. No one health care professional knows it all.

Since doctors practice what they learn, no wonder the typical MD treats you with drugs and surgery, while the typical ND talks to you about health and nutrition, and the typical chiropractor uses manipulation to help restore you to health.

Here's an easy way to separate the medical doctors who are truly trying to help you from the doctors that just run "patient mills". It's based on the astute observation of J. Apley who, back in 1978, wrote,

"Doctors who treat the **symptom** tend to give a prescription.

Doctors who treat the **patient** are more likely to offer guidance".

No matter what condition you have–whether its hearing loss, balance problems, tinnitus, or anything else wrong with your body, if you want to get better, you and your doctor need to root out the **source** of the problem, not just suppress the **symptoms** with drugs.

Take Prescription Drugs as a Last Resort, Not as Your First Line of Attack

Americans take a **lot** of prescription drugs. Doctors in the USA in 2008 prescribed a total of 1,505,200,000 prescriptions for just the 50 top prescription drugs. (And they prescribed untold millions more prescriptions for the hundreds of other drugs.) The retail value of these 1.5 billion prescriptions was a whopping $53,186,000,000.00![1]

Each year more and more people are damaging their ears from taking ototoxic drugs. Why? Simply this. People are taking more and more drugs, and the law of averages says that the more you take, the greater your chances of having adverse side effects.

The scary thing is that 44 of these top 50 prescription drugs (88%) can be ototoxic and damage your ears in some way (and all of them also have numerous other side effects).

Dr. John Abramson of the Harvard Medical School, when asked, "Are most Americans overmedicated?" replied, "They sure are!" He further explained, "It is no secret that **Americans take many drugs unnecessarily**, and when drugs are needed, people often take the wrong ones".[2]

So who's to blame—patients? doctors? or the drug industry? They all are! Here's why.

People: People want the magic pill that instantly gets rid of their physical problems, so they buy into the idea of "an injection for every infection", "a pill for every ill" and "a drug for every bug". They don't want to change their lifestyle, eating habits or exercise habits in order to get (and stay) well.

Doctors: Most doctors prescribe drugs because they think it's in their patients' best interest to do so because that is what they have been taught to believe. Where did they get this idea?...from the drug companies, of course. Doctors need to quit believing everything the drug companies tell them and look into all the different methods for healing people apart from drugs.

Drug Companies: Drug companies are in the business of making money, and they have found a cash cow that is making them billions of dollars.

There have been radical changes in the way that our medical knowledge is provided. Did you know that before 1980, most clinical research was publicly funded, but now most is funded directly by the drug and other medical industries, whose **primary** mission is to **maximize** the return on **investments** for investors (and thus not to cure people's illnesses— or they wouldn't need their drugs any more)? Remember, drug ads that tell you to "ask your doctor" about a particular drug have a single purpose—to sell more drugs, not to improve your health.[3]

Ninety percent of clinical trials now are commercially funded—as well as seventy-five percent of published clinical research.[4] I think these figures, while shocking, are still much too conservative. Did you know that when a pharmaceutical company sponsors a study, the odds are **five** times greater that the findings will favor its product?[5]

Furthermore, drug and medical industries fund 70% of continuing education lectures and seminars, which are among the activities that doctors are required to attend in order to maintain their licenses to practice. Wherever doctors turn for sources of information, drug companies dominate.[6]

Did you catch that? Your doctor's **primary** source of information is ultimately from the drug companies, and the drug companies are **primarily** in the business of making **money** for their investors, not making you well.

So where does that leave you? If you want to get healthy, you need to do your homework **before** you decide whether to take a drug for a given condition, or whether you should look for a alternate solution that is not harmful to your ears (and the rest of your body).

You need to ask yourself, "Are natural therapies a better alternative to some drugs?" If you look at the data rather than listen to the drug ads, you will see that natural alternatives, such as improved diet and routine exercise, often are **far more effective** than drugs at achieving real health improvements such as less heart disease and longer life.[7]

Now, here comes the kicker. Many patients prefer pills because they're easier. (In other words, people are **lazy** when it comes to protecting their health.) There is no question that many people would rather take a pill than change their lifestyle.

If the pills worked, it would simply be a question of how you want to spend your money. The problem is that the "magic" of the pills often is empowered by your cultural beliefs, but without a genuine scientific basis. **About two-thirds of your health is determined by the way you live your life**, and—for better or worse—no pills can change that.[8]

Therefore, you want to be sure that any drug you take is **absolutely necessary** before you take it, if you truly value your health. Drugs should always be your **last** resort, not your first line of attack.

Instead of worrying whether a certain drug is ototoxic or not, you should be questioning whether that drug is really necessary or not, and be actively looking for better alternatives.

In my own life I have always followed this principle. I keep my drug usage to an absolute minimum. For example, in the last 30 years, I can only remember getting two prescriptions—one was an antibiotic for an infection that I couldn't kill using natural methods, and the other was for a bad case of sciatic pain. Even then, I only took two of the pills, not the whole bottle. Apart from that, the only drug I take occasionally, is the pain-killer the dentist gives me before working on a live tooth. I **never** touch over-the-counter medications either.

It's tragic that people typically ignore the basic things that will help them the most to stay healthy such as getting adequate exercise, eating a healthy diet, watching their weight and getting plenty of rest. People typically refuse to do these things because they take effort and they want effortless health—hence they pop pills instead of doing those things that really make a difference.

Get Off the Drug Treadmill

When you take a drug, often you get side effects. When you complain to your doctor about the side effects, instead of taking you off the drug, he often just prescribes another drug to suppress the side effects of the first drug. Unfortunately, this second drug then produces even more side effects, so you have to take a third drug. Soon you are popping a handful of drugs 3 or 4 times a day—and your health steadily deteriorates.

Here is a fictitious (yet still true to life) example. Let's say you are depressed so you go to your doctor. He prescribes **Quetiapine** (*Seroquel*). That works for your depression, but it gives you hyperglycemia (high blood sugar and you start to develop diabetes). Your doctor then puts you on **Rosiglitazone** (*Avandia*) for your diabetes. One of the side effects of **Rosiglitazone** is increased LDL cholesterol (the bad kind of cholesterol), which in turn increases your blood pressure, and thus your risk for heart attacks. As a result, your doctor puts you on **Diltiazem** (*Cardizem*) a CALCIUM CHANNEL BLOCKER to bring down your blood pressure. But the **Diltiazem** increases your high blood sugar even more, so your doctor puts you on **Olmesartan** (*Benicar*) to try to bring down your high blood sugar. The **Olmesartan** increases the risk that you will die of a heart attack or stroke. At the same time, the **Diltiazem** you are now taking causes you to have GastroEsophageal Reflux Disease (GERD), so your doctor prescribes **Esomeprazole** (*Nexium*) a PROTON-PUMP INHIBITOR to try to control your acid reflux.

By now these drugs have affected your ears. You suffer from horrible bilateral tinnitus, which exacerbates your initial depression. You now feel like a zombie, you look like a walking cadaver and you hope for an early death to put you out of your misery. This is what can happen when you get on the drug treadmill and blindly take one drug after another.

At some point you have to say, "Enough is enough!" You need to stop popping pills and get off this drug treadmill, if you ever hope to regain your health.

Although this particular example is fictitious, it is representative of the miseries multitudes of people go through as one drug is added to another drug as their health deteriorates. When they can't stand it anymore and want to do something about it, they may contact me to see if I can help them.

In case you think this scenario is far-fetched, guess again. Each of these drugs do indeed cause such side effects.

One of the side effects of both **Quetiapine** and **Diltiazem** is hyperglycemia—they cause high blood sugar where none existed before—according to the PDR.

Rosiglitazone substantially increases your bad, low-density LDL cholesterol levels resulting in increased heart attacks. In fact, studies have revealed that the risk for heart attacks among people taking **Rosiglitazone** was 40% higher than for those taking other diabetes medications—yet it is still on the market (although restricted) at this time.[9] In fact, **Rosiglitazone** is now believed to have caused more than 83,000 heart attacks between 1999 and 2007![10]

Olmesartan also increases your risk of heart attacks and strokes. Here is more background on this drug. The "FDA is evaluating data from two clinical trials in which patients with Type 2 diabetes taking the blood pressure medication, **Olmesartan** (*Benicar*), an ANGIOTENSIN II RECEPTOR BLOCKER, had a **higher rate of death** from a cardiovascular cause compared to patients taking a placebo".

Notice that! **Olmesartan**, a high-blood pressure medication, causes death more often in those taking it, than in those who have high blood pressure but don't take it!

This report admits, "An unexpected finding observed in both trials was a greater number of deaths from a cardiovascular cause (heart attack, sudden death, or stroke) in the *Benicar*-treated patients compared to placebo".[11]

Now the reason you supposedly take a high blood pressure medication is to **prevent** heart attacks, strokes and sudden death—yet this drug apparently actually **causes** them—based on the results of not just one, but two, long-term studies.

After hearing this, any normal person would conclude that taking the drug could be dangerous to their health and quit taking it, yet does the FDA reach the same conclusion? Not on your life (and it is **your** life they are talking about)!

Here's what they say. The "FDA's review is ongoing and the Agency has **not** concluded that *Benicar* increases the risk of death". (Yet the two studies they reviewed showed just the opposite.)

So what is their recommendation? You're not going to believe it. The "FDA currently believes that the benefits of *Benicar* in patients with high blood pressure **continue to outweigh its potential risks**".[12]

What I want to know is what **benefits** are they talking about—since the supposed benefits of high-blood pressure medication are to **reduce** the risk of heart attacks, strokes and sudden death—and these studies clearly show that taking this drug results in **more** heart attacks, strokes and sudden death! Why ever would you want to take such a drug?

Diltiazem, and indeed all the CALCIUM CHANNEL BLOCKERS have a different nefarious side effect. They can cause GastroEsophageal Reflux Disease (GERD), and that "requires" still another drug for treatment.

Drugs that can result in GERD include not only the CALCIUM CHANNEL BLOCKERS (**Amlodipine**, **Diltiazem**, **Felodipine**, **Nicardipine**, etc.) but also the BETA BLOCKERS (**Acebutolol**, **Atenolol**, **Betaxolol**, **Carteolol**, etc.), some ANTIDEPRESSANTS and some ANTI-ANXIETY DRUGS.

Thus, when doctors prescribe drugs to treat conditions such as high blood pressure, heart disease, depression and anxiety, the drugs they prescribe can cause GERD where none existed before.

The statistics are alarming. "The number of people hospitalized for conditions related to GastroEsophageal Reflux Disease (GERD) doubled between 1998 and 2005". At the present time, "more than 20 million Americans have GERD".[13] Burgeoning drug use in the above classes of drugs no doubt is largely responsible for this enormous increase in GERD.

Here's how these drugs cause GERD. "When you eat or drink, food and liquid move from your mouth to your esophagus where a valve, called the lower esophageal sphincter (LES), relaxes to allow the food and liquid to pass into your stomach. The lower esophageal sphincter then squeezes shut to keep stomach contents from backing up (a process known as reflux) into your esophagus".[14]

As long as this valve stays tightly shut, you don't have a problem. However, if you take any of the above drugs, you need to be aware that these (and other) drugs actually reduce lower esophageal sphincter (LES) pressure (that is, they relax this muscle located at the top of your stomach). As a result, the contents of your stomach can then back up into your esophagus, eventually resulting in GERD.

When this happens, your doctor prescribes yet another drug such as the PROTON PUMP INHIBITOR **Esomeprazole** (*Nexium*) to try to control your GERD. Surprise, **Esomeprazole**—the little purple pill—has a number of side effects, including ototoxic side effects such as ataxia, dizziness, ear pain, tinnitus and vertigo.

Thus, when you use even more drugs to "cure" the side effects of other drugs, you can end up increasing the risk of damage to your ears (not to mention the rest of your body).

The way to prevent this is to find a health care professional who will treat your original underlying problem without causing all these other escalating side effects and health problems.

Enough is enough. Get off the drug treadmill while you still can.

Don't Take Drugs for Minor Ailments—Tough It Out Instead

Americans have become a nation of wimps. For every little ache and pain, they either turn to the medicine cabinet, or they run to the doctor for some drug or pain killer. The problem is, these drugs and pain killers can damage your ears and the rest of your body too.

Often, all you need to do is just let nature take its course. The problem will heal itself naturally in a day or two, or a week or two. Perhaps you just need to get extra rest, or take it easy, or have a massage, or put ice on it, or heat on it—things like that—rather than take drugs.

For example, don't be like so many women who take hormone replacement therapy (HRT) for their hot flashes—and later find out that the drugs they took caused unexpected nasty side effects. One lady, with the wisdom of hindsight, after she had lost most of her hearing to HRT, wrote, "[in retrospect] my life would have been much easier if I'd just withstood the hot flashes and not medicated them away!"

So often people take drugs for essentially minor problems. However, the side effects of the drugs cause major problems. Having trouble sleeping at times is a minor problem. Breaking your hip is a major problem. So don't let ototoxic drugs break your hips. I'm serious. Each year 32,000 older adults suffer hip fractures, **attributable to drug-induced falls**, resulting in more than 1,500 deaths. That's a **lot** of broken hips each year just from taking ototoxic drugs.[15]

In one study, the main categories of drugs responsible for the falls leading to hip fractures were sleeping pills and minor tranquilizers (30%), anti-psychotic drugs (52%) and antidepressants (17%). All of these drugs are often prescribed unnecessarily, especially in older adults.[16]

Specifically notice the above sentence. Doctors commonly **unnecessarily** prescribe these drugs for what are essentially minor problems. The result is major problems such as hip fractures and death.

Therefore, if you want to keep your "pins" under you as you age, go easy on the drugs! Herbals may work just as well or better, and won't compromise your balance.

Make Your Doctor Prove That the Benefits Will Far Outweigh the Side Effects

A new poll in Consumer Reports Magazine revealed that one in six Americans who have ever taken a prescription drug experienced a side effect that was serious enough to send them to the hospital![17] One in six! Considering the percentage of people in this country who are on some form of daily prescription medication (remember, it's over 50 percent now), this is a stunning statistic. That's 16 percent of the people who've ever taken a prescription medicine!

Since there are around 300 million people in the USA, and since 90% or more of the population have taken a prescription drug at some time in their lives, that works out to around 45 million people in the USA that have been hospitalized at one time or another by serious side effects from taking prescription drugs!

Remember, this poll is only talking about the "serious" side effects. Added to this are all the side effects that were not considered serious enough to go to the hospital. These side effects include many of the ototoxic side effects people also experience.

Thus, it appears that taking drugs ultimately may do more harm to your body than good. Therefore, **before** you take any drugs, make your doctor justify to you how the supposed benefits of taking the prescription will **far** outweigh the negative side effects. If he can't do that, you'll just be exchanging one problem for another, or more likely just adding more health issues to those you already have. As the cases in the previous section so powerfully testify, your doctor may be hard-pressed to do this.

Choose the Least Ototoxic Drug That Will Do the Job

If you want to avoid all ototoxic side effects of drugs, the obvious answer is, "Don't take ototoxic drugs in the first place". Use alternative medicine therapies instead.

However, if you do choose to use drugs that have ototoxic side effects, the wise solution is to choose the least ototoxic drug that will do the job.

The way to do this is to ask your doctor for a list of the drugs you could take for your condition that he feels will do the job. Then look up each of these drugs in Chapter 14 to see what their side effects are, how likely they are to occur and how severe these side effects might be. Next, list the drugs in order from the least ototoxic to the most ototoxic. From this list, choose the drug that has the fewest side effects.

Also, choose a drug that has side effects with which you are prepared to live (if you should be unlucky enough to get them). For example, if you already have bad tinnitus, you may decide not to take any drugs that have tinnitus as a side effect, but you are prepared to live with a drug that has some dizziness as a side effect. If you want to preserve your remaining hearing, you may choose to stay away from any drugs that have hearing loss as a side effect.

Important: While you are looking at the ototoxic side effects of the various drugs on your list, you must **not** neglect to look up in some authoritative drug book, or on-line drug website, **all** the other side effects of that drug. This book only deals with your ears, but you must consider your **whole** body, not just your ears. What is the ultimate benefit if you protect your ears, but severely damage your heart in the process. If your body dies, your ears won't hear anything either!

Take the Lowest Dose for the Shortest Possible Time

Once you have decided on which drug or drugs you are prepared to take, ask your doctor to prescribe the **lowest** dose that will treat your condition. This is because many drugs do not exhibit ototoxic side effects at very low doses, but such side effects may become apparent at higher doses. Thus, by keeping the dose low, you can often protect your ears from ototoxic side effects.

A number of people have told me that the original dose their doctor put them on did not affect their ears in any way, but when their doctor increased their dose, they soon noticed problems with their ears.

For example, one lady told me her existing tinnitus became noticeably louder when her doctor put her on a higher dose of **Irbesartan**. When she complained to her doctor, he reduced the dose to its old level again, and her tinnitus returned to its previous level.

Furthermore, ask your doctor to prescribe any drug for the **shortest** effective time possible. This is because some ototoxic drugs do not damage your ears in the short term, but the longer you take the drug, the more likely it is to damage your ears. By taking a given drug for only two weeks, for example, you may avoid all ototoxic side effects, whereas taking the same drug for several months may cause serious damage to your ears.

Use Herbals Instead of Prescription Drugs

In order to protect your ears (and the rest of your body) from drug side effects, you need to use the mildest medication that will do the job, not a harsh medication that stomps rough-shod over your body.

For example, a lady asked me, "Do you have an opinion on which antidepressants are the safest for our ears—e.g. *Pamelor, Zoloft, Lexapro, Celexa*, etc. Is there one that is significantly less ototoxic than the others?"

In my reply to her, I explained that personally I wouldn't use any of the above drugs. Why? Because there is a much safer alternative—the herbal, St. John's Wort.

You see, numerous studies have shown that St. John's Wort is at least as effective as prescription drugs in treating mild to moderate cases of depression, but it does not have the harsh action on your body that prescription anti-depressants have.

Here's some more good news. St. John's Wort is not known to be ototoxic in the least. Thus, you can take it for as long as you need to without fear of causing hearing loss, aggravating your tinnitus, making your hyperacusis worse or wrecking your balance. In addition, it doesn't have all the other bad side effects the above drugs have either.

St. John's Wort really works. My wife takes it as needed, and has never had any ototoxic (or other) side effects like she had with prescription drugs. I know a number of others that have had the same experience.

If you do decide to try St. John's Wort, first run it by your doctor or pharmacist because St. John's Wort is known to interact with various medications. You don't want to cause problems due to interactions between St. John's Wort and any other drugs you might be taking.

Also, be sure it says on the bottle that it is standardized to 0.3% (or to 0.5%) hypericin. (Hypericin is the active ingredient.) When you use a standardized formulation, you know exactly how much of the active ingredient you are getting. Otherwise, the active ingredient may vary all over the place, and you don't want that.

Here is another example of substituting a herbal for an ototoxic drug. This time it is a safer alternative to anti-anxiety drugs.

A lady explained: "I have been suffering from tinnitus for several years, and it drives me crazy when I'm trying to get to sleep. I have tried everything from counting sheep to meditation. I have been to an ear, nose and throat specialist, and to my local doctor and I have been told I will just have to live with it. I was on *Prozac* for a few years. I ended up on just half a tablet, but I found it made me feel flat and I didn't like it so I went off it. Is there anything I could take to stop me feeling anxious, especially when I'm trying to go to sleep? It seems *Prozac* could have made my tinnitus worse, is this correct? Does *Effexor* make tinnitus worse?"

Doctors often prescribe drugs such as **Fluoxetine** (*Prozac*) and **Venlafaxine** (*Effexor*) to help you reduce the anxiety you feel towards your tinnitus. These drugs can work for some people, but for others, they actually make their tinnitus worse.

For example, **Fluoxetine** can cause tinnitus in about 2% of the people taking it. Since multitudes of people take *Prozac*, this is a pretty significant number of people. **Venlafaxine** is no better. In fact, it causes tinnitus in about 3% of the people taking it.

There are safer alternatives to taking these prescription drugs. For example, if I were anxious about my tinnitus and had trouble sleeping because of it, I'd choose a herbal that has a relaxing, calming effect.

There are a number of herbs that have been used for hundreds of years—long before drugs hit the market—to reduce anxiety and promote sleep, and they did (and still do) work. You seldom hear about them, but if you are concerned about ototoxic (and other) side effects, they are a good place to start.

My choice of a herb that reduces anxiety, calms you down and helps you sleep is Valerian (*Valeriana officinalis*). You can get it at health food stores, or from a herbalist or a naturopathic doctor (ND).

Caution: as with St. John's Wort and other herbals, you should not mix herbals and prescription drugs without first talking to your doctor or pharmacist about any drug interactions. For example, in this case you wouldn't want to take *Prozac* and Valerian at the same time since the combined action of both may be too much for your body.

Build Up Your Body So You Won't Need to Take Drugs

Practice living a healthy life-style so you don't get sick in the first place, or build up your health, if you are already "sick". By building up your body, you'll discover that you no longer will need to take drugs. This advice is so obvious, but many people seem to miss it, or choose not to practice it because it means changing their diet and lifestyle, and that is just too much effort.

There are a number of ways you can build up and keep your body healthy. Diet and exercise are two very important ones. You also need to ensure that you keep your immune system robust, so it can fight off any infections before they can take hold.

Diet

As most people know, but few practice, eating the right foods goes a long ways towards keeping your body healthy, whereas eating too much junk food causes all sorts of problems. That is why diet and nutrition should be at the top of your list of things you do to keep yourself healthy so you won't have to take any drugs and medications.

Here's an example of how this can work out in practice. Millions of people take anti-inflammatory drugs (typically Non-Steroidal Anti-Inflammatory Drugs [NSAIDS]) to reduce pain and inflammation in their bodies. Unfortunately, these drugs have numerous side effects, and can also damage their ears.

Non-steroidal anti-inflammatory drugs include the:

1.   ACETIC ACIDS such as **Diclofenac** (*Voltaren*) and **Ketorolac** (*Toradol*).

2.   COX-2 INHIBITORS such as **Celecoxib** (*Celebrex*) and **Valdecoxib** (*Bextra*).

3.   FENAMATES such as **Mefenamic acid** (*Ponstel*).

4.   OXICAMS such as **Meloxicam** (*Mobic*).

5.   PROPIONIC ACIDS such as **Ibuprofen** (*Advil*) and **Naproxen** (*Aleve*).

6.   SALICYLATES such as **Acetylsalicylic acid** (*Aspirin*) and **Mesalamine** (*Asacol*).[18]

These drugs can have numerous ototoxic side effects. Some of the more common ototoxic side effects of NSAIDs include ear pain, hearing loss, tinnitus, and vestibular (balance) side effects such as ataxia, dizziness and vertigo.

People have asked me how they can both control the pain/inflammation they experience, and yet not suffer from these ototoxic side effects. The good news is that changes in diet go a long way towards reducing inflammation (and thus the need for such drugs).

Note: inflammation is not a "minor" problem, but is a "well- known contributor to chronic health conditions such as heart disease, diabetes, cancer and dementia".[19]

In order to reduce inflammation you need to greatly reduce your intake of foods that cause inflammation. According to nutrition expert Dr. Andrew Rubman, ND, the 10 worst inflammatory foods include:[20]

1.   Desserts made with lots of sugar (cookies, candy, ice cream and so on).

2.   Sweetened cereals.

3.   "White" carbohydrates (white bread, white rice, white potatoes, English muffins, etc.).

4.   Non-diet soft drinks.

5.   Anything containing high-fructose corn syrup.

6.   Processed meats (bologna, salami, hotdogs, sausage and others made with preservatives and additives).

7.   French fries, potato chips and other fried snack foods.

8.   Fast foods, most specifically the ones that are high-fat, high-calorie, high simple carbohydrate—which describes most of the inexpensive offerings at quick-serve restaurants.

9.   Margarine, because it contains processed sterols called stanols that have been implicated in both atherosclerosis and various fatty-deposit diseases.

10.   Organ meats such as liver, because these often contain undesirable products including antibiotics, fertilizer and other unwanted residues.

At the same time, you want to include (or greatly increase) your intake of the 10 best anti-inflammatory foods. Dr. Rubman's choices include:

1.   Wild salmon, mackerel and other omega-3-fatty-acid-rich fish.

2.   Berries.

3.   Green, leafy vegetables (e.g., spinach and kale).

4.   Cruciferous vegetables (broccoli, Brussels sprouts, cabbage, etc.).

5.   Deeply pigmented produce, such as sweet potatoes, eggplant and pomegranates… along with carrots, plums, oranges, peppers, peas and red grapes.

6.   Nuts.

7.   Whole grains.

8.   Tea—specifically black, green and white teas.

9.   Cold-pressed fresh oils, including avocado, flaxseed and olive oils in particular.

10.   Spices (specifically, garlic, ginger, turmeric, saffron).

Incidentally, wolfing your food down also increases the inflammation index of the foods you eat, so slow down and chew your food completely before swallowing.

Since making drastic lifestyle changes is difficult and prone to failure for many people, start by consciously choosing to replace **one** of the foods in the "worst" list with **one** of the foods in the "best" list. As you continue to do this, over time you will realize you have almost eliminated the worst inflammatory foods from your diet—and surprise—you'll notice you feel ever so much better in the process, and thus likely won't need to take anti-inflammatory drugs anymore. (And likely a lot of your other health problems will have improved too.)

Boost Your Immune System

Millions of people take antibiotics each year to kill infections in their bodies. The truth is, your body's immune system can handle most of these infectious agents if it is working properly.

Recurrent infections are a sign that your immune system is not functioning properly. Therefore, if you get infections easily, you need to boost your immune system. If you boost your immune system, you will likely find that your susceptibility to infections will drop dramatically. Two herbal preparations that help boost your immune system are Echinacea and Astragalus.

Echinacea (*Echinacea angustifolia, E. purpurea, E. pallida*) is a powerful immune-system booster. A typical dosage is up to nine 300 to 400 mg. capsules per day. (If you are allergic to asters and ragweeds, you may also be allergic to Echinacea. Also, don't use if you have an autoimmune disease.)[21] Astragalus (*Astragalus membranaceus*) is a herbal you can take long-term if you are prone to recurrent infections. A typical dosage is eight or nine 400 to 500 mg. capsules a day.[22]

Take probiotics—bacterial cultures—such as *Lactobacillus acidophilus*. Some naturopathic doctors explain that your intestinal tract comprises almost **half** of the functionality of your immune system. So having healthy intestinal flora helps keep you healthy, and your immune system robust.

It is important that every time you take an antibiotic, you also take more probiotic cultures since antibiotics kill off the "good guys" in your intestinal tract, thus shooting down your immune system, and thus leaving you open to further infections.

Just be sure any product you buy contains a minimum of 2.5 billion live organisms per gram. You can also eat live-culture yogurt or kefir to get the same benefits.

Boost Your Intake of Vitamins, Minerals and Enzymes

In Chapter 8 and the section "Now the Good News" you learned that loud noise produces free radicals that can zap the hair cells in your inner ears and cause them to die. With the death of each hair cell, a bit more of your hearing dies too.

Various ototoxic drugs also produce free radicals in your inner ears. You can fight these free radicals the same way you do when loud noise produces them.

The above-mentioned section in Chapter 8 shows you how to fight this free radical assault on your inner ears by taking the powerful antioxidant N-acetyl-cysteine (NAC) which your body converts to glutathione. You also learned your inner ears need adequate supplies of the vitamins A, C and E and the minerals magnesium and zinc in order to maintain good ear health.

While you are at it, make sure you supplement your diet with all the other vitamins and minerals you need in order to maintain your whole body in good health.

Exercise

In order to be healthy, your body needs exercise—the more the better. Few people get enough exercise for optimal health. Far too many people have sedentary jobs, and they are "couch potatoes" at home. This leads to poor health, and before you know it, your doctor is prescribing more drugs for whatever ails you.

Therefore, build some exercise into your daily routine. For example, each afternoon I take my dog and we go for a brisk walk in the fresh air in the country. (Fortunately, a mile in any direction from where I live is "in the country". This is one advantage to deliberately choosing to live in a small town.) We typically walk for a mile or two. It doesn't take us long—about half an hour. That gets the blood circulating again before I return to my desk.

Furthermore, I'm the only one on my street that uses a walk-behind lawnmower. The rest relax on their riding mowers while I work up a sweat mowing my grass. In order to get even more exercise, I deliberately mow up and down the hill rather than mow across the slope.

Exercise can also help cut down on your need for anti-anxiety drugs and sleeping pills. If you are anxious, instead of taking anti-anxiety drugs, why not try a vigorous exercise program. A vigorous exercise program will work off that extra nervous energy and make you healthily tired, resulting in a good night's sleep without the need for taking sleeping pills or anti-anxiety drugs.

These are just some of the many things you can do to help protect yourself from the ototoxic, and other, side effects of drugs. Keep your eyes and mind open for other strategies you can implement that also will help restore your body to health without drugs. I look forward to the day you too will have a spring in your step, a glow to your cheeks and a song in your heart.

---

1   AARP Bulletin, October, 2009.
2   *Are You Taking Too Many Medications*, 2007.
3   *Are You Taking Too Many Medications*, 2007.
4   *Are You Taking Too Many Medications*, 2007.

5   *Are You Taking Too Many Medications*, 2007.
6   *Are You Taking Too Many Medications*, 2007.
7   *Are You Taking Too Many Medications*, 2007.
8   *Are You Taking Too Many Medications*, 2007.
9   *Avandia—How Dangerous Is It Really?,* 2010.
10   *Diabetes Health Warning*, 2010.
11   *FDA MedWatch – Benicar (Olmesartan) Ongoing Safety Review*, June 11, 2010.
12   *FDA MedWatch – Benicar (Olmesartan) Ongoing Safety Review*, June 11, 2010.
13   Minocha, 2010.
14   Minocha, 2010.
15   Dancer, 2007. Quoting an article in the *American Family Physician*.
16   *Worst Pills Best Pills News*, September, 2007.
17   *Don't be a silent victim of a drug's side effects*, 2008.
18   Included here are just one or two representative drugs under each sub-class. For the full listing, see Table 14-1, sections 1.1 to 1.1.16.
19   *10 Best and Worst Foods for You,* 2010.
20   *10 Best and Worst Foods for You,* 2010.
21   White, 2000. p. 221.
22   White, 2000. p. 221.

Chapter 14

Ototoxic Drug Listings

222   (see **Acetylsalicylic acid**)

282   (see **Acetylsalicylic acid**)

282 MEP   (see **Acetylsalicylic acid**)

292   (see **Acetylsalicylic acid**)

3TC   (see **Lamivudine**)

5-Aminosalicylic acid   (see **Mesalamine**)

5-ASA   (see **Mesalamine**)

692   (see **Acetylsalicylic acid**)

Abatacept

Pronunciation guide: ah-BAY-tah-sept

Drug classification: Tumor necrosis factor modifiers (see section 14.36 in Table 14-1)

Brand names: *Orencia*

Ototoxic effects:
    Cochlear:
        Hearing loss: <1% (CPS)
        Tinnitus: <1% (CPS)

Vestibular:
    Dizziness: 2.6-4.6% [0.9% above placebo results] (CPS)
    Vertigo: <1% (CPS)
Outer/Middle Ear:
    Middle ear pressure: <1% (CPS)
    Otitis externa: 1.7% [placebo 0] (CPS)
    Otitis media: 1.1-1.3% (CPS)
Outer/Middle Ear:
    Ear disorder: <1% (CPS)

Risk assessment: Class 2

Abelcet (see **Amphotericin B**)

Abilify (see **Aripiprazole**)

Abobotulinum Toxin A

Pronunciation guide: a-boe-BOT-yoo-line-um TOKS-in

Drug classification: NEUROTOXINS (see section 53.40 in Table 14-1)

Brand names: *Dysport*

Ototoxic effects:
    Vestibular:
        Dizziness: (PDR)
        Vertigo: (PDR)

Risk assessment: Class 1

Acamprosate

Pronunciation guide: ah-kam-PRO-sate

Drug classification: MISCELLANEOUS DRUGS (see section 46 in Table 14-1)

Brand names: *Campral*

Ototoxic effects:
    Cochlear:
        Hearing loss: 0.1-1% (CPS, PDR)
        Tinnitus: 0.1-1% (CPS, PDR)
    Vestibular:
        Dizziness: 3-4% [<1% above placebo results] (CPS, PDR)
        Vertigo: 0.1-1% (CPS, PDR)

Risk assessment: Class 2

Notes:

This drug is being tested as a treatment for tinnitus. One early study shows promise, but it still does have adverse side effects as noted above.

AccuNeb   (see **Albuterol**)

Accupril   (see **Quinapril**)

Accuretic   (see **Quinapril**)

Accutane   (see **Isotretinoin**)

Acebutolol

Pronunciation guide: ah-see-BYOO-toe-lawl

Drug classification: BETA-ADRENERGIC-BLOCKING DRUGS (BETA-BLOCKERS) (see section 20.8.12 in Table 14-1)

Brand names: *Apo-Acebutolol, Monitan, Rhotral, Sectral*

Ototoxic effects:
  Cochlear:
    Tinnitus: (CPS)
  Vestibular:
    Dizziness: 2-4% (CPS, PDR)
    Vertigo: (CPS)

Risk assessment: Class 1

Aceclofenac

Pronunciation guide: AH-see-kloe-fen-ack

Drug classification: ACETIC ACIDS (see section 1.1.1 in Table 14-1)

Brand names: *Preservex*

Ototoxic effects:
  Cochlear:
    Tinnitus: (BNF)
  Vestibular:
    Dizziness: [101] (BNF)
    Vertigo: (BNF)

Risk assessment: Class 1

Acemetacin

Pronunciation guide: ah-see-MET-ah-sin

Drug classification: ACETIC ACIDS (see section 1.1.1 in Table 14-1)

Brand names: *Emflex, Rantudil Retard*

Ototoxic effects:
  Cochlear:
    Hearing disorder: [102]
    Tinnitus: [103] (San, She)
  Vestibular:
    Dizziness: (BNF)
    Vertigo: (BNF)

Risk assessment: Class 2

Notes:

Acemetacin is a prodrug of **Indomethacin**. Your body converts **Acemetacin** into **Indomethacin**. As such you could expect it to have similar ototoxic side effects as **Indomethacin**. (See the generic drug **Indomethacin** for its specific ototoxic properties.)

Aceon   (see **Perindopril**)

Acetadote   (see **Acetylcysteine**)

Acetaminophen (Paracetamol, APAP)

Pronunciation guide: ah-seet-ah-MIN-oh-fen

Drug classification: ANALGESIC DRUGS (PAINKILLERS) (see section 1 in Table 14-1)

Brand names: *Children's Tylenol* [1], *Parafon Forte* [2], *Tylenol, Tylenol Aches & Strains* [2], *Tylenol Flu Medication* [3]

Ototoxic effects:
  Cochlear:
    Hearing loss: [4]

Risk assessment: Class 5 when taken in large doses for long periods of time. Class 2 when taken regularly at normal doses for more than 1 year.

Notes:

[1] *Children's Tylenol* is a combination of **Acetaminophen** and **Pseudoephedrine**. (See the generic drug **Pseudoephedrine** for its specific ototoxic properties.)

[2] *Parafon Forte and Tylenol Aches & Strains* are both combinations of **Acetaminophen** and **Chlorzoxazone**. (See the generic drug **Chlorzoxazone** for its specific ototoxic properties.)

[3] *Tylenol Flu Medication* is a combination of **Acetaminophen**, **Diphenhydramine** and **Pseudoephedrine**. (See the generic drugs **Diphenhydramine** and **Pseudoephedrine** for their specific ototoxic properties.)

Acetaminophen is better known in Europe as **Paracetamol** or **APAP** (N-acetyl-para-amino-phenol).

Acetaminophen is one of the ingredients in a number of compound drugs. As always, check the labels and then look up each drug listed to see its ototoxic properties.

[4]A recent study revealed that **Acetaminophen** is very ototoxic. Cochlear cultures exposed to **Acetaminophen** began dying after about 24 hours, and by 96 hours, 100% of the hair cells had died. That's how ototoxic **Acetaminophen** really is![104]

People can develop progressive, irreversible hearing loss from taking "extremely high doses of **Acetaminophen** for a little as 2 months, or after taking clinically acceptable doses for as long as 10 years".[105] At regular dosages (e.g.: up to 4 pills a day), when taken two or more times a week for more than a year, **Acetaminophen** can cause hearing loss. For example, in a study of 26,917 men between the ages of 40 and 75 at the beginning of the study, men that used **Acetaminophen** at least twice a week had a 22% increased risk of hearing loss. However, when only men under the age of 50 were considered, the risk factor skyrocketed to 99%.[106]

It is thought that **Acetaminophen** depletes glutathione, a powerful natural antioxidant that helps protect our hearing from the effects of free radicals that are produced when our ears are exposed to loud noise,[107] to prescription drugs and to various chemicals. When glutathione levels are reduced, the free radicals floating around in the cochlea zap (kill) the hair cells, resulting in some degree of sensorineural hearing loss.

Acetaminophen can cause profound hearing loss when ingested in large doses (e.g. 15 to 75 pills a day) over several weeks or months. Taken by itself, these large doses would kill the liver, and thus the person, before hearing loss became apparent. However, when taken in combination with **Hydrocodone** (e.g. *Vicodin*), the **Hydrocodone** somehow protects the liver. As a result, the person doesn't die and eventually massive hearing loss becomes apparent.[108] For further information on how **Acetaminophen** and **Hydrocodone** work together to cause massive hearing loss, see the explanation under the drug **Hydrocodone**.

Also, see Chapter 2 "Ototoxic Drugs—What Are They?", the section entitled "The Story of Vicodin" in Chapter 5 and Chapter 7, "We 'Hear' With Our Eyes" for further information on **Acetaminophen**.

Acetazolamide

Pronunciation guide: ah-seet-ah-ZOLE-ah-mide

Drug classification: DIURETICS—CARBONIC ANHYDRASE INHIBITORS (see section 30.5.1 in Table 14-1)

Brand names: *Diamox*

Ototoxic effects:
    Cochlear:
        Hearing disorder: (CPS, PDR)
        Hearing loss: (PDR)
        Tinnitus: (CPS, PDR)
    Vestibular:
        Ataxia: (CPS, NDH)
        Dizziness: (BNF, CPS)

Risk assessment: Class 2

Notes:

See Chapter 7, "We 'Hear' With Our Eyes" for further information on this drug.

Acetazone Forte C8   (see **Chlorzoxazone**)

Acetylcysteine

Pronunciation guide: ah-SEET-ill-SIS-teen

Drug classification: ACETAMINOPHEN ANTIDOTES (see section 66.1.1 in Table 14-1)

Brand names: *Acetadote, Mucomyst*

Ototoxic effects:
    Vestibular:
        Ataxia: (DFC)
    Outer/Middle Ear:
        Earache/ear pain: 1% (DFC)

Risk assessment: Class 1

Notes:

Ataxia is a symptom of acute toxicity (overdose).

Acetylsalicylic acid (Aspirin)

Pronunciation guide: ah-SEE-till-sal-ih-SILL-ick ASS-id

Drug classification: SALICYLATES (see section 1.1.16 in Table 14-1)

Brand names: *222*[1], *282*[1], *282 MEP*[2], *292*[1], *692*[3], *Aggrenox*[4], *Alka-Seltzer, Anacin*[5], *ASA, Asasantine*[4], *Ascriptin, Aspirin*[6], *Aspirin Backache*[7], *Bayer Aspirin, BC Powder*[8], *Bufferin, Cepastat, Coated Aspirin, Darvon Compound-65*[9], *Debrox, Easprin, Ecotrin Enteric-coated Aspirin, Entrophen, Excedrin Back & Body*[10], *Excedrin Extra Strength*[10], *Excedrin Migraine*[10], *MSD Enteric coated ASA, Norgesic*[11], *Robaxisal*[12], *St. Joseph Aspirin, Vanquish Extra Strength Pain Reliever*[13]

Ototoxic effects:
    Cochlear:
        Hearing loss: >10% (NDH, PDR)
        Tinnitus: >10% (NDH, PDR)
    Vestibular:
        Dizziness: <5% (CPS, PDR)
        Vertigo: (CPS, PDR)
    Outer/Middle Ear:
        Earache/ear pain: (CPS)
        Ears feel "plugged": 1% (CPS)

Risk assessment: Class 2

Notes:

[1] *222, 282* and *292* are combinations of **ASA** (**Aspirin**), **Caffeine** and **Codeine**. (See the generic drugs **Caffeine** and **Codeine** for their specific ototoxic properties.)

[2] *282 MEP* is a combination of **ASA** (**Aspirin**) and **Meprobamate**. (See the generic drug **Meprobamate** for its specific ototoxic properties.)

[3] *692* is a combination of **ASA** (**Aspirin**), **Caffeine** and **Propoxyphene**. (See the generic drugs **Caffeine** and **Propoxyphene** for their specific ototoxic properties.)

[4] *Asasantine* and *Aggrenox* are both combinations of **ASA** (**Aspirin**) and **Dipyridamole**. (See the generic drug **Dipyridamole** for its specific ototoxic properties.)

[5] *Anacin* is a combination of **ASA** (**Aspirin**) and **Caffeine**. (See the generic drug **Caffeine** for its specific ototoxic properties.)

[6] *Aspirin* is a brand name of the Bayer Company in Canada. **Acetylsalicylic acid** (**ASA**) is the generic name. At the same time, **Aspirin** is also an official generic drug name designation in the United States.

[7] *Aspirin Backache* is a combination of **ASA** (**Aspirin**) and **Methocarbamol**. (See the generic drug **Methocarbamol** for its specific ototoxic properties.)

[8] *BC Powder* is a combination of **ASA** (**Aspirin**), Salicylamide and **Caffeine**. (See the generic drug **Caffeine** for its specific ototoxic properties.)

[9] *Darvon Compound-65* is a combination of **ASA** (**Aspirin**), **Caffeine** and **Propoxyphene**. (See the generic drugs **Caffeine** and **Propoxyphene** for their specific ototoxic properties.)

[10] *Excedrin* is a combination of **ASA** (**Aspirin**), **Acetaminophen** and **Caffeine**. (See the generic drugs **Acetaminophen** and **Caffeine** for their specific ototoxic properties.)

[11] *Norgesic* is a combination of **ASA** (**Aspirin**), **Orphenadrine** and **Caffeine**. (See the generic drugs **Caffeine** and **Orphenadrine** for their specific ototoxic properties.)

[12] *Robaxisal* is a combination of **ASA** (**Aspirin**), **Methocarbamol** and sometimes **Codeine**. (See the generic drugs **Methocarbamol** and **Codeine** for their specific ototoxic properties.)

[13] *Vanquish Extra Strength Pain Reliever* is a combination of **ASA** (**Aspirin**), **Acetaminophen** and **Caffeine** (PDR-N). (See the generic drugs **Acetaminophen** and **Caffeine** for their specific ototoxic properties.)

There are many other **ASA** (**Aspirin**) brand names and compounds too numerous to list here. The ones listed here are a few of the more common ones.

If your ears begin to ring or buzz (tinnitus), or if hearing loss occurs, consult your doctor before you take any more **ASA** (**Aspirin**) (CPS, PDR). If you already have the typical high-frequency hearing loss, you may have difficulty perceiving tinnitus. In such cases, you can't rely on the presence of tinnitus to warn you of damage to your ears from this drug (PDR). Tinnitus does not usually begin until your **ASA** (**Aspirin**) serum level is 19.6 mg/L (200 mcg/ml) or higher [109] (PDR). Plasma levels above 30 mg/L (300 mcg/ml) are clearly toxic (PDR). Taking 6 to 8 *Aspirin* a day can cause ringing in your ears and temporary hearing loss.[110]

SALICYLATE ototoxicity generally appears as a high-pitched or hissing tinnitus accompanied by hearing loss. Sometimes it will also affect your balance.[111] If you are taking **ASA (Aspirin)** and notice you now have tinnitus, hearing loss and/or dizziness, this indicates that your blood SALICYLATE concentrations are reaching or exceeding the upper limit of the therapeutic range (CP2). These three symptoms most frequently indicate chronic **ASA (Aspirin)** intoxication. They usually occur in people taking large doses, or doses for a long time. Also, increased serum levels of **ASA (Aspirin)** can result in SALICYLATE toxicity (salicylism). Symptoms of salicylism include nausea, vomiting, headaches, tinnitus, hearing loss, mental dullness, confusion, quickened pulse and increased respirations.[112]

High doses of **ASA (Aspirin)** typically produce both a flat hearing loss of up to 40 dB in both ears and some reduction in speech discrimination. As a general rule, the greater the blood serum levels of **ASA (Aspirin)**, the worse the resulting tinnitus and/or hearing loss (CP2, CPS). Usually, but not always, the hearing loss and accompanying tinnitus are completely reversible within 24 to 72 hours after you stop taking **ASA (Aspirin)**, although permanent hearing loss can occur.[113] There have been reports of permanent sudden sensorineural hearing loss (SSHL) and tinnitus from taking **ASA (Aspirin)**.[114]

Salicylate-induced hearing loss involves bilateral loss of pure tone sensitivity for all sound frequencies. Hearing losses generally range from 20-40 dB. Hearing loss occurs initially at a serum salicylate concentration of about 200 mcg/ml and increases with increasing concentrations. Maximum hearing loss occurs most frequently at a serum salicylate concentration of about 400 mcg/ml (AHF).

Using **ASA (Aspirin)** regularly over time can increase your risk of hearing loss. For example, in one study of 26,917 men between the ages of 40 and 75 at the beginning of the study, men that used **ASA (Aspirin)** at least twice a week had a 22% increased risk of hearing loss over men who were not regular users of **ASA (Aspirin)**. However, when only men under the age of 50 were considered, the risk factor for hearing loss jumped to 33%.[115]

Taking **ASA (Aspirin)** results in abnormal outer hair cell function and decreased cochlear blood flow.[116]

I have an anecdotal report in my files of a lady who had been taking very large doses of **ASA (Aspirin)** for headaches. This had been going on for about five years. She had put her hearing loss down to other causes, never thinking the **ASA (Aspirin)** was the culprit. However, when I suggested that taking **ASA (Aspirin)** could be causing much of her hearing loss, she stopped taking it. Just six days after she stopped taking **ASA (Aspirin)**, she wrote, "I have noticed that I am hearing better now. I have the TV volume set at level 18 instead of the usual 24. The ringing in my ears is still there but it is not as bad". Three days later she added, "Today when someone was talking behind me, I heard every word he said. My hearing still isn't perfect but it is better than it was".

You are at greater risk of **ASA** ototoxicity if you take high doses, are elderly or are dehydrated. The incidence of ototoxicity is about 1%.[117]

SALICYLATES such as **ASA (Aspirin)** can increase the effects of other ototoxic drugs (e.g. **Vancomycin**). You should avoid taking **ASA (Aspirin)** at the same time or following any ototoxic drugs because hearing loss may occur and may progress to deafness even after the medication is stopped. Although these effects may be reversible, they are usually permanent (CPS). That's the bad news.

The good news is that researchers have recently discovered that **ASA** (**Aspirin**) may actually help protect our ears from the damaging effects of taking AMINOGLYCOSIDE antibiotics such as **Streptomycin**, **Gentamicin** and **Neomycin**.

Here is how it works. AMINOGLYCOSIDE antibiotics bind iron in our bodies. When they do this, they produce free radicals that can damage or kill cells. The tiny hair cells in our inner ears are particularly vulnerable to free radical damage. When these hair cells die, the result is permanent hearing loss. **ASA** (**Aspirin**) quickly breaks down in our bodies to produce Salicylate, a compound that soaks up any extra iron and thereby prevents the AMINOGLYCOSIDES from forming free radicals.

The results in animal studies are impressive. Guinea pigs receiving **Gentamicin** alone had severe hearing loss of up to 70 dB and almost complete destruction of the outer hair cells in their cochlea. In contrast, guinea pigs given both **Gentamicin** and **ASA** (**Aspirin**) had minor hearing loss of less than 20 dB and minimal hair cell damage.[118] Current research is now determining if **ASA** (**Aspirin**) affords the same protection in humans. Let's hope it does!

Note: **ASA** (**Aspirin**) is still ototoxic and can damage your ears as shown earlier. However, if the choice is between relatively minor ear damage while taking a necessary course of AMINOGLYCOSIDE antibiotics and **ASA** (**Aspirin**) in order to save your life, as opposed to major ear damage from taking the same antibiotics without the protection **ASA** (**Aspirin**) seems to afford, the choice seems obvious.

See Chapter 2 "Ototoxic Drugs—What Are They," Chapter 4 "Are You at Risk," Chapter 5 "Here's How the System Works," Chapter 7, "We 'Hear' With Our Eyes," Chapter 8, "The Sinister Partnership Between Ototoxic Agents and Noise" and Chapter 9, "Aminoglycoside Antibiotics are the Ototoxic 'Bad boys'" for further information on this drug.

Achromycin   (see **Tetracycline**)

Aciphex   (see **Rabeprazole**)

Acitretin

Pronunciation guide: ah-sih-TREE-tin

Drug classification: VITAMIN A ANALOGS (see section 23.4 in Table 14-1)

Brand names: *Soriatane*

Ototoxic effects:
    Cochlear:
        Hearing loss: <1% (CPS, PDR)
        Tinnitus: 1-10% (CPS, PDR)
    Vestibular:
        Ataxia: <1% (CPS, PDR)
        Dizziness: <1% (CPS, PDR)
    Outer/Middle Ear:
        Earache/ear pain: 1-10% (CPS, PDR)
        Increased ear wax: 1-10% (CPS, PDR)

       Otitis externa: <1% (CPS, PDR)
       Otitis media: <1% (DFC, PDR)

Risk assessment: Class 2

Aclasta   (see **Zoledronic acid**)

Acthar   (see **Corticotropin**)

Actifed   (see **Pseudoephedrine**)

Actimmune   (see **Interferon gamma-1b**)

Actinomycin-D   (see **Dactinomycin**)

Actiq   (see **Fentanyl**)

Activelle   (see **Norethindrone**)

Actonel   (see **Risedronate**)

Acyclovir   (see **Valacyclovir**)

Adacel   (see **Tetanus vaccine**)

Adalat   (see **Nifedipine**)

Adalimumab

Pronunciation guide: ay-dah-LIM-yoo-mab

Drug classification: MONOCLONAL ANTIBODIES (see section 7.17.8 in Table 14-1)

Brand names: *Humira, Trudexa*

Ototoxic effects:
    Cochlear:
        Hearing loss: <0.1% [1, 2]
        Tinnitus: 0.1-1% [1, 2, 3]
    Vestibular:
        Dizziness: 1-10% [1]
        Vertigo: 0.1-1% [2]
    Outer/Middle Ear:
        Ear ache/Ear pain: 0.1-1% [1, 2]

Risk assessment: Class 2

Notes:

    [1] **Adalimumab** can cause dizziness (including vertigo), tinnitus, ear discomfort (including pain and swelling) and hearing loss.[119]

[2] **Adalimumab** can cause dizziness, ear or hearing problems, tinnitus and vertigo[120]

[3] I have an anecdotal report in my files of a man who was put on **Adalimumab** 40 mg. shots every two weeks. His tinnitus was bad during this time, but he attributed it to stress. Recently, he had an injection after not having had one for about a month. He explains, "Coincidently, my tinnitus was getting better during that period. A few hours after the shot my tinnitus acted up again, and has been very loud 24/7".

I have an anecdotal report in my files of a man who reported: "I started taking *Humira* 40 mg. Approximately 4 weeks after the first shot, I started having severe vertigo and dizziness along with tinnitus. My balance has been an issue ever since. After taking **Adalimumab** injections for 17 months I decided to stop taking the injections. Since stopping the injections, my symptoms have gradually subsided, although I am not completely free of them".

Adapin   (see **Doxepin**)

Adcirca   (see **Tadalafil**)

Adenocard   (see **Adenosine**)

Adenoscan   (see **Adenosine**)

Adenosine

Pronunciation guide: ah-DEN-oh-seen

Drug classification: Anti-arrhythmics (Heart rhythm regulators) (see section 20.4 in Table 14-1)

Brand names: *Adenocard, Adenoscan*

Ototoxic effects:
    Vestibular:
        Dizziness: 1-12% (CPS, PDR)
    Outer/Middle Ear:
        Earache/ear pain: <1% (CPS, PDR)

Risk assessment: Class 1

Adipex-P   (see **Phentermine**)

Adriamycin   (see **Doxorubicin**)

Adrucil   (see **Fluorouracil**)

Advagraf   (see **Tacrolimus**)

Advair Diskus   (see **Fluticasone**)

Advicor   (see **Lovastatin**)

Advil   (see **Ibuprofen**)

Advil Cold & Sinus   (see **Ibuprofen**)

Aerobid   (see **Flunisolide**)

Aerosporin   (see **Polymyxin B**)

Afloxan   (see **Proglumetacin**)

Agalsidase alfa

Pronunciation guide: ah-GAL-sih-dase AL-fah

Drug classification: ENZYMES (see section 32.1 in Table 14-1)

Brand names: *Replagal*

Ototoxic effects:
    Cochlear:
        Hearing loss: (CPS)
        Tinnitus: (CPS)
    Vestibular:
        Dizziness: (CPS)
        Vertigo: 1.8% (CPS)
    Outer/Middle Ear:
        Earache/ear pain: (CPS)

Risk assessment: Class 2

Agalsidase beta

Pronunciation guide: ah-GAL-sih-dase BAY-tah

Drug classification: ENZYMES (see section 32.1 in Table 14-1)

Brand names: *Fabrazyme*

Ototoxic effects:
    Cochlear:
        Hearing loss: (DFC, PDR)
        Tinnitus: 8% [5% above placebo results] (PDR)
    Vestibular:
        Ataxia: (PDR)
        Dizziness: 5-21% [<11% above placebo results] (CPS, PDR)
        Vertigo: 1-4% (CPS, PDR)

Risk assessment: Class 2

Aggrenox   (see **Acetylsalicylic acid**)

Agrylin   (see **Anagrelide**)

Airomir   (see **Albuterol**)

AK-Pentolate   (see **Cyclopentolate**)

Alacol   (see **Dextromethorphan**)

Alatrofloxacin   (see **Trovafloxacin**)

Albamycin-T   (see **Novobiocin**)

Albendazole

Pronunciation guide: al-BEN-dah-zole

Drug classification: ANTHELMINTIC DRUGS (see section 7.1 in Table 14-1)

Brand names: *Albenza*

Ototoxic effects:
    Vestibular:
        Dizziness: 1% (DFC, PDR)
        Vertigo: 1% (DFC, PDR)

Risk assessment: Class 1

Albenza   (see **Albendazole**)

Albert Pentoxifylline   (see **Pentoxifylline**)

Albert Tiafen   (see **Tiaprofenic acid**)

Albuterol (Salbutamol)

Pronunciation guide: al-BYOO-ter-ole (sal-BYOO-tah-mole)

Drug classification: BRONCHODILATORS—BETA ADRENERGIC AGONISTS (see section 63.4 in Table 14-1)

Brand names: *AccuNeb, Airomir, Asmavent, ProAir HFA, Proventil, Ventolin, Volmax*

Ototoxic effects:
    Cochlear:
        Tinnitus: <3% (CPS, PDR)
    Vestibular:
        Ataxia: <3% (CPS, PDR)
        Dizziness: 1-7% [placebo 0] (CPS, PDR)
        Vertigo: (CPS, PDR)

Outer/Middle Ear:
    Earache/ear pain: <3% (AHF, PDR)
    Otitis media: 0.9-4.3% [placebo 0] (AHF, PDR)
Unspecified/General Ear Conditions:
    Ear disorder: <3% (AHF, PDR)

Risk assessment: Class 2

Alclofenac

Pronunciation guide: al-KLOE-fen-ak

Drug classification: ACETIC ACIDS (see section 1.1.1 in Table 14-1)

Brand names: *Mervan*

Ototoxic effects:
    Cochlear:
        Tinnitus: (San, She)
    Unspecified/General Ear Conditions:
        Ototoxicity: (San)

Risk assessment: Class 2

Aldactazide (see **Spironolactone**)

Aldactone (see **Spironolactone**)

Aldesleukin

Pronunciation guide: al-dess-LOO-kin

Drug classification: CYTOKINES (see section 14.12 in Table 14-1)

Brand names: *Proleukin*

Ototoxic effects:
    Vestibular:
        Ataxia: (PDR)
        Dizziness: 11% (PDR)

Risk assessment: Class 1

Aldoclor (see **Chlorothiazide**)

Aldoril (see **Hydrochlorothiazide**)

Alemtuzumab

Pronunciation guide: ah-lem-TOO-zoo-mab

Drug classification: MONOCLONAL ANTIBODIES (see section 7.17.8 in Table 14-1)

Brand names: *Campath, MabCampath*

Ototoxic effects:
    Cochlear:
        Hearing loss: (CPS, PDR)
    Vestibular:
        Ataxia: (PDR)
        Dizziness: 1-12% (CPS, PDR)
        Vertigo: 3% (CPS)
    Outer/Middle Ear:
        Otitis media: (PDR)

Risk assessment: Class 2

Alendronate

Pronunciation guide: ah-LEN-droh-nate

Drug classification: BISPHOSPHONATES (see section 50.1.1 in Table 14-1)

Brand names: *Fosamax, Fosavance* [1]

Ototoxic effects:
    Cochlear:
        Tinnitus: [2, 3, 4]
    Vestibular:
        Dizziness: 0.1–1.0% [placebo 0] (CPS, PDR)
        Vertigo: (CPS, PDR)

Risk assessment: Class 2

Notes:

[1] *Fosavance* is a combination of **Alendronate** and **Cholecalciferol**. (See the generic drug **Cholecalciferol** for its specific ototoxic properties.)

[2] I have an anecdotal report in my files of a man whose physician thought his tinnitus resulted from taking **Alendronate**.

[3] I have an anecdotal report in my files of a woman whose tinnitus was thought to have resulted from taking **Alendronate**.

[4] I have an anecdotal report in my files of a man whose tinnitus was "raging again" a few hours after he took **Alendronate**.

Alertec   (see **Modafinil**)

Aleve   (see **Naproxen**)

Alfacalcidol   (see **Ergocalciferal**)

Alferon N   (see **Interferon alfa-n3**)

Alfuzosin

Pronunciation guide: al-foo-ZOE-sin

Drug classification: ALPHA ADRENERGIC BLOCKING DRUGS (see section 20.8.1 in Table 14-1)

Brand names: *Xatral*

Ototoxic effects:
    Vestibular:
        Dizziness: 5.7% [2.9% above placebo results] (CPS)
        Vertigo: 0.1-1% (CPS)

Risk assessment: Class 1

Alglucosidase alfa

Pronunciation guide: al-gloo-KOE-sih-dase al-fah

Drug classification: ENZYMES (see section 32.1 in Table 14-1)

Brand names: *Myozyme*

Ototoxic effects:
    Cochlear:
        Hearing loss: [1] <11.9% (CPS)
    Vestibular:
        Dizziness: 6.7% (CPS)
    Outer/Middle Ear:
        Earache/ear pain: 5.1% (CPS)
        Otitis media: 40.7% (CPS, DFC)
        Otorrhagia: 5.1% (CPS)

Risk assessment: Class 3

Notes:

[1] Hearing loss may be conductive or sensorineural. Hearing loss seems more related to the high incidence of middle ear infections in the people with Pompe's Disease taking **Alglucosidase alfa**, rather than from the **Alglucosidase** therapy itself (CPS).

Alinia   (see **Nitazoxanide**)

Aliskiren

Pronunciation guide: ah-LIS-keh-ren

Drug classification: RENIN INHIBITORS (see section 20.8.36 in Table 14-1)

Brand names: *Rasilez*

Ototoxic effects:
    Vestibular:
        Vertigo: <1% (CPS)

Risk assessment: Class 1

Alka-Seltzer   (see **Acetylsalicylic acid**)

Allegra   (see **Fexofenadine**)

Allegra-D   (see **Fexofenadine**)

Aller-Chlor   (see **Chlorpheniramine**)

Allopurinol

Pronunciation guide: al-oh-PURE-ih-nole

Drug classification: XANTHINE OXIDASE INHIBITORS (see section 46.10 in Table 14-1)

Brand names: *Zyloprim*

Ototoxic effects:
    Cochlear:
        Tinnitus: <1% (AHF, PDR)
    Vestibular:
        Ataxia: (CPS)
        Dizziness: <1% (CPS, PDR)
        Vertigo: <1% (CPS, PDR)

Risk assessment: Class 1

Notes:
    See Chapter 7, "We 'Hear' With Our Eyes" for further information on this drug.

Almogran   (see **Almotriptan**)

Almotriptan

Pronunciation guide: al-moh-TRIP-tan

Drug classification: SEROTONIN-RECEPTOR AGONISTS (see section 53.32 in Table 14-1)

Brand names: *Almogran*, *Axert*

Ototoxic effects:
    Cochlear:
        Hyperacusis: 0.1-1% (DFC, PDR)
        Tinnitus: 0.1-1% (DFC, PDR)
    Vestibular:
        Ataxia: <0.1% (PDR)
        Dizziness: >1% (NDH, PDR)
        Nystagmus: <0.1% (DFC, PDR)
        Vertigo: 0.1-1% (DFC, PDR)

Outer/Middle Ear:
   Earache/ear pain: 0.1-1% (DFC, PDR)
   Otitis media: <0.1% (DFC, PDR)

Risk assessment: Class 2

Alosetron

Pronunciation guide: ah-LOSS-eh-tron

Drug classification: SEROTONIN-RECEPTOR ANTAGONISTS (see section 34.1.4 in Table 14-1)

Brand names: *Lotronex*

Ototoxic effects:
   External/Middle Ear:
      Otitis: (PDR)
   Unspecified/General Ear Conditions:
      Ear disorder: <0.1% (PDR)

Risk assessment: Class 1

Aloxi   (see **Palonosetron**)

Alprazolam

Pronunciation guide: al-PRAH-zoe-lam

Drug classification: BENZODIAZEPINES (see section 60.12.8 in Table 14-1)

Brand names: *Xanax*, *Xanax TS*

Ototoxic effects:
   Cochlear:
      Hyperacusis: [1, 2]
      Tinnitus: 6.6% (CPS, PDR)
   Vestibular:
      Ataxia: (CPS, PDR)
      Dizziness: 0.8-2.5% [<1% above placebo results] (CPS, PDR)
      Vertigo: (BNF, NDH)

Risk assessment: Class 2

Notes:

[1] If you stop taking **Alprazolam** "cold turkey" instead of weaning off it very slowly, you may experience tinnitus and/or hyperacusis. As one lady explained, "I have seen countless people that have stopped taking *Xanax* develop tinnitus, hyperacusis or both".

[2] I have an anecdotal report in my files of a man that wrote, "When I first acquired hyperacusis/tinnitus my ENT put me on *Xanax*. It was a godsend for about a year. At that point the interdose withdrawals [short half-life] of the medication were too much for me to put up with. I'd take 3 tablets a day, and after about 4 hours of taking a tablet I'd start getting increased hyperacusis".

Long term use of **Alprazolam** can result in various ototoxic side effects. As one lady explained, "About 15 years ago I started having panic attacks and began taking *Xanax* (**Alprazolam**) at 1.5 mg/day and have been on it ever since. Two years ago I had some really bad panic attacks so my doctor doubled my *Xanax* medication to 3 mg/day. Now everything is out of control for some reason. In the past year or two, in spite of the increased dose, things have been getting much worse to the point I don't feel normal any more. My hearing is a lot worse, I have vertigo and balance problems. I feel unsteady on my feet. My ears are ringing. They are also supersensitive to sounds [hyperacusis]. As a result, I can't wear a hearing aid in one ear anymore".

Caution: Eating grapefruit or drinking grapefruit juice during the time you are taking this drug may make the listed side effects worse than shown here.

See Chapter 4 "Are You at Risk?", Chapter 10 "Beware of Benzodiazepines—Don't Let This Nasty Time-Bomb Ambush You and Your Ears" and Chapter 11, "Grapefruit Juice and Ototoxic Drugs" for further information on this drug.

Altace   (see **Ramipril**)

Altocor   (see **Lovastatin**)

Altretamine

Pronunciation guide: al-TRET-ah-meen

Drug classification: ALKYLATING DRUGS (see section 14.1 in Table 14-1)

Brand names: *Hexalen*

Ototoxic effects:
Vestibular:
Ataxia: (AHF, PDR)
Dizziness: (AHF, PDR)
Vertigo: (AHF, PDR)

Risk assessment: Class 1

Alumadrine   (see **Phenylpropanolamine**)

Amantadine

Pronunciation guide: ah-MAN-tah-deen

Drug classification: ANTI-VIRAL DRUGS (see section 7.17 in Table 14-1)

Brand names: *Symmetrel*

Ototoxic effects:
Vestibular:
Ataxia: 1-5% (CPS, PDR)
Dizziness: 5-10% (CPS, PDR)

Risk assessment: Class 2

Notes:

Ataxia may be a sign of **Amantadine** overdose (PDR).

See Chapter 7, "We 'Hear' With Our Eyes" for further information on this drug.

Ambien   (see **Zolpidem**)

Ambien CR   (see **Zolpidem**)

AmBisome   (see **Amphotericin B**)

Amen   (see **Medroxyprogesterone**)

Amerge   (see **Naratriptan**)

Americaine Otic   (see **Benzocaine**)

Amezinium

Pronunciation guide: ah-meh-ZIN-ee-um

Drug classification: SYMPATHOMIMETIC DRUGS (see section 17.16 in Table 14-1)

Brand names: *Tenfortan*

Ototoxic effects:
Cochlear:
Tinnitus: (She)

Risk assessment: Class 1

Amicar   (see **Aminocaproic acid**)

Amikacin

Pronunciation guide: am-ih-KAY-sin

Drug classification: AMINOGLYCOSIDES (see section 7.4.1 in Table 14-1)

Brand names: *Amikin*

Ototoxic effects:
Cochlear:
Hearing loss: (CPS, PDR)
Tinnitus: (CPS, PDR)
Vestibular:
Ataxia: (CPS)
Dizziness: (CPS, PDR)
Loss of balance: (CPS, PDR)
Nystagmus: (CPS, PDR)
Vertigo: (CPS, PDR)

Outer/Middle Ear:
    Feeling of fullness in ears: (CPS, PDR)
Unspecified/General Ear Conditions:
    Ototoxicity: (CPS)

Risk assessment: Class 5

Notes:

If you are taking **Amikacin**, you should be under close medical observation. The incidence of ototoxicity in **Amikacin** is up to 13.9%.[121]

You have a greater chance of having vestibular (balance) problems and permanent hearing loss in both ears if you have pre-existing kidney damage, or if you have normal kidney function but are being treated at higher doses and/or for longer periods than those recommended (CPS, PDR).

Therefore, before taking **Amikacin**, tell your doctor if you have any of these risk factors—pre-existing hearing loss, ear damage from previously prescribed drugs, impaired kidney function, advanced age or dehydration (CPS, PDR). Any of these risk factors may make your ears more susceptible to damage from **Amikacin** than would be expected in the general population.

The side effects of **Amikacin** can result in hearing loss, loss of balance or both. **Amikacin** primarily affects auditory function. Cochlear damage includes high-frequency hearing loss and usually occurs before clinical hearing loss can be detected. Initially, high-frequency audiometric testing is the only way to detect hearing loss (CPS, PDR).

Be aware that hearing loss (and other ear damage) may develop without warning while you are taking **Amikacin** (PDR). In order to reduce the chances of ototoxicity, you should only take **Amikacin** for 7 to 10 days. Your doctor should stop this medication if there is no definite clinical response within 3 to 5 days of therapy.[122]

Since hearing loss from taking **Amikacin** is often permanent, you need your hearing checked both **before** and **during** treatment (serial high-frequency audiograms) in order that your doctor may take appropriate action to minimize the risk of permanent hearing loss (CPS). This is particularly true if you already have any hearing or balance problems or problems with your kidneys (PDR).

You should know that you may not have any symptoms such as hearing loss or vertigo while you are taking **Amikacin** to warn you that you are damaging your ears. Total or partial hearing loss in both ears, or disabling vertigo may not show up until several weeks after you have stopped taking **Amikacin**. Such damage to your ears is usually permanent. Because of this risk, if you detect any signs of hearing loss, dizziness, tinnitus or feeling of fullness in your ears, stop taking **Amikacin** and immediately notify your doctor (PDR). If you have any of these signs, your doctor should strongly consider stopping treatment immediately or adjust the dosage (CPS, PDR).

The risk of permanent hearing loss and kidney damage increases when you take **Amikacin** at the same time as rapidly-acting diuretic (water pills), nephrotoxic (kidney-damaging) or ototoxic (ear damaging) drugs. You can quickly lose your hearing if you have poor kidney function and are treated at the same time with **Amikacin** and one of the rapidly-acting diuretic drugs given intravenously such as **Ethacrynic acid**, **Furosemide** or **Mannitol** (CPS).

You should not use other neurotoxic (nerve damaging) or nephrotoxic (kidney damaging) drugs, particularly **Amphotericin B**, **Bacitracin**, Cephaloridine, **Cisplatin**, **Colistin**, **Paromomycin**, **Polymyxin B**, **Vancomycin**, **Viomycin**, or other AMINOGLYCOSIDE antibiotics at the same time as, or following, taking **Amikacin** (PDR).

See Chapter 9, "Aminoglycoside Antibiotics are the Ototoxic 'Bad boys'" for further information on this drug.

Amikin   (see **Amikacin**)

Amiloride

Pronunciation guide: a-MILL-oh-ride

Drug classification: DIURETICS—POTASSIUM-SPARING (see section 30.5.8 in Table 14-1)

Brand names: *Apo-Amiloride, Midamor, Moduret* [1], *Moduretic* [1]

Ototoxic effects:
Cochlear:
Tinnitus: <1% (CPS, PDR)
Vestibular:
Dizziness: 1-8% (CPS, PDR)
Vertigo: <1% (CPS, PDR)

Risk assessment: Class 2

Notes:

[1] *Moduret* and *Moduretic* are combinations of **Amiloride** and **Hydrochlorothiazide**. (See the generic drug **Hydrochlorothiazide** for its specific ototoxic properties.)

Aminocaproic acid

Pronunciation guide: ah-mee-noe-kah-PROE-ik ASS-id

Drug classification: ANTI-FIBRINOLYTIC DRUGS (see section 36.4 in Table 14-1)

Brand names: *Amicar*

Ototoxic effects:
Cochlear:
Hearing loss: (AHF, PDR)
Tinnitus: (CPS, PDR)
Vestibular:
Dizziness: (CPS, PDR)

Risk assessment: Class 2

Aminoglutethimide

Pronunciation guide: ah-mee-noe-gloo-TETH-ih-mide

Drug classification: Non-steroidal aromatase inhibitors (see section 14.24 in Table 14-1)

Brand names: *Cytadren*

Ototoxic effects:
  Vestibular:
    Ataxia: (BNF, CPS)
    Dizziness: (BNF, CPS)
    Vertigo: (CPS)

Risk assessment: Class 1

Aminopyrine

Pronunciation guide: ah-mee-noe-PYE-reen

Drug classification: Analgesic drugs (Painkillers) (see section 1 in Table 14-1)

Brand names: *Ampyrone*, *Dipyrone*

Ototoxic effects:
  Cochlear:
    Hearing loss: (NTP)
    Tinnitus: (NTP)
  Vestibular:
    Dizziness: (NTP)

Risk assessment: Class 2

Notes:

  In the USA, the FDA has removed this drug from use. It was formerly used in both human and veterinary medicine.

Aminosalicylic acid   (see **Mesalamine**)

Aminosidine   (see **Paromomycin**)

Amiodarone

Pronunciation guide: am-ee-OH-dah-rohn

Drug classification: Anti-arrhythmics (Heart Rhythm Regulators) (see section 20.4 in Table 14-1)

Brand names: *Cordarone*, *Novo-Amiodarone*, *Pacerone*

Ototoxic effects:
  Cochlear:
    Tinnitus: <1% (CPS)

Vestibular:
    Ataxia: 4-9% (CPS, PDR)
    Dizziness: 4-9% (CPS, PDR)
    Nystagmus: (AHF)
    Vertigo: (BNF, CPS)

Risk assessment: Class 2

Notes:

Vertigo occurs frequently at the beginning of therapy when high doses are used (CPS).

Caution: Eating grapefruit or drinking grapefruit juice during the time you are taking this drug may make the listed side effects worse than shown here.

See Chapter 11, "Grapefruit Juice and Ototoxic Drugs" for further information on this drug.

Amitiza   (see **Lubiprostone**)

Amitriptyline

Pronunciation guide: ah-mee-TRIP-tih-leen

Drug classification: TRICYCLIC ANTI-DEPRESSANTS (see section 60.1.8 in Table 14-1)

Brand names: *Elavil, Elavil Plus* [1], *Etrafon* [1], *Limbitrol* [2], *Triavil* [1]

Ototoxic effects:
    Cochlear:
        Hearing disorder: [3]
        Hearing loss: [5]
        Hyperacusis: [6]
        Tinnitus: (CPS, PDR)
    Vestibular:
        Ataxia: (CPS, PDR)
        Dizziness: (CPS, PDR)
        Nystagmus: [4] (CPS)
        Vertigo: (CPS)

Risk assessment: Class 3

Notes:

[1] *Elavil Plus, Etrafon* and *Triavil* are combinations of **Amitriptyline** and **Perphenazine.** (See the generic drug **Perphenazine** for its specific ototoxic properties.)

[2] *Limbitrol* is a combination of **Amitriptyline** and **Chlordiazepoxide**. (See the generic drug **Chlordiazepoxide** for its specific ototoxic properties.)

[3] There is a report of a change in the ability to perceive tones.[123]

[4] Nystagmus may be a symptom of **Amitriptyline** overdose (CPS).

I have an anecdotal report in my files of a woman who has "screaming tinnitus" whenever she takes **Amitriptyline**. Her tinnitus changes in both sounds and pitch. She also hears different sounds in each ear, sometimes more than one at a time.

In another anecdotal report in my files, a man began taking **Amitriptyline** which resulted in severe tinnitus. When he stopped taking the drug, he joyfully reported that 12 days later his tinnitus went away.

Also in my files, a lady reported annoying tinnitus occurring when her doctor put her on double her previous dose of **Amitriptyline**.

[5] In yet another anecdotal report in my files, a man reported distorted hearing, hearing loss and tinnitus after taking his first 40 mg. dose of **Amitriptyline** after being on it for 2 weeks at 10, 20 and 30 mg.

[6] I have an anecdotal report in my files of a woman who had been taking **Amitriptyline** for 12 years. She writes, "Lately I have noticed several symptoms which I'm sure are linked to this drug. I suddenly started getting chronic ear infections in my left ear at least once every couple of months, and this has continued for the last few years. I also have terrible tinnitus, worse in the problem left ear, and what I believe is hyperacusis. I find watching the television even at low volumes causes my ears to have a full feeling and my tinnitus to increase quite severely".

See Chapter 4 "Are You at Risk?" for further information on this drug.

Amlodipine

Pronunciation guide: am-LOE-dih-peen

Drug classification: CALCIUM-CHANNEL-BLOCKING DRUGS (CALCIUM BLOCKERS) (see section 20.8.16 in Table 14-1)

Brand names: *Caduet* [1], *Exforge* [2], *Exforge HCT* [3], *Lotrel* [4], *Norvasc*

Ototoxic effects:
    Cochlear:
        Tinnitus: 0.1-2% (CPS, PDR)
    Vestibular:
        Ataxia: <0.1% (CPS, PDR)
        Dizziness: 1.1-4.5% [<2.9% above placebo results] (CPS, PDR)
        Vertigo: 0.1-2% (CPS, PDR)
    Outer/Middle Ear:
        Earache/ear pain: (PDR)

Risk assessment: Class 2

Notes:

[1] *Caduet* is a combination of **Amlodipine** and **Atorvastatin**. (See the generic drug **Atorvastatin** for its specific ototoxic properties.)

[2] *Exforge* is a combination of **Amlodipine** and **Valsartan**. (See the generic drug **Valsartan** for its specific ototoxic properties.)

[3] *Exforge HCT* is a combination of **Amlodipine, Valsartan and Hydrochlorothiazide**. (See the generic drugs **Valsartan** and **Hydrochlorothiazide** for their specific ototoxic properties.)

[4] *Lotrel* is a combination of **Amlodipine** and **Benazepril**. (See the generic drug **Benazepril** for its specific ototoxic properties.)

Caution: Eating grapefruit or drinking grapefruit juice during the time you are taking this drug may make the listed side effects worse than shown here. Taking **Amlodipine** with grapefruit juice can increase the potency of **Amlodipine** up to 16%.

See Chapter 11, "Grapefruit Juice and Ototoxic Drugs" for further information on this drug.

Ammonul   (see **Sodium phenylacetate**)

Amobarbital

Pronunciation guide: am-oh-BAR-bi-tal

Drug classification: BARBITURATES (see section 60.12.4 in Table 14-1)

Brand names: *Amytal*

Ototoxic effects:
  Vestibular:
      Dizziness: (CPS, Med)
      Vertigo: (CPS)

Risk assessment: Class 1

Amoebriz   (see **Mebendazole**)

Amonafide (Nafidimide)

Pronunciation guide: ah-MON-ah-fide (nah-FIH-dih-mide)

Drug classification: ANTI-NEOPLASTICS (ANTI-CANCER DRUGS) (see section 14 in Table 14-1)

Brand names: *Quinamed*

Ototoxic effects:
  Cochlear:
      Tinnitus: 1-10% [1] (San, She)
  Vestibular:
      Dizziness: 1-10% [1]

Risk assessment: Class 2

Notes:

  [1] Can cause tinnitus and dizziness.[124]

Amoxapine

Pronunciation guide: ah-MOX-ah-peen

Drug classification: TRICYCLIC ANTI-DEPRESSANTS (see section 60.1.8 in Table 14-1)

Brand names: *Asendin*

Ototoxic effects:
    Cochlear:
        Tinnitus: <1% (CPS, PDR)
    Vestibular:
        Ataxia: >1% (PDR)
        Dizziness: >1% (CPS, PDR)

Risk assessment: Class 1

Amphotec   (see **Amphotericin B**)

Amphotericin B

Pronunciation guide: am-foe-TER-ih-sin

Drug classification: ANTI-FUNGAL ANTIBIOTICS (see section 7.10 in Table 14-1)

Brand names: *Abelcet, AmBisome, Amphotec, Fungizone*

Ototoxic effects:
    Cochlear:
        Hearing loss: (CPS, PDR)
        Tinnitus: 1-5% (DFC, PDR)
    Vestibular:
        Dizziness: 7-10.3% (CPS, PDR)
        Vertigo, transient: (CPS, PDR)
    Unspecified/General Ear Conditions:
        Ear disorder: (DFC, PDR)

Risk assessment: Class 2

Notes:

    See Chapter 4 "Are You at Risk?" for further information on this drug.

Ampicillin

Pronunciation guide: am-pih-SILL-in

Drug classification: PENICILLINS (see section 7.4.40 in Table 14-1)

Brand names: *Ampicin*

Ototoxic effects:
    Unspecified/General Ear Conditions:
        Ototoxicity: (CPS)

Risk assessment: Class 1 (Class 4 in high doses)

Notes:

    Ampicillin may be ototoxic when given intravenously in very high doses (CPS).

    See Chapter 4 "Are You at Risk?" for further information on this drug.

Ampicin (see **Ampicillin**)

Ampigen SB (see **Sultamicillin**)

Ampyrone (see **Aminopyrine**)

Amrix (see **Cyclobenzaprine**)

Amtolmetin

Pronunciation guide: am-TOLE-met-in

Drug classification: ACETIC ACIDS (see section 1.1.1 in Table 14-1)

Brand names: *Artromed, Eufans*

Ototoxic effects:
　　Cochlear:
　　　　Tinnitus: (She)

Risk assessment: Class 1

Amytal (see **Amobarbital**)

Anacin (see **Acetylsalicylic acid**)

Anafranil (see **Clomipramine**)

Anagrelide

Pronunciation guide: a-NAG-re-lied

Drug classification: PLATELET INHIBITOR DRUGS (see section 36.24 in Table 14-1)

Brand names: *Agrylin*

Ototoxic effects:
　　Cochlear:
　　　　Tinnitus: 1-5% (CPS, PDR)
　　Vestibular:
　　　　Dizziness: 14.5-15.4% (CPS, PDR)
　　Unspecified/General Ear Conditions:
　　　　Ear disorder: (CPS)

Risk assessment: Class 2

Anaprox (see **Naproxen**)

Ancobon (see **Flucytosine**)

Andante (see **Bunazosin**)

Androcur　(see **Cyproterone**)

Androderm　(see **Testosterone**)

AndroGel　(see **Testosterone**)

Anexate　(see **Flumazenil**)

Angeliq　(see **Estradiol**)

Anistreplase

Pronunciation guide: an-EYE-strep-lace

Drug classification: Coagulation drugs (see section 36.16 in Table 14-1)

Brand names: *Eminase*

Ototoxic effects:
　　Vestibular:
　　　　Dizziness: <10% (CPS, PDR)
　　　　Vertigo: <10% (CPS, PDR)

Risk assessment: Class 1

Ansaid　(see **Flurbiprofen**)

Antabuse　(see **Disulfiram**)

Antihelmycin　(see **Hygromycin B**)

Antihemophilic factor

Pronunciation guide: an-tee-hee-moe-FILL-ik FAK-tor

Drug classification: Anti-fibrinolytic drugs (see section 36.4 in Table 14-1)

Brand names: *Helixate*, *Kogenate*

Ototoxic effects:
　　Vestibular:
　　　　Dizziness: (NDH, PDR)
　　Outer/Middle Ear:
　　　　Otitis media: (PDR)

Risk assessment: Class 1

Antipyrine　(see **Benzocaine**)

Antivert　(see **Meclizine**)

Antizol   (see **Fomepizole**)

Antrypol   (see **Suramin**)

Anzemet   (see **Dolasetron**)

APAP   (see **Acetaminophen**)

Aplenzin   (see **Bupropion**)

Apo-Acebutolol   (see **Acebutolol**)

Apo-Amiloride   (see **Amiloride**)

Apo-Beclomethasone   (see **Beclomethasone**)

Apo-Bromocriptine   (see **Bromocriptine**)

Apo-Butorphanol   (see **Butorphanol**)

Apo-Carvedilol   (see **Carvedilol**)

Apo-Cetirizine   (see **Cetirizine**)

Apo-Clorazepate   (see **Clorazepate**)

Apo-Diltiaz   (see **Diltiazem**)

Apo-Divalproex   (see **Divalproex**)

Apo-Doxepin   (see **Doxepin**)

Apo-Etodolac   (see **Etodolac**)

Apo-Fenofibrate   (see **Fenofibrate**)

Apo-Feno-Micro   (see **Fenofibrate**)

Apo-Flavoxate   (see **Flavoxate**)

Apo-Floctafenine   (see **Floctafenine**)

Apo-Fluconazole   (see **Fluconazole**)

Apo-Fluvoxamine   (see **Fluvoxamine**)

Apo-Gabapentin   (see **Gabapentin**)

Apo-Hydro   (see **Hydrochlorothiazide**)

Apo-Indapamide   (see **Indapamide**)

Apo-Keto   (see **Ketoprofen**)

Apo-Ketorolac   (see **Ketorolac**)

Apo-Lisinopril   (see **Lisinopril**)

Apo-Loratadine   (see **Loratadine**)

Apo-Lovastatin   (see **Lovastatin**)

Apo-Mefenamic   (see **Mefenamic acid**)

Apo-Methazolamide   (see **Methazolamide**)

Apo-Midazolam   (see **Midazolam**)

Apo-Misoprostol   (see **Misoprostol**)

Apo-Moclobemide   (see **Moclobemide**)

Apo-Nabumetone   (see **Nabumetone**)

Apo-Norflox   (see **Norfloxacin**)

Apo-Nortriptyline   (see **Nortriptyline**)

Apo-Oxaprozin   (see **Oxaprozin**)

Apo-Phenylbutazone   (see **Phenylbutazone**)

Apo-Pimozide   (see **Pimozide**)

Apo-Prazo   (see **Prazosin**)

Apo-Selegiline   (see **Selegiline**)

Apo-Sotalol   (see **Sotalol**)

Apo-Temazepam   (see **Temazepam**)

Apo-Tenoxicam   (see **Tenoxicam**)

Apo-Timol   (see **Timolol**)

Apo-Trimethoprim   (see **Trimethoprim**)

Apo-Valproic   (see **Valproic acid**)

Aprepitant (and Fosaprepitant)

Pronunciation guide: ah-PRE-pit-ant, foss-ah-PRE-pit-ant

Drug classification: P/Neurokinin-1 receptor antagonists (see section 34.1.1 in Table 14-1)

Brand names: *Emend, Emend IV*

Ototoxic effects:
    Cochlear:
        Tinnitus: 3.7% [same as placebo results] (NDH, PDR)
    Vestibular:
        Dizziness: 6.6% [2.2% above placebo results] (NDH, PDR)

Risk assessment: Class 1

Notes:

    Fosaprepitant is very similar to **Aprepitant** and has essentially the same ototoxic side effects.

Apresazide   (see **Hydrochlorothiazide**)

Apri 28   (see **Ethinyl estradiol**)

Apriso   (see **Mesalamine**)

Aralen   (see **Chloroquine**)

Arava   (see **Leflunomide**)

Arcoxia   (see **Etoricoxib**)

Arelix   (see **Piretanide**)

Arestin   (see **Minocycline**)

Aricept   (see **Donepezil**)

Aripiprazole

Pronunciation guide: air-eh-PIP rah-zole

Drug classification: Antipsychotic drugs (see section 60.8 in Table 14-1)

Brand names: *Abilify*

Ototoxic effects:
    Cochlear:
        Hearing loss: 0.01-0.1% (PDR)
        Tinnitus: 0.1-1% (DFC, PDR)
    Vestibular:
        Ataxia: 0.1-1% (NDH, PDR)
        Dizziness: 8-11% [3% above placebo results] (NDH, PDR)
        Vertigo: 0.1-1% (DFC, PDR)
    Outer/Middle Ear:
        Earache/ear pain: 0.1-1% (NDH, PDR)
        Otitis externa: (DFC)
        Otitis media: (DFC)

Risk assessment: Class 2

Aristocort   (see **Triamcinolone**)

Arixtra   (see **Fondaparinux**)

Arranon   (see **Nelarabine**)

Arsenic trioxide

Pronunciation guide: ARE-seh-nik try-OX-side

Drug classification: ANTI-NEOPLASTICS (ANTI-CANCER DRUGS) (see section 14 in Table 14-1)

Brand names: *Trisenox*

Ototoxic effects:
    Cochlear:
        Tinnitus: 5% (DFC, PDR)
    Vestibular:
        Dizziness: 23% (DFC, PDR)
    Outer/Middle Ear:
        Earache/ear pain: 8% (DFC, PDR)

Risk assessment: Class 2

Artemether/Lumefantrine

Pronunciation guide: are-TEM-eth-er/loo-MEH-fan-treen

Drug classification: ANTI-MALARIAL DRUGS (see section 7.14.8 in Table 14-1)

Brand names: *Coartem*

Ototoxic effects:
    Cochlear:
        Tinnitus: <3% (PDR)

Vestibular:
    Ataxia: <3% (PDR)
    Dizziness: 4-39% (PDR)
    Nystagmus: <3% (PDR)
    Vertigo: 3% (PDR)

Risk assessment: Class 2

Arthrotec   (see **Diclofenac**)

Articaine

Pronunciation guide: ARE-tih-kane

Drug classification: AMIDES (see section 4.1 in Table 14-1)

Brand names: *Septocaine, Ultracaine*[1]

Ototoxic effects: [125]
    Cochlear:
        Tinnitus: (CPS)
    Vestibular:
        Dizziness: <1% (CPS, DFC)
    Outer/Middle Ear:
        Earache/ear pain: <1% (DFC)

Risk assessment: Class 1

Notes:

[1] *Ultracaine* is a combination of **Articaine** and Epinephrine. (**Articaine** is the ototoxic agent.)

Artromed   (see **Amtolmetin**

ASA   (see **Acetylsalicylic acid**)

Asacol   (see **Mesalamine**)

Asasantine   (see **Acetylsalicylic acid**)

Ascarel   (see **Pyrantel**)

Ascriptin   (see **Acetylsalicylic acid**)

Asendin   (see **Amoxapine**)

Asmanex   (see **Mometasone**)

Asmavent   (see **Albuterol**)

Aspirin   (see **Acetylsalicylic acid**)

Aspirin Backache   (see **Acetylsalicylic acid**)

Astelin   (see **Azelastine**)

Astromicin

Pronunciation guide: ass-troe-MY-sin

Drug classification: AMINOGLYCOSIDES (see section 7.4.1 in Table 14-1)

Brand names: *Fortimicin* [1]

Ototoxic effects:
  Cochlear:
    Hearing loss: 0.1% [2]
    Tinnitus: 0.1% [2]
  Vestibular:
    Vertigo: 0.1% [2]
    Vestibular disorder: [2]
  Outer/Middle Ear:
    Feeling of fullness in ears: [2]

Risk assessment: Class 4

Notes:

[1] *Fortimicin* is a fairly new drug. Actually, there is a whole family of them numbered A, B, C, D and KE. These drugs are used in Japan and the Far East.

[2] As reported by the manufacturer, Kyowa Hakko Kogyo Co, Ltd. in Japan.[126]

You should not take **Astromicin** if you have had previous ear damage from taking any AMINOGLYCOSIDE antibiotic, or if you already have a hearing loss. You are at greater risk if you are elderly, if you have kidney problems, if you take this drug for a long time or if you take it in high doses. If any of these risk factors apply to you, you should have your hearing tested. Note that AMINOGLYCOSIDE-induced hearing loss normally begins in the high frequencies and works its way down the hearing frequency spectrum[127].

See Chapter 9, "Aminoglycoside Antibiotics are the Ototoxic 'Bad boys'" for further information on this drug.

Atabrine   (see **Quinacrine**)

Atacand   (see **Candesartan**)

Atacand HCT   (see **Candesartan**)

Atacand Plus   (see **Candesartan**)

Atarax   (see **Hydroxyzine**)

Atenolol

Pronunciation guide: ah-TEN-oh-lawl

Drug classification: Beta-adrenergic-blocking drugs (Beta-Blockers) (see section 20.8.12 in Table 14-1)

Brand names: *Tenolin, Tenoretic* [1], *Tenormin, Venapulse*

Ototoxic effects:
 Cochlear:
  Hearing loss: [128]
  Tinnitus: <1% (CPS)
 Vestibular:
  Ataxia: <1% (CPS)
  Dizziness: 3-13% [<7% above placebo results] (CPS, PDR)
  Vertigo: 2% [1.5-1.8% above placebo results] (CPS, PDR)

Risk assessment: Class 2

Notes:

[1] *Tenoretic* is a combination of **Atenolol** and **Chlorthalidone**. (See the generic drug **Chlorthalidone** for its specific ototoxic properties.)

I have an anecdotal report in my files from Peggy who was prescribed **Atenolol** and suffered serious ototoxic side effects. She writes, "In Dec. of 1998, I was given **Atenolol** for some little irregular heart-beats. Within a few days, my perfectly normal ears started to give me all kinds of noise, roaring and muffledness. Within a week, I woke up one morning stone cold deaf in one ear. I had pressure in my head so extreme that it felt like my head was stuffed with bricks. The hearing in my other ear was distorted".

I have another anecdotal report in my files of a man who got tinnitus "some years after my doctor prescribed **Atenolol** for high blood pressure. I have thought for some time that this beta blocker may be the cause of my tinnitus".

In a somewhat similar anecdotal report in my files a lady reported, "I started taking **Atenolol** in November, 2005. In June, 2007, out of nowhere, tinnitus kicked in and never left. I am suspicious that it may be the beta blocker".

In another anecdotal report in my files, a man explained, "In November I was given **Atenolol**. By December I had vertigo, right ear hearing loss, short term memory problems and anxiety issues. In January I switched to **Metoprolol** and the **Atenolol** side effects went away except of the hearing loss".

In yet another anecdotal report in my files a man wrote, "I have been taking **Atenolol** for about 3 years with no ill effects—until recently. Over the last month the hearing in my left ear has come and gone—and now there is a constant ringing. I went off the **Atenolol** for about a week and my hearing returned about 75%. I took another 25 mg. of **Atenolol** this morning and the ringing returned along with the associated loss of hearing in my left ear".

See Chapter 5 "Here's How the System Works" for further information on this drug.

Ativan   (see **Lorazepam**)

Atomoxetine

Pronunciation guide: at-oh-MOX-ah-teen

Drug classification: SELECTIVE NOREPINEPHRINE REUPTAKE INHIBITORS (see section 60.1.24 in Table 14-1)

Brand names: *Strattera*

Ototoxic effects:
   Vestibular:
      Dizziness: 5-6% [<4% above placebo results] (AHF, CPS)
   Outer/Middle Ear:
      Otitis: 1-3% [<2% above placebo results] (CPS, NDH)

Risk assessment: Class 1

Atorvastatin

Pronunciation guide: ah-TOR-vah-stah-tin

Drug classification: HMG-COA REDUCTASE INHIBITORS (see section 20.12.8 in Table 14-1)

Brand names: *Lipitor*

Ototoxic effects:
   Cochlear:
      Hearing loss: <2% (PDR)
      Tinnitus: <2% (CPS, PDR)
   Vestibular:
      Dizziness: >2% (CPS, PDR)

Risk assessment: Class 2

Notes:

   Caution: Eating grapefruit or drinking grapefruit juice during the time you are taking this drug may make the listed side effects worse than shown here. In fact, taking **Atorvastatin** with grapefruit juice can increase the potency of **Atorvastatin** by as much as 250%.

   See Chapter 2 "Ototoxic Drugs—What Are They?" and Chapter 11, "Grapefruit Juice and Ototoxic Drugs" for further information on this drug.

Atovaquone/Proguanil

Pronunciation guide: ah-TOE-vah-kwon pro-goo-AH-nil

Drug classification: ANTI-PROTOZOALS (see section 7.14 in Table 14-1)

Brand names: *Malarone, Mepron*

Ototoxic effects:
    Cochlear:
        Tinnitus: (She)
    Vestibular:
        Dizziness: 3-8% (CPS, PDR)

Risk assessment: Class 1

Atretol   (see **Carbamazepine**)

Atriance   (see **Nelarabine**)

Atripla   (see **Efavirenz**)

Atrohist   (see **Pyrilamine**)

Atrohist Plus   (see **Phenylpropanolamine**)

AtroPen   (see **Atropine**)

Atropine

Pronunciation guide: AH-troe-peen

Drug classification: ANTI-CHOLINERGIC DRUGS (see section 17.1 in Table 14-1)

Brand names: *AtroPen, Atropisol, Donnatal* [1]

Ototoxic effects:
    Vestibular:
        Ataxia: <10% (NDH)
        Dizziness: >10% (NDH, PDR)
    Unspecified/General Ear Conditions:
        Ototoxicity: [129] (San)

Risk assessment: Class 2

Notes:

[1] *Donnatal* is a combination of **Atropine**, **Hyoscyamine**, **Phenobarbital** and **Scopolamine**. (See the generic drugs **Hyoscyamine**, **Phenobarbital** and **Scopolamine** for their specific ototoxic properties.)

See Chapter 7, "We 'Hear' With Our Eyes" for further information on this drug.

Atropisol   (see **Atropine**)

Atrovent   (see **Ipratropium**)

Attenuvax   (see **Measles vaccine**)

Auranofin

Pronunciation guide: ore-RAIN-oh-fin

Drug classification: ANTI-RHEUMATIC DRUGS (see section 46.1 in Table 14-1)

Brand names: *Ridaura*

Ototoxic effects:
　　Cochlear:
　　　　Tinnitus: (Ka8)
　　Unspecified/General Ear Conditions:
　　　　Ototoxicity: [130] (Str)

Risk assessment: Class 2

Aureomycin　(see **Chlortetracycline**)

Avalide　(see **Irbesartan**)

Avamys　(see **Fluticasone**)

Avapro　(see **Irbesartan**)

Avastin　(see **Bevacizumab**)

AVC　(see **Sulfanilamide**)

Avelox　(see **Moxifloxacin**)

Aventyl　(see **Nortriptyline**)

Avinza　(see **Morphine**)

Avlosulfon　(see **Dapsone**)

Avonex　(see **Interferon beta-1a**)

Axert　(see **Almotriptan**)

Axocet　(see **Butalbital**)

Azactam　(see **Aztreonam**)

Azapropazone

Pronunciation guide: ah-zah-PROE-pah-zone

Drug classification: NON-STEROIDAL ANTI-INFLAMMATORY DRUGS (NSAIDs) (see section 1.1 in Table 14-1)

Brand names: *Rheumox*

Ototoxic effects:
    Cochlear:
        Tinnitus: (BNF)
    Vestibular:
        Dizziness: (BNF)
        Vertigo: [131] (BNF)

Risk assessment: Class 1

Azatadine

Pronunciation guide: ah-ZAH-tah-deen

Drug classification: H$_1$ RECEPTOR ANTAGONISTS (see section 10.1 in Table 14-1)

Brand names: *Optimine*, *Rynatan*[1], *Trinalin*[1]

Ototoxic effects:
    Cochlear:
        Tinnitus: (CPS, PDR)
    Vestibular:
        Ataxia: (CPS)
        Dizziness: (CPS, PDR)
        Labyrinthitis, acute: (PDR)
        Vertigo: (PDR)

Risk assessment: Class 1

Notes:

[1] *Rynatan* and *Trinalin* are both combinations of **Azatadine** and **Pseudoephedrine**. (See the generic drug **Pseudoephedrine** for its specific ototoxic properties.)

Azelastine

Pronunciation guide: ah-ZELL-ass-teen

Drug classification: H$_1$ RECEPTOR ANTAGONISTS (see section 10.1 in Table 14-1)

Brand names: *Astelin*

Ototoxic effects:
    Vestibular:
        Dizziness: 2% [0.6% above placebo results] (PDR)
        Vertigo: <2% (PDR)

Risk assessment: Class 1

Azilect   (see **Rasagiline**)

Azithromycin

Pronunciation guide: ay-zih-throw-MYE-sin

Drug classification: MACROLIDE ANTIBIOTICS (see section 7.4.32 in Table 14-1)

Brand names: *Zithromax*

Ototoxic effects:
    Cochlear:
        Hearing loss: <1% (CPS, PDR)
        Tinnitus: <1% (CPS, PDR)
    Vestibular:
        Dizziness: 1.1-3.9% (CPS, PDR)
        Vertigo: <1% (CPS, PDR)

Risk assessment: Class 3

Notes:

Hearing loss may be reversible (CP2).

Hearing loss has been reported in some people receiving long-term high-dose **Azithromycin** (i. e., 500 – 600 mg. daily for up to 9 months) (AHF).

Hearing loss generally develops within 1½ to 20 weeks. If the hearing loss is temporary, hearing typically returns within 5 weeks after stopping the **Azithromycin** (AHF).

I have an anecdotal report in my files of a woman with a serious infection who was given mega-doses of **Azithromycin** (8 grams per day). As a result, her hearing dropped to almost nothing.

I have another anecdotal report in my files of a woman who got tinnitus after taking **Azithromycin** for a sinus infection.

I have an anecdotal report in my files of a man who had an eye infection and used eye drops containing **Azithromycin** for 3 weeks. He was told to rub the solution on the top and bottom eyelids of his right eye. During this time, he noticed a blocked feeling in his right ear. Subsequent hearing testing revealed he had lost the hearing in his right ear.

Azosemide

Pronunciation guide: ah-ZOE-seh-mide

Drug classification: DIURETICS—LOOP (see section 30.5.4 in Table 14-1)

Brand names: —

Ototoxic effects:
    Unspecified/General Ear Conditions:
        Ototoxicity: [132]

Risk assessment: Not enough information to rate

AZT (see **Zidovudine**)

Aztreonam

Pronunciation guide: AZ-tree-oh-nam

Drug classification: MONOBACTAMS (see section 7.4.12.4 in Table 14-1)

Brand names: *Azactam*

Ototoxic effects:
 Cochlear:
  Hearing loss: (AHF)
  Tinnitus: <1% (DFC, PDR)
 Vestibular:
  Dizziness: <1% (DFC, PDR)
  Vertigo: <1% (DFC, PDR)

Risk assessment: Class 2

Azulfidine   (see **Sulfasalazine**)

B6   (see **Pyridoxine**)

Bacampicillin

Pronunciation guide: bak-am-pih-SILL-in

Drug classification: PENICILLINS (see section 7.4.40 in Table 14-1)

Brand names: *Penglobe*

Ototoxic effects:
 Vestibular:
  Dizziness: 0.6-1.2% (CPS)
  Vertigo: 0.6-1.2% (CPS)

Risk assessment: Class 1

Baciguent   (see **Bacitracin**)

Bacitracin

Pronunciation guide: bass-ih-TRAY-sin

Drug classification: BACITRACINS (see section 7.4.4 in Table 14-1)

Brand names: *Baciguent*

Ototoxic effects:
 Unspecified/General Ear Conditions:
  Ototoxicity: (Str)

Risk assessment: Not enough information to rate

Backache Caplets (see **Magnesium salicylate**)

Baclofen

Pronunciation guide: BAK-low-fen

Drug classification: SKELETAL MUSCLE RELAXANTS (see section 53.36 in Table 14-1)

Brand names: *Lioresal*

Ototoxic effects:
    Cochlear:
        Tinnitus: 0.1-1% (CPS, PDR)
    Vestibular:
        Ataxia: <10% (CPS, PDR)
        Dizziness: 1.7-15% (CPS, PDR)
        Nystagmus: <10% (CPS, PDR)
        Vertigo: (AHF)

Risk assessment: Class 2

Bactrim (see **Trimethoprim**)

Bactroban (see **Mupirocin**)

Balamine (see **Dextromethorphan**)

Balsalazide (see **Mesalamine**)

Banzel (see **Rufinamide**)

Baycol (see **Cerivastatin**)

Bayer Aspirin (see **Acetylsalicylic acid**)

BC Powder (see **Acetylsalicylic acid**)

BCNU (see **Carmustine**)

Beclomethasone

Pronunciation guide: beh-kloe-METH-ah-sone

Drug classification: GLUCOCORTICOIDS (see section 40.1.4 in Table 14-1)

Brand names: *Apo-Beclomethasone, Beconase, Vancenase, Vanceril*

Ototoxic effects:
    Cochlear:
        Tinnitus: 2-3% [placebo 0] (PDR)

Vestibular:
> Dizziness: (CPS)

Outer/Middle Ear:
> Burning/stinging: (CPS)
> Earache/ear pain: <2% (DFC, PDR)

Risk assessment: Class 2

Notes:

Stinging and burning have been reported rarely when the medication has gained access to the middle ear (CPS).

Beconase   (see **Beclomethasone**)

Benadryl   (see **Diphenhydramine**)

Benazepril

Pronunciation guide: ben-AH-zah-pril

Drug classification: ANGIOTENSIN-CONVERTING ENZYME (ACE) INHIBITORS (see section 20.8.8 in Table 14-1)

Brand names: *Lotensin, Lotensin HCT* [1]

Ototoxic effects:
Cochlear:
> Tinnitus: 0.3-1% (CPS, PDR)

Vestibular:
> Dizziness: 3.6-6.3% [1.2-2.9% above placebo results] (CPS, PDR)
> Vertigo: 1.1%-1.5% [0.6% above placebo results] (CPS, PDR)

Risk assessment: Class 2

Notes:

[1]*Lotensin HCT* is a combination of **Benazepril** and **Hydrochlorothiazide**. (See the generic drug **Hydrochlorothiazide** for its specific ototoxic properties.)

Bendectin   (see **Doxylamine**)

Bendroflumethiazide

Pronunciation guide: ben-droh-floo-meh-THYE-ah-zide

Drug classification: THIAZIDE-RELATED DIURETIC (see section 30.5.12 in Table 14-1)

Brand names: *Corzide* [1]

Ototoxic effects:
Cochlear:
> Hearing loss: (Eps)
> Tinnitus: (Eps)

Vestibular:
    Dizziness: (DFC, PDR)
    Vertigo: (DFC, PDR)

Risk assessment: Class 2

Notes:

[1] *Corzide* is a combination of **Nadolol** and **Bendroflumethiazide**. (See the generic drug **Nadolol** for its specific ototoxic properties.)

BenGay   (see **Methyl salicylate**)

Benicar   (see **Olmesartan**)

Benoral   (see **Benorilate**)

Benorilate (Benorylate)

Pronunciation guide: be-NOE-ril-ate

Drug classification: SALICYLATES (see section 1.1.16 in Table 14-1)

Brand names: *Benoral*

Ototoxic effects:
    Cochlear:
        Tinnitus: [133] (Ka7, San)
    Vestibular:
        Dizziness: (BNF)
        Vertigo: (BNF)
    Unspecified/General Ear Conditions:
        Ototoxicity: (San)

Risk assessment: Class 2

Benorylate   (see **Benorilate**)

Benoxaprofen

Pronunciation guide: ben-OX-ah-pro-fen

Drug classification: PROPIONIC ACIDS (see section 1.1.13 in Table 14-1)

Brand names: *Oraflex*

Ototoxic effects:
    Cochlear:
        Tinnitus: (Ka7)

Risk assessment: Class 1

Benzalkonium

Pronunciation guide: ben-zal-KOE-nee-um

Drug classification: ANTI-BACTERIAL DRUGS (see section 7.4 in Table 14-1)

Brand names: *Ony-clear*, *Zephiran*

Ototoxic effects:
Unspecified/General Ear Conditions:
Ototoxicity: (Str)

Risk assessment: Not enough information to rate

Notes:

Ototoxicity can occur when **Benzalkonium** is applied to the middle ear in concentrations of only 0.1%.[134]

Benzethonium

Pronunciation guide: ben-zeth-OH-nee-um

Drug classification: ANTI-BACTERIAL DRUGS (see section 7.4 in Table 14-1)

Brand names: *Buro-sol*, *VoSoL*

Ototoxic effects:
Unspecified/General Ear Conditions:
Ototoxicity: [135]

Risk assessment: Not enough information to rate

Benzocaine

Pronunciation guide: BEN-zoe-kane

Drug classification: ESTERS (see section 4.4 in Table 14-1)

Brand names: *Americaine Otic*, *Tympagesic* [1]

Ototoxic effects:
Outer/Middle Ear:
Burning/stinging: (PDR, USP)

Risk assessment: Class 1

Notes:

[1] *Tympagesic* is a combination of **Phenylephrine**, **Antipyrine** and **Benzocaine**. (See the generic drug **Phenylephrine** for its specific ototoxic properties.) **Antipyrine** (an-tee-PYE-reen) in combination with **Benzocaine** may cause tinnitus (PDR). **Antipyrine** is an ANALGESIC DRUG (PAINKILLER) (see section 1 in Table 14-1).

Benzocaine can cause burning, stinging, redness, oozing sores in ear canal if you have contact dermatitis and/or hypersensitivity to **Benzocaine** (PDR, USP).

Benztropine

Pronunciation guide: BENZ-troe-peen

Drug classification: ANTI-CHOLINERGIC DRUGS (see section 17.1 in Table 14-1)

Brand names: *Cogentin*

Ototoxic effects:
    Vestibular:
        Ataxia: (CPS)
        Dizziness: (CPS)

Risk assessment: Class 1

Bepridil

Pronunciation guide: BEH-prih-dill

Drug classification: CALCIUM-CHANNEL-BLOCKING DRUGS (CALCIUM BLOCKERS) (see section 20.8.16 in Table 14-1)

Brand names: *Vascor*

Ototoxic effects:
    Cochlear:
        Tinnitus: 6.5% [4.2% above placebo results] (PDR)
    Vestibular:
        Dizziness: 11.6-27.2% [4.8-20.4% above placebo results] (PDR)
        Vertigo: 0.5-2% (PDR)

Risk assessment: Class 2

Betagan   (see **Levobunolol**)

Betaloc   (see **Metoprolol**)

Betamethasone

Pronunciation guide: bay-tah-METH-ah-sone

Drug classification: GLUCOCORTICOIDS (see section 40.1.4 in Table 14-1)

Brand names: *Betnesol, Celestone, Diproderm, Lotrisone*[1], *Repetabs, Soluspan*

Ototoxic effects:
    Vestibular:
        Dizziness: (Med)
        Vertigo: (CPS, PDR)
    Outer/Middle Ear:
        Burning/stinging: (CPS)

Risk assessment: Class 1

Notes:

[1] *Lotrisone* is a combination of **Betamethasone** and Clotrimazole. (**Betamethasone** is the ototoxic agent.)

Burning and stinging have been reported rarely when the medication has gained access to the middle ear (CPS).

See Chapter 12, "Potpourri" for further information on this drug.

Betapace　(see **Sotalol**)

Betasept　(see **Chlorhexidine**)

Betaseron　(see **Interferon beta-1b**)

Betaxolol

Pronunciation guide: beh-TAX-oh-lawl

Drugclassification:Beta-adrenergic-blockingdrugs(Beta-Blockers)(seesection20.8.12 in Table 14-1)

Brand names: *Betoptic, Kerlone*

Ototoxic effects:
　Cochlear:
　　Hearing loss: <2% (PDR)
　　Tinnitus: <2% (PDR)
　Vestibular:
　　Ataxia: <2% (PDR)
　　Dizziness: (AHF, PDR)
　　Labyrinthine disorder: <2% (PDR)
　　Vertigo: <2% (AHF, PDR)
　Outer/Middle Ear:
　　Earache/ear pain: <2% (PDR)

Risk assessment: Class 3

Notes:

I have an anecdotal report in my files of a man who explained: "I've had tinnitus for 18 years. I recently did a 2-month trial of **Betaxolol**, and as I got into the higher doses, noticed that sometimes my constant hissing tinnitus would sharpen into a shrill, louder, more noxious whistle. I then discovered that tinnitus is a rare adverse effect of **Betaxolol**, and tapered off as fast as I could (2 weeks). I've been off 6 weeks now, yet this new obnoxious form of tinnitus has continued.

Betaxon　(see **Levobetaxolol**)

Betimol　(see **Timolol**)

Betnesol   (see **Betamethasone**)

Betoptic   (see **Betaxolol**)

Bevacizumab

Pronunciation guide: beh-vah-SIZZ-yoo-mab

Drug classification: MONOCLONAL ANTIBODIES (see section 7.17.8 in Table 14-1)

Brand names: *Avastin*

Ototoxic effects:
    Cochlear:
        Hearing loss: (CPS)
    Vestibular:
        Ataxia: (CPS, NDH)
        Dizziness: 19-26% [<6% above placebo results] (NDH, PDR)
        Vertigo: (CPS)
    Outer/Middle Ear:
        Otitis media: (CPS)
    Unspecified/General Ear Conditions:
        Ear disorder: (CPS)

Risk assessment: Class 2

Bexarotene

Pronunciation guide: bex-AIR-oh-teen

Drug classification: RETINOIDS (see section 14.28 in Table 14-1)

Brand names: *Targretin*

Ototoxic effects:
    Vestibular:
        Ataxia: <10% (DFC, PDR)
        Dizziness: <10% (DFC, PDR)
    Outer/Middle Ear:
        Earache/ear pain: <10% (DFC, PDR)
        Otitis externa: <10% (DFC, PDR)

Risk assessment: Class 2

Bextra   (see **Valdecoxib**)

Bexxar   (see **Tositumomab**)

Bezafibrate

Pronunciation guide: bee-zah-FYE-brate

Drug classification: FIBRATES (see section 20.12.4 in Table 14-1)

Brand names: *Bezalip*

Ototoxic effects:
    Vestibular:
        Dizziness: 2.3% [placebo 0] (BNF, CPS)
        Vertigo: (BNF)

Risk assessment: Class 1

Bezalip   (see **Bezafibrate**)

Biarison   (see **Proquazone**)

Biaxin   (see **Clarithromycin**)

Bicillin   (see **Penicillin**)

Biltricide   (see **Praziquantel**)

Biphentin   (see **Methylphenidate**)

Biquin   (see **Quinidine**)

Bismuth subsalicylate

Pronunciation guide: BIS-muth sub-sah-LISS-ah-late

Drug classification: SALICYLATES (see section 1.1.16 in Table 14-1)

Brand names: *Helidac* [1], *Maalox Total Stomach Relief*, *Pepto-Bismol Original*

Ototoxic effects:
    Cochlear:
        Hearing loss: (PDR-N)
        Tinnitus: (PDR-N, She)
    Vestibular:
        Ataxia: <1% (PDR)
        Dizziness: <1% (PDR)
        Vertigo: <1% (PDR)

Risk assessment: Class 2

Notes:

[1] *Helidac* is a combination of **Bismuth subsalicylate**, **Metronidazole** and **Tetracycline**. (See the generic drugs **Metronidazole** and **Tetracycline** for their specific ototoxic properties.)

Ringing in the ears (tinnitus) may occur if *Pepto-Bismol* is taken with other SALICYLATES such as **Aspirin** (PDR-H).

High doses may cause salicylism (NDH). Symptoms of salicylism include nausea, vomiting, headaches, tinnitus, hearing loss, mental dullness, confusion, quickened pulse and increased respirations.

Bisoprolol

Pronunciation guide: bis-OH-proe-lol

Drug classification: BETA-ADRENERGIC-BLOCKING DRUGS (BETA-BLOCKERS) (see section 20.8.12 in Table 14-1)

Brand names: *Monocor, Zebeta, Ziac* [1]

Ototoxic effects:
    Cochlear:
        Hearing loss: (PDR)
        Tinnitus: 1.4% (CPS, PDR)
    Vestibular:
        Dizziness: 3.2-5.1% [1.4-3.4% above placebo results] (CPS, PDR)
        Vertigo: (CPS, PDR)
    Outer/Middle Ear:
        Earache/ear pain: 1.2-2.1% (CPS, PDR)

Risk assessment: Class 2

Notes:

[1] *Ziac* is a combination of **Bisoprolol** and **Hydrochlorothiazide**. (See the generic drug **Hydrochlorothiazide** for its specific ototoxic properties.)

Bitolterol

Pronunciation guide: by-TALL-ter-ohl

Drug classification: BRONCHODILATORS—BETA ADRENERGIC AGONISTS (see section 63.4 in Table 14-1)

Brand names: *Tornalate*

Ototoxic effects:
    Vestibular:
        Dizziness: 4% (PDR)
        Vertigo: <1% (PDR)

Risk assessment: Class 1

Bivax   (see **Rubella & mumps vaccine**)

Blenoxane   (see **Bleomycin**)

Bleomycin

Pronunciation guide: blee-oh-MYE-sin

Drug classification: ANTI-NEOPLASTICS (ANTI-CANCER DRUGS) (see section 14 in Table 14-1)

Brand names: *Blenoxane*

Ototoxic effects:
    Cochlear:
        Hearing loss: (Eps)
        Tinnitus: (Ka8)
    Unspecified/General Ear Conditions:
        Ototoxicity: [136] (Ka8)

Risk assessment: Class 2

Blocadren   (see **Timolol**)

Bonamine   (see **Meclizine**)

Bondormin   (see **Brotizolam**)

Bonine   (see **Meclizine**)

Boniva   (see **Ibandronate**)

Bortezomib

Pronunciation guide: bore-TEZ-uh-mib

Drug classification: ANTI-NEOPLASTICS (ANTI-CANCER DRUGS) (see section 14 in Table 14-1)

Brand names: *Velcade*

Ototoxic effects:
    Cochlear:
        Hearing loss: (AHF, PDR)
    Vestibular:
        Ataxia: (CPS, PDR)
        Dizziness: <1-23% (AHF, PDR)
        Vertigo: (DFC, PDR)

Risk assessment: Class 2

Notes:

    Hearing loss may be bilateral and permanent. One patient experienced severe permanent bilateral hearing loss after receiving 4 cycles of **Bortezomib** (AHF, PDR).

Bosentan

Pronunciation guide: bow-SEN-tan

Drug classification: ENDOTHELIN RECEPTOR ANTAGONISTS (see section 20.8.24 in Table 14-1)

Brand names: *Tracleer*

Ototoxic effects:
    Cochlear:
        Tinnitus: <1% (CPS)
    Vestibular:
        Vertigo: <1% (CPS)
    Outer/Middle Ear:
        Otitis: 2% (CPS)

Risk assessment: Class 1

Botox   (see **Botulinum Toxin Type A**)

Botox Cosmetic   (see **Botulinum Toxin Type A**)

Botulinum Toxin Type A (Clostridium botulinum Toxin Type A)

Pronunciation guide: BOT-yoo-line-um TOKS-in

Drug classification: NEUROTOXINS (see section 53.40 in Table 14-1)

Brand names: *Botox*, *Botox Cosmetic*, *Xeomin*

Ototoxic effects:
    Cochlear:
        Hearing loss: [1] (CPS, PDR)
        Tinnitus: (CPS, PDR)
    Vestibular:
        Dizziness: 5% [3% above placebo results] (CPS, PDR)
        Nystagmus: (DFC, PDR)
        Vertigo: (CPS, PDR)

Risk assessment: Class 3

Notes:

[1] In my files, I have three anecdotal reports of hearing loss resulting from *Botox* injections. In addition to profound hearing loss in one ear, one man also experienced tinnitus and vertigo.

Botulinum Toxin Type B

Pronunciation guide: BOT-yoo-line-um TOKS-in

Drug classification: NEUROTOXINS (see section 53.40 in Table 14-1)

Brand names: *Myobloc*

Ototoxic effects:
    Cochlear:
        Tinnitus: >2% (DFC, PDR)
    Vestibular:
        Dizziness: 3-6% [1-4% above placebo results] (DFC, PDR)
        Vertigo: >2% (DFC, PDR)

Outer/Middle Ear:
    Otitis media: <2% (DFC, PDR)

Risk assessment: Class 2

Brethaire   (see **Terbutaline**)

Bretylate   (see **Bretylium**)

Bretylium

Pronunciation guide: bre-TIE-lee-um

Drug classification: ANTI-ARRHYTHMICS (HEART RHYTHM REGULATORS) (see section 20.4 in Table 14-1)

Brand names: *Bretylate*

Ototoxic effects:
    Vestibular:
        Dizziness: 0.7% (CPS, DFC)
        Vertigo: 0.7% (CPS, DFC)

Risk assessment: Class 1

Brevicon   (see **Ethinyl estradiol**)

Brexidol   (see **Piroxicam**)

Bricanyl   (see **Terbutaline**)

Bromocriptine

Pronunciation guide: broe-moe-KRIP-teen

Drug classification: DOPAMINE RECEPTOR AGONISTS (see section 53.16.1 in Table 14-1)

Brand names: *Apo-Bromocriptine, Parlodel*

Ototoxic effects:
    Cochlear:
        Hearing loss: (Eps)
    Vestibular:
        Ataxia: (CPS, PDR)
        Dizziness: 8-17% (DFC, PDR)
        Vertigo: <1% (CPS, PDR)

Risk assessment: Class 2

Bromodiphenhydramine   (see **Diphenhydramine**)

Bromopheniramine   (see **Dextromethorphan**)

Brotizolam

Pronunciation guide: broe-TIE-zoh-lam

Drug classification: BENZODIAZEPINES (see section 60.12.8 in Table 14-1)

Brand names: Bondormin

Ototoxic effects:
 Cochlear:
  Tinnitus: (San, She)
 Vestibular:
  Ataxia: [137]
 Unspecified/General Ear Conditions:
  Ototoxicity: (San)

Risk assessment: Class 2

Notes:

 See Chapter 10 "Beware of Benzodiazepines—Don't Let This Nasty Time-Bomb Ambush You and Your Ears" for further information on this drug.

Budesonide

Pronunciation guide: byoo-DESS-oh-nide

Drug classification: GLUCOCORTICOIDS (see section 40.1.4 in Table 14-1)

Brand names: *Entocort EC*, *Pulmicort*, *Rhinocort*, *Symbicort*

Ototoxic effects:
 Vestibular:
  Dizziness: 7% [2% above placebo results] (CPS, PDR)
  Vertigo: <5% (NDH, PDR)
 Outer/Middle Ear:
  Earache/ear pain: 1-3% (AHF, PDR)
  Otitis: 2-5% [<1% above placebo results] (NDH, PDR)
  Otitis externa: 1-3% (AHF, PDR)
  Otitis media: 1.3-12% (<1% above placebo results) (AHF, PDR)

Risk assessment: Class 2

Bufferin   (see **Acetylsalicylic acid**)

Bumetanide

Pronunciation guide: byoo-MET-ah-nide

Drug classification: DIURETICS—LOOP (see section 30.5.4 in Table 14-1)

Brand names: *Bumex, Burinex*

Ototoxic effects:
    Cochlear:
        Hearing loss: 0.5-1.1% (CPS, PDR)
        Tinnitus: (BNF)
    Vestibular:
        Dizziness: 1.1% (CPS, PDR)
        Vertigo: 0.1% (CPS, PDR)
    Outer/Middle Ear:
        Earache/ear pain: 0.1% (CPS, PDR)

Risk assessment: Class 2

Notes:

Hearing loss is often temporary when **Bumetanide** is used alone and there are no other contributing factors.[138]

See Chapter 4 "Are You at Risk?" for further information on this drug.

Bumex (see **Bumetanide**)

Bunazosin

Pronunciation guide: bun-ah-ZOE-sin

Drug classification: ALPHA ADRENERGIC BLOCKING DRUGS (see section 20.8.1 in Table 14-1)

Brand names: *Andante, Dentantol*

Ototoxic effects:
    Cochlear:
        Tinnitus: (San, She)
    Unspecified/General Ear Conditions:
        Ototoxicity: (San)

Risk assessment: Class 2

Buphenyl (see **Sodium phenylbutyrate**)

Bupivacaine

Pronunciation guide: byoo-PIV-ah-kane

Drug classification: AMIDES (see section 4.1 in Table 14-1)

Brand names: *Marcaine, Sensorcaine*

Ototoxic effects:
    Cochlear:
        Hyperacusis: (CPS)
        Tinnitus: (CPS, PDR)
    Vestibular:
        Dizziness: (CPS, PDR)

Risk assessment: Class 1

Buprenex   (see **Buprenorphine**)

Buprenorphine

Pronunciation guide: byoo-pree-NOR-feen

Drug classification: OPIATE AGONIST DRUGS (see section 1.4.1 in Table 14-1)

Brand names: *Buprenex, Suboxone* [1]*, Temgesic*

Ototoxic effects:
    Cochlear:
        Hearing loss: <1% (CPS)
        Tinnitus: <1% (CPS, PDR)
    Vestibular:
        Ataxia: (AHF, PDR)
        Dizziness/vertigo: 5-10% (CPS, PDR)
        Vertigo: <1% (CPS, NDH)
    Outer/Middle Ear:
        Earache/ear pain: 1.7% (CPS)
        Otitis media: <1% (CPS)
    Unspecified/General Ear Conditions:
        Ear disorder: <1% (CPS)

Risk assessment: Class 2

Notes:

[1] *Suboxone* is a combination of **Buprenorphine** and Naloxone. (**Buprenorphine** is the ototoxic agent.)

Bupropion

Pronunciation guide: byoo-PROE-pee-on

Drug classification: DOPAMINE REUPTAKE INHIBITORS (see section 53.24 in Table 14-1)

Brand names: *Aplenzin, Wellbutrin, Wellbutrin SR, Wellbutrin XL, Zyban*

Ototoxic effects:
    Cochlear:
        Auditory disorder: 5.3% [2.1% above placebo results] (NDH, PDR)
        Hearing loss: <1% (CPS, PDR)
        Hyperacusis: <1% (CPS)
        Tinnitus: 1-6% [1-4% above placebo results] (CPS, PDR)
    Vestibular:
        Ataxia: >1% (CPS, PDR)
        Dizziness: 7-22.3% [1-7% above placebo results] (CPS, PDR)
        Vertigo: 0.1-1% (CPS, PDR)

Outer/Middle Ear:
Earache/ear pain: <1% (CPS)

Risk assessment: Class 4

Notes:

I have an anecdotal report in my files of a lady that began taking **Bupropion** for her depression. It solved her depression, but she noticed her hearing dropping. The longer she was on the **Bupropion**, the worse her hearing got. She stopped taking the **Bupropion** because as she said, "I'd rather be depressed than totally deaf!" To be sure it was the **Bupropion** that was causing the hearing loss, she tried taking it again, and by that same evening she had more hearing loss, so she quit taking it altogether.

I have an anecdotal report in my files of a person who explained, "I have had horrific tinnitus since starting *Wellbutrin*. I am on a lower dose now and the tinnitus is manageable".

I have an anecdotal report in my files of a lady who "developed an abrupt onset of severe ataxia and tinnitus upon beginning **Bupropion**. The gait disturbance [ataxia] has been debilitating".

I have another anecdotal report in my files of a lady that was taking **Bupropion** for 2 years when one day she woke up with tinnitus and hearing loss in one ear. She is now experiencing hearing loss in her other ear also.

Burinex   (see **Bumetanide**)

Buro-sol   (see **Benzethonium**)

Buserelin

Pronunciation guide: BYOO-ser-rel-in

Drug classification: Anti-neoplastics (Anti-cancer drugs) (see section 14 in Table 14-1)

Brand names: *Suprefact, Suprefact Depot*

Ototoxic effects:
Cochlear:
Hearing disorder: <1% (BNF, CPS)
Tinnitus: <1% (CPS)
Vestibular:
Dizziness: 1-15% (BNF, CPS)
Vertigo: <1% (CPS)
Outer/Middle Ear:
Earache/ear pain: <1% (CPS)
Unspecified/General Ear Conditions:
Ear disorder: <5% (CPS)

Risk assessment: Class 2

BuSpar   (see **Buspirone**)

Buspirone

Pronunciation guide: byoo-SPYE-rone

Drug classification: Anxiolytics (see section 60.12.1 in Table 14-1)

Brand names: *BuSpar*

Ototoxic effects:
 Cochlear:
  Auditory disorder: <0.1% (CPS, PDR)
  Hyperacusis: 0.1-1% (CPS, PDR)
  Tinnitus: >1% (CPS, PDR)
 Vestibular:
  Ataxia: (CPS, PDR)
  Dizziness: 12% [9% above placebo results] (CPS, PDR)

Risk assessment: Class 2

Busulfan

Pronunciation guide: byoo-SUL-fan

Drug classification: Alkylating drugs (see section 14.1 in Table 14-1)

Brand names: *Myleran*

Ototoxic effects:
 Vestibular:
  Dizziness: >10% (AHF, NDH)
 Unspecified/General Ear Conditions:
  Ear disorder: (AHF, NDH)

Risk assessment: Class 1

Notes:
 See Chapter 7, "We 'Hear' With Our Eyes" for further information on this drug.

Butabarbital

Pronunciation guide: byoo-ta-BAR-bi-tal

Drug classification: Barbiturates (see section 60.12.4 in Table 14-1)

Brand names: *Secbutabarbital*

Ototoxic effects:
 Vestibular:
  Dizziness: (CPS [1], Med)
  Vertigo: (CPS [1])

Risk assessment: Class 1

Notes:

[1] General comment for this class of drugs—not necessarily specific to this drug.

Butalbital

Pronunciation guide: byoo-TAL-bi-tal

Drug classification: BARBITURATES (see section 60.12.4 in Table 14-1)

Brand names: *Axocet* [1], *Esgic-Plus* [2], *Fioricet* [2], *Fioricet with Codeine* [3], *Fiorinal, Fiorinal-C* [4], *Fiorinal with Codeine* [4], *Phrenilin* [1], *Phrenilin Forte* [1], *Phrenilin with Caffeine and Codeine* [5], *Sedapap* [1]

Ototoxic effects:
Cochlear:
Tinnitus: 0.1-1% (CPS, PDR)
Vestibular:
Dizziness: 2.6% (CPS, PDR)
Vertigo: 0.1-1% (PDR)
Outer/Middle Ear:
Earache/ear pain: 0.1-1% (PDR)

Risk assessment: Class 2

Notes:

[1] *Axocet, Phrenilin* and *Sedapap* are combinations of **Butalbital** and **Acetaminophen**. (The the generic drug **Acetaminophen** for its ototoxic properties.)

[2] *Esgic-Plus* and *Fioricet* are combinations of **Butalbital, Acetaminophen & Caffeine**. (See the generic drugs **Acetaminophen** and **Caffeine** for their specific ototoxic properties.)

[3] *Fioricet with Codeine* is a combination of **Butalbital, Acetaminophen, Caffeine & Codeine**. (See the generic drugs **Acetaminophen, Caffeine** and **Codeine** for their specific ototoxic properties.)

[4] *Fiorinal-C* and *Fiorinal with Codeine* are combinations of **Butalbital, ASA (Aspirin), Caffeine & Codeine**. (See the generic drugs **ASA, Caffeine** and **Codeine** for their specific ototoxic properties.)

[5] *Phrenilin with Caffeine and Codeine* is a combination of **Butalbital, Acetaminophen, Caffeine & Codeine**. (See the generic drugs **Acetaminophen, Caffeine** and **Codeine** for their specific ototoxic properties.)

Note that not every side effect shown above occurs with every drug combination.

Butorphanol

Pronunciation guide: byoo-TOR-fah-nole

Drug classification: OPIATE AGONIST/ANTAGONIST DRUGS (see section 1.4.4 in Table 14-1)

Brand names: *Apo-Butorphanol, Stadol, Stadol NS*

Ototoxic effects:
    Cochlear:
        Hearing loss: 6% (CPS)
        Hyperacusis: 0.1-1% (CPS)
        Tinnitus: 0.1-9% (CPS, PDR)
    Vestibular:
        Ataxia: 0.1-1% (CPS)
        Dizziness: 4.8-85% [<75% above placebo results] (CPS, PDR)
        Vertigo: 6-9% [5-8% above placebo results] (CPS, PDR)
    Outer/Middle Ear:
        Earache/ear pain: 0.1-3% (CPS, PDR)
    Unspecified/General Ear Conditions:
        Ear disorder: 6% (CPS)

Risk assessment: Class 4

Bystolic   (see **Nebivolol**)

Cabergoline

Pronunciation guide: kah-BER-go-leen

Drug classification: Dopamine receptor agonists (see section 53.16.1 in Table 14-1)

Brand names: *Dostinex*

Ototoxic effects:
    Vestibular:
        Dizziness: 15-17% [10% above placebo results] (CPS, PDR)
        Vertigo: 1-4% [placebo 0] (CPS, PDR)

Risk assessment: Class 1

Cadithro   (see **Roxithromycin**)

Caduet   (see **Amlodipine**)

Caelyx   (see **Doxorubicin**)

Cafergot   (see **Ergotamine**)

Caffedrine   (see **Caffeine**)

Caffeine

Pronunciation guide: kaf-FEEN

Drug classification: Psychostimulants (see section 60.20 in Table 14-1)

Brand names: *Caffedrine*

Ototoxic effects:
    Cochlear:
        Tinnitus: (AHF, DFC)
    Vestibular:
        Dizziness: (Med)
        Vertigo: (CPS)

Risk assessment: Class 1

Notes:

Caffeine can cause tinnitus or make your existing tinnitus worse.

Apart from prescription and non-prescription drugs, **Caffeine** is found in coffee, tea (see **Camellia sinensis** in the ototoxic herbals section), some soft drinks (colas) and chocolate. It has the same side effects in these as it does in prescription drugs.

See Chapter 11, "Grapefruit Juice and Ototoxic Drugs" for further information on this drug.

Calan   (see **Verapamil**)

Calcitonin

Pronunciation guide: kal-sih-TOE-nin

Drug classification: PARATHYROID DRUGS (see section 40.42.4 in Table 14-1)

Brand names: *Miacalcin*

Ototoxic effects:
    Cochlear:
        Hearing loss: <1% (DFC, PDR)
        Tinnitus: <1% (DFC, PDR)
    Vestibular:
        Dizziness: 1-3% (DFC, PDR)
        Vertigo: <1% (DFC, PDR)
    Outer/Middle Ear:
        Earache/ear pain: <1% (DFC, PDR)
        Feeling of fullness in ears: (CPS)

Risk assessment: Class 2

Calcitriol   (see **Ergocalciferal**)

Caldine   (see **Lacidipine**)

Campath   (see **Alemtuzumab**)

Campral   (see **Acamprosate**)

Camptosar   (see **Irinotecan**)

Canakinumab

Pronunciation guide: kah-nah-KIN-yoo-mab

Drug classification: MONOCLONAL ANTIBODIES (see section 7.17.8 in Table 14-1)

Brand names: *Ilaris*

Ototoxic effects:
    Vestibular:
        Vertigo: 9-14% (PDR)

Risk assessment: Class 2

Candesartan

Pronunciation guide: kan-dah-SAR-tan

Drug classification: ANGIOTENSIN-2-RECEPTOR ANTAGONISTS (see section 20.8.4 in Table 14-1)

Brand names: *Atacand, Atacand HCT* [1], *Atacand Plus* [1]

Ototoxic effects:
    Cochlear:
        Tinnitus: 0.5-1% (CPS, PDR)
    Vestibular:
        Dizziness: 2.5-4% [0.2-1.7% above placebo results] (CPS, PDR)
        Vertigo: 0.5-1% (CPS, PDR)
    Outer/Middle Ear:
        Otitis: <1% (CPS)

Risk assessment: Class 2

Notes:

[1] *Atacand HCT* and *Atacand Plus* are combinations of **Candesartan** and **Hydrochlorothiazide**. (See the generic drug **Hydrochlorothiazide** for its specific ototoxic properties.)

Capastat (see **Capreomycin**)

Capecitabine

Pronunciation guide: kap-ah-SEET-ah-been

Drug classification: ANTI-METABOLITE DRUGS (see section 14.8 in Table 14-1)

Brand names: *Xeloda*

Ototoxic effects:
    Cochlear:
        Hearing loss: (CPS)

Vestibular:
- Ataxia: 0.4-0.5% (CPS, PDR)
- Equilibrium disorder: (AHF, PDR)
- Dizziness: 0.2-12% (CPS, PDR)
- Vertigo: (CPS, PDR)

Outer/Middle Ear:
- Earache/ear pain: (CPS)
- Ears blocked: (CPS)
- Otitis media: (CPS)

Risk assessment: Class 2

Capoten   (see **Captopril**)

Capozide   (see **Captopril**)

Capozide 25   (see **Captopril**)

Capreomycin

Pronunciation guide: kap-ree-oh-MY-sin

Drug classification: AMINOGLYCOSIDES (see section 7.4.1 in Table 14-1)

Brand names: *Capastat*

Ototoxic effects:
Cochlear:
- Hearing loss: 11% (AHF, PDR)
- Tinnitus: (AHF, PDR)

Vestibular:
- Dizziness: (AHF, PDR)
- Vertigo: (AHF, PDR)

Risk assessment: Class 4

Notes:

11% of the 722 people in one **Capreomycin** study had a slight hearing loss of 5-10 dB at 4,000 to 8,000 Hz. Only 3% had a more obvious hearing loss (PDR).

Hearing loss can be permanent, but tends to be temporary. Also, hearing loss tends not to get worse after you stop taking **Capreomycin**.[139] (PDR)

You are particularly at risk for hearing loss if you have kidney problems, if you are dehydrated or if you are taking any other ototoxic drugs at the same time as you take **Capreomycin** (PDR).

See Chapter 4 "Are You at Risk?" and Chapter 9, "Aminoglycoside Antibiotics are the Ototoxic 'Bad boys'" for further information on this drug.

Captopril

Pronunciation guide: KAP-toe-pril

Drug classification: Angiotensin-converting enzyme (ACE) inhibitors (see section 20.8.8 in Table 14-1)

Brand names: *Capoten, Capozide, Capozide 25*[1]

Ototoxic effects:
    Cochlear:
        Tinnitus:[2]
    Vestibular:
        Ataxia: 0.1-0.2% (CPS, PDR)
        Dizziness: 0.5-2% [same as placebo] (CPS, PDR)

Risk assessment: Class 1

Notes:

[1] *Capozide 25* is a combination of **Captopril** and **Hydrochlorothiazide**. (See the generic drug **Hydrochlorothiazide** for its specific ototoxic properties.)

[2] Medications that commonly cause tinnitus or make tinnitus worse include ACE inhibitors, such as **Captopril** (*Capoten*).[140]

Carac   (see **Fluorouracil**)

Carafate   (see **Sucralfate**)

Carbamazepine

Pronunciation guide: kar-bah-MAZ-eh-peen

Drug classification: Anti-convulsant drugs (see section 53.12 in Table 14-1)

Brand names: *Atretol, Carbatrol, Equetro, Taro-Carbamazepine, Tegretol*

Ototoxic effects:
    Cochlear:
        Auditory hallucinations: 0.01-0.1% (CPS)
        Hearing loss:[1] 0.01-0.1% (CPS)
        Hyperacusis: 0.01-0.1% (CPS, PDR)
        Tinnitus: 0.01-0.1% (CPS, PDR)
    Vestibular:
        Ataxia: 5-15% [placebo 0] (CPS, PDR)
        Dizziness: 10-44% [<32% above placebo results] (NDH, PDR)
        Nystagmus: 0.1-1% (CPS, PDR)
        Vertigo: >10% (CPS, NDH)
    Outer/Middle Ear:
        Earache/ear pain: <5% (PDR)

Risk assessment: Class 3

Notes:

[1] One patient experienced temporary hearing loss (30–40 dB) for about three weeks following an overdose (36 g) of **Carbamazepine**.[141]

I have an anecdotal report in my files of a man that used *Tegretol* for 10 years. He believes that it caused his loss of hearing in the high frequencies in his left ear. He also suffers from mild to moderate tinnitus, and more recently, fullness in that ear.

Caution: Eating grapefruit or drinking grapefruit juice during the time you are taking this drug may make the listed side effects worse than shown here. In fact, taking **Carbamazepine** with grapefruit juice can increase the potency of **Carbamazepine** by as much as 40%.

See Chapter 7, "We 'Hear' With Our Eyes" and Chapter 11, "Grapefruit Juice and Ototoxic Drugs" for further information on this drug.

Carbatrol   (see **Carbamazepine**)

Carbex   (see **Selegiline**)

Carbidopa   (see **Levodopa**)

Carbocaine   (see **Mepivacaine**)

Carbolith   (see **Lithium**)

Carboplatin

Pronunciation guide: KAR-boh-plah-tin

Drug classification: ALKYLATING DRUGS (see section 14.1 in Table 14-1)

Brand names: *Paraplatin*

Ototoxic effects:
   Cochlear:
      Hearing loss: 12-15% (CPS)
      Tinnitus: 1% (CPS)
   Vestibular:
      Dizziness: (NDH)
   Unspecified/General Ear Conditions:
      Ototoxicity: 12-13% (BNF, PDR)

Risk assessment: Class 5

Notes:

15% of the people taking **Carboplatin** now have a hearing loss in the frequencies between 4,000 and 8,000 Hz (CPS).

The ototoxic effects of **Carboplatin** affect up to 50% of the people taking it.[142]

If you already have a hearing loss as a result of taking **Cisplatin**, your hearing loss may worsen even more if you take **Carboplatin** in the future (CPS).

Carboprost

Pronunciation guide: KAR-boe-prost

Drug classification: PROSTAGLANDIN ANALOGS (see section 40.36.1 in Table 14-1)

Brand names: *Hemabate* [1]

Ototoxic effects:
    Cochlear:
        Tinnitus: (DFC)
    Vestibular:
        Dizziness: (DFC)
        Vertigo: (DFC)

Risk assessment: Class 1

Notes:

[1] *Hemabate* is a combination of **Carboprost** and Tromethamine. (**Carboprost** is the ototoxic agent.)

Carbromal

Pronunciation guide: kar-BROE-mall

Drug classification: ANXIOLYTICS, SEDATIVES & HYPNOTICS (see section 60.12 in Table 14-1)

Brand names: *Pelidorm*

Ototoxic effects:
    Vestibular:
        Ataxia: (NTP)

Risk assessment: Class 1

Cardene   (see **Nicardipine**)

Cardif   (see **Nitrendipine**)

Cardioquin   (see **Quinidine**)

Cardizem   (see **Diltiazem**)

Cardovar BD   (see **Trimazosin**)

Cardura   (see **Doxazosin**)

Cardura-2   (see **Doxazosin**)

Carisoprodol

Pronunciation guide: kar-eye-soe-PROE-dol

Drug classification: SKELETAL MUSCLE RELAXANTS (see section 53.36 in Table 14-1)

Brand names: *Soma, Soma Compound*[1], *Soma Compound with Codeine*[2]

Ototoxic effects:
Vestibular:
Ataxia: (CPS, PDR)
Dizziness: (CPS, PDR)
Nystagmus:[3] (AHF)
Vertigo: (CPS, PDR)

Risk assessment: Class 1

Notes:

[1] *Soma Compound* is a combination of **Carisoprodol** and **Acetylsalicylic acid** (**Aspirin**). (See the generic drug **Acetylsalicylic acid** for its specific ototoxic properties.)

[2] *Soma Compound with Codeine* is a combination of **Carisoprodol**, **Acetylsalicylic acid** (**Aspirin**) and **Codeine**. (See the generic drugs **Acetylsalicylic acid** and **Codeine** for their specific ototoxic properties.)

[3] Acute overdose can cause nystagmus (AHF).

See Chapter 7, "We 'Hear' With Our Eyes" for further information on this drug.

Carmustine (BCNU)

Pronunciation guide: kar-MUS-teen

Drug classification: ALKYLATING DRUGS (see section 14.1 in Table 14-1)

Brand names: *Gliadel*

Ototoxic effects:
Vestibular:
Ataxia: 2-6% [<4% above placebo results] (NDH, PDR)
Dizziness: 2-5% [~same as placebo] (AHF, PDR)
Equilibrium disorder: (AHF)

Risk assessment: Class 1

Carnitor   (see **Levocarnitine**)

Carprofen

Pronunciation guide: kar-PROE-fen

Drug classification: PROPIONIC ACIDS (see section 1.1.13 in Table 14-1)

Brand names: *Rimadyl*

Ototoxic effects:
  Cochlear:
    Tinnitus: (Ka7)
  Vestibular:
    Ataxia: [1]
    Vestibular dysfunction: [1]

Risk assessment: Class 1

Notes:

[1] Dogs given **Carprofen** may exhibit signs of ataxia and vestibular dysfunction.[143]

In North America, this drug is currently only used in veterinary medicine.

Carteolol

Pronunciation guide: KAR-tee-oh-lawl

Drugclassification:Beta-adrenergic-blockingdrugs(Beta-Blockers)(seesection20.8.12 in Table 14-1)

Brand names: *Cartrol*

Ototoxic effects:
  Cochlear:
    Tinnitus: >1% (PDR)
  Vestibular:
    Dizziness: >1% (NDH, PDR)

Risk assessment: Class 1

Cartia XT   (see **Diltiazem**)

Cartrol   (see **Carteolol**)

Carvedilol

Pronunciation guide: kar-VAH-dah-lawl

Drugclassification:Beta-adrenergic-blockingdrugs(Beta-Blockers)(seesection20.8.12 in Table 14-1)

Brand names: *Apo-Carvedilol, Coreg*

Ototoxic effects:
  Cochlear:
    Hearing loss: <0.1% (CPS, PDR)
    Tinnitus: 0.1-1% (CPS, PDR)
  Vestibular:
    Dizziness: 2.0-32.4% [0.6-13.2% above placebo results] (CPS, PDR)
    Vertigo: 1.4% [0.3% above placebo results] (CPS, PDR)

Risk assessment: Class 2

Notes:

Caution: Eating grapefruit or drinking grapefruit juice during the time you are taking this drug may make the listed side effects worse than shown here. In fact, taking **Carvedilol** with grapefruit juice can increase the potency of **Carvedilol** by as much as 16%.

See Chapter 11, "Grapefruit Juice and Ototoxic Drugs" for further information on this drug.

Cataflam   (see **Diclofenac**)

Catapres   (see **Clonidine**)

CCNU   (see **Lomustine**)

CDDP   (see **Cisplatin**)

Ceclor   (see **Cefaclor**)

CeeNU   (see **Lomustine**)

Cefaclor

Pronunciation guide: SEF-ah-klor

Drug classification: CEPHALOSPORINS (see section 7.4.8 in Table 14-1)

Brand names: *Ceclor*

Ototoxic effects:
    Vestibular:
        Dizziness: 0.1-1% (CPS, PDR)
        Vertigo: (PDR)
    Outer/Middle Ear:
        Earache/ear pain: 0.1-1% (PDR)
        Otitis media: 0.1-1% (PDR)

Risk assessment: Class 1

Cefadroxil

Pronunciation guide: sef-ah-DROX-ill

Drug classification: CEPHALOSPORINS (see section 7.4.8 in Table 14-1)

Brand names: *Duricef*

Ototoxic effects:
    Vestibular:
        Dizziness: (CPS, NDH)
        Vertigo: (CPS)

Risk assessment: Class 1

Cefpodoxime

Pronunciation guide: SEF-pod-OX-eem

Drug classification: CEPHALOSPORINS (see section 7.4.8 in Table 14-1)

Brand names: *Vantin*

Ototoxic effects:
    Cochlear:
        Tinnitus: <1% (PDR)
    Vestibular:
        Dizziness: <1% (PDR)
        Vertigo: <1% (PDR)

Risk assessment: Class 1

Cefprozil

Pronunciation guide: sef-PRO-zil

Drug classification: CEPHALOSPORINS (see section 7.4.8 in Table 14-1)

Brand names: *Cefzil*

Ototoxic effects:
    Cochlear:
        Tinnitus: (AHF)
    Vestibular:
        Dizziness: 1% (CPS, PDR)
        Vestibular disorder: [1]

Risk assessment: Class 1

Notes:

    [1] In my files, I have an anecdotal report of a man who was left with "documented bilateral vestibular nerve damage" from taking **Cefprozil**.

Ceftin   (see **Cefuroxime**)

Ceftriaxone

Pronunciation guide: sef-try-AX-own

Drug classification: CEPHALOSPORINS (see section 7.4.8 in Table 14-1)

Brand names: *Rocephin*

Ototoxic effects:
    Cochlear:
        Tinnitus: [1]

Vestibular:

Ataxia: <0.1% (CPS)

Dizziness: 0.1-1% (CPS, NDH)

Risk assessment: Class 1

Notes:

[1] In my files, I have an anecdotal report of a man that was given an injection of **Ceftriaxone**. The result was loud tinnitus for about 4 hours before his tinnitus returned to its normal level.

Cefuroxime

Pronunciation guide: seh-fyoor-OX-eem

Drug classification: CEPHALOSPORINS (see section 7.4.8 in Table 14-1)

Brand names: *Ceftin, Kefurox, Zinacef*

Ototoxic effects:

Cochlear:

Hearing loss: (CPS, PDR)

Vestibular:

Dizziness: 0.1-2% (CPS, PDR)

Risk assessment: Class 2

Notes:

Resulting hearing loss may be mild to severe (PDR).

"Mild to severe hearing loss has been reported in a few pediatric patients receiving **Cefuroxime** for the treatment of meningitis" (AHF).

Cefzil   (see **Cefprozil**)

Celebrex   (see **Celecoxib**)

Celecoxib

Pronunciation guide: sell-ah-COX-ib

Drug classification: COX-2 INHIBITORS (see section 1.1.4 in Table 14-1)

Brand names: *Celebrex*

Ototoxic effects:

Cochlear:

Hearing loss: 0.1-1.9% (CPS, PDR)

Tinnitus: 0.1-1.9% (CPS, PDR)

Vestibular:

Ataxia: <0.1% (CPS, PDR)

Dizziness: 2% [0.3% above placebo results] (CPS, PDR)

Labyrinthitis: 0.1-1% (PDR)
Vertigo: 0.1-1.9% (CPS, PDR)
Outer/Middle Ear:
Earache/ear pain: 0.1-1.9% (CPS, PDR)
Otitis media: 0.1-1.9% (CPS, PDR)
Unspecified/General Ear Conditions:
Ear disorder: 0.1-1.9% (CPS, PDR)

Risk assessment: Class 3

Notes:

I have an anecdotal report in my files of a woman who takes **Celecoxib** for her arthritis. When she takes it, her tinnitus gets louder, but her arthritis problems improve. So she chooses the tinnitus over the arthritis pain.

Celectol   (see **Celiprolol**)

Celestone   (see **Betamethasone**)

Celexa   (see **Citalopram**)

Celiprolol

Pronunciation guide: SEE-lee-proe-lol

Drug classification: BETA-ADRENERGIC-BLOCKING DRUGS (BETA-BLOCKERS) (see section 20.8.12 in Table 14-1)

Brand names: *Celectol*

Ototoxic effects:
Cochlear:
Tinnitus: (Ka7)
Vestibular:
Dizziness: [144]

Risk assessment: Class 1

CellCept   (see **Mycophenolate**)

Celontin   (see **Methsuximide**)

Celsentri   (see **Maraviroc**)

Cenestin   (see **Estradiol**)

Centrax   (see **Prozepam**)

Centrimide   (see **Cetrimide**)

Cepastat   (see **Acetylsalicylic acid**)

Cephalexin

Pronunciation guide: sef-ah-LEX-in

Drug classification: CEPHALOSPORINS (see section 7.4.8 in Table 14-1)

Brand names: *Keflex*

Ototoxic effects:
    Cochlear:
        Hearing loss: (CPS)
        Tinnitus: (CPS)
    Vestibular:
        Dizziness: (CPS, PDR)
        Vertigo: (CPS)

Risk assessment: Class 2

Notes:

    Young children have ended up with hearing loss, tinnitus and/or vertigo after taking **Cephalexin** (CPS).

    I have an anecdotal report in my files of a man who had a drop in his hearing when he began taking **Cephalexin**. His hearing returned when he stopped taking it.

    I have another anecdotal report in my files of a woman who suffered total permanent hearing loss after taking a ten-day course of **Cephalexin**. She now has a cochlear implant. From her symptoms it appears she may have had an allergic reaction to this drug. As a result its ototoxic side effects were particularly severe on her hearing.

    See Chapter 7, "We 'Hear' With Our Eyes" for further information on this drug.

Cerebyx   (see **Fosphenytoin**)

Cerivastatin

Pronunciation guide: SIR-iv-ah-sta-tin

Drug classification: HMG-CoA REDUCTASE INHIBITORS (see section 20.12.8 in Table 14-1)

Brand names: *Baycol*

Ototoxic effects:
    Vestibular:
        Dizziness: 2.1% [same placebo] (CPS, PDR)
        Vertigo: (CPS, PDR)

Risk assessment: Class 1

Notes:

    Caution: Eating grapefruit or drinking grapefruit juice during the time you are taking this drug may make the listed side effects worse than shown here.

See Chapter 11, "Grapefruit Juice and Ototoxic Drugs" for further information on this drug.

Certolizumab

Pronunciation guide: SERT-oh-LIZ-yoo-mab

Drug classification: MONOCLONAL ANTIBODIES (see section 7.17.8 in Table 14-1)

Brand names: *Cimzia*

Ototoxic effects:
    Vestibular:
        Dizziness: 1.8% [0.9% above placebo results] (CPS)
        Vertigo: <1% (CPS)

Risk assessment: Class 1

Cerumenex   (see **Triethanolamine**)

Cesamet   (see **Nabilone**)

Cetirizine

Pronunciation guide: seh-TEER-ih-zeen

Drug classification: PIPERAZINE DERIVATIVES (see section 10.8.1 in Table 14-1)

Brand names: *Apo-Cetirizine, Reactine, Zyrtec*

Ototoxic effects:
    Cochlear:
        Hearing loss: <2% (CPS, PDR)
        Tinnitus: <2% (CPS, PDR)
    Vestibular:
        Ataxia: <2% (CPS, PDR)
        Dizziness: 2% [0.8% above placebo results] (CPS, PDR)
        Vertigo: <2% (CPS, PDR)
    Outer/Middle Ear:
        Earache/ear pain: <2% (CPS, PDR)
    Unspecified/General Ear Conditions:
        Ototoxicity: <2% (CPS, PDR)

Risk assessment: Class 2

Cetrimide (Centrimide)

Pronunciation guide: SEH-trih-mide (SEN-trih-mide)

Drug classification: ANTI-BACTERIAL DRUGS (see section 7.4 in Table 14-1)

Brand names: *Resdan Dandruff Treatment, Xylonor* [1], *Ziacaine* [1]

Ototoxic effects:
  Unspecified/General Ear Conditions:
    Ototoxicity: (Str)

Risk assessment: Not enough information to rate

Notes:

  [1] *Xylonor* and *Ziacaine* are combinations of **Cetrimide** and **Lidocaine**. (See the generic drug **Lidocaine** for its specific ototoxic properties.)

Cetuximab

Pronunciation guide: seh-TUX-eh-mab

Drug classification: MONOCLONAL ANTIBODIES (see section 7.17.8 in Table 14-1)

Brand names: *Erbitux*

Ototoxic effects:
  Cochlear:
    Hearing loss: 1-3% (CPS)
    Tinnitus: 1-2% (CPS)
  Vestibular:
    Ataxia: 1% (CPS)
    Dizziness: 8% (CPS)
    Vertigo: 1-2% (CPS)
  Outer/Middle Ear:
    Earache/ear pain: 8% (CPS)
    Otitis externa: 8% (CPS)
    Otitis media: 2% (CPS)
  Unspecified/General Ear Conditions:
    Ear disorder: 1-2% (CPS)

Risk assessment: Class 2

Cevimeline

Pronunciation guide: seh-vih-MEH-leen

Drug classification: CHOLINERGIC AGONIST DRUGS (see section 17.12.1 in Table 14-1)

Brand names: *Evoxac*

Ototoxic effects:
  Cochlear:
    Hearing loss: <1% (DFC, PDR)
    Tinnitus: <1% (DFC, PDR)
  Vestibular:
    Ataxia: <1% (PDR)
    Vertigo: 1-3% (NDH, PDR)

Outer/Middle Ear:
    Earache/ear pain: 1-3% (NDH, PDR)
    Otitis media: 1-3% (NDH, PDR)

Risk assessment: Class 2

Champix   (see **Varenicline**)

Chantix   (see **Varenicline**)

Chemet   (see **Succimer**)

Chibroxin   (see **Norfloxacin**)

Children's Tylenol   (see **Acetaminophen**)

Chirocaine   (see **Levobupivacaine**)

Chlophedianol

Pronunciation guide: kloe-feh-DIE-ah-nole

Drug classification: ANTITUSSIVE DRUGS (see section 63.1 in Table 14-1)

Brand names: *Ulone*

Ototoxic effects:
    Vestibular:
        Vertigo: (CPS)

Risk assessment: Class 1

Notes:

    You may experience vertigo when you take large doses of **Chlophedianol** (CPS).

Chloral hydrate

Pronunciation guide: KLOR-al HYE-drate

Drug classification: ANXIOLYTICS, SEDATIVES & HYPNOTICS (see section 60.12 in Table 14-1)

Brand names: *Welldorm*

Ototoxic effects:
    Vestibular:
        Ataxia: (AHF, CPS)
        Dizziness: (AHF, DFC)
        Vertigo: (AHF, CPS)
    Outer/Middle Ear:
        Middle ear pressure: (CPS)

Risk assessment: Class 1

Notes:

There are reports of increased middle ear pressure in some infants and children taking **Chloral hydrate** (CPS).

Chlorambucil

Pronunciation guide: klor-AM-byoo-sill

Drug classification: ALKYLATING DRUGS (see section 14.1 in Table 14-1)

Brand names: *Leukeran*

Ototoxic effects:
Vestibular:
Ataxia: (CPS, PDR)

Risk assessment: Class 1

Chloramphenicol

Pronunciation guide: klor-am-FEN-ih-kole

Drug classification: CHLORAMPHENICOLS (see section 7.4.16 in Table 14-1)

Brand names: *Chloromycetin, Diochloram, Pentamycetin*

Ototoxic effects:
Cochlear:
Hearing loss: [1]
Tinnitus: (Ka8)
Unspecified/General Ear Conditions:
Ototoxicity: [145, 146]

Risk assessment: Class 2

Notes:

[1] **Chloramphenicol** was first reported to be ototoxic in 1959 after a patient was given high systemic doses of this drug.[147]

Do not use an otic preparation containing **Chloramphenicol** if you have a perforated eardrum (CPS).

When **Chloramphenicol** is taken alone, it supposedly is not very ototoxic. However, the synergistic effect of noise while taking this drug shoots the risk way up![148]

See Chapter 7, "We 'Hear' With Our Eyes" and Chapter 8, "The Sinister Partnership Between Ototoxic Agents and Noise" for further information on this drug.

Chlordiazepoxide

Pronunciation guide: klor-dye-az-uh-POX-ide

Drug classification: BENZODIAZEPINES (see section 60.12.8 in Table 14-1)

Brand names: *Librium*

Ototoxic effects:
    Cochlear:
        Tinnitus: (She)
    Vestibular:
        Ataxia: (NDH, PDR)
        Vertigo: (BNF)

Risk assessment: Class 1

Notes:

    See Chapter 10 "Beware of Benzodiazepines—Don't Let This Nasty Time-Bomb Ambush You and Your Ears" for further information on this drug.

Chlorhexidine

Pronunciation guide: klor-HEX-ih-deen

Drug classification: ANTI-BACTERIAL DRUGS (see section 7.4 in Table 14-1)

Brand names: *Betasept, Hibiclens, Hibistat*

Ototoxic effects:
    Cochlear:
        Hearing loss: (AHF, PDR)

Risk assessment: normally Class 1 (can be Class 4—see note below)

Notes:

    Chlorhexidine can cause hearing loss and deafness if it penetrates the middle ear through a perforated eardrum (AHF, PDR).

    Chlorhexidine is used to sterilize the external ear before ear surgery. Surgeons need to be aware that if any gets absorbed into the middle ear, it can cause both severe sensorineural hearing loss and vestibular problems.[149, 150]

Chloromycetin   (see **Chloramphenicol**)

Chloroprocaine

Pronunciation guide: klor-oh-PROE-kane

Drug classification: ESTERS (see section 4.4 in Table 14-1)

Brand names: *Nesacaine*

Ototoxic effects:
    Cochlear:
        Tinnitus: (CPS, PDR)
    Vestibular:
        Dizziness: (CPS, PDR)

Risk assessment: Class 1

Chloroquine

Pronunciation guide: KLOR-oh-kwin

Drug classification: Anti-malarial drugs (see section 7.14.8 in Table 14-1)

Brand names: *Aralen*

Ototoxic effects:
Cochlear:
Hearing loss: (CPS, PDR)
Tinnitus: (CPS, PDR)
Vestibular:
Dizziness: (NDH)
Vertigo: (CPS, NDH)
Unspecified/General Ear Conditions:
Ototoxicity: (NDH)

Risk assessment: Class 4

Notes:

If you already have a hearing loss and take **Chloroquine**, you may end up with even worse hearing and/or tinnitus. Also, if you take **Chloroquine** for a long time and/or in high doses, you are at greater risk for a hearing loss (PDR).

Hearing loss, which is usually permanent, has been reported after prolonged therapy with high dosages of **Chloroquine**. Hearing loss may not show up until several weeks after **Chloroquine** therapy (AHF).

Hearing loss caused by **Chloroquine** may progress or even develop after you have stopped taking it (CPS).

Note: sometimes severe and permanent hearing losses occur after just taking small doses of **Chloroquine** (CPS).

I have an anecdotal report in my files of a man who took **Chloroquine** as a precautionary measure while travelling in South Africa. He took one pill a week for 4 weeks. Two hours after taking the 4th pill, he experienced "extremely increased tinnitus" and vertigo. The vertigo went away over a period of a few months, but he still has the increased tinnitus now some 10 years later. Fortunately, he did not experience any hearing loss.

See Chapter 7, "We 'Hear' With Our Eyes" and Chapter 9, "Aminoglycoside Antibiotics are the Ototoxic 'Bad boys'" for further information on this drug.

Chlorothiazide

Pronunciation guide: klor-oh-THYE-ah-zide

Drug classification: Diuretics—thiazide-related (see section 30.5.12 in Table 14-1)

Brand names: *Aldoclor*[1], *Diuril, Sodium Diuril, Supres*[1]

Ototoxic effects:
> Vestibular:
>> Dizziness: (CPS, PDR)
>> Vertigo: (CPS, PDR)

Risk assessment: Class 1

Notes:

> [1] *Aldoclor* and *Supres* are combinations of **Chlorothiazide** and **Methyldopa**. (See the generic drug **Methyldopa** for its specific ototoxic properties.)

Chlorpheniramine

Pronunciation guide: klor-fen-IR-ah-meen

Drug classification: H_1 RECEPTOR ANTAGONISTS (see section 10.1 in Table 14-1)

Brand names: *Aller-Chlor, Chlor-Trimeton, Chlor-Tripolon, Chlor-Tripolon Decongestant* [1],

De-Congestine [2]

Ototoxic effects:
> Cochlear:
>> Tinnitus: (BNF, CPS)
> Vestibular:
>> Ataxia: (CP2, CPS)
>> Dizziness: (CP2, CPS)
>> Labyrinthitis: (CPS)
>> Vertigo: (CPS)

Risk assessment: Class 2

Notes:

> [1] In the USA, *Chlor-Tripolon Decongestant* is a combination of **Chlorpheniramine** and **Phenylpropanolamine**. (See the generic drug **Phenylpropanolamine** for its specific ototoxic properties.) However in Canada, *Chlor-Tripolon Decongestant* is a combination of **Chlorpheniramine** and **Pseudoephedrine**. (See the generic drug **Pseudoephedrine** for its specific ototoxic properties.)

> [2] *De-Congestine* is a combination of **Chlorpheniramine** and **Pseudoephedrine**. (See the generic drug **Pseudoephedrine** for its specific ototoxic properties.)

There are numerous drug preparations that use **Chlorpheniramine** as one of their compounds. They are too numerous to mention here. As always, check the labels and then look up each drug listed to see its ototoxic properties.

Dexchlorpheniramine (dex-klor-fen-EAR-ah-meen) (*Polaramine*) is a form of **Chlorpheniramine** and likely has similar ototoxic properties. Suss lists it as being ototoxic (rarely).[151]

See Chapter 7, "We 'Hear' With Our Eyes" for further information on **Chlorpheniramine** and **Dexchlorpheniramine**.

Chlorphenoxamine

Pronunciation guide: klor-fen-OX-ah-meen

Drug classification: H₁ RECEPTOR ANTAGONISTS (see section 10.1 in Table 14-1)

Brand names: *Spirbon* [1], *Systral C* [2]

Ototoxic effects:
    Cochlear:
        Tinnitus: (San, She)

Risk assessment: Class 1

Notes:

[1] *Spirbon* is a combination of **Chlorphenoxamine**, Emetine and **Ephedrine**. (See the generic drug **Ephedrine** for its specific ototoxic properties.)

[2] *Systral C* is a combination of **Chlorphenoxamine** and **Caffeine**. (See the generic drug **Caffeine** for its specific ototoxic properties.)

Chlortetracycline

Pronunciation guide: klor-teh-trah-SYE-kleen

Drug classification: TETRACYCLINES (see section 7.4.60 in Table 14-1)

Brand names: *Aureomycin*

Ototoxic effects:
    Cochlear:
        Hearing loss: [1]

Risk assessment: Class 2

Notes:

Chlortetracycline is closely related to **Tetracycline** so you could expect it to have much the same ototoxic properties as **Tetracycline**. (See **Tetracycline** for its specific ototoxic properties.)

[1] I have an anecdotal report in my files of a man that took **Chlortetracycline** for a strep throat. The **Chlortetracycline** cured his strep throat, but left him with a permanent hearing loss.

See Chapter 7, "We 'Hear' With Our Eyes" for further information on **Chlortetracycline**.

Chlorthalidone

Pronunciation guide: KLOR-thal-ih-doan

Drug classification: DIURETICS—THIAZIDE-RELATED (see section 30.5.12 in Table 14-1)

Brand names: *Hygroton, Thalitone*

Ototoxic effects:
  Cochlear:
    Hearing loss: (Eps)
    Tinnitus: (Eps)
  Vestibular:
    Dizziness: 1-10% (CPS, PDR)
    Vertigo: (CPS, PDR)

Risk assessment: Class 2

Notes:

  See Chapter 7, "We 'Hear' With Our Eyes" for further information on this drug.

Chlor-Trimeton (see **Chlorpheniramine**)

Chlor-Tripolon (see **Chlorpheniramine**)

Chlor-Tripolon Decongestant (see **Chlorpheniramine**)

Chlor-Tripolon N.D. (see **Loratadine**)

Chlorzoxazone

Pronunciation guide: klor-ZOX-ah-zone

Drug classification: SKELETAL MUSCLE RELAXANTS (see section 53.36 in Table 14-1)

Brand names: *Acetazone Forte C8* [1], *Flectadol* [2], *Tafirol Flex* [2]

Ototoxic effects:
  Vestibular:
    Dizziness: 6% (CPS, PDR)
    Vertigo: >1% (CPS)

Risk assessment: Class 1

Notes:

  [1] *Acetazone Forte C8* is a combination of **Chlorzoxazone**, **Acetaminophen** and **Codeine**. (See the generic drugs **Acetaminophen** and **Codeine** for their specific ototoxic properties.)

  [2] *Flectadol* and *Tafirol Flex* are combinations of **Chlorzoxazone** and **Acetaminophen**. (See the generic drug **Acetaminophen** for its specific ototoxic properties.)

Cholecalciferol (see **Ergocalciferal**)

Cholestyramine

Pronunciation guide: koe-LESS-tir-ah-meen

Drug classification: BILE ACID SEQUESTRANTS (see section 20.12.1 in Table 14-1)

Brand names: *Questran*

Ototoxic effects:
    Cochlear:
        Tinnitus: (CPS, PDR)
    Vestibular:
        Dizziness: >10% (NDH, PDR)
        Vertigo: >10% (NDH, PDR)

Risk assessment: Class 2

Choline magnesium trisalicylate

Pronunciation guide: KOE-leen mag-NEE-see-um try-sah-LISS-ih-late

Drug classification: SALICYLATES (see section 1.1.16 in Table 14-1)

Brand names: *Trilisate*

Ototoxic effects:
    Cochlear:
        Hearing loss: <2% (CPS, PDR)
        Tinnitus: 10.2% (CPS, PDR)
    Vestibular:
        Dizziness: <2% (CPS, PDR)

Risk assessment: Class 3

Notes:

    Choline magnesium trisalicylate can cause permanent tinnitus and hearing loss (PDR).

    If you get tinnitus, your doctor should reduce your dosage (CPS, PDR).

Choloxin   (see **Dextrothyroxine**)

Chronovera   (see **Verapamil**)

Cialis   (see **Tadalafil**)

Cicatrin   (see **Neomycin**)

Ciclesonide

Pronunciation guide: sih-KLEH-son-ide

Drug classification: GLUCOCORTICOIDS (see section 40.1.4 in Table 14-1)

Brand names: *Omnaris*

Ototoxic effects:
    Outer/Middle Ear:
        Earache/ear pain: 2.2% [1.6% above placebo results] (AHF, NDH)

Risk assessment: Class 1

Cidecin   (see **Daptomycin**)

Cidofovir

Pronunciation guide: sye-DOE-foh-veer

Drug classification: Anti-retroviral protease inhibitors (see section 7.17.1.1 in Table 14-1)

Brand names: *Vistide*

Ototoxic effects:
    Cochlear:
        Hearing loss: (DFC, PDR)
        Hyperacusis: (DFC, PDR)
        Tinnitus: (DFC, PDR)
    Vestibular:
        Ataxia: (NDH, PDR)
        Dizziness: (NDH, PDR)
        Vertigo: (PDR)
    Outer/Middle Ear:
        Earache/ear pain: (DFC, PDR)
        Otitis externa: (DFC, PDR)
        Otitis media: (DFC, PDR)
    Unspecified/General Ear Conditions:
        Ear disorder: (DFC, PDR)

Risk assessment: Class 3

Notes:

When you take **Cidofovir**, you may experience hearing loss and tinnitus within 24 to 48 hours. After you stop taking **Cidofovir**, your hearing may improve and your tinnitus may lessen, but you will likely be left with some permanent hearing loss and tinnitus (CP2).

Cidomycin   (see **Gentamicin**)

Cilazapril

Pronunciation guide: sih-LAY-zah-pril

Drug classification: Angiotensin-converting enzyme (ACE) inhibitors (see section 20.8.8 in Table 14-1)

Brand names: *Inhibace*

Ototoxic effects:
    Cochlear:
        Tinnitus: <1% (CPS)

Vestibular:
    Ataxia: <1% (CPS)
    Dizziness: 3-8.2% [1.7% above placebo results] (CPS)
    Vertigo: <1% (CPS)
Outer/Middle Ear:
    Ears feel "plugged up": <0.1% (CPS)

Risk assessment: Class 2

Cilostazol

Pronunciation guide: sill-AHS-tah-zoll

Drug classification: PLATELET INHIBITOR DRUGS (see section 36.24 in Table 14-1)

Brand names: *Pletal*

Ototoxic effects:
    Cochlear:
        Tinnitus: <2% (PDR)
    Vestibular:
        Dizziness: 9-10% [3-4% above placebo results] (NDH, PDR)
        Vertigo: 1-3% [<2% above placebo results] (NDH, PDR)
    Outer/Middle Ear:
        Earache/ear pain: <2% (PDR)

Risk assessment: Class 2

Notes:

Caution: Eating grapefruit or drinking grapefruit juice during the time you are taking this drug may make the listed side effects worse than shown here.

See Chapter 11, "Grapefruit Juice and Ototoxic Drugs" for further information on this drug.

Cimzia   (see **Certolizumab**)

Cinnarizine

Pronunciation guide: sin-NAH-rih-zeen

Drug classification: PIPERAZINES (see section 10.8 in Table 14-1)

Brand names: *Stugeron*

Ototoxic effects:
    Cochlear:
        Tinnitus: (She)

Risk assessment: Class 1

Cinobac   (see **Cinoxacin**)

Cinoxacin

Pronunciation guide: sin-OX-ah-sin

Drug classification: QUINOLONES (see section 7.4.48 in Table 14-1)

Brand names: *Cinobac*

Ototoxic effects:
    Cochlear:
        Tinnitus: <1% (DFC, RXL)
    Vestibular:
        Dizziness: 1% (DFC, RXL)

Risk assessment: Class 1

Cipralex   (see **Escitalopram**)

Cipro   (see **Ciprofloxacin**)

Cipro XL   (see **Ciprofloxacin**)

Ciprodex   (see **Ciprofloxacin**)

Ciprofibrate

Pronunciation guide: sip-proe-FYE-brate

Drug classification: FIBRATES (see section 20.12.4 in Table 14-1)

Brand names: *Modalim*

Ototoxic effects:
    Vestibular:
        Dizziness: (BNF)
        Vertigo: (BNF)

Risk assessment: Class 1

Ciprofloxacin

Pronunciation guide: sih-proe-FLOX-ah-sin

Drug classification: QUINOLONES (see section 7.4.48 in Table 14-1)

Brand names: *Cipro, Cipro XL, Ciprodex* [1], *Ciproxin*

Ototoxic effects:
    Cochlear:
        Hearing disorder: (BNF)
        Hearing loss: [2] <1% (CPS, PDR)
        Tinnitus: <1% (CPS, PDR)

Vestibular:
    Ataxia: <1% (CPS, PDR)
    Dizziness: 1-2% (CPS, PDR)
    Nystagmus: <1% (CPS, PDR)
    Vertigo: <1% (AHF, PDR)
Outer/Middle Ear:
    Earache/ear pain: 0.4-3% (CPS, PDR)
    Otitis externa: 0.4-1.5% (PDR)

Risk assessment: Class 4

Notes:

[1] *Ciprodex* is a combination of **Ciprofloxacin** and **Dexamethasone**. (See the generic drug **Dexamethasone** for its specific ototoxic properties.)

[2] Hearing loss is often at the higher frequencies. Hearing loss may be temporary (CPS).

The CPS also lists the following side effects: ear precipitate (residue) (0.5%), ear puritis (1.5%) and ear debris (0.6%) These side effects indicate external ear infections (Otitis externa). In addition, the CPS lists ear congestion (0.4%) which likely indicates middle ear infections (Otitis media).

I have an anecdotal report in my files of a man who lost a lot of his hearing when he took **Ciprofloxacin** for an infection. His hearing problem started with "weird" tinnitus about the time the infection was going away. The tinnitus eventually stopped but his hearing did not improve.

I have another anecdotal report in my files of a woman who only took **Ciprofloxacin** for three days. After that she had "horrible vertigo," ringing in her ears and hearing loss.

I have yet another anecdotal report in my files of a woman who lost her hearing in one ear after taking **Ciprofloxacin** for 3 days. She wrote, "I went to the doctor with a sinus infection. He gave me a prescription for **Ciprofloxacin**. I took one pill that evening (Wednesday), then took one the next morning and evening for the next three days, a total of 7 pills in all. By the time I took the 7th pill Saturday evening I had this awful popping, ringing, crackling sound in my left ear, and was deaf in that ear. My hearing has not returned at all, and that was a month ago now".

I have an anecdotal report in my files of a man that took a two-week course of **Ciprofloxacin** for prostatitis. He writes, "I took the first dose of *Ciproxin* later that same day, and then another dose that same night. At approximately 1:30 AM that very night, I was suddenly awoken from my sleep by a loud ringing in my ears—the like and severity of which I had never experienced before. I was completely unable to sleep that night. I managed to see out the two weeks, but it was perhaps the most distressing and uncomfortable two weeks of my life that I can ever recall. I only managed to sleep for perhaps 30 minutes each day on average. The loud ringing in the ears never went away. Ever since that course of *Ciproxin* I have suffered repeated 'attacks' of tinnitus. In the 6 months since I took it, I have had probably 6 or more of these episodes, and at their worst they are of the same severity as the original attack. The only saving grace appears to be that the attacks are usually shorter lived, and I have the token 'comfort' of (thus far) knowing that they generally subside within a few days".

In another anecdotal report in my files, a woman also only took **Ciprofloxacin** for three days which resulted in "profound bilateral hearing loss, tinnitus and inner ear damage that affects my balance".

In yet another anecdotal report in my files a woman took **Ciprofloxacin** for slight diarrhea while she was pregnant (4 months along). Her baby was born with bilateral severe hearing loss (60 – 90 dB in both ears).

See Chapter 7, "We 'Hear' With Our Eyes" for further information on this drug.

Ciproxin   (see **Ciprofloxacin**)

Cisapride

Pronunciation guide: SIS-ah-pride

Drug classification: PROKINETIC DRUGS (see section 34.24 in Table 14-1)

Brand names: *Prepulsid, Propulsid*

Ototoxic effects:
 Vestibular:
  Dizziness/vertigo: 1.2% (CPS)

Risk assessment: Class 1

Notes:

Caution: Eating grapefruit or drinking grapefruit juice during the time you are taking this drug may make the listed side effects worse than shown here. In fact, taking **Cisapride** with grapefruit juice can increase the potency of **Cisapride** by as much as 39%.

See Chapter 11, "Grapefruit Juice and Ototoxic Drugs" for further information on this drug.

Cisplatin (CDDP)

Pronunciation guide: SIS-plah-tin

Drug classification: ALKYLATING DRUGS (see section 14.1 in Table 14-1)

Brand names: *Platinol*

Ototoxic effects:
 Cochlear:
  Hearing loss: 24-100% (CPS, PDR)
  Tinnitus: 9-31% (CPS, PDR)
 Vestibular:
  Ataxia: (AHF)
  Vertigo: (AHF, CPS)
  Vestibular disorder: (CPS, PDR)
 Outer/Middle Ear:
  Earache/ear pain: (AHF)
 Unspecified/General Ear Conditions:
  Ototoxicity: (AHF, BNF)

Risk assessment: Class 5

Notes:

> **Cisplatin** is very likely the most ototoxic of all known drugs.[152] It is known to cause significant and permanent hearing loss in many people. High doses can cause profound hearing loss.[153]
>
> A couple of studies revealed that the incidence of hearing loss in people taking **Cisplatin** ranges from 3% to 100%! [154] Another study showed that approximately 40% end up with hearing losses from taking **Cisplatin**.[155]
>
> Up to 31% of the people receiving **Cisplatin** lose their hearing and/or get tinnitus with their very first dose. This first dose can produce severe hearing loss or deafness. Sensorineural hearing loss usually occurs in both ears (bilateral) (CPS, PDR), but it can occur in just one ear (AHF). Hearing loss tends to become more frequent and more severe with repeated doses (CPS, PDR).
>
> Hearing loss associated with **Cisplatin** is almost always permanent and progressive. Rarely does hearing recover.[156] **Cisplatin** attacks the very high frequencies first, then progresses to the high frequencies (4,000 to 8,000 Hz) where it becomes apparent. **Cisplatin**-induced hearing loss decreases your ability to hear and understand normal speech (CPS, PDR).
>
> Hearing loss occurs in about 24% of patients receiving the usual doses of **Cisplatin**. High-frequency loss on audiograms has been reported in up to 74-100% of patients receiving cumulative doses of 200 mg/m^2 or more of **Cisplatin** (AHF).
>
> Hearing loss appears to be most severe in older adults and in children, especially young children. People with preexisting hearing loss may be more susceptible to **Cisplatin**-induced ototoxicity (AHF).
>
> **Cisplatin** causes a permanent hearing loss in the speech frequencies in about 7% of the people taking it according to one study.[157] Hearing loss often begins three to four days into treatment, or it might not appear until several weeks or months after you have taken your last dose[158] This is because **Cisplatin** irreversibly binds to plasma proteins and can still be detected up to six months after you complete drug therapy.[159]. **Cisplatin** damages both the auditory neurons and the auditory hair cells. The damage begins in the outer hair cells and may progress to the inner hair cells.[160]
>
> Tinnitus may accompany a hearing loss due to **Cisplatin**, or may be present without any apparent hearing loss. Typically, the tinnitus goes away within a few weeks of stopping **Cisplatin** therapy.[161]
>
> You should have audiograms done before beginning **Cisplatin** therapy, and between successive doses (CPS, PDR). Also, you should have audiograms done 6 to 8 weeks after your final treatment, and whenever you notice a drop in your hearing or an increase in your tinnitus. Your audiogram should cover not only the conventional frequencies up to 8,000 Hz, but also the high frequencies between 8,000 and 20,000 Hz.[162]
>
> After you have had **Cisplatin** therapy, you should avoid loud noise for up to six months[163] in order to avoid even more hearing loss from the synergistic effects of **Cisplatin** and noise.

There are a number of factors that can put you at higher risk of **Cisplatin** ototoxicity. You are more at risk if you have taken high doses, or have taken several courses of **Cisplatin** therapy. **Cisplatin** ototoxicity also occurs more frequently and severely in children. **Cisplatin** ototoxicity can be much worse if you take **Cisplatin** along with an AMINOGLYCOSIDE antibiotic and a LOOP DIURETIC such as **Furosemide**—a typical combination used to treat cancer.[164] You are also more at risk if you have had radiation on your head or ear, or if you have low serum albumin and other factors.[165] Other factors associated with increased risk include: you are either very young or very old, you are dehydrated, you are taking other ototoxic drugs at the same time and you have kidney problems (CPS, PDR).[166]

Strangely enough, some research indicates that you are even at greater risk if you have brown eyes as compared to blue eyes.[167]

Unfortunately doctors (and society in general) commonly underestimate the detrimental social and emotional effects of **Cisplatin** therapy in real life. Hearing loss compounds the already stressful social isolation experienced by many cancer patients.[168]

New research indicates that taking a combination of D-methionine and Brain Derived Neurotrophic Factor (BDNF) may protect both your hair cells and your neurons from the ototoxic effects of **Cisplatin** therapy (Med).

Another new discovery is that N-acetyl-cysteine (NAC), a form of the amino acid cysteine and produced by the body, can help prevent ototoxicity caused by **Cisplatin**. NAC is a powerful anti-oxidant.

Researchers believe that NAC prevents ototoxicity by binding to the **Cisplatin** platinum molecules and rendering them inactive. NAC is a free-radical scavenger. It also boosts levels of a powerful intracellular antioxidant called glutathione.[169]

A recent discovery (Nov. 2009) reveals that if you have variations in the thiopurine methyltransferase [TMPT] gene and the catechol-O-methyltransferase gene [COMT], you have a 98% chance of becoming deaf after having **Cisplatin** infused.[170] There are also other factors, as yet undiscovered, that cause **Cisplatin**-induced hearing loss in some people that do not have these genetic variations.

See Chapter 2 "Ototoxic Drugs—What Are They," Chapter 4 "Are You at Risk," Chapter 6 "The Shocking Truth about Hearing Testing and Ototoxic Drugs," Chapter 8, "The Sinister Partnership Between Ototoxic Agents and Noise" and Chapter 12, "Potpourri" for further information on this drug.

Citalopram

Pronunciation guide: sih-TAL-oh-pram

Drug classification: SELECTIVE SEROTONIN REUPTAKE INHIBITORS (see section 60.1.32 in Table 14-1)

Brand names: *Celexa*

Ototoxic effects:
    Cochlear:
        Tinnitus: 0.1-1% (CPS, PDR)

Vestibular:
    Ataxia: 0.1-1% (CPS, PDR)
    Dizziness: 2.3% [>1% above placebo results] (CPS, PDR)
    Vertigo: 0.1-1% (CPS, PDR)
Outer/Middle Ear:
    Earache/ear pain: 0.1-1% (CPS)
    Otitis media: (CPS)

Risk assessment: Class 2

Citanest   (see **Prilocaine**)

Clarinex   (see **Desloratadine**)

Clarithromycin

Pronunciation guide: klar-ITH-roe-mye-sin

Drug classification: MACROLIDE ANTIBIOTICS (see section 7.4.32 in Table 14-1)

Brand names: *Biaxin*

Ototoxic effects:
    Cochlear:
        Hearing disorder: (CPS)
        Hearing loss: 1-5% (CPS, PDR)
        Tinnitus: 2% (CPS, PDR)
    Vestibular:
        Dizziness: 2% (CPS, PDR)
        Vertigo: (CPS, PDR)
    Unspecified/General Ear Conditions:
        Ear disorder: (CPS)

Risk assessment: Class 3

Notes:

Hearing loss usually is reversible (CPS, PDR). In one study, between 2% and 5% of patients had deafness, ear disorder, partial transitory deafness and/or tinnitus (CPS).

Temporary hearing loss has been reported in a few patients receiving high (e.g., 2 g daily) dosages of **Clarithromycin** (AHF).

I have an anecdotal report in my files of a man who was prescribed **Clarithromycin** for a sinus infection. Two or three days later severe tinnitus started, and has never stopped since. In addition, he lost much of his residual hearing. (He did have a hearing loss before this episode.)

I have an anecdotal report in my files of another man that developed permanent, severe tinnitus from taking **Clarithromycin**. He wrote, "I took the 500 mg. sustained release tablet twice a day for two weeks. The amazing thing is that this drug seems to act the same way as the AMINOGLYCOSIDES do in that it displays delayed ototoxicity combined when combined with loud sound. Here's what happened. I developed tinnitus 4 days after finishing the drug. Three days later the tinnitus went away completely. Three days after that, I attended a Christmas Eve service and was exposed to 90 db of music for 25 minutes. The next day my ears were badly stuffed. The following day I had incredible tinnitus. The rest is history. Permanent damage which would have reversed if I had not been exposed to the sound".

Claritin   (see **Loratadine**)

Claritin Extra   (see **Loratadine**)

Claritin Liberator   (see **Loratadine**)

Claritin-D   (see **Loratadine**)

Clarus   (see **Isotretinoin**)

Clemastine

Pronunciation guide: KLEM-as-teen

Drug classification: H$_1$ RECEPTOR ANTAGONISTS (see section 10.1 in Table 14-1)

Brand names: *Tavist*

Ototoxic effects:
    Cochlear:
        Tinnitus: (Med, PDR)
    Vestibular:
        Dizziness: (CPS, PDR)
        Vertigo: (PDR)

Risk assessment: Class 1

Cleocin   (see **Clindamycin**)

Climara   (see **Estradiol**)

Clindamycin

Pronunciation guide: klin-dah-MYE-sin

Drug classification: LINCOMYCINS (see section 7.4.24 in Table 14-1)

Brand names: *Cleocin, Dalacin*

Ototoxic effects:
    Cochlear:
        Tinnitus: [171]
    Vestibular:
        Dizziness: <1% (CPS, PDR)
        Vertigo: <1% (CPS, PDR)

Risk assessment: Class 1

Clinoril   (see **Sulindac**)

Clobazam

Pronunciation guide: KLO-bah-zam

Drug classification: Benzodiazepines (see section 60.12.8 in Table 14-1)

Brand names: *Frisium*

Ototoxic effects:
    Vestibular:
        Ataxia: 3.9% (BNF, CPS)
        Dizziness: 1.8% (CPS)
        Nystagmus: (CPS)
        Vertigo: (BNF)

Risk assessment: Class 2

Notes:

    See Chapter 10 "Beware of Benzodiazepines—Don't Let This Nasty Time-Bomb Ambush You and Your Ears" for further information on this drug.

Clomid   (see **Clomiphene**)

Clomiphene

Pronunciation guide: KLOE-mih-feen

Drug classification: Estrogen agonist—antagonists (see section 40.16 in Table 14-1)

Brand names: *Clomid, Milophene, Serophene*

Ototoxic effects:
    Cochlear:
        Hearing loss: (PDR)
        Tinnitus: (CPS, PDR)
    Vestibular:
        Dizziness: <1% (CPS, PDR)
        Vertigo: <1% (DFC, PDR)

Risk assessment: Class 2

Notes:

    Abnormalities in unborn children have included deafness (PDR).

    See Chapter 7, "We 'Hear' With Our Eyes" for further information on this drug.

Clomipramine

Pronunciation guide: kloe-MIH-prah-meen

Drug classification: TRICYCLIC ANTI-DEPRESSANTS (see section 60.1.8 in Table 14-1)

Brand names: *Anafranil*

Ototoxic effects:
    Cochlear:
        Auditory Hallucinations: [172]
        Hearing loss: 0.1-1% (AHF, PDR)
        Hyperacusis: 0.1-1% (AHF, PDR)
        Tinnitus: 4-6% [placebo 0] (CPS, PDR)
    Vestibular:
        Ataxia: 0.1-1% (CPS, PDR)
        Dizziness: 41-54% [27-40% above placebo results] (CPS, PDR)
        Nystagmus: <0.1% (AHF, PDR)
        Vertigo: >1% (CPS, PDR)
        Vestibular disorder: 2% (AHF, DFC)
    Outer/Middle Ear:
        Earache/ear pain: 0.1-1% (AHF, PDR)
        Otitis media: 4% (AHF, DFC)

Risk assessment: Class 3

Notes:

> Caution: Eating grapefruit or drinking grapefruit juice during the time you are taking this drug may make the listed side effects worse than shown here. In fact, taking **Clomipramine** with grapefruit juice can increase the potency of **Clomipramine** by as much as 300%.

> I have an anecdotal report in my files of a woman who took **Clomipramine** and began experiencing tinnitus and hearing loss. She went to her doctor and got off the drug. Later, she wrote, "I've been off the **Clomipramine** now for 2 weeks, and I have noticed that my tinnitus has diminished noticeably, and I can hear better. Sound is not so muffled anymore". Fourteen days later, she wrote, "My ears still have a tiny bit of ring, but I probably always had it," so she is back to normal regarding her tinnitus, although she still has other problems related to taking the **Clomipramine**.

> I have another anecdotal report in my files of a man that was taking **Clomipramine** for depression. As his dose increased, so did his tinnitus.

> See Chapter 11, "Grapefruit Juice and Ototoxic Drugs" for further information on this drug.

Clonazepam

Pronunciation guide: kloe-NAZ-eh-pam

Drug classification: BENZODIAZEPINES (see section 60.12.8 in Table 14-1)

Brand names: *Klonopin, Rivotril*

Ototoxic effects:
    Vestibular:
        Ataxia: 1-30% [placebo 0] (CPS, PDR)
        Dizziness: 1-12% [1-8% above placebo results] (CPS, PDR)
        Nystagmus: (CPS, PDR)
        Vertigo: (CPS, PDR)
    Outer/Middle Ear:
        Earache/ear pain: 0.1-1% (PDR)
        Otitis: 0.1-1% (PDR)

Risk assessment: Class 2

Notes:

    See Chapter 4 "Are You at Risk?" and Chapter 10 "Beware of Benzodiazepines—Don't Let This Nasty Time-Bomb Ambush You and Your Ears" for further information on this drug.

Clonidine

Pronunciation guide: KLOE-nih-deen

Drug classification: CENTRALLY ACTING ANTIADRENERGIC DRUGS (see section 20.8.20 in Table 14-1)

Brand names: *Catapres, Clorpres*[1]*, Combipres*[1]*, Dixarit, Duraclon*

Ototoxic effects:
    Cochlear:
        Auditory hallucinations: 5.3% (CPS, PDR)
        Tinnitus: 5.3% [placebo 0] (DFC, PDR)
    Vestibular:
        Dizziness: 13.2-16% [<8.9% above placebo results] (CPS, PDR)
        Vertigo: (PDR)

Risk assessment: Class 3

Notes:

    [1] *Clorpres* and *Combipres* are combinations of **Clonidine** and **Chlorthalidone**. (See the generic drug **Chlorthalidone** for its specific ototoxic properties.)

Clopidogrel

Pronunciation guide: cloe-PID-oh-grel

Drug classification: PLATELET INHIBITOR DRUGS (see section 36.24 in Table 14-1)

Brand names: *Plavix*

Ototoxic effects:
    Vestibular:
        Dizziness: 2.4-6.2% (NDH, PDR)
        Vertigo: 1-2.5% (BNF, PDR)

Risk assessment: Class 1

Clopixol (see **Zuclopenthixol**)

Clorazepate

Pronunciation guide: klor-AZ-ee-pate

Drug classification: BENZODIAZEPINES (see section 60.12.8 in Table 14-1)

Brand names: *Apo-Clorazepate, Novo-Clopate, Tranxene*

Ototoxic effects:
    Cochlear:
        Tinnitus: (Eps)
    Vestibular:
        Ataxia: (CP2, PDR)
        Dizziness: (CP2, PDR)
        Vertigo: (BNF, CP2)

Risk assessment: Class 1

Notes:
    See Chapter 10 "Beware of Benzodiazepines—Don't Let This Nasty Time-Bomb Ambush You and Your Ears" for further information on this drug.

Clorpres (see **Clonidine**)

Clostridium botulinum Toxin Type A (see **Botulinum Toxin Type A**)

Clozapine

Pronunciation guide: KLOE-zah-peen

Drug classification: ANTIPSYCHOTIC DRUGS (see section 60.8 in Table 14-1)

Brand names: *Clozaril, Gen-Clozapine*

Ototoxic effects:
    Cochlear:
        Auditory hallucinations: (AHF)
    Vestibular:
        Ataxia: 1% (CPS, PDR)
        Dizziness/vertigo: 19-27% (AHF, PDR)
        Nystagmus: <1% (CPS, PDR)
        Vertigo: (AHF)
    Unspecified/General Ear Conditions:
        Ear disorder: <1% (CPS, PDR)

Risk assessment: Class 2

Clozaril (see **Clozapine**)

Co-Actifed (see **Pseudoephedrine**)

Coartem   (see **Artemether/Lumefantrine**)

Coated Aspirin   (see **Acetylsalicylic acid**)

Codeine

Pronunciation guide: koe-DEEN

Drug classification: Opiate agonist drugs (see section 1.4.1 in Table 14-1)

Brand names: *Codeine Contin*

Ototoxic effects:
    Cochlear:
        Tinnitus: (AHF, NTP)
    Vestibular:
        Dizziness: (CPS, PDR)
        Labyrinthitis: (NTP)
        Nystagmus: (CPS)
        Vertigo: (BNF, CPS)
        Vestibular disorder: (CPS)

Risk assessment: Class 2

Notes:
    See Chapter 7, "We 'Hear' With Our Eyes" for further information on this drug.

Codeine Contin   (see **Codeine**)

Cogentin   (see **Benztropine**)

Cognex   (see **Tacrine**)

Colazal   (see **Mesalamine**)

Colestid   (see **Colestipol**)

Colestipol

Pronunciation guide: koe-LESS-tih-pole

Drug classification: Bile acid sequestrants (see section 20.12.1 in Table 14-1)

Brand names: *Colestid*

Ototoxic effects:
    Vestibular:
        Dizziness: 0.1-1% (CPS, PDR)
        Vertigo: 0.1-1% (CPS)

Risk assessment: Class 1

Colistimethate   (see **Colistin**)

Colistin (Colistimethate, Polymyxin E)

Pronunciation guide: KOL-iss-tin (kol-liss-tih-METH-ate, pol-ee-MIX-in)

Drug classification: Polypeptides (see section 7.4.44 in Table 14-1)

Brand names: *Coly-Mycin M, Coly-Mycin S, Cortisporin TC* [1]

Ototoxic effects:
    Vestibular:
        Ataxia: (CPS, PDR)
        Dizziness: (CPS, PDR)
        Nystagmus: (AHF, PDR)
        Vertigo: (CPS, PDR)
    Unspecified/General Ear Conditions:
        Ototoxicity: [173] (BNF)

Risk assessment: Class 2

Notes:

[1] *Cortisporin TC* is a combination of **Colistin**, **Hydrocortisone**, **Neomycin**, and Thonzonium. (See the generic drugs **Hydrocortisone** and **Neomycin** for their specific ototoxic properties.)

Colistimethate is a close derivative of **Colistin** and is treated here as essentially the same drug as **Colistin**.

"**Colistin** is highly ototoxic when administered topically. However, no ototoxicity has been reported with systemic administration of this drug".[174]

See Chapter 7, "We 'Hear' With Our Eyes" for further information on **Colistin**.

Colocort   (see **Hydrocortisone**)

Coly-Mycin M   (see **Colistin**)

Coly-Mycin S   (see **Colistin**)

Combigan   (see **Timolol**)

Combipres   (see **Clonidine**)

Combivent   (see **Ipratropium**)

Combivir   (see **Zidovudine**)

Compound W   (see **Salicylic acid**)

Comtan   (see **Entacapone**)

Comvax   (see **Haemophilus vaccine**)

Concerta   (see **Methylphenidate**)

Copaxone   (see **Glatiramer**)

Coptin   (see **Sulfadiazine**)

Cordarone   (see **Amiodarone**)

Coreg   (see **Carvedilol**)

Corgard   (see **Nadolol**)

Coricidin D   (see **Phenylpropanolamine**)

Cortef   (see **Hydrocortisone**)

Cortenema   (see **Hydrocortisone**)

Corticotropin

Pronunciation guide: KOR-tih-koh-troe-pin

Drug classification: ADRENOCORTICOTROPHIC HORMONES (ACTH) (see section 40.1.1 in Table 14-1)

Brand names: *Acthar*

Ototoxic effects:
    Cochlear:
        Tinnitus: [175]
    Vestibular:
        Dizziness: (CP2)
        Vertigo: (AHF, DFC)

Risk assessment: Class 1

Notes:

   Corticotropin is a natural ADRENOCORTICOTROPHIC HORMONE (ACTH).

Cortisone

Pronunciation guide: KOR-tih-sone

Drug classification: GLUCOCORTICOIDS (see section 40.1.4 in Table 14-1)

Brand names: *Cortone*

Ototoxic effects:
    Vestibular:
        Vertigo: (CPS, PDR)

Risk assessment: Class 1

Cortisporin   (see **Neomycin**)

Cortisporin TC   (see **Colistin**)

Cortone   (see **Cortisone**)

Cortrosyn   (see **Cosyntropin**)

Corzide   (see **Bendroflumethiazide**)

Cosmegen   (see **Dactinomycin**)

Cosopt   (see **Timolol**)

Cosyntropin

Pronunciation guide: koe-sin-TROW-pin

Drug classification: ADRENOCORTICOTROPHIC HORMONES (ACTH) (see section 40.1.1 in Table 14-1)

Brand names: *Cortrosyn* [1], *Synacthen Depot* [2]

Ototoxic effects:
    Cochlear:
        Tinnitus: [176]
    Vestibular:
        Dizziness: [177] (CPS)
        Vertigo: (CPS)

Risk assessment: Class 1

Notes:

[1] **Cosyntropin** (*Cortrosyn*) **for injection** is a combination of **Cosyntropin** and **Mannitol**. (See the generic drug **Mannitol** for its specific ototoxic properties.)

[2] *Synacthen Depot* is a combination of **Cosyntropin** and Zinc hydroxide. (**Cosyntropin** is the ototoxic agent.)

Cosyntropin is a synthetic ADRENOCORTICOTROPHIC HORMONE (ACTH) and may cause tinnitus.

Co-Trimoxazole   (see **Trimethoprim**)

Covera-HS   (see **Verapamil**)

Coversyl   (see **Perindopril**)

Coversyl Plus   (see **Perindopril**)

Cozaar   (see **Losartan**)

Crestor   (see **Rosuvastatin**)

Crixivan   (see **Indinavir**)

Cromolyn sodium (Sodium cromoglycate)

Pronunciation guide: KROE-moh-lynn SOE-dee-um

Drug classification: Respiratory anti-inflammatory drugs (see section 63.8 in Table 14-1)

Brand names: *Gastrocrom, Intal*

Ototoxic effects:
    Cochlear:
        Tinnitus: (PDR)
    Vestibular:
        Dizziness: <0.01% (CPS, PDR)
        Vertigo: <0.001% (CPS, PDR)

Risk assessment: Class 1

Cubicin   (see **Daptomycin**)

Cuprimine   (see **Penicillamine**)

Cyanocobalamin (Vitamin B$_{12}$)

Pronunciation guide: sye-an-oh-koe-BAL-ah-min

Drug classification: Vitamins (see section 75.4 in Table 14-1)

Brand names: *Nascobal*

Ototoxic effects:
    Vestibular:
        Ataxia: 4% (CP2, PDR)
        Dizziness: 12% (PDR)

Risk assessment: Class 1

Cyclen   (see **Ethinyl estradiol**)

Cyclizine

Pronunciation guide: SYE-klih-zeen

Drug classification: Piperazines (see section 10.8 in Table 14-1)

Brand names: *Marzine*

Ototoxic effects:
    Cochlear:
        Auditory hallucinations: (CPS)
        Tinnitus: (CPS)
    Vestibular:
        Vertigo: (CPS)

Risk assessment: Class 1

Notes:
    See Chapter 7, "We 'Hear' With Our Eyes" for further information on this drug.

Cyclobenzaprine

Pronunciation guide: sye-kloe-BEN-zah-preen

Drug classification: SKELETAL MUSCLE RELAXANTS (see section 53.36 in Table 14-1)

Brand names: *Amrix, Flexeril, Novo-Cycloprine*

Ototoxic effects:
    Cochlear:
        Tinnitus: <1% (CPS, PDR)
    Vestibular:
        Ataxia: <1% (CPS, PDR)
        Dizziness: 3-19% [1-4% above placebo results] (CPS, PDR)
        Vertigo: <1% (CPS, PDR)

Risk assessment: Class 2

Cyclomen　　(see **Danazol**)

Cyclopentolate

Pronunciation guide: sye-kloe-PEN-toe-late

Drug classification: ANTI-CHOLINERGIC DRUGS (see section 17.1 in Table 14-1)

Brand names: *AK-Pentolate*

Ototoxic effects:
    Vestibular:
        Ataxia: (AHF, DFC)

Risk assessment: Class 1

Cyclophosphamide

Pronunciation guide: sye-kloe-FOSS-fah-mide

Drug classification: ALKYLATING DRUGS (see section 14.1 in Table 14-1)

Brand names: *Cytoxan, Neosar, Procytox*

Ototoxic effects:
    Vestibular:
        Dizziness: (AHF, CPS)
    Unspecified/General Ear Conditions:
        Ototoxicity: (Str)

Risk assessment: Class 2

Cycloserine

Pronunciation guide: sye-kloe-SER-een

Drug classification: ANTI-TUBERCULOSIS DRUGS (see section 7.7.1 in Table 14-1)

Brand names: *Seromycin*

Ototoxic effects:
    Vestibular:
        Dizziness: (AHF, BNF)
        Vertigo: (NDH, PDR)

Risk assessment: Class 1

Notes:

    See Chapter 7, "We 'Hear' With Our Eyes" for further information on this drug.

Cyclosporine

Pronunciation guide: SYE-kloe-spore-een

Drug classification: IMMUNOSUPPRESSANT DRUGS (see section 43 in Table 14-1)

Brand names: *Gengraf, Neoral, Restasis, Sandimmune, SangCya*

Ototoxic effects:
    Cochlear:
        Hearing loss: 1-3% (AHF, PDR)
        Tinnitus: 1-3% (AHF, PDR)
    Vestibular:
        Ataxia: (CP2, CPS)
        Dizziness: 1-8% [3-5% above placebo results] (AHF, PDR)
        Vertigo: 1-3% (AHF, PDR)
        Vestibular disorder: 1-3% (AHF, PDR)
    Unspecified/General Ear Conditions:
        Ear disorder: <5% [placebo 0] (AHF, PDR)

Risk assessment: Class 3

Notes:

    Caution: Eating grapefruit or drinking grapefruit juice during the time you are taking this drug may make the listed side effects worse than shown here. In fact, taking **Cyclosporine** with grapefruit juice can increase the potency of **Cyclosporine** by as much as 300%.

See Chapter 11, "Grapefruit Juice and Ototoxic Drugs" for further information on this drug.

Cycrin   (see **Medroxyprogesterone**)

Cylert   (see **Pemoline**)

Cymbalta   (see **Duloxetine**)

Cyproheptadine

Pronunciation guide: sih-proe-HEP-tah-deen

Drug classification: H_1 RECEPTOR ANTAGONISTS (see section 10.1 in Table 14-1)

Brand names: *Periactin*

Ototoxic effects:
Cochlear:
Tinnitus: (CPS, PDR)
Vestibular:
Dizziness: (CPS, PDR)
Labyrinthitis, acute: (PDR)
Vertigo: (CPS, PDR)

Risk assessment: Class 1

Notes:
See Chapter 7, "We 'Hear' With Our Eyes" for further information on this drug.

Cyproterone

Pronunciation guide: SYE-proe-teh-rone

Drug classification: STEROID ANTI-NEOPLASTICS (see section 14.32 in Table 14-1)

Brand names: *Androcur*

Ototoxic effects:
Vestibular:
Ataxia: (CPS)
Dizziness: (CP2, CPS)
Unspecified/General Ear Conditions:
Ear disorder: (CPS)

Risk assessment: Class 1

Cystagon   (see **Cysteamine**)

Cysteamine

Pronunciation guide: sis-TEE-ah-meen

Drug classification: Miscellaneous drugs (see section 46 in Table 14-1)

Brand names: *Cystagon*

Ototoxic effects:
    Cochlear:
        Hearing loss: (DFC)
    Vestibular:
        Ataxia: (DFC)
        Dizziness: (DFC)

Risk assessment: Class 2

Cytadren (see **Aminoglutethimide**)

Cytarabine

Pronunciation guide: sye-TARE-ah-been

Drug classification: Anti-neoplastics (Anti-cancer drugs) (see section 14 in Table 14-1)

Brand names: *Cytosar, DepoCyt*

Ototoxic effects:
    Cochlear:
        Hearing loss: (AHF)
    Vestibular:
        Ataxia: 1-11% (CPS, PDR)
        Dizziness: 18-21% (CPS, PDR)

Risk assessment: Class 2

Cytosar (see **Cytarabine**)

Cytotec (see **Misoprostol**)

Cytovene (see **Ganciclovir**)

Cytoxan (see **Cyclophosphamide**)

Dactinomycin

Pronunciation guide: dak-tih-noe-MYE-sin

Drug classification: Anti-neoplastics (Anti-cancer drugs) (see section 14 in Table 14-1)

Brand names: *Actinomycin-D, Cosmegen*

Ototoxic effects:
    Unspecified/General Ear Conditions:
        Ototoxicity: [178] (Str)

Risk assessment: Not enough information to rate

Dalacin　(see **Clindamycin**)

Dalalone DP　(see **Dexamethasone**)

Dalgan　(see **Dezocine**)

Dalmane　(see **Flurazepam**)

Danazol

Pronunciation guide: DA-na-zole

Drug classification: ANDROGENS (MALE SEX HORMONES) (see section 40.4 in Table 14-1)

Brand names: *Cyclomen, Danocrine*

Ototoxic effects:
　Vestibular:
　　　Dizziness: (CPS, PDR)
　　　Vertigo: (BNF, CPS)

Risk assessment: Class 1

Danocrine　(see **Danazol**)

Dantrium　(see **Dantrolene**)

Dantrolene

Pronunciation guide: DAN-troe-leen

Drug classification: SKELETAL MUSCLE RELAXANTS (see section 53.36 in Table 14-1)

Brand names: *Dantrium*

Ototoxic effects:
　Cochlear:
　　　Auditory hallucinations: (AHF)
　Vestibular:
　　　Dizziness: (AHF)

Risk assessment: Class 1

Dapsone

Pronunciation guide: DAP-sone

Drug classification: ANTI-LEPROSY DRUGS (see section 7.14.4 in Table 14-1)

Brand names: *Avlosulfon*

Ototoxic effects:
    Cochlear:
        Tinnitus: <1% (AHF, PDR)
    Vestibular:
        Dizziness: (CPS)
        Vertigo: <1% (AHF, PDR)

Risk assessment: Class 1

Daptacel   (see **Tetanus vaccine**)

Daptomycin

Pronunciation guide: dap-toe-MYE-sin

Drug classification: LIPOPEPTIDES (see section 7.4.28 in Table 14-1)

Brand names: *Cidecin, Cubicin*

Ototoxic effects:
    Cochlear:
        Hearing loss: [179]
        Tinnitus: <1% (CPS, PDR)
    Vestibular:
        Dizziness: 2.2-5.8% [0.2% above placebo results] (NDH, PDR)
        Vertigo: <1% (DFC, PDR)

Risk assessment: Class 2

Daranide   (see **Dichlorphenamide**)

Darunavir

Pronunciation guide: duh-ROO-nah-veer

Drug classification: ANTI-RETROVIRAL PROTEASE INHIBITORS (see section 7.17.1.1 in Table 14-1)

Brand names: *Prezista*

Ototoxic effects:
    Vestibular:
        Vertigo: (DFC, NDH)

Risk assessment: Class 1

Darvon   (see **Propoxyphene**)

Darvon Compound-65   (see **Acetylsalicylic acid**)

Darvon-N   (see **Propoxyphene**)

Dasatinib

Pronunciation guide: duh-SAH-tih-nib

Drug classification: TYROSINE KINASE INHIBITORS (see section 14.40 in Table 14-1)

Brand names: *Sprycel*

Ototoxic effects:
  Cochlear:
      Tinnitus: 1-10% (CPS, DFC)
  Vestibular:
      Dizziness: 1-14% (AHF, CPS)
      Vertigo: 1-10% (CPS, DFC)

Risk assessment: Class 2

Daunorubicin (Liposomal daunorubicin)

Pronunciation guide: daw-nah-ROO-bih-sin (lih-poe-SOE-mal daw-noe-ROO-bih-sin)

Drug classification: ANTHRACYCLINES (see section 14.4 in Table 14-1)

Brand names: *DaunoXome* [1]

Ototoxic effects:
  Cochlear:
      Hearing loss: <5% (NDH, PDR)
      Tinnitus: <5% (NDH, PDR)
  Vestibular:
      Ataxia: <5% (NDH, PDR)
      Dizziness: 8-9% (NDH, PDR)
  Outer/Middle Ear:
      Earache/ear pain: <5% (NDH, PDR)

Risk assessment: Class 2

Notes:

  [1] *DaunoXome* is a combination of **Daunorubicin** and Liposome. (**Daunorubicin** is the ototoxic agent.)

DaunoXome   (see **Daunorubicin**)

Daypro   (see **Oxaprozin**)

DCM   (see **Dichloromethotrexate**)

Deanxit   (see **Melitracen**)

Debrox   (see **Acetylsalicylic acid**)

Decadron   (see **Dexamethasone**)

Decadron with Xylocaine   (see **Dexamethasone**)

Declomycin   (see **Demeclocycline**)

De-Congestine   (see **Chlorpheniramine**)

Deferasirox

Pronunciation guide: deh-fah-RASS-ih-rocks

Drug classification: HEAVY METAL ANTAGONISTS/CHELATING AGENTS (see section 66.4 in Table 14-1)

Brand names: *Exjade*

Ototoxic effects:
    Cochlear:
        Auditory disturbance: [1] (NDH, PDR)
        Hearing loss: 0.1-1% (CPS, PDR)
    Vestibular:
        Dizziness: 0.7-1.9% (CPS, PDR)
        Vertigo: 0.6-3.8% (CPS)
    Outer/Middle Ear:
        Earache/ear pain: 2.1-4.7% (CPS)
        Otitis: 5.4-9.1% (CPS, PDR)

Risk assessment: Class 2

Notes:

   [1] In this case "Auditory disturbance" is defined as a high-frequency hearing loss (PDR).

Deferoxamine (Desferroxamine)

Pronunciation guide: dee-fer-OX-ah-meen (des-fer-ROX-ah-meen)

Drug classification: HEAVY METAL ANTAGONISTS/CHELATING AGENTS (see section 66.4 in Table 14-1)

Brand names: *Desferal*

Ototoxic effects:
    Cochlear:
        Hearing disorder: (CPS)
        Hearing loss: (CPS, PDR)
        Tinnitus: (CPS, PDR)
    Vestibular:
        Dizziness: (CPS, PDR)

Risk assessment: Class 2

Notes:

Deferoxamine can cause high-frequency sensorineural hearing loss. This hearing loss is more likely to occur if you exceed dosage guidelines. In most cases, both hearing loss and tinnitus are reversible if you immediately stop taking **Deferoxamine**. However, in some cases, you may end up with permanent hearing loss/tinnitus (CPS, PDR). Therefore, if hearing loss occurs, stop taking **Deferoxamine** in order to increase the chance that your hearing will come back (CPS).

It is interesting that **Deferoxamine**, at low concentrations, when taken with **Gentamicin**, helps to protect the inner ear from **Gentamicin** ototoxicity.[180]

See Chapter 9, "Aminoglycoside Antibiotics are the Ototoxic 'Bad boys'" for further information on this drug.

Definity   (see **Perflutren**)

Dehydral   (see **Methenamine**)

Delavirdine

Pronunciation guide: dell-ah-VUR-deen

Drug classification: PIPERAZINES (see section 10.8 in Table 14-1)

Brand names: *Rescriptor*

Ototoxic effects:
    Cochlear:
        Tinnitus: <2% (CPS, PDR)
    Vestibular:
        Ataxia: <5% (AHF)
        Dizziness: 1.4-4.2% (CPS, PDR)
        Nystagmus: <2% (CPS, PDR)
        Vertigo: <2% (CPS, PDR)
    Outer/Middle Ear:
        Earache/ear pain: <2% (CPS, PDR)
        Otitis media: (AHF, PDR)

Risk assessment: Class 2

Delta-9-tetrahydrocannabinol   (see **Dronabinol**)

Deltasone   (see **Prednisone**)

Demadex   (see **Torsemide**)

Demeclocycline (Demethylchlortetracycline)

Pronunciation guide: dem-eh-kloe-SYE-kleen (de-meth-ill-klor-tet-rah-SYE-kleen)

Drug classification: TETRACYCLINES (see section 7.4.60 in Table 14-1)

Brand names: *Declomycin*

Ototoxic effects:
   Cochlear:
       Tinnitus: (PDR)
   Vestibular:
       Dizziness: (PDR)

Risk assessment: Class 1

Demerol   (see **Meperidine**)

Demethylchlortetracycline   (see **Demeclocycline**)

Demulen   (see **Ethinyl estradiol**)

Dentantol   (see **Bunazosin**)

Depacon   (see **Valproate**)

Depakene   (see **Valproic acid**)

Depakote   (see **Divalproex**)

Depen   (see **Penicillamine**)

DepoCyt   (see **Cytarabine**)

Depo-Medrol   (see **Methylprednisolone**)

Depo-Medrol with Lidocaine   (see **Lidocaine**)

Depo-Provera   (see **Medroxyprogesterone**)

Deprenyl   (see **Selegiline**)

Deproic   (see **Valproic acid**)

Deserpidine

Pronunciation guide: deh-SER-pih-deen

Drug classification: RAUWOLFIA ALKALOIDS (see section 20.8.32 in Table 14-1)

Brand names: *Enduronyl, Harmonyl, Oreticyl*

Ototoxic effects:
   Vestibular:
       Dizziness: (Med+)

Unspecified/General Ear Conditions:
    Ototoxicity: (San)

Risk assessment: Not enough information to rate

Desferal   (see **Deferoxamine**)

Desferroxamine   (see **Deferoxamine**)

Desipramine

Pronunciation guide: dess-IP-rah-meen

Drug classification: TRICYCLIC ANTI-DEPRESSANTS (see section 60.1.8 in Table 14-1)

Brand names: *Norpramin, Pertofrane*

Ototoxic effects:
    Cochlear:
        Hyperacusis: (CPS)
        Tinnitus: <1% (CPS, PDR)
    Vestibular:
        Ataxia: <1% (CPS, PDR)
        Dizziness: 1-10% (CPS, PDR)

Risk assessment: Class 2

Desloratadine

Pronunciation guide: dess-lor-AT-ah-deen

Drug classification: H_1 RECEPTOR ANTAGONISTS (see section 10.1 in Table 14-1)

Brand names: *Clarinex*

Ototoxic effects:
    Vestibular:
        Dizziness: 4% [1% above placebo results] (PDR)
    Outer/Middle Ear:
        Otitis media: 6.1% [4.5% above placebo results] (PDR)

Risk assessment: Class 1

Desogestrel—Ethinyl estradiol   (see **Ethinyl estradiol**)

Desvenlafaxine

Pronunciation guide: dess-ven-lah-FAX-in

Drug classification: SELECTIVE SEROTONIN & NOREPINEPHRINE REUPTAKE INHIBITORS (see section 60.1.28 in Table 14-1)

Brand names: *Pristiq*

Ototoxic effects:
    Cochlear:
        Tinnitus: 1-2% [1% above placebo results] (NDH, PDR)
    Vestibular:
        Dizziness: 10-16% [5-11% above placebo results] (NDH, PDR)

Risk assessment: Class 1

Desyrel   (see **Trazodone**)

Detrol   (see **Tolterodine**)

Dexacort   (see **Dexamethasone**)

Dexamethasone

Pronunciation guide: dex-ah-METH-ah-sone

Drug classification: GLUCOCORTICOIDS (see section 40.1.4 in Table 14-1)

Brand names: *Dalalone DP*, *Decadron*, *Decadron with Xylocaine* [1], *Dexacort*, *Hexadrol*

Ototoxic effects:
    Cochlear:
        Hearing loss: (NTP)
    Vestibular:
        Ataxia: (PDR)
        Dizziness: (Med)
        Nystagmus: (PDR)
        Vertigo: (CPS, PDR)

Risk assessment: Class 2

Notes:

[1] *Decadron Phosphate with Xylocaine* is a combination of **Dexamethasone** and **Lidocaine**. (See the generic drug **Lidocaine** for its specific ototoxic properties.)

Dexamethasone is being used to reduce severe hearing loss in children with bacterial meningitis (Haemophilus influenzae type b meningitis). However, watch out! It makes the hearing loss even worse if it is used on nonbacterial forms of meningitis; on patients who have already received antibiotics; and in those who do not receive treatment immediately.[181]

Dexchlorpheniramine   (see **Chlorpheniramine**)

Dexfenfluramine

Pronunciation guide: dex-fen-FLURE-ah-meen

Drug classification: ANOREXIANTS (see section 60.20.1 in Table 14-1)

Brand names: *Redux*

Ototoxic effects:
    Cochlear:
        Hearing loss: [1] (PDR)
        Tinnitus: 0.1-1% (PDR)
    Vestibular:
        Ataxia: 0.1-1% (PDR)
        Dizziness: 5.5% [1.5% above placebo results] (PDR, USP)
        Vertigo: 3.1% [1.4% above placebo results] (PDR, USP)

Risk assessment: Class 2

Notes:

[1] Includes transitory hearing loss and cochlear infarctions (inner ear strokes) (PDR).

Dexilant   (see **Dexlansoprazole**)

Dexketoprofen

Pronunciation guide: dex-kee-toe-PROE-fen

Drug classification: PROPIONIC ACIDS (see section 1.1.13 in Table 14-1)

Brand names: *Keral*

Ototoxic effects:
    Cochlear:
        Tinnitus: (BNF)
    Vestibular:
        Dizziness: (BNF)
        Vertigo: (BNF)

Risk assessment: Class 1

Dexlansoprazole

Pronunciation guide: dex-lanz-AH-pray-zol

Drug classification: PROTON PUMP INHIBITORS (see section 34.8.4 in Table 14-1)

Brand names: *Dexilant*, *Kapidex*

Ototoxic effects:
    Cochlear:
        Tinnitus: <1% (PDR)
    Vestibular:
        Dizziness: <2% (PDR)
        Vertigo: <2% (PDR)
    Outer/Middle Ear:
        Earache/ear pain: <2% (PDR)

Risk assessment: Class 2

Dextromethorphan

Pronunciation guide: dex-troe-meth-OR-fan

Drug classification: ANTIHISTAMINES (see section 10 in Table 14-1)

Brand names: *Alacol* [1], *Balamine* [2]

Ototoxic effects:
    Cochlear:
        Auditory hallucinations: [3]
    Vestibular:
        Ataxia: (AHF, PDR)
        Dizziness: (AHF, PDR)
        Nystagmus: (AHF, PDR)

Risk assessment: Class 1

Notes:

[1] *Alacol* is a combination of **Dextromethorphan**, **Phenylephrine** and **Bromopheniramine**. (See the generic drug **Phenylephrine** for its ototoxic properties.) **Bromopheniramine** [broe-moe-fen-EER-ah-meen] likely has similar ototoxic side effects as **Pheniramine**—namely dizziness and tinnitus. (See the generic drug **Pheniramine** for its specific ototoxic properties.)

[2] *Balamine* is a combination of Carbinoxamine, **Pseudoephedrine** and **Dextromethorphan**. (See the generic drug **Pseudoephedrine** for its specific ototoxic properties.)

Ataxia and nystagmus are symptoms of **Dextromethorphan** overdose (PDR).

[3] Higher doses of **Dextromethorphan** can cause auditory hallucinations.[182]

Dextrothyroxine

Pronunciation guide: dex-troe-thye-ROX-een

Drug classification: ANTI-LIPEMICS (see section 20.12 in Table 14-1)

Brand names: *Choloxin*

Ototoxic effects:
    Cochlear:
        Tinnitus: (CPS)
    Vestibular:
        Dizziness: (CPS)

Risk assessment: Class 1

Dezocine

Pronunciation guide: DEZ-oh-seen

Drug classification: OPIATE AGONIST DRUGS (see section 1.4.1 in Table 14-1)

Brand names: *Dalgan*

Ototoxic effects:
  Cochlear:
      Tinnitus: <1% (PDR)
  Vestibular:
      Dizziness/vertigo: 1-3% (PDR)
  Outer/Middle Ear:
      Ears feel "plugged up": <1% (PDR)

Risk assessment: Class 1

DHE   (see **Dihydroergotamine**)

Diamicron   (see **Gliclazide**)

Diamicron MR   (see **Gliclazide**)

Diamox   (see **Acetazolamide**)

Diane-35   (see **Ethinyl estradiol**)

Diastat   (see **Diazepam**)

Diazemuls   (see **Diazepam**)

Diazepam

Pronunciation guide: die-AZ-eh-pam

Drug classification: BENZODIAZEPINES (see section 60.12.8 in Table 14-1)

Brand names: *Diastat, Diazemuls, Dizac, Valium*

Ototoxic effects:
  Cochlear:
      Hearing loss: [1,2]
      Tinnitus: (She)
  Vestibular:
      Ataxia: 3-8% [2% above placebo results] (CPS, PDR)
      Dizziness: 3% [1% above placebo results] (CPS, PDR)
      Nystagmus: (CPS, PDR)
      Vertigo: 2% (CPS, PDR)

Risk assessment: Class 2

Notes:

[1] I have an anecdotal report in my files of a man who had a drop in his hearing while he was taking **Diazepam**. His hearing returned about a week after he stopped taking it. Apparently **Diazepam** reduces blood flow to the brain, and this could account for his hearing loss.

[2] In my files I also have a letter from an audiologist. He wrote, "I have seen patients who have used **Diazepam** for extended periods of time (over 10 years) develop auditory neuropathies and other brain-level hearing abnormalities".

Caution: Eating grapefruit or drinking grapefruit juice during the time you are taking this drug may make the listed side effects worse than shown here. In fact, taking **Diazepam** with grapefruit juice can increase the potency of **Diazepam** by as much as 320%.

See Chapter 4 "Are You at Risk?", Chapter 10 "Beware of Benzodiazepines—Don't Let This Nasty Time-Bomb Ambush You and Your Ears" and Chapter 11, "Grapefruit Juice and Ototoxic Drugs" for further information on this drug.

Diazoxide

Pronunciation guide: die-az-OX-ide

Drug classification: VASODILATORS (see section 20.8.40 in Table 14-1)

Brand names: *Hyperstat*

Ototoxic effects:
    Cochlear:
        Hearing loss: (CPS, PDR)
        Tinnitus: (AHF, CPS)
    Vestibular:
        Dizziness: 2% (CPS, PDR)

Risk assessment: Class 2

Notes:

Hearing loss may be transitory (CPS, PDR).

Dibekacin

Pronunciation guide: dih-BEH-kay-sin

Drug classification: AMINOGLYCOSIDES (see section 7.4.1 in Table 14-1)

Brand names: *Panimycin*

Ototoxic effects:
    Cochlear:
        Hearing loss: <0.1% [1]
        Tinnitus: <0.1% [1]
    Vestibular:
        Vertigo: <0.1% [1]
    Unspecified/General Ear Conditions:
        Ototoxicity: [183]

Risk assessment: Class 4

Notes:

[1] Ototoxic side effects such as hearing loss, tinnitus and vertigo may occur. If you take

this drug your doctor should carefully monitor you for ototoxic side effects. If adverse ototoxic reactions occur, you should discontinue this drug if possible.[184]

You should have serial audiograms done to watch for hearing loss. You are particularly at risk from the ototoxic side effects of **Dibekacin** if you have kidney problems, if you are elderly, if you take this drug for a long time or if you take this drug in higher than normal doses.[185]

See Chapter 9, "Aminoglycoside Antibiotics are the Ototoxic 'Bad boys'" for further information on this drug.

Dicetel   (see **Pinaverium**)

Dichloromethotrexate (DCM)

Pronunciation guide: die-klor-oh-meth-oh-TREX-ate

Drug classification: ANTI-METABOLITE DRUGS (see section 14.8 in Table 14-1)

Brand names: —

Ototoxic effects:
  Cochlear:
      Auditory disorder: [1]
      Hearing loss: [186]
  Vestibular:
      Vestibular disorder: [1]

Risk assessment: Class 4

Notes:

[1] Causes permanent damage to both the cochlear (hearing) and vestibular (balance) systems. This drug is not marketed in the USA.[187]

Dichlorphenamide

Pronunciation guide: die-klor-FEN-ah-mide

Drug classification: DIURETICS—CARBONIC ANHYDRASE INHIBITORS (see section 30.5.1 in Table 14-1)

Brand names: *Daranide*

Ototoxic effects:
  Cochlear:
      Tinnitus: (PDR)
  Vestibular:
      Ataxia: (PDR)
      Dizziness: (PDR)

Risk assessment: Class 1

Diclectin   (see **Doxylamine**)

Diclofenac

Pronunciation guide: die-KLOE-fen-ack

Drug classification: ACETIC ACIDS (see section 1.1.1 in Table 14-1)

Brand names: *Arthrotec* [1], *Cataflam, Novo-Difenac, Pennsaid, Voltaren, Voltaren Rapide, Voltaren SR*

Ototoxic effects:
    Cochlear:
        Hearing loss: <1% (CPS, PDR)
        Tinnitus: 1-10% (AHF, PDR)
    Vestibular:
        Dizziness: 2-5.3% (CPS, PDR)
        Vertigo: 1% (CPS, PDR)
    Outer/Middle Ear:
        Earache/ear pain: <1% (CPS)

Risk assessment: Class 2

Notes:

[1]*Arthrotec* is a combination of **Diclofenac** and **Misoprostol**. (See the generic drug **Misoprostol** for its specific ototoxic properties.)

Hearing loss may be temporary or permanent (PDR).

I have an anecdotal report in my files of an elderly woman who took **Diclofenac** for 15 days. On day 16 she complained of severe tinnitus. On day 17 she had severe vertigo lasting 4 days. She also had severe hearing loss in her right ear.

See Chapter 2 "Ototoxic Drugs—What Are They?" for further information on this drug.

Diclofensine

Pronunciation guide: die-KLOE-fen-seen

Drug classification: DOPAMINE REUPTAKE INHIBITORS (see section 53.24 in Table 14-1)

Brand names: —

Ototoxic effects:
    Cochlear:
        Tinnitus: (Ka7)

Risk assessment: Class 1

Didanosine

Pronunciation guide: dye-DAN-oh-seen

Drug classification: ANTI-RETROVIRAL REVERSE TRANSCRIPTASE INHIBITORS (see section 7.17.1.4 in Table 14-1)

Brand names: *Videx*

Ototoxic effects:
> Cochlear:
>> Hearing loss: <1% (CPS)
>> Tinnitus: <1% (CPS)
> Vestibular:
>> Ataxia: <1% (CPS)
>> Dizziness: 1-7% (CPS, NDH)
> Outer/Middle Ear:
>> Earache/ear pain: 1-11% (CPS)
>> Otitis externa: <1% (CPS)
>> Otitis media: 1-11% (CPS)
> Unspecified/General Ear Conditions:
>> Ear disorder: <1% (CPS)

Risk assessment: Class 2

Diflucan   (see **Fluconazole**)

Diflunisal

Pronunciation guide: dye-FLOO-nih-sal

Drug classification: SALICYLATES (see section 1.1.16 in Table 14-1)

Brand names: *Dolobid*

Ototoxic effects:
> Cochlear:
>> Hearing loss: (CPS, PDR)
>> Tinnitus: 1-3% (CPS, PDR)
> Vestibular:
>> Dizziness: 1-3% (CPS, PDR)
>> Vertigo: <1% (CPS, PDR)

Risk assessment: Class 2

Digoxin

Pronunciation guide: dih-JOX-in

Drug classification: CARDIAC GLYCOSIDES (see section 20.4.1 in Table 14-1)

Brand names: *Lanicor*, *Lanoxicaps*, *Lanoxin*

Ototoxic effects:
> Vestibular:
>> Dizziness: 6% [1% above placebo results] (NDH, PDR)
>> Vertigo:[188] (NDH)
> Unspecified/General Ear Conditions:
>> Ototoxicity: (Str)

Risk assessment: Class 2

Notes:

> See Chapter 7, "We 'Hear' With Our Eyes" for further information on this drug.

Dihydroergotamine (DHE)

Pronunciation guide: die-hye-droe-er-GOT-ah-meen

Drug classification: ERGOT ALKALOIDS (see section 17.4 in Table 14-1)

Brand names: *DHE, Migranal*

Ototoxic effects:
  Cochlear:
      Tinnitus: 0.1-1% (PDR)
  Vestibular:
      Ataxia: <0.1% (PDR)
      Dizziness: 4% [2% above placebo results] (CPS, PDR)
      Vertigo: 0.1-1% (PDR)
  Outer/Middle Ear:
      Earache/ear pain: 0.1-1% (PDR)

Risk assessment: Class 2

Dihydrostreptomycin   (see **Streptomycin**)

Dihydrotachysterol   (see **Ergocalciferal**)

Dilacor   (see **Diltiazem**)

Dilantin   (see **Phenytoin**)

Dilaudid   (see **Hydromorphone**)

Dilaudid-HP   (see **Hydromorphone**)

Dilevalol

Pronunciation guide: die-LEH-vah-lole

Drug classification: BETA-ADRENERGIC-BLOCKING DRUGS (BETA-BLOCKERS) (see section 20.8.12 in Table 14-1)

Brand names: —

Ototoxic effects:
  Cochlear:
      Tinnitus: (San, She)

Risk assessment: Class 1

Diltiazem

Pronunciation guide: dill-TYE-ah-zem

Drug classification: CALCIUM-CHANNEL-BLOCKING DRUGS (CALCIUM BLOCKERS) (see section 20.8.16 in Table 14-1)

Brand names: *Apo-Diltiaz*, *Cardizem*, *Cartia XT*, *Dilacor*, *Novo-Diltazem*, *Tiazac*, *Tiazac XC*

Ototoxic effects:
Cochlear:
Tinnitus: 1% [placebo 0] (CPS, PDR)
Vestibular:
Ataxia: <1% (CPS, PDR)
Dizziness: 3-10% [placebo 0] (CPS, PDR)
Vertigo: <1% (CPS, PDR)
Outer/Middle Ear:
Earache/ear pain: <1% (AHF, PDR)
Otitis media: <1% (AHF, PDR)

Risk assessment: Class 2

Dimenhydrinate

Pronunciation guide: dye-men-HYE-drih-nate

Drug classification: ANTI-CHOLINERGIC DRUGS (see section 17.1 in Table 14-1)

Brand names: *Dramamine*

Ototoxic effects:
Cochlear:
Tinnitus: (AHF)
Vestibular:
Ataxia: (AHF)
Dizziness: (AHF, NDH)
Vertigo: (NDH)

Risk assessment: Class 1

Dinoprostone

Pronunciation guide: dye-noe-PROST-ohn

Drug classification: PROSGLANDINS (see section 40.36 in Table 14-1)

Brand names: *Prostin E2*

Ototoxic effects:
Cochlear:
Hearing loss: (AHF, PDR)

Vestibular:
    Dizziness: (CPS, PDR)

Risk assessment: Class 2

Diochloram   (see **Chloramphenicol**)

Diodoquin   (see **Iodoquinol**)

Diovan   (see **Valsartan**)

Diovan HCT   (see **Valsartan**)

Dipentum   (see **Olsalazine**)

Diphenhydramine

Pronunciation guide: die-fen-HYE-drah-meen

Drug classification: H_1 RECEPTOR ANTAGONISTS (see section 10.1 in Table 14-1)

Brand names: *Benadryl, Nytol, Simply Sleep*

Ototoxic effects:
    Cochlear:
        Tinnitus: (PDR)
    Vestibular:
        Ataxia: (AHF, CPS)
        Dizziness: (CPS, PDR)
        Labyrinthitis, acute: (PDR)
        Vertigo: (CPS, PDR)

Risk assessment: Class 2

Notes:

Bromodiphenhydramine (broe-moe-die-fen-HYE-dra-meen) (see section 10.1 in Table 14-1) is a form of **Diphenhydramine** so you could expect it to have similar ototoxic side effects. **Bromodiphenhydramine** can apparently cause ototoxicity and tinnitus (San, She).

Caution: Eating grapefruit or drinking grapefruit juice during the time you are taking this drug may make the listed side effects worse than shown here.

See Chapter 7, "We 'Hear' With Our Eyes" and Chapter 11, "Grapefruit Juice and Ototoxic Drugs" for further information on **Diphenhydramine**.

Diphenidol

Pronunciation guide: die-FEN-ih-dol

Drug classification: ANTI-EMETICS (see section 34.1 in Table 14-1)

Brand names: *Vontrol*

Ototoxic effects:
   Cochlear:
      Auditory hallucinations: (AHF)
   Vestibular:
      Dizziness: (AHF)

Risk assessment: Class 1

Diphenylhydantoin   (see **Phenytoin**)

Diphenylhydrazine

Pronunciation guide: die-fen-ill-HIE-drah-zeen

Drug classification: H_1 RECEPTOR ANTAGONISTS (see section 10.1 in Table 14-1)

Brand names: —

Ototoxic effects:
   Unspecified/General Ear Conditions:
      Ototoxicity: (Str)

Risk assessment: Not enough information to rate

Diphtheria, tetanus & pertussis vaccine   (see **Tetanus vaccine**)

Diprivan   (see **Propofol**)

Diproderm   (see **Betamethasone**)

Diprosalic   (see **Salicylic acid**)

Dipyridamole

Pronunciation guide: dye-peer-IH-duh-mohl

Drug classification: PLATELET INHIBITOR DRUGS (see section 36.24 in Table 14-1)

Brand names: *Persantine*

Ototoxic effects:
   Cochlear:
      Tinnitus: 0.1% (CPS, DFC)
   Vestibular:
      Ataxia: (CPS, PDR)
      Dizziness: 11.8-13.6% [5.2% above placebo results] (CPS, PDR)
      Vertigo: 0.03% (CPS, DFC)
   Outer/Middle Ear:
      Earache/ear pain: 0.1% (CPS, DFC)

Risk assessment: Class 2

Notes:

Symptoms of acute **Dipyridamole** toxicity include ataxia in animals (PDR). It will likely affect people the same way.

Dipyrone (see **Aminopyrine**)

Dirithromycin

Pronunciation guide: die-rith-roe-MY-sin

Drug classification: MACROLIDE ANTIBIOTICS (see section 7.4.32 in Table 14-1)

Brand names: *Dynabac*

Ototoxic effects:
Cochlear:
Hearing loss: (PDR)
Tinnitus: 0.1-1% (PDR)
Vestibular:
Dizziness/vertigo: 2.1-2.3% (PDR)

Risk assessment: Class 2

Notes:

Dirithromycin is converted during absorption in the intestine into Erythromycylamine. As such, it is very similar to **Erythromycin**. **Erythromycin** is known to cause hearing loss (PDR). (See **Erythromycin** for its specific ototoxic properties.)

Disalcid (see **Salsalate**)

Disopyramide

Pronunciation guide: dye-soe-PEER-ah-mide

Drug classification: ANTI-ARRHYTHMICS (HEART RHYTHM REGULATORS) (see section 20.4 in Table 14-1)

Brand names: *Rythmodan*

Ototoxic effects:
Vestibular:
Dizziness: 1-10% (CPS, NDH)
Vertigo: 1-10% (CPS)

Risk assessment: Class 1

Disulfiram

Pronunciation guide: dye-SUL-fih-ram

Drug classification: SYNTHETIC ALCOHOL DEHYDROGENASE INHIBITORS (see section 66.8 in Table 14-1)

Brand names: *Antabuse*

Ototoxic effects:
Vestibular:
Ataxia: (AHF)
Vertigo: (AHF)

Risk assessment: Class 1

Notes:

See Chapter 7, "We 'Hear' With Our Eyes" for further information on this drug.

Diucardin   (see **Hydroflumethiazide**)

Diupres   (see **Reserpine**)

Diuretin   (see **Sodium salicylate**)

Diuril   (see **Chlorothiazide**)

Divalproex

Pronunciation guide: die-VAL-pro-ex

Drug classification: ANTI-CONVULSANT DRUGS (see section 53.12 in Table 14-1)

Brand names: *Apo-Divalproex, Depakote, Epiject, Epival, Novo-Divalproex*

Ototoxic effects:
Cochlear:
Hearing loss: 1-5% (CPS, PDR)
Tinnitus: 1-7% [<6% above placebo results] (CPS, PDR)
Vestibular:
Ataxia: 8% [7% above placebo results] (CPS, PDR)
Dizziness: 5.2-25% [<12% above placebo results] (CPS, PDR)
Nystagmus: 7-8% [6-7% above placebo results] (CPS, PDR)
Vertigo: 1-5% (CPS, PDR)
Outer/Middle Ear:
Earache/ear pain: 1-5% (CPS, PDR)
Otitis media: 1-5% (CPS, PDR)
Unspecified/General Ear Conditions:
Ear disorder: 1-5% (CPS, PDR)

Risk assessment: Class 4

Notes:

Hearing loss may be either temporary or permanent (CPS, PDR).

I have an anecdotal report in my files of a man who took **Divalproex**. This drug left him with permanent bilateral tinnitus.

Dixarit   (see **Clonidine**)

Dixeran   (see **Melitracen**)

Dizac   (see **Diazepam**)

Doan's Analgesic Caplets   (see **Magnesium salicylate**)

Docetaxel

Pronunciation guide: daws-eh-TAX-ell

Drug classification: MITOTIC INHIBITORS (see section 14.16 in Table 14-1)

Brand names: *Taxotere*

Ototoxic effects:
   Cochlear:
      Hearing loss: [1] 1.2-12.7% (NDH, PDR)
   Vestibular:
      Dizziness: 2.3-15.9% (PDR)

Risk assessment: Class 4

Notes:

   [1] Listed as "altered hearing" in the NDH.

   Rare cases of ototoxicity, hearing disorders and/or hearing loss have been reported (DFC, PDR).

Dodd's Pills   (see **Sodium salicylate**)

Dolasetron

Pronunciation guide: doe-LAZ-eh-tron

Drug classification: SEROTONIN-RECEPTOR ANTAGONISTS (see section 34.1.4 in Table 14-1)

Brand names: *Anzemet*

Ototoxic effects:
   Cochlear:
      Tinnitus: <0.1% (DFC, PDR)
   Vestibular:
      Ataxia: <0.1% (DFC, PDR)
      Dizziness: 1.3-5.5% [<4.4% above placebo results] (CPS, PDR)
      Vertigo: 0.3-2% (CPS, PDR)

Risk assessment: Class 2

Dolobid   (see **Diflunisal**)

Donepezil

Pronunciation guide: doe-NEP-ah-zill

Drug classification: CHOLINESTERASE INHIBITORS (see section 53.4.1 in Table 14-1)

Brand names: *Aricept*

Ototoxic effects:
   Cochlear:
      Hearing loss: 0.1-1% (CPS, PDR)
      Tinnitus: 0.1-1% (CPS, PDR)
   Vestibular:
      Ataxia: 1-2% (CPS, PDR)
      Dizziness: 2-8% [<2% above placebo results] (DFC, PDR)
      Nystagmus: 0.1-1% (CPS, PDR)
      Vertigo: 1-2% (CPS, PDR)
   Outer/Middle Ear:
      Earache/ear pain: 0.1-1% (CPS, PDR)
      Otitis externa: 0.1-1% (CPS, PDR)
      Otitis media: 0.1-1% (CPS, PDR)

Risk assessment: Class 2

Notes:

   Caution: Eating grapefruit or drinking grapefruit juice during the time you are taking this drug may make the listed side effects worse than shown here.

   See Chapter 11, "Grapefruit Juice and Ototoxic Drugs" for further information on this drug.

Donnatal   (see **Atropine**)

Doral   (see **Quazepam**)

Doribax   (see **Doripenem**)

Doripenem

Pronunciation guide: door-ih-PEN-em

Drug classification: CARBAPENEMS (see section 7.4.12.1 in Table 14-1)

Brand names: *Doribax*

Ototoxic effects:
   Vestibular:
      Dizziness: 0.1-1% (CPS)
      Vertigo: 0.1-1% (CPS)

Risk assessment: Class 1

Dormonoct   (see **Loprazolam**)

Dostinex   (see **Cabergoline**)

Dosulepin   (see **Dothiepin**)

Dothiepin (Dosulepin)

Pronunciation guide: doe-THIGH-ah-pin (doe-SOO-leh-pin)

Drug classification: TRICYCLIC ANTI-DEPRESSANTS (see section 60.1.8 in Table 14-1)

Brand names: *Prothiaden*

Ototoxic effects:
    Cochlear:
        Tinnitus: [1]
    Vestibular:
        Ataxia: [1]
        Dizziness: [1, 189]

Risk assessment: Class 1

Notes:

    [1] Can cause ataxia, dizziness and tinnitus.[190]

Doxazosin

Pronunciation guide: dox-AY-zoe-sin

Drug classification: ALPHA ADRENERGIC BLOCKING DRUGS (see section 20.8.1 in Table 14-1)

Brand names: *Cardura, Cardura-2*

Ototoxic effects:
    Cochlear:
        Auditory Hallucinations: [191]
        Hearing loss: <1% (CPS)
        Hyperacusis: [1]
        Tinnitus: [1] 0.5-1.3% [<0.7% above placebo results] (CPS, PDR)
    Vestibular:
        Ataxia: 1% [placebo 0] (CPS, PDR)
        Dizziness: 14.6-20.7% [6.6-10% above placebo results] (CPS, PDR)
        Vertigo: 2-3% [1% above placebo results] (CPS, PDR)
    Outer/Middle Ear:
        Earache/ear pain: 0.5-1% (CPS, PDR)
        Otitis media: <1% (CPS)

Risk assessment: Class 3

Notes:

[1] I have an anecdotal report in my files of a lady that took **Doxazosin** for 26 days. By day 18 she had severe tinnitus. Fortunately, 6 weeks after stopping the **Doxazosin**, her severe tinnitus had dropped by about 80%. In addition to the tinnitus, she also developed severe hyperacusis, which has not gone away yet. She also reported that her doctor had had two other patients that also developed severe tinnitus from taking **Doxazosin**. In one case it took 9 months for the tinnitus to fade away; in the other, it took a full year.

Doxepin

Pronunciation guide: DOX-eh-pin

Drug classification: TRICYCLIC ANTI-DEPRESSANTS (see section 60.1.8 in Table 14-1)

Brand names: *Adapin, Apo-Doxepin, Sinequan*

Ototoxic effects:
   Cochlear:
       Tinnitus: (CPS, PDR)
   Vestibular:
       Ataxia: (NDH, PDR)
       Dizziness: >10% (NDH, PDR)
       Vertigo: (CPS)

Risk assessment: Class 1

Notes:

   See Chapter 7, "We 'Hear' With Our Eyes" for further information on this drug.

Doxil   (see **Doxorubicin**)

Doxorubicin (Liposomal doxorubicin)

Pronunciation guide: dox-oh-ROO-bih-sin (lih-poe-SOE-mal dox-oh-ROO-bih-sin)

Drug classification: ANTHRACYCLINES (see section 14.4 in Table 14-1)

Brand names: *Adriamycin, Caelyx* [1], *Doxil* [1], *Myocet* [1]

Ototoxic effects:
   Cochlear:
       Tinnitus: <1% (CPS, PDR)
   Vestibular:
       Ataxia: <1% (CPS, PDR)
       Dizziness: 1-5% (CPS, PDR)
       Nystagmus: <1% (CPS)
       Vertigo: <1% (CPS, PDR)
   Outer/Middle Ear:
       Otitis media: <1% (CPS, PDR)

Risk assessment: Class 2

Notes:

[1] *Caelyx*, *Doxil* and *Myocet* are combinations of **Doxorubicin** and Liposome. **Doxorubicin** is the ototoxic agent.

Doxycycline

Pronunciation guide: dox-ih-SYE-kleen

Drug classification: TETRACYCLINES (see section 7.4.60 in Table 14-1)

Brand names: *Vibra-Tabs*

Ototoxic effects:
 Cochlear:
  Hearing loss: [1, 2]
  Tinnitus: (CPS)

Risk assessment: Class 2

Notes:

Doxycycline is one of the TETRACYCLINES and likely has many of the same ototoxic properties **Tetracycline** has. (See the generic drug **Tetracycline** for its specific ototoxic properties.)

[1] I have an anecdotal report in my files of a man who lost much of his hearing after taking **Doxycycline** for a urinary tract infection.

[2] I have another anecdotal report in my files of a man who, after taking a 10-day course of **Doxycycline** used to treat a cold, reported, "the hearing in my already-impaired right ear suddenly reduced to virtually zero and remains there".

Doxylamine

Pronunciation guide: doks-ILL-ah-meen

Drug classification: H_1 RECEPTOR ANTAGONISTS (see section 10.1 in Table 14-1)

Brand names: *Bendectin*[1], *Diclectin*[1], *Mersyndol with Codeine*[2]

Ototoxic effects:
 Cochlear:
  Tinnitus: (NTP)
 Vestibular:
  Dizziness: (CPS, NTP)
  Vertigo: (CPS)

Risk assessment: Class 1

Notes:

[1] *Bendectin and Diclectin* are combinations of **Doxylamine** and **Pyridoxine**. (See the generic drug **Pyridoxine** for its specific ototoxic properties.)

[2] *Mersyndol with Codeine* is a combination of **Acetaminophen**, **Codeine** and **Doxylamine**. (See the generic drugs **Acetaminophen** and **Codeine** for their specific ototoxic properties.)

Dramamine (see **Dimenhydrinate**)

Drisdol (see **Ergocalciferal**)

Dristan Sinus (see **Ibuprofen**)

Dronabinol (Delta-9-tetrahydrocannabinol)

Pronunciation guide: droe-NAB-ih-nol (DEL-tah nine TET-rah-hye-droe-kan-nah-BIH-nall)

Drug classification: SEROTONIN-RECEPTOR ANTAGONISTS (see section 34.1.4 in Table 14-1)

Brand names: *Marinol, Sativex*

Ototoxic effects:
    Cochlear:
        Tinnitus: 0.3-1% (CPS, PDR)
    Vestibular:
        Ataxia: 4% [placebo 0] (CPS, PDR)
        Dizziness: 12-32.6% [7-22.9% above placebo results] (CPS, PDR)
        Equilibrium disorder: 2.4% [1.2% above placebo results] (CPS)
        Vertigo: 4.2-5% [2.9-3% above placebo results] (CPS)

Risk assessment: Class 2

Notes:

See **Cannabis sativa** in the ototoxic herbals section for additional information on the natural version (marijuana) of this drug and its specific ototoxic properties.)

Drospirenone—Ethinyl estradiol (see **Ethinyl estradiol**)

DTP Adsorbed (see **Tetanus vaccine**)

Duloxetine

Pronunciation guide: doh-LOCKS-ah-teen

Drug classification: SELECTIVE SEROTONIN & NOREPINEPHRINE REUPTAKE INHIBITORS (see section 60.1.28 in Table 14-1)

Brand names: *Cymbalta*

Ototoxic effects:
    Cochlear:
        Tinnitus: 0.1-1% (CPS, PDR)

Vestibular:
Ataxia: 0.01-1% (PDR, RXL)
Dizziness: 10-17% [<11% above placebo results] (NDH, PDR)
Vertigo: >1% (CPS, PDR)
Outer/Middle Ear:
Earache/ear pain: 0.1-1% (CPS, PDR)

Risk assessment: Class 1

Notes:

Tinnitus may start after you stop taking **Duloxetine** (CPS).

DuoFilm   (see **Salicylic acid**)

DuoTrav   (see **Travoprost**)

Duraclon   (see **Clonidine**)

Duragesic   (see **Fentanyl**)

Duralith   (see **Lithium**)

Duranest   (see **Etidocaine**)

Duricef   (see **Cefadroxil**)

Dyazide   (see **Triamterene**)

Dyclone   (see **Dyclonine**)

Dyclonine

Pronunciation guide: DIE-kloe-neen

Drug classification: LOCAL ANESTHETICS (see section 4.10 in Table 14-1)

Brand names: *Dyclone*

Ototoxic effects:
Cochlear:
Tinnitus: (PDR)
Vestibular:
Dizziness: (PDR)

Risk assessment: Class 1

Dynabac   (see **Dirithromycin**)

Dynacin   (see **Minocycline**)

DynaCirc   (see **Isradipine**)

Dynastat   (see **Parecoxib**)

Dyrenium   (see **Triamterene**)

Dysport   (see **Abobotulinum Toxin A**)

E.E.S.   (see **Erythromycin**)

Easprin   (see **Acetylsalicylic acid**)

Ebixa   (see **Memantine**)

EC-Naprosyn   (see **Naproxen**)

Ecotrin Enteric-coated Aspirin   (see **Acetylsalicylic acid**)

Eculizumab

Pronunciation guide: ek-yoo-LIZ-yoo-mab

Drug classification: MONOCLONAL ANTIBODIES (see section 7.17.8 in Table 14-1)

Brand names: *Soliris*

Ototoxic effects:
    Cochlear:
        Tinnitus: <1% (CPS)
    Vestibular:
        Dizziness: 6.7-8.2% (CPS)
        Vertigo: <1% (CPS)

Risk assessment: Class 2

Edecrin   (see **Ethacrynic acid**)

Edluar   (see **Zolpidem**)

Edronax   (see **Reboxetine**)

Efavirenz

Pronunciation guide: eff-ah-VYE-renz

Drug classification: ANTI-RETROVIRAL REVERSE TRANSCRIPTASE INHIBITORS (see section 7.17.1.4 in Table 14-1)

Brand names: *Atripla*[1], *Sustiva*

Ototoxic effects:
> Cochlear:
>> Tinnitus: <2% (CPS, PDR)
>
> Vestibular:
>> Ataxia: <2% (CPS, PDR)
>> Dizziness: 2-28.1% (CPS, PDR)
>> Equilibrium disorder: (CPS, PDR)
>> Vertigo: <2% (CPS, PDR)

Risk assessment: Class 2

Notes:

> [1] *Atripla* is a combination of **Efavirenz**, Emtricitabine and Tenofovir. (**Efavirenz** is the ototoxic agent.)

Effexor   (see **Venlafaxine**)

Effexor XL   (see **Venlafaxine**)

Eflornithine

Pronunciation guide: eh-FLOR-nih-theen

Drug classification: ANTI-PROTOZOALS (see section 7.14 in Table 14-1)

Brand names: *Vaniqa*

Ototoxic effects:
> Vestibular:
>> Dizziness: 1.3-1.5% (DFC, PDR)
>> Vertigo: 0.1-1% (DFC, PDR)
>
> Unspecified/General Ear Conditions:
>> Ototoxicity: (CP2)

Risk assessment: Class 2

Efudex   (see **Fluorouracil**)

ELA-Max   (see **Lidocaine**)

Elaprase   (see **Idursulfase**)

Elavil   (see **Amitriptyline**)

Elavil Plus   (see **Amitriptyline**)

Eldepryl   (see **Selegiline**)

Eletriptan

Pronunciation guide: ell-ah-TRIP-tan

Drug classification: Serotonin-receptor agonists (see section 53.32 in Table 14-1)

Brand names: *Relpax*

Ototoxic effects:
  Cochlear:
    Tinnitus: 0.1-1% (CPS, DFC)
  Vestibular:
    Ataxia: 0.1-1% (BNF, CPS)
    Dizziness: 2.4-7.2% [<4.4% above placebo results] (AHF, CPS)
    Vertigo: 0.2-1.8% [<1.3% above placebo results] (CPS, NDH)
  Outer/Middle Ear:
    Earache/ear pain: 0.1-1% (CPS, DFC)
    Otitis media: <0.1% (CPS, DFC)
  Unspecified/General Ear Conditions:
    Ear disorder: <0.1% (CPS, DFC)

Risk assessment: Class 2

Elidel   (see **Pimecrolimus**)

Eligard   (see **Leuprolide**)

Elmiron   (see **Pentosan**)

Elocon   (see **Mometasone**)

Eloxatin   (see **Oxaliplatin**)

Emadine   (see **Emedastine**)

Embeda   (see **Morphine**)

Emedastine

Pronunciation guide: em-eh-DAS-teen

Drug classification: H_1 receptor antagonists (see section 10.1 in Table 14-1)

Brand names: *Emadine*

Ototoxic effects:
  Cochlear:
    Tinnitus: (San, She)

Risk assessment: Class 1

Emend   (see **Aprepitant**)

Emend IV   (see **Aprepitant**)

Emflex   (see **Acemetacin**)

Eminase   (see **Anistreplase**)

Emla   (see **Lidocaine**)

Emsam   (see **Selegiline**)

E-Mycin   (see **Erythromycin**)

Enalapril (Enalaprilat)

Pronunciation guide: eh-NAH-leh-pril (eh-NAH-leh-pril-at)

Drug classification: ANGIOTENSIN-CONVERTING ENZYME (ACE) INHIBITORS (see section 20.8.8 in Table 14-1)

Brand names: *Lexxel*[1], *Vaseretic*[2], *Vasotec*

Ototoxic effects:
 Cochlear:
  Hearing loss: [3] 0.5-1% (AHF, CPS)
  Tinnitus: 0.5-1% (CPS, PDR)
 Vestibular:
  Ataxia: 0.5-1% (CPS, PDR)
  Dizziness: 4.3-8.6% [4.3-7.3% above placebo results] (CPS, PDR)
  Vertigo: <0.5-1.6% [0.4% above placebo results] (CPS, PDR)

Risk assessment: Class 2

Notes:

[1] *Lexxel* is a combination of **Enalapril** and **Felodipine**. (See the generic drug **Felodipine** for its specific ototoxic properties.)

[2] *Vaseretic* is a combination of **Enalapril** and **Hydrochlorothiazide**. (See the generic drug **Hydrochlorothiazide** for its specific ototoxic properties.)

Enalapril and **Enalaprilat** are closely related chemically. In fact, your body converts **Enalapril** to **Enalaprilat**. Therefore, you experience the same side effects for both these drugs (CPS, PDR).

[3] Hearing loss is temporary (AHF).

Enalaprilat   (see **Enalapril**)

Enbrel   (see **Etanercept**)

Enduron   (see **Methyclothiazide**)

Enduronyl (see **Deserpidine**)

Enfuvirtide

Pronunciation guide: en-foo-VEER-tide

Drug classification: Anti-retroviral HIV fusion inhibitors (see section 7.17.1.12 in Table 14-1)

Brand names: *Fuzeon*

Ototoxic effects:
Vestibular:
Vertigo: 3.6% [3% above placebo results] (CPS)
Outer/Middle Ear:
Otitis: 2.2% [1% above placebo results] (CPS)

Risk assessment: Class 1

Engerix-B (see **Hepatitis B vaccine**)

Enoxacin

Pronunciation guide: eh-NOX-ah-sin

Drug classification: Quinolones (see section 7.4.48 in Table 14-1)

Brand names: *Penetrex*

Ototoxic effects:
Cochlear:
Tinnitus: 0.1-1% (CP2, PDR)
Vestibular:
Ataxia: <0.1% (PDR)
Dizziness/vertigo: 3% (PDR)
Nystagmus: (PDR)
Vertigo: (CP2)

Risk assessment: Class 1

Entacapone

Pronunciation guide: en-tah-KAP-own

Drug classification: Anti-parkinsonian drugs (see section 53.16 in Table 14-1)

Brand names: *Comtan*

Ototoxic effects:
Vestibular:
Ataxia: 1.2% [0.7% above placebo results] (CPS)
Dizziness: 7.5-10% [1.5% above placebo results] (CPS, NDH)

Risk assessment: Class 1

Entacyl   (see **Piperazine**)

Entocort EC   (see **Budesonide**)

Entrophen   (see **Acetylsalicylic acid**)

Ephedrine

Pronunciation guide: eh-FED-rin

Drug classification: Bronchodilators—beta adrenergic agonists (see section 63.4 in Table 14-1)

Brand names: *Marax* [1]

Ototoxic effects:
    Cochlear:
        Auditory hallucinations: (AHF)
    Vestibular:
        Dizziness: (CPS, NDH)
        Vertigo: (NTP, PDR)

Risk assessment: Class 1

Notes:

    [1] *Marax* is a combination of **Ephedrine** and **Theophylline**. (See the generic drug **Theophylline** for its specific ototoxic properties.)

    See Chapter 7, "We 'Hear' With Our Eyes" for further information on this drug.

Epiject   (see **Divalproex**)

Epival   (see **Divalproex**)

Epivir   (see **Lamivudine**)

Epoetin alfa

Pronunciation guide: eh-poe-EH-tin

Drug classification: Hematopoietic agents (see section 36.20 in Table 14-1)

Brand names: *Eprex*

Ototoxic effects:
    Vestibular:
        Dizziness: 9-10% [same as placebo] (CPS)
        Vertigo: 1-5% (CPS)
    Outer/Middle Ear:
        Earache/ear pain: 1-5% (CPS)
        Otitis: 5.1% [3.5% above placebo results] (CPS)
        Otitis media: 1-5% (CPS)

Risk assessment: Class 2

Eprex   (see **Epoetin alfa**)

Eprosartan

Pronunciation guide: ep-roe-SAR-tan

Drug classification: ANGIOTENSIN-2-RECEPTOR ANTAGONISTS (see section 20.8.4 in Table 14-1)

Brand names: *Teveten, Teveten HCT* [1]

Ototoxic effects:
    Cochlear:
        Tinnitus: <1% (CPS, PDR)
    Vestibular:
        Ataxia: <1% (CPS, PDR)
        Dizziness: >1.8-4.1% [0.2-2.5% above placebo results] (CPS, PDR)
        Vertigo: <1% (CPS, PDR)
    Outer/Middle Ear:
        Otitis externa: <1% (CPS, PDR)
        Otitis media: <1% (CPS, PDR)

Risk assessment: Class 2

Notes:

[1] *Teveten HCT* is a combination of **Eprosartan** and **Hydrochlorothiazide**. (See the generic drug **Hydrochlorothiazide** for its specific ototoxic properties.)

Equetro   (see **Carbamazepine**)

Erbitux   (see **Cetuximab**)

Ergamisol   (see **Levamisole**)

Ergocalciferal (Vitamin D$_2$)

Pronunciation guide: er-goe-kal-SIH-fer-all

Drug classification: VITAMINS (see section 75.4 in Table 14-1)

Brand names: *Drisdol, Ostoforte, Vitamin D$_2$*

Ototoxic effects:
    Cochlear:
        Tinnitus: (CPS)
    Vestibular:
        Ataxia: (CPS)
        Vertigo: (BNF, CPS)

Risk assessment: Class 1

Notes:

There are various forms of Vitamin D including **Ergocalciferal** (Vitamin D$_2$), **Alfacalcidol**, **Calcitriol**, **Cholecalciferol** (Vitamin D$_3$) and **Dihydrotachysterol** (BNF, CPS). (See also **Paricalcitol**.)

Overdoses can result in hypercalcemia and symptoms such as ataxia, tinnitus and vertigo (CPS).

Ergometrine   (see **Ergonovine**)

Ergonovine (Ergometrine)

Pronunciation guide: er-goe-NOE-veen

Drug classification: ERGOT ALKALOIDS (see section 17.4 in Table 14-1)

Brand names: *Ergotrate*

Ototoxic effects:
    Cochlear:
        Tinnitus: (AHF, Med)
    Vestibular:
        Dizziness: (AHF, CPS)
        Vertigo: (CPS)

Risk assessment: Class 1

Ergotamine

Pronunciation guide: er-GOT-ah-meen

Drug classification: ERGOT ALKALOIDS (see section 17.4 in Table 14-1)

Brand names: *Cafergot* [1]

Ototoxic effects:
    Vestibular:
        Dizziness: 1-10% (CPS)
        Vertigo: (AHF, BNF)

Risk assessment: Class 1

Notes:

[1] *Cafergot* is a combination of **Ergotamine** and **Caffeine**. (See the generic drug **Caffeine** for its specific ototoxic properties.)

Ergotrate   (see **Ergonovine**)

Ertapenem

Pronunciation guide: er-tah-PEN-em

Drug classification: CARBAPENEMS (see section 7.4.12.1 in Table 14-1)

Brand names: *Invanz*

Ototoxic effects:
Vestibular:
Dizziness: 1.5-2.1% (NDH, PDR)
Vertigo: >0.1% (DFC, PDR)
Outer/Middle Ear:
Otitis: (DFC)

Risk assessment: Class 1

Eryc   (see **Erythromycin**)

Ery-Ped   (see **Erythromycin**)

Ery-Tab   (see **Erythromycin**)

Erythrocin   (see **Erythromycin**)

Erythromycin

Pronunciation guide: ER-ith-roe-MYE-sin

Drug classification: MACROLIDE ANTIBIOTICS (see section 7.4.32 in Table 14-1)

Brand names: *E.E.S., E-Mycin, Eryc, Ery-Ped, Ery-Tab, Erythrocin, Ilosone, Ilotycin, PCE, Pediazole*[1]

Ototoxic effects:
Cochlear:
Hearing loss: (CPS, PDR)
Hyperacusis: [2]
Tinnitus: (CPS, PDR)
Vestibular:
Ataxia: (CPS, PDR)
Dizziness: (CPS, PDR)
Vertigo: (CPS, PDR)

Risk assessment: Class 2

Notes:

[1] *Pediazole* is a combination of **Erythromycin** and **Sulfisoxazole**. (See the generic drug **Sulfisoxazole** for its specific ototoxic properties.)

Erythromycin was introduced in 1952. However, reports that it was ototoxic didn't surface until 21 years later in 1973.[192]

Erythromycin can cause hearing loss, according to a group of Spanish research physicians.[193] Generally, hearing loss occurs in people with kidney problems who are receiving high doses (CPS, PDR). In rare instances (involving intravenous administration) the hearing loss is permanent (PDR). Hearing loss from **Erythromycin** occurs in both children and adults. The evidence suggests that it occurs when you take high doses (2 g to 4 g/day [AHF]) for two weeks or so.[194] (There are also anecdotal reports of permanent hearing loss from taking **Erythromycin** orally.)

Hearing losses due to **Erythromycin** appear to occur in the speech frequencies at the same time they appear in the high frequencies. This makes it relatively easy to detect a hearing loss due to this drug.[195] Hearing loss can occur almost immediately after taking **Erythromycin**.[196] The good news is that when you stop taking **Erythromycin**, improvement generally comes rapidly since hearing loss is typically temporary. Hearing usually returns to "normal" in 1 to 30 days after stopping the drug.[197]

There have been isolated reports of reversible hearing loss occurring chiefly in patients with renal insufficiency, and in patients receiving high doses of **Erythromycin** (PDR). In rare instances involving I.V. use, the ototoxic effect has been permanent (DFC).

[2] I have an anecdotal report in my files of a man that lost his hearing in one ear after he took a course of **Erythromycin**. In addition he experienced hyperacusis, balance problems and "horrific bilateral tinnitus". His condition appears to be permanent as this had happened five years ago at the time he wrote to me.

Caution: Eating grapefruit or drinking grapefruit juice during the time you are taking this drug may make the listed side effects worse than shown here.

See Chapter 2 "Ototoxic Drugs—What Are They," Chapter 3 "Ototoxic Side Effects and Your Ears," Chapter 4 "Are You at Risk," Chapter 5 "Here's How the System Works," Chapter 7, "We 'Hear' With Our Eyes," Chapter 9, "Aminoglycoside Antibiotics are the Ototoxic 'Bad boys'" and Chapter 11, "Grapefruit Juice and Ototoxic Drugs" for further information on this drug.

Escitalopram

Pronunciation guide: ess-sih-TAL-oh-pram

Drug classification: SELECTIVE SEROTONIN REUPTAKE INHIBITORS (see section 60.1.32 in Table 14-1)

Brand names: *Cipralex*, *Lexapro*

Ototoxic effects:
Cochlear:
Auditory hallucinations: 0.1-1% (CPS, PDR)
Hearing loss: 0.1-1% (CPS)
Tinnitus: 1.1% [0.4% above placebo results] (CPS, PDR)
Vestibular:
Ataxia: (PDR)
Dizziness: 4-13.5% [2-7.7% above placebo results] (CPS, PDR)
Nystagmus: (PDR)
Vertigo: 1.0-1.4% [<0.8% above placebo results] (CPS, PDR)
Outer/Middle Ear:
Earache/ear pain: >1% (NDH, PDR)

Unspecified/General Ear Conditions:
 Ear disorder: 0.1-1% (CPS)
 Meniere's disease: (CPS)
 Perforated eardrum: (CPS)

Risk assessment: Class 2

Esgic-Plus   (see **Butalbital**)

Esidrix   (see **Hydrochlorothiazide**)

Esimil   (see **Hydrochlorothiazide**)

Eskalith   (see **Lithium**)

Esomeprazole

Pronunciation guide: ess-oh-MEE-pray-zol

Drug classification: PROTON PUMP INHIBITORS (see section 34.8.4 in Table 14-1)

Brand names: *Nexium*

Ototoxic effects:
 Cochlear:
  Tinnitus: <1% (PDR)
 Vestibular:
  Ataxia: [1] (PDR)
  Dizziness: <2.5% (CPS, PDR)
  Vertigo: <1% (CPS, PDR)
 Outer/Middle Ear:
  Earache/ear pain: <1% (PDR)
  Otitis media: 1.5% (CPS, PDR)

Risk assessment: Class 2

Notes:

[1] Overdose can cause ataxia (PDR).

I have an anecdotal report in my files of a man who took **Esomeprazole** and 6 to 8 weeks later had sudden tinnitus in one ear, and a week after that, in his other ear also. He explains, "I think I'm going crazy with 2 different tones that will not stop!"

Estazolam

Pronunciation guide: ess-TAZ-oh-lam

Drug classification: BENZODIAZEPINES (see section 60.12.8 in Table 14-1)

Brand names: *ProSom*

Ototoxic effects:
    Cochlear:
        Hearing loss: <0.1% (PDR)
        Tinnitus: 0.1-1% (PDR)
    Vestibular:
        Ataxia: < 0.1% (PDR)
        Dizziness: 7% [4% above placebo results] (PDR)
        Nystagmus: <0.1% (PDR)
    Outer/Middle Ear:
        Earache/ear pain: 0.1-1% (PDR)

Risk assessment: Class 2

Notes:

    See Chapter 10 "Beware of Benzodiazepines—Don't Let This Nasty Time-Bomb Ambush You and Your Ears" for further information on this drug.

Estraderm   (see **Estradiol**)

Estradiol

Pronunciation guide: ess-trah-DYE-ole

Drug classification: ESTROGENS (see section 40.20 in Table 14-1)

Brand names: *Angeliq* [1], *Cenestin, Climara, Estraderm, Estring, Femtran, Premarin,*

    Vivelle-dot

Ototoxic effects:
    Cochlear:
        Hearing loss: [2, 198]
        Tinnitus: [3] 0.5-1% [placebo 0] (CPS)
    Vestibular:
        Dizziness: <11% [1% above placebo results] (CPS, PDR)
        Vertigo: (CPS, PDR)
    Outer/Middle Ear:
        Ear pain: [4] 1-2% [placebo 0] (CPS)
        Otitis: 2.9% [same as placebo] (PDR)
        Otitis media: 1-3% (CPS, PDR)

Risk assessment: Class 2

Notes:

    [1] *Angeliq* is a combination of **Estradiol** and Drospirenone. (**Estradiol** is the ototoxic agent.)

    [2] **Warning**: If you have otosclerosis, read this. You should not use **Estradiol** if you have a worsening of your otosclerosis, or if your "otosclerosis deteriorates during pregnancy"[199] as you may experience a further drop in your hearing.[200] If you do decide to take **Estradiol** and have otosclerosis, you should be under "close medical supervision".

Furthermore, you should weigh the long term benefits against the risks to your hearing.[201] (See also comments under **Estriol** below.)

[3] I have an anecdotal report in my files of a woman that wrote, "I started HRT (hormone replacement therapy) and within 10 days my ear started "drumming" (one of the many tinnitus sounds).

[4] I also have an anecdotal report in my files of a woman who wrote, "I have recently started taking HRT (hormone replacement therapy—estrogen only—via a transdermal patch) for the past 11 weeks. Since starting HRT, I have had a constant pain deep inside my left ear, with intermittent nerve pain radiating behind the ear. It can happen anytime and last from 1 minute to 1 hour to all day. My doctor examined my ear but cannot find anything wrong. I decided to stop the HRT for one week. The pain subsided quite dramatically. My doctor suggested I start a lower dose. With the lower dose, the pain is mild compared to what it was".

Estradiol-17 beta

Pronunciation guide: ess-trah-DYE-ole

Drug classification: ESTROGENS (see section 40.20 in Table 14-1)

Brand names: *Vagifem*

Ototoxic effects:
    Vestibular:
        Dizziness: <5% (CPS)
    Outer/Middle Ear:
        Ear pain: <5% (CPS)
    Unspecified/General Ear Conditions:
        Ear disorder: <5% (CPS)

Risk assessment: Class 1

Estramustine   (see **Mechlorethamine**)

Estring   (see **Estradiol**)

Estriol

Pronunciation guide: ESS-tree-ole

Drug classification: ESTROGENS (see section 40.20 in Table 14-1)

Brand names: *Synapause-E3*

Ototoxic effects:
    Cochlear:
        Hearing loss: [1]

Risk assessment: Class 2 (but Class 4 if you have otosclerosis)

Notes:

[1] **Warning**: If you have otosclerosis and especially if you had a drop in your hearing from worsening otosclerosis during your pregnancies, then taking **Estriol** (hormone replacement therapy—HRT) may cause your otosclerosis to flare up again with a consequent drop in your hearing. You should not take **Estriol** if you have "a history of a manifestation or deterioration of otosclerosis during pregnancy".[202]

I have an anecdotal report in my files of a woman who was placed on **Estriol** causing her otosclerosis to flare up, and immediately she had a marked increase in her tinnitus. Soon after, her husband noticed that she was losing more of her hearing. Her doctor never warned her about this serious side effect.

A small study funded by the National Institutes of Health suggests that women who undergo hormone replacement therapy (HRT) run the risk of hearing loss. In addition to the hearing loss, women on HRT process sound 30% less effectively than those who do not take this drug. This would be most noticeable in noisy surroundings where you are trying to listen to one particular person.[203]

Eszopiclone

Pronunciation guide: ess-ZOP-ah-klone

Drug classification: HYPNOTIC DRUGS (see section 60.16 in Table 14-1)

Brand names: *Lunesta*

Ototoxic effects:
    Cochlear:
        Hyperacusis: 0.1-0.01% (DFC, PDR)
        Tinnitus: 0.1-1% (DFC, PDR)
    Vestibular:
        Ataxia: 0.1-1% (DFC, PDR)
        Dizziness: 5-7% [1-3% above placebo results] (NDH, PDR)
        Nystagmus: 0.1-1% (DFC, PDR)
        Vertigo: 0.1-1% (DFC, PDR)
        Vestibular disorder: 0.1-1% (DFC, PDR)
    Outer/Middle Ear:
        Earache/ear pain: 0.1-1% (DFC, PDR)
        Otitis externa: 0.1-1% (DFC, PDR)
        Otitis media: 0.1-1% (DFC, PDR)

Risk assessment: Class 2

Etanercept

Pronunciation guide: ee-TAN-er-sept

Drug classification: TUMOR NECROSIS FACTOR MODIFIERS (see section 14.36 in Table 14-1)

Brand names: *Enbrel*

Ototoxic effects:
    Cochlear:
        Tinnitus: 1% [placebo 0] (CPS)
    Vestibular:
        Dizziness: 3-5% [2-4% above placebo results] (CPS)
        Vertigo: 1% [placebo 0] (CPS)
    Outer/Middle Ear:
        Otitis media: <1% (CPS)
    Outer/Middle Ear:
        Ear disorder: <1% (CPS)

Risk assessment: Class 2

Ethacrynic acid

Pronunciation guide: eth-uh-KRIH-nik ASS-id

Drug classification: DIURETICS—LOOP (see section 30.5.4 in Table 14-1)

Brand names: *Edecrin*

Ototoxic effects:
    Cochlear:
        Hearing loss: (CPS, PDR)
        Tinnitus: (CPS, PDR)
    Vestibular:
        Vertigo: (CPS, PDR)
    Outer/Middle Ear:
        Feeling of fullness in ears: (CPS, PDR)

Risk assessment: Class 4

Notes:

Warning: You can get severe, permanent hearing loss from taking **Ethacrynic acid**.[204]

Ototoxicity was first reported in 1966.[205] The incidence of hearing loss is about 0.7%.[206]

Ototoxicity due to **Ethacrynic acid** seems to develop more gradually and takes longer to recover from than the other LOOP DIURETICS.[207]

You are more likely to have side effects such as hearing loss, tinnitus, vertigo and a sense of fullness in the ears if you have severe kidney problems. These symptoms are normally associated with intravenous administration, and with higher doses than recommended. Hearing loss is usually temporary and lasts from 1 to 24 hours. However, some people end up with permanent hearing loss. A number of these people were also receiving other ototoxic drugs at the same time (CPS, PDR).

Ethacrynic acid may increase the ototoxic potential of other drugs such as the AMINOGLYCOSIDE antibiotics and some CEPHALOSPORIN antibiotics. As a result, you should avoid taking them both at the same time (CPS, PDR).

See Chapter 4 "Are You at Risk?" and Chapter 12, "Potpourri" for further information on this drug.

Ethinyl estradiol

(including)

Desogestrel—**Ethinyl estradiol**
Drospirenone—**Ethinyl estradiol**
Etonogestrel—Ethinyl estradiol
Levonorgestrel—Ethinyl estradiol
Norethindrone—Ethinyl estradiol
Norgestimate—**Ethinyl estradiol**

Pronunciation guide: ETH-in-il es-trah-DIE-ole, DAY-soh-jest-rul, nor-JES-tih-mate

Drug classification: CONTRACEPTIVES (see section 40.12 in Table 14-1)

Brand names: *Apri 28,* *Brevicon*[1]*, Cyclen*[2]*, Demulen*[3]*, Diane-35*[4]*, Linessa 28*[5]*, Loestrin* [1]*, Marvelon*[5]*, Minestrin* [1]*, Mircette*[5]*, Necon 1/35*[1]*, NuvaRing*[6]*, Ortho*[1]*, Ortho 7/7/7* [1]*, Ortho-Cept*[5]*, Seasonale*[7]*, Select*[1]*, Select 1/35* [1]*, Synphasic*[1]*, Tri-Cyclen*[2]*, Triquilar 28* [7]*, Yasmin 28*[8]*, Yaz*[8]

Ototoxic effects:
Cochlear:
Auditory disorder:[9] (CPS)
Hearing disorder: (CPS)
Tinnitus: <1% (CPS)
Vestibular:
Dizziness: 1-5% (CPS, PDR)
Labyrinthitis: <1% (CPS)
Vertigo: 1-5% (CPS)
Outer/Middle Ear:
Earache/ear pain: 1-5% (CPS)
Ears blocked: <1% (CPS)
Eustachian tube disorder: <1% (CPS)
Otitis externa:<1% (CPS)
Otitis media: <1% (CPS)
Outer/Middle Ear:
Ear disorder: <1% (CPS)

Risk assessment: Class 2

Notes:

[1] *Brevicon, Loestrin, Minestrin, Necon 1/35, Ortho, Ortho 7/7/7, Select, Select 1/35* and *Synphasic* are combinations of **Norethindrone** and **Ethinyl estradiol**. (See the generic drug **Norethindrone** for its specific ototoxic properties.)

[2] *Cyclen* and *Tri-Cyclen* are combinations of Norgestimate and **Ethinyl estradiol**. (**Ethinyl estradiol** is the ototoxic agent.)

[3] *Demulen* is a combination of Ethynodiol and **Ethinyl estradiol**. (**Ethinyl estradiol** is the ototoxic agent.)

[4] *Diane-35* is a combination of **Cyproterone** and **Ethinyl estradiol**. (See the generic drug **Cyproterone** for its specific ototoxic properties.)

[5] *Linessa 28*, *Marvelon*, *Mircette* and *Ortho-Cept* are combinations of Desogestrel and **Ethinyl estradiol**. (**Ethinyl estradiol** is the ototoxic agent.)

[6] *NuvaRing* is a combination of **Etonogestrel** and **Ethinyl estradiol**. (See the generic drug **Etonogestrel** for its specific ototoxic properties.)

[7] *Seasonale* and *Triquilar 28* are combinations of **Levonorgestrel** and **Ethinyl estradiol**. (See the generic drug **Levonorgestrel** for its specific ototoxic properties.)

[8] *Yasmin 28* and *Yaz* are combinations of Drospirenone and **Ethinyl estradiol**. (**Ethinyl estradiol** is the ototoxic agent.)

[9] See the PROGESTINS—**Medroxyprogesterone** and **Norelgestromin**—for more information on auditory disorders (including hearing loss) as **Norgestimate** is also a PROGESTIN and likely causes similar ear problems.

Ethionamide

Pronunciation guide: eh-thy-ON-ah-mide

Drug classification: ANTI-TUBERCULOSIS DRUGS (see section 7.7.1 in Table 14-1)

Brand names: *Trecator*

Ototoxic effects:
Vestibular:
Dizziness: (AHF, PDR)
Unspecified/General Ear Conditions:
Ototoxicity: (San)

Risk assessment: Not enough information to rate

Notes:
See Chapter 7, "We 'Hear' With Our Eyes" for further information on this drug.

Ethmozine   (see **Moricizine**)

Ethopropazine (Phenopropazine)

Pronunciation guide: eth-oh-PROE-pah-zeen (fen-oh-PROE-pah-zeen)

Drug classification: PHENOTHIAZINES (see section 60.8.1 in Table 14-1)

Brand names: *Parsitan*

Ototoxic effects:
Vestibular:
Ataxia: (CPS)
Dizziness: (CPS)

Risk assessment: Class 1

Ethosuximide

Pronunciation guide: eth-oh-SUX-ih-mide

Drug classification: ANTI-CONVULSANT DRUGS (see section 53.12 in Table 14-1)

Brand names: *Zarontin*

Ototoxic effects:
   Vestibular:
       Ataxia: (CPS, PDR)
       Dizziness: (CPS, PDR)

Risk assessment: Class 1

Notes:
   See Chapter 7, "We 'Hear' With Our Eyes" for further information on this drug.

Ethotoin

Pronunciation guide: ETH-oh-toyn

Drug classification: ANTI-CONVULSANT DRUGS (see section 53.12 in Table 14-1)

Brand names: *Peganone*

Ototoxic effects:
   Vestibular:
       Ataxia: (AHF, PDR)
       Dizziness: (DFC, PDR)
       Nystagmus: (DFC, PDR)

Risk assessment: Class 1

Etidocaine

Pronunciation guide: eh-TIH doe-kane

Drug classification: AMIDES (see section 4.1 in Table 14-1)

Brand names: *Duranest*

Ototoxic effects:
   Cochlear:
       Tinnitus: (PDR)
   Vestibular:
       Dizziness: (PDR)

Risk assessment: Class 1

Etodolac

Pronunciation guide: ee-toe-DOE-lak

Drug classification: ACETIC ACIDS (see section 1.1.1 in Table 14-1)

Brand names: *Apo-Etodolac, Lodine, Ultradol*

Ototoxic effects:
    Cochlear:
        Hearing loss: <1% (CPS, PDR)
        Tinnitus: 1-3% (CPS, PDR)
    Vestibular:
        Dizziness: 3-9% (CPS, PDR)
        Vertigo: <1% (CPS, PDR)
    Outer/Middle Ear:
        Earache/ear pain: <1% (CPS)
        Middle ear pressure: <1% (CPS)

Risk assessment: Class 2

Etonogestrel

Pronunciation guide: eh-toe-noe-JESS-trel

Drug classification: CONTRACEPTIVES (see section 40.12 in Table 14-1)

Brand names: *Implanon*

Ototoxic effects:
    Vestibular:
        Dizziness: 7.2% (PDR)
    Outer/Middle Ear:
        Otitis media: <5% (PDR)

Risk assessment: Class 1

Etonogestrel—Ethinyl estradiol (see **Ethinyl estradiol**)

Etoposide

Pronunciation guide: eh-toe-POE-side

Drug classification: ANTI-NEOPLASTICS (ANTI-CANCER DRUGS) (see section 14 in Table 14-1)

Brand names: *Toposar, VePesid*

Ototoxic effects:
    Vestibular:
        Vertigo (transient): (AHF)

Risk assessment: Class 1

Etoricoxib

Pronunciation guide: EE-tore-ih-kox-ib

Drug classification: COX-2 INHIBITORS (see section 1.1.4 in Table 14-1)

Brand names: *Arcoxia*

Ototoxic effects:
    Cochlear:
        Tinnitus: (BNF)
     Vestibular:
        Dizziness: (BNF)
        Vertigo: (BNF)

Risk assessment: Class 1

Etrafon   (see **Amitriptyline**)

Etravirine

Pronunciation guide: eh-trah-VIH-reen

Drug classification: ANTI-RETROVIRAL REVERSE TRANSCRIPTASE INHIBITORS (see section 7.17.1.4 in Table 14-1)

Brand names: *Intelence*

Ototoxic effects:
    Vestibular:
        Vertigo: <1% (NDH, PDR)

Risk assessment: Class 1

Etretinate

Pronunciation guide: eh-TRET-ih-nate

Drug classification: ANTI-PSORIASIS DRUGS (see section 23.1 in Table 14-1)

Brand names: *Tegison*

Ototoxic effects:
    Cochlear:
        Hearing loss: <1% (PDR)
    Vestibular:
        Dizziness: 1-10% (PDR)
    Outer/Middle Ear:
        Earache/ear pain: 1-10% (PDR)
        Otitis externa: 1-10% (PDR)
        Otitis media: <1% (PDR)

Risk assessment: Class 2

Notes:

    See Chapter 7, "We 'Hear' With Our Eyes" for further information on this drug.

Eufans   (see **Amtolmetin**)

Euglucon   (see **Glyburide**)

Evista   (see **Raloxifene**)

Evoxac   (see **Cevimeline**)

Evra   (see **Norelgestromin**)

Exbenzol   (see **Mebendazole**)

Excedrin Back & Body   (see **Acetylsalicylic acid**)

Excedrin Extra Strength   (see **Acetylsalicylic acid**)

Excedrin Migraine   (see **Acetylsalicylic acid**)

Exelon   (see **Rivastigmine**)

Exforge   (see **Amlodipine**)

Exforge HCT   (see **Amlodipine**)

Exjade   (see **Deferasirox**)

Extavia   (see **Interferon beta-1b**)

Extramycin   (see **Sisomicin**)

Exubera   (see **Insulin, human**)

Fabrazyme   (see **Agalsidase beta**)

Famotidine

Pronunciation guide: fah-MOE-tih-deen

Drug classification: H_2 RECEPTOR ANTAGONISTS (see section 10.4 in Table 14-1)

Brand names: *Novo-Famotidine, Pepcid, Pepcid AC*

Ototoxic effects:
  Cochlear:
    Tinnitus: 0.1% (CPS, PDR)
  Vestibular:
    Dizziness: 0.1-1.3% (CPS, PDR)
    Vertigo: (NDH)

Outer/Middle Ear:
    Earache/ear pain: <0.1% (CPS)
    Eustachian tube disorder: <0.1% (CPS)

Risk assessment: Class 1

Fanapt   (see **Iloperidone**)

Fanapta   (see **Iloperidone**)

Fansidar   (see **Sulfadoxine—Pyrimethamine**)

Fareston   (see **Toremifene**)

Farlutal   (see **Medroxyprogesterone**)

Fasigyn   (see **Tinidazole**)

Faslodex   (see **Fulvestrant**)

Febuxostat

Pronunciation guide: feh-BUKS-oh-stat

Drug classification: Xanthine oxidase inhibitors (see section 46.10 in Table 14-1)

Brand names: *Uloric*

Ototoxic effects:
    Cochlear:
        Hearing loss: <1% (PDR)
        Tinnitus: <1% (PDR)
    Vestibular:
        Ataxia: <1% (PDR)
        Dizziness: >1% (<0.5% above placebo results] (PDR)
        Vertigo: <1% (PDR)

Risk assessment: Class 2

Felbamate

Pronunciation guide: FELL-bah-mate

Drug classification: Anti-convulsant drugs (see section 53.12 in Table 14-1)

Brand names: *Felbatol*

Ototoxic effects:
    Cochlear:
        Hearing loss: (AHF, PDR)

Vestibular:
> Ataxia: 3.5-6.5% [2.8-3.5% above placebo results] (AHF, PDR)
> Dizziness: 18.4% [4.4% above placebo results] (AHF, PDR)
> Nystagmus: (DFC, PDR)

Outer/Middle Ear:
> Otitis Media: 3.4-9.7% [placebo 0] (AHF, PDR)

Risk assessment: Class 2

Felbatol   (see **Felbamate**)

Feldene   (see **Piroxicam**)

Felodipine

Pronunciation guide: fell-OH-dih-peen

Drug classification: CALCIUM-CHANNEL-BLOCKING DRUGS (CALCIUM BLOCKERS) (see section 20.8.16 in Table 14-1)

Brand names: *Plendil, Renedil*

Ototoxic effects:
Vestibular:
> Dizziness: 0.5% [0.2% above placebo results] (CPS, PDR)
> Dizziness/vertigo: 4.6% (CPS)

Risk assessment: Class 1

Notes:

Caution: Eating grapefruit or drinking grapefruit juice during the time you are taking this drug may make the listed side effects worse than shown here. In fact, taking **Felodipine** with grapefruit juice can increase the potency of **Felodipine** by as much as 600%.

See Chapter 11, "Grapefruit Juice and Ototoxic Drugs" for further information on this drug.

Femara   (see **Letrozole**)

Femtran   (see **Estradiol**)

Fenbufen

Pronunciation guide: fen-BYOO-fen

Drug classification: PROPIONIC ACIDS (see section 1.1.13 in Table 14-1)

Brand names: *Lederfen*

Ototoxic effects:
Cochlear:
> Tinnitus: [208] (BNF)

Vestibular:
>   Dizziness: [209] (BNF)
>   Vertigo: (BNF)

Risk assessment: Class 1

Fenofibrate

Pronunciation guide: fee-noh-FYE-brate

Drug classification: FIBRATES (see section 20.12.4 in Table 14-1)

Brand names: *Apo-Fenofibrate*, *Apo-Feno-Micro*, *Lipidil*, *Tricor*

Ototoxic effects:
>   Cochlear:
>   Tinnitus: (PDR)
>   Vestibular:
>   Dizziness: >10% (NDH, PDR)
>   Vertigo: (DFC, PDR)
>   Outer/Middle Ear:
>   Earache/ear pain: (NDH, PDR)
>   Otitis media: (DFC, PDR)

Risk assessment: Class 2

Fenoprofen

Pronunciation guide: FEN-oh-proe-fen

Drug classification: PROPIONIC ACIDS (see section 1.1.13 in Table 14-1)

Brand names: *Nalfon*

Ototoxic effects:
>   Cochlear:
>   Hearing loss: 1.6% [placebo 0] (CPS, PDR)
>   Tinnitus: 4.5% [4.1% above placebo results] (CPS, PDR)
>   Vestibular:
>   Ataxia: (CPS)
>   Dizziness: 6.5% [0.9% above placebo results] (CPS, PDR)
>   Vertigo: (BNF)

Risk assessment: Class 3

Notes:

If you have to take this drug, you might want to keep the duration as short as possible since "during short term studies, the incidence of adverse reactions was remarkably lower than that seen in longer-term studies" (PDR).

Fentanyl

Pronunciation guide: FEN-tah-nil

Drug classification: OPIATE AGONIST DRUGS (see section 1.4.1 in Table 14-1)

Brand names: *Actiq, Duragesic, Fentora, Ionsys, ratio-Fentanyl*

Ototoxic effects:
    Hearing loss: <1% (DFC, PDR)
    Tinnitus: >1% (DFC, PDR)
  Vestibular:
    Ataxia: 1-5% (PDR)
    Dizziness: 3-16% [2% above placebo results] (CPS, PDR)
    Equilibrium disorder: (PDR)
    Vertigo: 1-4% (CPS, PDR)
  Outer/Middle Ear:
    Earache/ear pain: <1% (DFC, PDR)
  Unspecified/General Ear Conditions:
    Ear disorder: >1% (DFC, PDR)

Risk assessment: Class 2

Notes:

Hearing loss may be temporary or permanent (PDR).

Fentora   (see **Fentanyl**)

Feprazone (Methrazone)

Pronunciation guide: FEH-prah-zone (METH-rah-zone)

Drug classification: NON-STEROIDAL ANTI-INFLAMMATORY DRUGS (NSAIDs) (see section 1.1 in
    Table 14-1)

Brand names: *Zepelin*

Ototoxic effects:
  Cochlear:
    Tinnitus: (Ka7)

Risk assessment: Class 1

Ferrlecit   (see **Sodium ferric gluconate**)

Fexofenadine

Pronunciation guide: fex-oh-FEN-ah-deen

Drug classification: H_1 RECEPTOR ANTAGONISTS (see section 10.1 in Table 14-1)

Brand names: *Allegra, Allegra-D*[1]

Ototoxic effects:
    Cochlear:
        Tinnitus: [2] (CPS)
    Vestibular:
        Ataxia: [2] (CPS)
        Dizziness: 1.9-2.2% [<1.6% above placebo results] (CPS, PDR)
    Outer/Middle Ear:
        Earache/ear pain: (CPS)
        Otitis media: 2.4-4.3% [1.1-2.4% above placebo results] (AHF, PDR)

Risk assessment: Class 2

Notes:

[1] *Allegra-D* is a combination of **Fexofenadine** and **Pseudoephedrine**. (See the generic drug **Pseudoephedrine** for its specific ototoxic properties.)

[2] Symptoms of overdose (CPS).

Caution: Eating grapefruit or drinking grapefruit juice during the time you are taking this drug may make the listed side effects worse than shown here.

See Chapter 11, "Grapefruit Juice and Ototoxic Drugs" for further information on this drug.

Fioricet　　(see **Butalbital**)

Fioricet with Codeine　　(see **Butalbital**)

Fiorinal　　(see **Butalbital**)

Fiorinal with Codeine　　(see **Butalbital**)

Fiorinal-C　　(see **Butalbital**)

Flagyl　　(see **Metronidazole**)

Flavoxate

Pronunciation guide: flah-VOX-ate

Drug classification: ANTI-CHOLINERGIC DRUGS (see section 17.1 in Table 14-1)

Brand names: *Apo-Flavoxate, Urispas*

Ototoxic effects:
    Vestibular:
        Dizziness: (NDH)
        Vertigo: (CPS, PDR)

Risk assessment: Class 1

Flecainide

Pronunciation guide: FLEH-kay-nide

Drug classification: ANTI-ARRHYTHMICS (HEART RHYTHM REGULATORS) (see section 20.4 in Table 14-1)

Brand names: *Tambocor*

Ototoxic effects:
  Cochlear:
    Hearing loss: <1% (CPS)
    Tinnitus: 1-3% (CPS, PDR)
  Vestibular:
    Ataxia: 1-3% (CPS, PDR)
    Dizziness: 18.9-37% (CPS, PDR)
    Nystagmus: <1% (CPS, PDR)
    Vertigo: 1-3% (NDH, PDR)

Risk assessment: Class 2

Flectadol   (see **Chlorzoxazone**)

Flexeril   (see **Cyclobenzaprine**)

Floctafenine

Pronunciation guide: flok-tah-FEN-een

Drug classification: FENAMATES (see section 1.1.7 in Table 14-1)

Brand names: *Apo-Floctafenine, Idarac*

Ototoxic effects:
  Cochlear:
      Tinnitus: (CPS)
    Vestibular:
      Dizziness: (CPS)

Risk assessment: Class 1

Flomax   (see **Tamsulosin**)

Florazole   (see **Metronidazole**)

Florinef   (see **Fludrocortisone**)

Flovent   (see **Fluticasone**)

Floxicam   (see **Isoxicam**)

Floxin   (see **Ofloxacin**)

Floxuridine

Pronunciation guide: flox-YOOR-ih-deen

Drug classification: ANTI-METABOLITE DRUGS (see section 14.8 in Table 14-1)

Brand names: *FUDR*

Ototoxic effects:
    Vestibular:
        Ataxia: (AHF, CP2)
        Nystagmus: (AHF, PDR)
        Vertigo: (AHF)

Risk assessment: Class 1

Fluarix   (see **Influenza vaccine**)

Fluconazole

Pronunciation guide: floo-KON-ah-zole

Drug classification: ANTI-FUNGAL ANTIBIOTICS (see section 7.10 in Table 14-1)

Brand names: *Apo-Fluconazole, Diflucan*

Ototoxic effects:
    Vestibular:
        Dizziness: 0.2-1% (CPS, PDR)
        Vertigo: 0.2-1% (CPS)

Risk assessment: Class 1

Flucytosine

Pronunciation guide: floo-SYE-toe-seen

Drug classification: ANTI-FUNGAL ANTIBIOTICS (see section 7.10 in Table 14-1)

Brand names: *Ancobon*

Ototoxic effects:
    Cochlear:
        Hearing loss: (AHF, PDR)
    Vestibular:
        Ataxia: (AHF, PDR)
        Vertigo: (AHF, PDR)

Risk assessment: Class 2

Fludara   (see **Fludarabine**)

Fludarabine

Pronunciation guide: floo-DAR-ah-been

Drug classification: ANTI-METABOLITE DRUGS (see section 14.8 in Table 14-1)

Brand names: *Fludara*

Ototoxic effects:
    Cochlear:
        Auditory hallucinations: <6% (AHF)
        Hearing loss: 2-6% (CPS, PDR)

Risk assessment: Class 3

Fludrocortisone

Pronunciation guide: floo-droe-KOR-tih-sone

Drug classification: MINERALOCORTICOIDS (see section 40.1.8 in Table 14-1)

Brand names: *Florinef*

Ototoxic effects:
    Vestibular:
        Vertigo: (CPS, PDR)

Risk assessment: Class 1

Flulaval   (see **Influenza vaccine**)

Flumadine   (see **Rimantadine**)

Flumazenil

Pronunciation guide: floo-MAZ-eh-nil

Drug classification: BENZODIAZEPINE ANTAGONISTS (see section 66.1.4 in Table 14-1)

Brand names: *Anexate, Romazicon*

Ototoxic effects:
    Cochlear:
        Hearing loss: <1% (DFC, PDR)
        Hyperacusis: <1% (DFC, PDR)
        Tinnitus: <1% (DFC, PDR)
    Vestibular:
        Ataxia: (PDR)
        Dizziness: 1.2-9% (AHF, PDR)
        Vertigo: <1% (CPS, PDR)

Risk assessment: Class 2

Notes:

    Hearing loss may be temporary (PDR).

Flunarizine

Pronunciation guide: floo-NAR-ih-zeen

Drug classification: PIPERAZINES (see section 10.8 in Table 14-1)

Brand names: *Sibelium*

Ototoxic effects:
    Vestibular:
        Dizziness/vertigo: (CPS)

Risk assessment: Class 1

Flunisolide

Pronunciation guide: floo-NISS-oh-lide

Drug classification: GLUCOCORTICOIDS (see section 40.1.4 in Table 14-1)

Brand names: *Aerobid, Nasarel*

Ototoxic effects:
    Vestibular:
        Dizziness: 3-9% (NDH, PDR)
        Vertigo: 1-3% (DFC, PDR)
    Outer/Middle Ear:
        Earache/ear pain: 1-3% (DFC, PDR)
        Otitis: 3-9% (DFC, PDR)

Risk assessment: Class 2

Flunitrazepam

Pronunciation guide: floo-nih-TRA-zeh-pam

Drug classification: BENZODIAZEPINES (see section 60.12.8 in Table 14-1)

Brand names: *Rohypnol*

Ototoxic effects:
    Vestibular:
        Ataxia: (BNF)
        Vertigo: (BNF)

Risk assessment: Class 1

Notes:

    See Chapter 10 "Beware of Benzodiazepines—Don't Let This Nasty Time-Bomb Ambush You and Your Ears" for further information on this drug.

Fluoroplex   (see **Fluorouracil**)

Fluorouracil

Pronunciation guide: flure-oh-YOOR-ah-sill

Drug classification: Anti-metabolite drugs (see section 14.8 in Table 14-1)

Brand names: *Adrucil, Carac, Efudex, Fluoroplex*

Ototoxic effects:
    Vestibular:
        Ataxia: (AHF, NDH)
        Nystagmus: (NDH, PDR)

Risk assessment: Class 1

Fluoxetine

Pronunciation guide: floo-OX-eh-teen

Drug classification: Selective serotonin reuptake inhibitors (see section 60.1.32 in Table 14-1)

Brand names: *Novo-Fluoxetine, Prozac, Sarafem*

Ototoxic effects:
    Cochlear:
        Hearing loss: <0.1% (CPS, PDR)
        Hyperacusis: <0.1% (CPS, PDR)
        Tinnitus: 2% [placebo 0] (CPS, PDR)
    Vestibular:
        Ataxia: 0.1-1% (CPS, PDR)
        Dizziness: 5.7-14% [0.9-6% above placebo results] (CPS, PDR)
        Nystagmus: <0.1% (CPS, PDR)
        Vertigo: 0.1-1% (CPS, PDR)
    Outer/Middle Ear:
        Earache/ear pain: >1% (CPS, PDR)

Risk assessment: Class 3

Notes:

In my files I have an anecdotal report of a woman who had taken **Fluoxetine** for several years. Then she stopped taking it. Within months she noticed that her hearing had noticeably improved. Later she began taking **Fluoxetine** once more and noticed that her hearing was definitely getting worse so she stopped taking it. Again, after several months her hearing improved.

Another hard of hearing woman had taken **Fluoxetine** for five years. She told me that she noticed a significant increase in her hearing three weeks after she stopped taking **Fluoxetine**.

Also in my files I have an anecdotal report of a man who had been taking **Fluoxetine** for 3 months. About 6 weeks later he began to notice a bit of hearing loss. Three weeks later he writes, "it became obvious that my hearing was rapidly diminishing in both ears".

In my files I have an anecdotal report of a woman who began to take **Fluoxetine** and within two months, she noticed that she now had tinnitus.

Another anecdotal report in my files tells of a woman who had taken **Fluoxetine** for 7 years. Nine months after stopping the **Fluoxetine** she writes, "I am still experiencing a feeling of imbalance accompanied by a feeling of fullness in my ears and tinnitus". She has been to an ENT and found she had lost some hearing. Her neurologist thinks her problems are likely a result of the **Fluoxetine**.

Symptoms of **Fluoxetine** overdose may include ataxia and vertigo (PDR).

See Chapter 2 "Ototoxic Drugs—What Are They?" for further information on this drug.

Flurazepam

Pronunciation guide: flure-AZ-eh-pam

Drug classification: BENZODIAZEPINES (see section 60.12.8 in Table 14-1)

Brand names: *Dalmane*

Ototoxic effects:
    Cochlear:
        Tinnitus: (She)
    Vestibular:
        Ataxia: (CPS, PDR)
        Dizziness: (CPS, PDR)
        Vertigo: (BNF)

Risk assessment: Class 1

Notes:

See Chapter 10 "Beware of Benzodiazepines—Don't Let This Nasty Time-Bomb Ambush You and Your Ears" for further information on this drug.

Flurbiprofen

Pronunciation guide: flure-BIH-proe-fen

Drug classification: PROPIONIC ACIDS (see section 1.1.13 in Table 14-1)

Brand names: *Ansaid, Froben*

Ototoxic effects:
    Cochlear:
        Hearing loss: <1% (DFC, RXL)
        Tinnitus: 1.2% (CP2, CPS)

Vestibular:
    Ataxia: 0.1-1% (CPS, DFC)
    Dizziness: 1.6% (CP2, CPS)
    Vertigo: 0.6% (BNF, CPS)
    Vestibular disorder: <0.1% (CPS)
Outer/Middle Ear:
    Earache/ear pain: 0.3% (CPS)
Unspecified/General Ear Conditions:
    Ear disorder: 0.2% (CPS)

Risk assessment: Class 2

Notes:

Hearing loss is temporary (RXL).

FluShield   (see **Influenza vaccine**)

Fluticasone

Pronunciation guide: FLOO-tih-kah-sone

Drug classification: Glucocorticoids (see section 40.1.4 in Table 14-1)

Brand names: *Advair Diskus* [1], *Avamys*, *Flovent*

Ototoxic effects:
Vestibular:
    Dizziness: 1-4% [2-4% above placebo results] (AHF, PDR)
Outer/Middle Ear:
    Earache/ear pain: 1-3% (DFC, PDR)
    Otitis media: 1-3% (DFC, PDR)

Risk assessment: Class 1

Notes:

[1] *Advair Diskus* is a combination of **Fluticasone** and **Salmeterol**. (See the generic drug **Salmeterol** for its specific ototoxic properties.)

I have an anecdotal report in my files of a lady who explained, "My doctor prescribed *Avamys* to tackle my ongoing sinus problem. On the third day I started to feel a bit nauseous. By the fifth day I had a couple of mild bouts of dizziness, and on day six I was distinctly dizzy and way too nauseous. I stopped using it, and after 24 hours my dizziness and nausea were gone".

Fluvastatin

Pronunciation guide: floo-vah-STA-tin

Drug classification: HMG-CoA reductase inhibitors (see section 20.12.8 in Table 14-1)

Brand names: *Lescol*

Ototoxic effects:
    Vestibular:
        Ataxia: (PDR)
        Dizziness: (CPS, PDR)
        Vertigo: (CPS, PDR)

Risk assessment: Class 1

Fluviral S/F   (see **Influenza vaccine**)

Fluvoxamine

Pronunciation guide: floo-VOX-ah-meen

Drug classification: SELECTIVE SEROTONIN REUPTAKE INHIBITORS (see section 60.1.32 in Table 14-1)

Brand names: *Apo-Fluvoxamine, Luvox, Novo-Fluvoxamine*

Ototoxic effects:
    Cochlear:
        Hearing loss: 0.1-1% (CPS, PDR)
        Hyperacusis: 0.1-1% (CPS)
        Tinnitus: 0.1-1% (CPS, PDR)
    Vestibular:
        Ataxia: 0.1-1% (CPS, PDR)
        Dizziness: 9.4-14.8% [1.3-5% above placebo results] (CPS, PDR)
        Vertigo: >1% (CPS, PDR)
    Outer/Middle Ear:
        Earache/ear pain: 0.1-1% (CPS, PDR)
        Otitis media: 0.1-1% (DFC, PDR)

Risk assessment: Class 2

Fluzone   (see **Influenza vaccine**)

Fomepizole

Pronunciation guide: foe-MEE-pih-zole

Drug classification: SYNTHETIC ALCOHOL DEHYDROGENASE INHIBITORS (see section 66.8 in Table 14-1)

Brand names: *Antizol*

Ototoxic effects:
    Cochlear:
        Tinnitus: <3% (CPS, DFC)
    Vestibular:
        Dizziness: 6% (CPS, DFC)
        Nystagmus: <3% (CPS, DFC)
        Vertigo: <3% (CPS, DFC)

Risk assessment: Class 2

Fondaparinux

Pronunciation guide: fon-dah-PARE-ah-nucks

Drug classification: ANTI-THROMBOTIC DRUGS (see section 36.8 in Table 14-1)

Brand names: *Arixtra*

Ototoxic effects:
Vestibular:
Dizziness: 3.6% (CPS, PDR)
Vertigo: (BNF)

Risk assessment: Class 1

Forteo   (see **Teriparatide**)

Fortimicin   (see **Astromicin**)

Fortovase   (see **Saquinavir**)

Fosamax   (see **Alendronate**)

Fosaprepitant   (see **Aprepitant**)

Fosavance   (see **Alendronate**)

Foscarnet

Pronunciation guide: foss-KAR-net

Drug classification: ANTI-VIRAL DRUGS (see section 7.17 in Table 14-1)

Brand names: *Foscavir*

Ototoxic effects:
Cochlear:
Hearing loss: <1% (AHF, PDR)
Tinnitus: <1% (AHF, PDR)
Vestibular:
Ataxia: 1-5% (NDH, PDR)
Dizziness: >5% (NDH, PDR)
Nystagmus: <1% (PDR)
Vertigo: <1% (PDR)
Outer/Middle Ear:
Earache/ear pain: <1% (AHF, PDR)
Otitis: <1% (AHF, PDR)

Risk assessment: Class 3

Foscavir   (see **Foscarnet**)

Fosfomycin

Pronunciation guide: foss-foe-MY-sin

Drug classification: URINARY ANTI-INFECTIVES (see section 7.20 in Table 14-1)

Brand names: *Monurol*

Ototoxic effects:
Vestibular:
Dizziness: 1.3-2.3% (CPS, PDR)
Unspecified/General Ear Conditions:
Ear disorder: <1% (CPS, PDR)

Risk assessment: Class 1

Fosinopril

Pronunciation guide: foh-SIN-oh-pril

Drug classification: ANGIOTENSIN-CONVERTING ENZYME (ACE) INHIBITORS (see section 20.8.8 in Table 14-1)

Brand names: *Monopril, Monopril HCT* [1]

Ototoxic effects:
Cochlear:
Tinnitus: 0.5-2% (CPS, PDR)
Vestibular:
Dizziness: 3.2-11.9% [<6.5% above placebo results] (CPS, PDR)
Vertigo: 0.4-1% (CPS, PDR)
Outer/Middle Ear:
Earache/ear pain: <1% (CPS)

Risk assessment: Class 2

Notes:

[1] *Monopril HCT* is a combination of **Fosinopril** and **Hydrochlorothiazide**. (See the generic drug **Hydrochlorothiazide** for its specific ototoxic properties.)

Fosint   (see **Indoprofen**)

Fosphenytoin

Pronunciation guide: faws-FEN-ih-toe-in

Drug classification: ANTI-CONVULSANT DRUGS (see section 53.12 in Table 14-1)

Brand names: *Cerebyx*

Ototoxic effects:
    Cochlear:
        Hearing loss: 2.2% (CPS, PDR)
        Hyperacusis: 0.1-1% (CPS, PDR)
        Tinnitus: 8.9% (CPS, PDR)
    Vestibular:
        Ataxia: 8.4-11.1% (CPS, PDR)
        Dizziness: 5-31.1% (CPS, PDR)
        Nystagmus: 15.1-44.4% (CPS, PDR)
        Vertigo: 2.2% (CPS, PDR)
    Outer/Middle Ear:
        Earache/ear pain: 0.1-1% (CPS, PDR)

Risk assessment: Class 5

Notes:

Ataxia and nystagmus are signs of **Fosphenytoin** overdose. Nystagmus generally appears at about 20 mg/L and ataxia at around 30 mg/L (PDR).

Fosrenol   (see **Lanthanum**)

Fradiomycin   (see **Neomycin**)

Framycetin

Pronunciation guide: fram-EE-see-tin

Drug classification: AMINOGLYCOSIDES (see section 7.4.1 in Table 14-1)

Brand names: *Sofracort*[1], *Soframycin*[2]

Ototoxic effects:
    Unspecified/General Ear Conditions:
        Ototoxicity: [210] (BNF)

Risk assessment: Class 4

Notes:

[1] *Sofracort* is a combination of **Dexamethasone**, **Framycetin** and **Gramicidin**. (See the generic drugs **Dexamethasone** and **Gramicidin** for their specific ototoxic properties.)

[2] *Soframycin* is a combination of **Framycetin** and **Gramicidin**. See the generic drug **Gramicidin** for its specific ototoxic properties.)

See Chapter 9, "Aminoglycoside Antibiotics are the Ototoxic 'Bad boys'" for further information on this drug.

Frisium   (see **Clobazam**)

Froben   (see **Flurbiprofen**)

Frova   (see **Frovatriptan**)

Frovatriptan

Pronunciation guide: frow-vah-TRIP-tan

Drug classification: SEROTONIN-RECEPTOR AGONISTS (see section 53.32 in Table 14-1)

Brand names: *Frova*

Ototoxic effects:
  Cochlear:
      Hyperacusis: 0.1-1% (CPS, PDR)
      Tinnitus: >1% (NDH, PDR)
  Vestibular:
      Ataxia: 0.1-1%% (CPS, PDR)
      Dizziness: 8% [3% above placebo results] (NDH, PDR)
      Vertigo: 0.1-1%% (CPS, PDR)
  Outer/Middle Ear:
      Earache/ear pain: 0.1-1% (CPS, PDR)

Risk assessment: Class 2

Frusemide   (see **Furosemide**)

FUDR   (see **Floxuridine**)

Fulvestrant

Pronunciation guide: full-VES-trant

Drug classification: ESTROGEN ANTAGONISTS (see section 40.16.1 in Table 14-1)

Brand names: *Faslodex*

Ototoxic effects:
  Vestibular:
      Dizziness: 6.9% (NDH, PDR)
      Vertigo: <1% (PDR)

Risk assessment: Class 1

Fulvicin   (see **Griseofulvin**)

Fungizone   (see **Amphotericin B**)

Furadantin   (see **Nitrofurantoin**)

Furosemide (Frusemide)

Pronunciation guide: fur-OH-seh-mide (FROO-seh-mide)

Drug classification: DIURETICS—LOOP (see section 30.5.4 in Table 14-1)

Brand names: *Lasix*

Ototoxic effects:
    Cochlear:
        Hearing loss: (CPS, PDR)
        Tinnitus: (CPS, PDR)
    Vestibular:
        Ataxia: (NTP)
        Dizziness: (CPS, PDR)
        Vertigo: (CPS, PDR)
    Outer/Middle Ear:
        Feeling of fullness in ears: (DFC)

Risk assessment: Class 4

Notes:

Warning: If you take **Furosemide** you may end up with severe and permanent hearing loss.[211] However, if you take **Furosemide** by itself and do not have any other contributing factors, your hearing loss may be temporary. Hearing loss affects about 6.4% of the people taking **Furosemide**.[212]

Furosemide has been known to be ototoxic since 1970.[213]

You have a greater chance of hearing loss if you have severe kidney problems and take large doses of **Furosemide** intravenously at a rate exceeding 4 mg/minute. You are also at risk if you take doses exceeding several times the usual recommended dose, or if you are also receiving known ototoxic drugs such as AMINOGLYCOSIDE antibiotics, **Ethacrynic acid** or **Cisplatin** at the same time. Unless your life depends on it, you should avoid these drug combinations (CPS, PDR). In one study, 67% of the people taking **Furosemide** at the rate of 25 mg. per minute ended up with noticeable hearing loss.[214]

Several reports reveal that one result for children undergoing kidney transplants is that some of them end up with permanent hearing loss. In these cases, the onset of hearing loss is usually insidious and gradually progressive up to 6 months after **Furosemide** therapy stops (CPS). Furthermore, giving **Furosemide** injections to neonatal babies also often results in hearing loss (PDR).

If you are receiving high doses of SALICYLATES at the same time as **Furosemide**, as in rheumatic disease, you may experience SALICYLATE toxicity at lower doses because you can overload your kidneys (PDR).

See Chapter 1 "How to Effectively Use This Book," Chapter 4 "Are You at Risk," Chapter 7, "We 'Hear' With Our Eyes," Chapter 9, "Aminoglycoside Antibiotics are the Ototoxic 'Bad boys'" and Chapter 12, "Potpourri" for further information on this drug.

Fuzeon   (see **Enfuvirtide**)

Gabapentin

Pronunciation guide: GAB-ah-pen-tin

Drug classification: ANTI-CONVULSANT DRUGS (see section 53.12 in Table 14-1)

Brand names: *Apo-Gabapentin, Neurontin, Novo-Gabapentin*

Ototoxic effects:
  Cochlear:
      Hearing loss: 0.1-1% (AHF, PDR)
      Hyperacusis: <0.1% (AHF, PDR)
      Tinnitus: 0.1-1% (AHF, PDR)
  Vestibular:
      Ataxia: 3.3-12.5% [<6.9% above placebo results] (CPS, PDR)
      Dizziness: 2.5-28% [0.9-20.5% above placebo results] (CPS, PDR)
      Labyrinthitis: <0.1% (AHF, PDR)
      Nystagmus: 8.3-20.4% [4.3-16.4% above placebo results] (CPS, PDR)
      Vertigo: >1% (CPS, PDR)
      Vestibular disorder: <0.1% (DFC)
  Outer/Middle Ear:
      Earache/ear pain: 0.1-1% (AHF, PDR)
      Eustachian tube disorder: <0.1% (DFC)
      Feeling of fullness in ears: 0.1-1% (AHF, PDR)
      Otitis externa: <0.1% (AHF,PDR)
      Otitis media: 1.2% [placebo 0] (AHF, PDR)
      Perforated eardrum: <0.1% (AHF, PDR)

Risk assessment: Class 4

Notes:

I have an anecdotal report in my files of a woman who, after a year and a half on **Gabapentin**, now has a moderate to severe hearing loss. She strongly believes this loss resulted from taking **Gabapentin**.

I have another anecdotal report in my files of a woman who is suffering from hearing loss and explained that "the only possible cause" of her hearing loss was the **Gabapentin** she had been taking for the past 2+ years.

I have yet another anecdotal report in my files of a person who explained, "I have been taking **Gabapentin** for some time now for my epilepsy. My neurologist did not point out that this drug might produce tinnitus and other hearing/ear-related problems. Now I'm suffering from tinnitus in both ears, occasional dizziness and vertigo, and the odd spasm of ear pain. I have also noticed some hearing loss. I hope that coming off the **Gabapentin** will eliminate these problems, and that the damage to my ears won't be permanent".

I have still another anecdotal report in my files of a lady who took **Gabapentin** for 10 months, then tapered off the drug. Within a month of completing the taper, she developed "terrible hyperacusis," and the mild tinnitus she had became much worse. After 1 year, her hyperacusis is "much better", but not gone, and her tinnitus is somewhat better but still worse than prior to taking the **Gabapentin**.

See Chapter 7, "We 'Hear' With Our Eyes" for further information on this drug.

Gabitril   (see **Tiagabine**)

Gadodiamide

Pronunciation guide: gad-oh-DIE-ah-mide

Drug classification: MRI CONTRAST DRUGS (see section 26.1 in Table 14-1)

Brand names: *Omniscan*

Ototoxic effects:
    Cochlear:
        Tinnitus: <1% (CPS)
    Vestibular:
        Ataxia: (CPS)
        Dizziness: <3% (CPS)

Risk assessment: Class 1

Gadopentetate

Pronunciation guide: gad-oh-PEN-teh-tate

Drug classification: MRI CONTRAST DRUGS (see section 26.1 in Table 14-1)

Brand names: *Magnevist*

Ototoxic effects:
    Cochlear:
        Hearing disorder: (CPS)
        Tinnitus: (CPS)
    Vestibular:
        Dizziness: 1.5% (CPS)
        Nystagmus: (CPS)
    Outer/Middle Ear:
        Earache/ear pain: <2.8% (CPS)

Risk assessment: Class 2

Gadoteridol

Pronunciation guide: gad-oh-TER-ih-dol

Drug classification: MRI CONTRAST DRUGS (see section 26.1 in Table 14-1)

Brand names: *ProHance*

Ototoxic effects:
    Cochlear:
        Tinnitus: (She)
    Vestibular:
        Dizziness: (Med)

Risk assessment: Class 1

Gadoversetamide

Pronunciation guide: gad-oh-ver-SEH-tah-mide

Drug classification: MRI CONTRAST DRUGS (see section 26.1 in Table 14-1)

Brand names: *OptiMARK*

Ototoxic effects:
    Cochlear:
        Hyperacusis: (CPS)
        Tinnitus: <1% (CPS)
    Vestibular:
        Dizziness: 3.0-3.1% (CPS)
        Vertigo: <1% (CPS)
    Outer/Middle Ear:
        Earache/ear pain: <1% (CPS)

Risk assessment: Class 2

Galantamine

Pronunciation guide: gah-LAN-tah-meen

Drug classification: CHOLINESTERASE INHIBITORS (see section 17.12.4 in Table 14-1)

Brand names: *Reminyl*

Ototoxic effects:
    Cochlear:
        Tinnitus: 0.1-1% (CPS, DFC)
    Vestibular:
        Ataxia: 0.1-1% (CPS, PDR)
        Dizziness: 1-10% [1-6% above placebo results] (CPS, PDR)
        Vertigo: 0.1-1% (CPS, PDR)

Risk assessment: Class 2

Gallium nitrate

Pronunciation guide: GAL-lee-um NIE-trate

Drug classification: ANTI-NEOPLASTICS (ANTI-CANCER DRUGS) (see section 14 in Table 14-1)

Brand names: *Ganite*

Ototoxic effects:
    Cochlear:
        Hearing loss: <1% (DFC, PDR)
        Tinnitus: <1% (DFC, PDR)

Risk assessment: Class 2

Notes:

Doctors report rare cases of tinnitus and partial hearing loss in people who received high doses of **Gallium nitrate** in anticancer treatment (PDR).

Galsulfase

Pronunciation guide: gal-SUL-fase

Drug classification: ENZYMES (see section 32.1 in Table 14-1)

Brand names: *Naglazyme*

Ototoxic effects:
> Outer/Middle Ear:
>> Earache/ear pain: 42% [22% above placebo results] (DFC)
>> Otitis media: (DFC)

Risk assessment: Class 1

Gammagard   (see **Immune globulin**)

Gamunex   (see **Immune globulin**)

Ganciclovir

Pronunciation guide: gan-SYE-kloe-veer

Drug classification: ANTI-RETROVIRAL PROTEASE INHIBITORS (see section 7.17.1.1 in Table 14-1)

Brand names: *Cytovene*

Ototoxic effects:
> Cochlear:
>> Hearing loss: <1% (CPS, PDR)
>> Tinnitus: <1% (CPS, PDR)
> Vestibular:
>> Ataxia: <1% (CPS, PDR)
>> Dizziness: <1% (CPS, PDR)
>> Vertigo: <1% (CPS)
> Outer/Middle Ear:
>> Earache/ear pain: <1% (CPS, PDR)
> Unspecified/General Ear Conditions:
>> Ear disorder: (CPS)

Risk assessment: Class 2

Ganite   (see **Gallium nitrate**)

Gantanol   (see **Sulfamethoxazole**)

Gantrisin (see **Sulfisoxazole**)

Garamycin (see **Gentamicin**)

Garasone (see **Gentamicin**)

Gastrocrom (see **Cromolyn sodium**)

Gatifloxacin

Pronunciation guide: GAT-ih-flox-ah-sin

Drug classification: QUINOLONES (see section 7.4.48 in Table 14-1)

Brand names: *Tequin, Zymar*

Ototoxic effects:
  Cochlear:
      Tinnitus: 0.1-3% (CPS, PDR)
  Vestibular:
      Ataxia: <0.1% (CPS, PDR)
      Dizziness: 3% (CPS, PDR)
      Vertigo: 0.1-3% (CPS, PDR)
  Outer/Middle Ear:
      Earache/ear pain: <0.1% (CPS, PDR)

Risk assessment: Class 2

Gelatin

Pronunciation guide: JEL-ah-tin

Drug classification: MISCELLANEOUS DRUGS (see section 46 in Table 14-1)

Brand names: *Gelfoam*

Ototoxic effects:
  Outer/Middle Ear:
      Hearing loss: (CPS, PDR)

Risk assessment: Class 1

Notes:

  Doctors have reported conductive hearing loss in association with the use of *Gelfoam* during tympanoplasty (eardrum repair) (CPS, PDR).

Gelfoam (see **Gelatin**)

Gemfibrozil

Pronunciation guide: jem-FIH-broe-zil

Drug classification: FIBRATES (see section 20.12.4 in Table 14-1)

Brand names: *Lopid*

Ototoxic effects:
Vestibular:
Dizziness: 2.8% [same as placebo] (CPS, PDR)
Vertigo: 1.5% [0.2% above placebo results] (CPS, PDR)

Risk assessment: Class 1

Gen-Clozapine   (see **Clozapine**)

Gengraf   (see **Cyclosporine**)

Genotropin   (see **Somatropin**)

Gentamicin

Pronunciation guide: jen-tah-MYE-sin

Drug classification: AMINOGLYCOSIDES (see section 7.4.1 in Table 14-1)

Brand names: *Cidomycin, Garamycin, Garasone* [1]

Ototoxic effects:
Cochlear:
Hearing loss: (CPS, PDR)
Tinnitus: (CPS, PDR)
Vestibular:
Ataxia: (CPS, NDH)
Dizziness: (CPS, PDR)
Loss of balance: (CPS)
Oscillopsia: [2] (CPS)
Vertigo: (CPS, PDR)
Unspecified/General Ear Conditions:
Ototoxicity: (CPS, NDH)

Risk assessment: Class 5

Notes:

[1] *Garasone* is a combination of **Betamethasone** and **Gentamicin**. (See the generic drug **Betamethasone** for its specific ototoxic properties.)

[2] **Warning**: "As far as the vestibular (balance) system is concerned, there is **no** safe **Gentamicin** dose".[215] Of 36 patients with ear damage from **Gentamicin**, **every one** had gait ataxia and 50% had oscillopsia.[216] **Gentamicin** toxicity is the most common single known cause of bilateral vestibulopathy (balance problems in both ears), accounting for about 15% of all cases.[217]

Just taking ear drops containing **Gentamicin** can damage your ears, particularly if you have damaged ear drums. Federal officials in Canada recently received 20 reports of ear damage from taking **Gentamicin** ear drops. Commonly, the result is balance problems in both ears. For example, one man now has blurred vision when he moves his head. He cannot read signs when driving on a bumpy road, nor can he recognize people's faces when out walking. His oscillopsia resulted from taking a two-week course of ear drops prescribed by his doctor for a persistent ear infection. Ten days later he noticed his balance was off. That was nine years ago and he still suffers daily from oscillopsia.[218]

In the past and still today, **Gentamicin** has been responsible for the hearing loss of many people because it is relatively cheap to produce. This is particularly true in China. One study of hard of hearing children in China revealed that 123 of the 154 studied had lost their hearing from taking antibiotics. Of these 123 children, 60 of them had hearing problems due to taking **Gentamicin**.[219]

If you are being treated with **Gentamicin**, you should be under close clinical observation. Even when **Gentamicin** is used as drops in your ear canals for ear infections, your doctor needs to keep the possibility of ototoxicity in mind and monitor your ears accordingly. Also, your doctor should evaluate your auditory and vestibular function if you have kidney problems (CPS, PDR).

If possible, you should have serial audiograms taken (before you begin taking **Gentamicin**, during the treatment and after treatment is completed), particularly if you are at high-risk to ototoxic problems (PDR).

If you take **Gentamicin**, you may experience serious adverse side effects, both vestibular and auditory. Ototoxicity may not appear right away but can show up days, weeks or months after you have finished taking **Gentamicin**.

Gentamicin actually persists in your ears for between 80 days and a year after completing a course of this drug. Therefore, don't expect hearing loss (if you are lucky enough to have a temporary loss) to improve immediately. Recovery time may be as short as one week, or it could take 6 months.[220] However, you could reasonably expect that hearing restoration could take up to a year or more.[221]

Gentamicin primarily damages your vestibular (balance) system. In fact, it affects the vestibular system twice as often as it does the cochlear (hearing) system.[222]

The side effects of taking **Gentamicin** may include, dizziness, vertigo, ataxia, tinnitus (ringing or roaring sounds in your ears) and hearing loss (usually permanent). Initially, hearing loss usually occurs in the high frequencies. Hearing loss can sometimes be reversed if you recognize it soon enough. Therefore, your doctor should strongly consider discontinuing **Gentamicin** if you develop tinnitus, dizziness or hearing loss, except if you have a life-threatening condition (CPS, PDR).

Vestibular symptoms generally peak about three months after you stop taking **Gentamicin**. During the first three months after treatment, you may need to use either crutches, canes, walkers or wheelchairs. The good news is that you will rarely need them for more than a year.[223]

Ototoxic damage from **Gentamicin** may be reversible about 50% of the time. This means that if you lose your hearing as a result of taking **Gentamicin**, you have one chance in two that this hearing loss will be permanent.[224]

Ototoxicity occurs most often if you have kidney problems (especially if you require dialysis), or if you have normal kidney function, but are treated at higher doses, and/or for longer periods than recommended, if you are dehydrated, or if you have previously taken other ototoxic drugs such as **Streptomycin**, **Neomycin**, **Kanamycin**, etc. Also, understand that the toxic effects of these drugs may be cumulative (CPS, PDR).

Note: you should only take **Gentamicin** for 7 to 10 days.[225] However, ototoxic side effects can show up even if you only take **Gentamicin** for 5 to 7 days. The resulting side effects such as hearing loss, tinnitus, vertigo, loss of balance, oscillopsia and ataxia may be permanent (CPS).

Lynn Brown runs a web site called *Wobblers Anonymous* (http://www.wobblers.com) for people who have damaged or destroyed balance systems from taking **Gentamicin** (and some other ototoxic drugs).

The medical community would have you believe that such reactions are extremely rare. However, the evidence says otherwise. For example, the *Wobblers Anonymous* web site has received over 216,000 visits in the past nine years! That is a lot of activity for a supposedly rare side effect.

Even taking something as innocuous as antibiotic eye drops can have devastating effects on your balance system. For example, Lynn told me that six people in her group alone lost their balance just from taking eye drops containing **Gentamicin** following cataract surgery.

Many people, when they find the *Wobblers Anonymous* web site exclaim, as did one woman, "What a great surprise to find this web site and to realize that there are so many others suffering from vestibular damage. I was led to believe that **Gentamicin** toxicity was extremely rare!" This theme is repeated over and over throughout the guest book.

Reading the *Wobblers* guest-book comments is **very** revealing, not to mention both shocking and scary. You realize just how often the vestibular side effects of **Gentamicin** affect real people in very real (and devastating) ways. Here are a number of the hundreds of stories posted there lest you think these are rare occurrences. Vestibular damage is much more common than people and doctors realize. (If you want to, read all these stories for yourself in the guest book at www.wobblers.com.)

One man wrote, "I received **Gentamicin** in 1993 for endocarditis. Classic results: lost all balance control and my involuntary eye muscle control, as well as kidney damage and who knows what else.

Now it is very dangerous for me to use power tools or climb, so I can no longer work my trade in construction or carpentry. I fell a lot until I realized I wasn't going to get better.

This drug causes severe physical limitations, emotional trauma, loss of family interactions (I can't even take my grand-daughter by the hand and walk across the yard to the swing-set, let alone push her in it), loss of income and loss of independence in later years. The future doesn't look all that great".

A woman wrote, "After being given **Gentamicin** for 4 weeks, my balance is horribly affected".

Especially tragic are stories of children affected with permanent balance problems. For example, a teen-aged girl had ear surgery. The resulting infection spread, and she was on **Gentamicin** for 7 weeks. She wrote, "About 4 weeks into it I started experiencing all the spinning troubles and also the inability to walk correctly. I constantly looked intoxicated and had to rely on my friends to be my eyes".

She laments, "It saddens me to think that my life has now completely changed all because of a medicine that was supposed to help me".

A man wrote, "I have been a wobbler since January 1999. I am 55 years old and continue to stagger like an old drunk, even though I recently celebrated 22 years of sobriety".

One woman who had her balance destroyed from **Gentamicin** treatments laments, "I can't drive, for nothing stays still. Even while working on the computer everything bounces. I cannot let go of my walker".

Another lady relates, "I was given the drug from hell after having a hysterectomy. That was 4 years ago. I'm so nauseated and dizzy today—just like it had happened yesterday".

One woman explains, "I was damaged by **Gentamicin** in 2000. I have severe hearing loss, balance problems and vision impairments that exacerbate my balance problems".

Another lady writes, "I have been damaged from **Gentamicin** since April, 2000. I received **Gentamicin** after an infection from back surgery. I wasn't told anything about the side effects of this drug. After 3 weeks, I became a wobbler. I now have severe oscillopsia".

Don't expect your doctors and medical professionals to really understand about the ototoxic side effects of **Gentamicin** (or any other drug) as the following story attests.

A man wrote, "I've had **Gentamicin** toxicity for two years now. I was treated for six days for acute endocarditis and then sent home for home care and treated with **Gentamicin** for two more weeks. I was given a handout on side effects and what to look for.

When I told the home nurse that I was dizzy and felt nausea and my right ear had plugged up, she asked if I heard a ringing in the ear and I said no. She said it wasn't the medication because I would hear a ringing in the ear! She said I 'must have got water in the ear.'

The next day I started getting dizzier and vomiting. I called the pharmacist. I told him I was really dizzy and vomiting. He said I must have the flu. He asked if I heard a ringing in the ear. I said no, but my right ear had plugged up and all I can hear is my pulse. He said it wasn't the medication, and that I probably had congestion and the flu.

The next day I went to my primary doctor. I told him how I felt. He asked if I heard a ringing in the ear. I said no, but my ear feels plugged up. He looked in my ears and said, 'Your ears look fine.' I got sicker and could barely walk.

I went to urgent care and told the doctor my story. She said the vertigo was the result of a virus, and I would be like this for three days, but it might last a month. 'It's not the medication,' she said, 'because I would have to hear a ringing in the ears.' Finally, I went to an ENT. After two days of tests, he told me I had permanent damage to my inner ear due to **Gentamicin** toxicity.

The worst part is that my doctor released me to go back to work full time even though my eyesight bounces and is blurred. I walk like I'm drunk. My balance is bad and I trip a lot and sometimes fall. I wobble when I'm standing and have a weird feeling in my head with pressure that feels like a headache coming on".

This man ends with the warning, "Don't let the doctors tell you that you have to hear a ringing in your ears" in order to have **Gentamicin** ototoxicity. Tinnitus, while common, is only one of many ototoxic symptoms you could experience.

Here is another lady's story, "I have been a wobbler since 1995. I had a routine hysterectomy after which I had several complications. When I was finally able to get up and around, I found myself dizzy and falling down, especially in the dark, or even in dim light.

Seven years later, I still have lots of problems. Probably the worst thing is that I don't look like anything is wrong with me. However, anyone walking next to me can tell something is wrong. I cannot swim or dance or ride a bike. I still fall frequently. (You should see all the bruises!)"

Another lady relates, "I, too, am a victim of **Gentamicin**, which was prescribed while I was in the hospital fighting pneumonia. It's been about 8 months now. I can no longer walk without assistance. Can't dance, go to the beach or even go to the grocery store to buy food".

An attorney writes about the outcome of his taking **Gentamicin** (and **Vancomycin**—a common combination). "This has ruined my legal practice because I can't concentrate at the computer for extended periods and cannot read for extended periods. It looks like I'll be wobbling off into the future".

A lady explains, "I cannot drive any more. As a result I had to quit my job as it was an hour's drive away. My mental status is now foggy at best. I cannot see or walk in the dark. My life as I knew it has changed drastically".

Another lady relates: "My vision jumps. In the dark I have no balance. I have broken my ribs twice, and am now under care for a twisted ankle and a lot of bruised muscles".

A man who received **Gentamicin** and **Clindamycin** for a bone infection writes what his life is now like, "I enjoyed all sports and played them at a very competitive level. Now I can't play any of them. I have trouble walking on uneven surfaces, and can't recognize faces of people I know when I walk down the street. I often have moments of 'brain fog' where I forget a person's name, even while I'm talking to them, and I know them well".

A lady explains, "I cannot drive at all. Darkness and sunlight play a big part in my inability to walk. I used to love to read. Now if I read, I have to be laying down so that my head does not move. I cannot talk or chew without my vision bouncing. This sucks!"

"After taking **Gentamicin** for 13 days," another woman writes, "I started experiencing vertigo right after the drug was stopped. I still can't stand up, let alone walk without assistance. I have totally lost my independence and must rely on someone for all my needs. I am unable to focus visually, go for walks, bike, drive, or go anywhere on my own. My life has been totally shut down! To think that this constant dizziness and nausea and the loss of independence could be permanent is devastating. Travelling in a vehicle is sickening—there go our retirement plans! I want my life back!"

Yet another woman relates, "After surgery, I was put on **Gentamicin** for 6 weeks. Now I am a wobbler. I can't walk without a cane. I can't drive. I was declared totally disabled. I can't use a ceiling fan, or watch my grandchildren run and play. Riding in a car is my worst time, and I make a small trip into a nightmare for my husband".

Here is another anecdotal report I have in my files. A lady wrote, "My sister suffered vestibular damage from **Gentamicin** eye drops prescribed off-label for use in the ear (as a preventative for infection!). My sister has been diagnosed with vestibular damage, nystagmus, and oscillopsia; she experiences all the gamut of symptoms—the vertigo, dizziness, nausea, vomiting, and the ataxic gait. She even experiences motor function shut-down, and a loss of consciousness when in an environment that becomes too challenging for her brain—too much visual stimuli".

A wide range of drugs can increase your risk of hearing loss with **Gentamicin**. Such drugs include other AMINOGLYCOSIDES and **Polymyxin** antibiotics, **Vancomycin**, **Furosemide**, **Ethacrynic acid**, and **Cisplatin**.[226]

Avoid using potent LOOP DIURETICS such as **Ethacrynic acid** and **Furosemide** at the same time as **Gentamicin** since these drugs can cause, or enhance, ototoxicity. Note too, that when given intravenously, diuretics may cause fairly rapid rise in **Gentamicin** serum levels and thus make its ototoxic effects even worse (CPS, PDR).

If you have to take both **Gentamicin** and LOOP DIURETICS, take the LOOP DIURETIC first. When you have completed the LOOP DIURETIC therapy, then begin taking the **Gentamicin**. The reason for this is because research indicates that if **Gentamicin** is given first and then the LOOP DIURETIC, these drugs act synergistically. This just means that the resulting damage to your ears will be much more severe than if you took the LOOP DIURETIC first.[227]

Also, be aware that exposing your ears to loud noise while you are on **Gentamicin**—or even up to a year after to stop taking it—can make the ototoxic effects worse than if you are not around loud noise when taking this drug.[228]

Recent studies have shown that some people are particularly susceptible to the ototoxic effects of **Gentamicin**. This seems to be related to the 1555A>G mutation in the mitochondrial RNA (mitochondrial deletions in the 12S sub-unit). Researchers estimate that about 1% of the general population have this mutation.[229] This susceptibility is passed on genetically through the mother. People with this genetic defect account for about 17% of the reported cases of hearing loss resulting from taking **Gentamicin**. (This is true of other AMINOGLYCOSIDE antibiotics as well.)[230]

Here is some good news. Today, with a better understanding of how **Gentamicin** affects our ears, doctors can even use **Gentamicin** to help people with certain ear problems. Because of its ototoxic properties, **Gentamicin** is sometimes used to treat intractable vertigo in people with severe Meniere's disease. It sounds like an oxymoron, but if **Gentamicin** is used soon enough, it may preserve the person's remaining hearing while eliminating the vertigo.

This is because the sensory cells of the balance system are more sensitive to **Gentamicin** damage than are the cells of the hearing system. Therefore, doctors use a carefully-controlled dose to reduce vestibular function without affecting hearing. They stop treatment as soon as any hearing or vestibular damage can be measured, but before the cells in the vestibular system are completely destroyed. This leaves the person with balance but not vertigo.[231] However, in practice, it is very difficult to achieve this, without also causing some degree of hearing loss.

The current procedure is to inject the **Gentamicin** directly through the eardrum. In one study, the follow-up results showed that after two years the vertigo was still controlled in 90% of the people in this study.[232] Note however, that this treatment does not always work, and can even cause further problems.

Gentamicin Treatment for Vertigo

If you want to learn more about this treatment, order the book, *Please Make My World Stop Spinning!—The Agony of Meniere's Disease*. (See the back of this book for ordering information.)

In my files, I have an anecdotal report of a man who was given 5 injections of **Gentamicin** to stop the vertigo of Meniere's Disease, and now he still has the vertigo, but in addition he has hearing loss and oscillopsia.

Doctors have also tried injecting **Gentamicin** directly into the semi-circular canals in the vestibular system. However, this causes hearing loss in a high proportion of those having this procedure.[233]

Another thing you should know about **Gentamicin** is that veterinarians may use it in treating your pet's ear infections. Unfortunately, **Gentamicin** can affect your pet's hearing, just like it does your own. I know this first hand. Our dog Riley went completely deaf after being treated with *Otomax*, a **Gentamicin**-based ointment used for ear infections in pets. His hearing gradually returned after 3 or 4 weeks, but he still has a moderate hearing loss that makes him almost useless as a hearing ear dog. Other people have told me the same thing happened to their pet's hearing also.

See Chapter 4 "Are You at Risk," Chapter 8, "The Sinister Partnership Between Ototoxic Agents and Noise," Chapter 9, "Aminoglycoside Antibiotics are the Ototoxic 'Bad boys'" and Chapter 12, "Potpourri" for further information on this drug.

Geodon (see **Ziprasidone**)

Gin Pain Pills (see **Sodium salicylate**)

Glatiramer

Pronunciation guide: glah-TEER-ah-mer

Drug classification: MULTIPLE SCLEROSIS DRUGS (see section 53.28 in Table 14-1)

Brand names: *Copaxone*

Ototoxic effects:
  Cochlear:
    Hearing loss: >2% [same as placebo] (CPS, PDR)
    Tinnitus: >2% [same as placebo] (CPS, PDR)
  Vestibular:
    Ataxia: 0.1-1% (CPS, PDR)
    Dizziness: >2% [same as placebo] (CPS, PDR)
    Nystagmus: 4% [2.4% above placebo results] (CPS, PDR)
    Vertigo: 6% [1% above placebo results] (CPS, PDR)

Outer/Middle Ear:
    Earache/ear pain: 7-12% [<2.5% above placebo results] (CPS, PDR)
    Otitis externa: 0.1-1% (CPS, PDR)
    Otitis media: 3.7% [0.6% above placebo results] (CPS)

Risk assessment: Class 3

Gleevec   (see **Imatinib**)

Gliadel   (see **Carmustine**)

Glibenclamide   (see **Glyburide**)

Gliclazide

Pronunciation guide: GLIK-lah-zide

Drug classification: SULFONYLUREAS (see section 40.8.12 in Table 14-1)

Brand names: *Diamicron, Diamicron MR*

Ototoxic effects:
    Cochlear:
        Hearing loss: <1% (CPS)
        Tinnitus: <1% (CPS)
    Vestibular:
        Dizziness: 2.2-2.3% (CPS)
    Outer/Middle Ear:
        Otitis media: 0.8-1.1% (CPS)

Risk assessment: Class 2

Glipizide

Pronunciation guide: GLIP-ih-zide

Drug classification: SULFONYLUREAS (see section 40.8.12 in Table 14-1)

Brand names: *Glucotrol*

Ototoxic effects:
    Vestibular:
        Ataxia: <1% (AHF, PDR)
        Dizziness: 6.8% [1% above placebo results] (AHF, PDR)
        Vertigo: <1% (AHF, PDR)

Risk assessment: Class 1

Glisoxepide

Pronunciation guide: glis-OX-eh-pide

Drug classification: SULFONYLUREAS (see section 40.8.12 in Table 14-1)

Brand names: *Glucoben, Pro-Diaban*

Ototoxic effects:
    Cochlear:
        Tinnitus: (She)

Risk assessment: Class 1

Glucoben   (see **Glisoxepide**)

Gluco-K   (see **Potassium gluconate**)

Glucotrol   (see **Glipizide**)

Glumetza   (see **Metformin**)

Glyburide (Glibenclamide)

Pronunciation guide: GLYE-byoor-ide (GLIH-ben-klah-mide)

Drug classification: SULFONYLUREAS (see section 40.8.12 in Table 14-1)

Brand names: *Euglucon, ratio-Glyburide*

Ototoxic effects:
    Cochlear:
        Tinnitus: (CPS)
    Vestibular:
        Dizziness: (CPS)

Risk assessment: Class 1

Goserelin

Pronunciation guide: GOE-seh-rel-in

Drug classification: GONADOTROPINS (see section 40.24 in Table 14-1)

Brand names: *Zoladex*

Ototoxic effects:
    Cochlear:
        Hyperacusis: <1% (CPS)
    Vestibular:
        Dizziness: 5-6% (CPS, PDR)
        Vertigo: <1% (CPS)

Risk assessment: Class 1

Gramicidin

Pronunciation guide: gra-MIH-sih-din

Drug classification: ANTI-BACTERIAL DRUGS (see section 7.4 in Table 14-1)

Brand names: [1]

Ototoxic effects:
> Unspecified/General Ear Conditions:
>> Ototoxicity: (San)

Risk assessment: Not enough information to rate

Notes:

> [1] **Gramicidin** is used in antibiotic ointments, creams and solutions such as *Neosporin*. *Neosporin* is a combination of **Gramicidin**, **Neomycin** and **Polymyxin B**. (See information on *Neosporin* under the generic drug **Neomycin**)

Granisetron

Pronunciation guide: gran-IZ-eh-tron

Drug classification: SEROTONIN-RECEPTOR ANTAGONISTS (see section 34.1.4 in Table 14-1)

Brand names: *Kytril*

Ototoxic effects:
> Vestibular:
>> Dizziness: 0.1-5% (CPS, PDR)
>> Vertigo: <0.1% (CPS)

Risk assessment: Class 1

Grepafloxacin

Pronunciation guide: GREP-ah-flox-ah-sin

Drug classification: QUINOLONES (see section 7.4.48 in Table 14-1)

Brand names: *Raxar*

Ototoxic effects:
> Cochlear:
>> Hearing loss: <1% (CPS, PDR)
>> Tinnitus: <1% (CPS, PDR)
> Vestibular:
>> Dizziness: 2.1-5.4% (CPS, PDR)
>> Vertigo: <1% (CPS, PDR)

Risk assessment: Class 2

Griseofulvin

Pronunciation guide: gris-ee-oh-FULL-vin

Drug classification: ANTI-FUNGAL ANTIBIOTICS (see section 7.10 in Table 14-1)

Brand names: *Fulvicin, Grisovin*

Ototoxic effects:
    Cochlear:
        Hearing loss (transient): (AHF, NDH)
    Vestibular:
        Ataxia: (BNF)
        Dizziness: (CPS, PDR)
        Vertigo: (CPS)

Risk assessment: Class 2

Notes:

    See Chapter 7, "We 'Hear' With Our Eyes" for further information on this drug.

Grisovin   (see **Griseofulvin**)

Guanabenz

Pronunciation guide: GWAHN-ah-benz

Drug classification: CENTRALLY ACTING ANTIADRENERGIC DRUGS (see section 20.8.20 in Table 14-1)

Brand names: *Wytensin*

Ototoxic effects:
    Cochlear:
        Tinnitus: <3% (AHF)
    Vestibular:
        Ataxia: <3% (AHF, DFC)
        Dizziness: 12-17% [10% above placebo results] (AHF, DFC)

Risk assessment: Class 1

Guanfacine

Pronunciation guide: GWAHN-fah-seen

Drug classification: CENTRALLY ACTING ANTIADRENERGIC DRUGS (see section 20.8.20 in Table 14-1)

Brand names: *Tenex*

Ototoxic effects:
    Cochlear:
        Tinnitus: <3% (DFC, PDR)
    Vestibular:
        Dizziness: 1-15% [<4% above placebo results] (NDH, PDR)
        Vertigo: (DFC, PDR)

Risk assessment: Class 2

Guanidine

Pronunciation guide: GWAHN-ih-deen

Drug classification: CHOLINERGIC AGONIST DRUGS (see section 17.12.1 in Table 14-1)

Brand names: *Imidourea*

Ototoxic effects:
    Vestibular:
        Ataxia: (DFC)

Risk assessment: Class 1

Gusperimus

Pronunciation guide: gus-PEH-rih-mus

Drug classification: IMMUNOSUPPRESSANT DRUGS (see section 43 in Table 14-1)

Brand names: *Spanidin*

Ototoxic effects:
    Cochlear:
        Tinnitus: (San, She)

Risk assessment: Class 1

Habitrol   (see **Nicotine**)

Haemophilus vaccine

Pronunciation guide: hem-OFF-fil-us VAK-seen

Drug classification: VACCINES (see section 70.8 in Table 14-1)

Brand names: *Comvax* [1], *PedvaxHIB* [2]

Ototoxic effects:
    Outer/Middle Ear:
        Otitis media: 0.5-2.7% (CPS, PDR)

Risk assessment: Class 1

Notes:

[1] *Comvax* is a combination of **Haemophilus b conjugate**, Meningococcal protein conjugate and **Hepatitis B** (recombinant) vaccines). (See the generic drug **Hepatitis B vaccine** for its specific ototoxic properties.)

[2] *PedvaxHIB* is a combination of **Haemophilus b conjugate** and Meningococcal protein conjugate vaccines. (**Haemophilus vaccine** is the ototoxic agent.)

Halcion   (see **Triazolam**)

Haldol　(see **Haloperidol**)

Haloperidol

Pronunciation guide: hah-loe-PER-ih-dole

Drug classification: ANTIPSYCHOTIC DRUGS (see section 60.8 in Table 14-1)

Brand names: *Haldol*

Ototoxic effects:
　Vestibular:
　　Vertigo: (CPS, PDR)

Risk assessment: Class 1

Notes:
　See Chapter 7, "We 'Hear' With Our Eyes" for further information on this drug.

Harmonyl　(see **Deserpidine**)

Havrix　(see **Hepatitis A vaccine**)

HCTZ　(see **Hydrochlorothiazide**)

Helidac　(see **Bismuth subsalicylate**)

Helixate　(see **Antihemophilic factor**)

Hemabate　(see **Carboprost**)

Hepatitis A vaccine

Pronunciation guide: hep-ah-TIE-tiss AYE VAK-seen

Drug classification: VACCINES (see section 70.8 in Table 14-1)

Brand names: *Havrix, Vaqta*

Ototoxic effects:
　Vestibular:
　　Ataxia: (DFC)
　　Dizziness: (AHF, PDR)
　　Vertigo: <1% (AHF, PDR)
　Outer/Middle Ear:
　　Otitis: 1.0-3.2% (CPS, PDR)
　　Otitis media: 5.8-9.9% (CPS, PDR)

Risk assessment: Class 2

Hepatitis B vaccine

Pronunciation guide: hep-ah-TYE-tis BEE VAK-seen

Drug classification: Vaccines (see section 70.8 in Table 14-1)

Brand names: *Engerix-B, Recombivax HB, Twinrix* [1]

Ototoxic effects:
  Cochlear:
      Tinnitus: >1% (CPS, PDR)
  Vestibular:
      Dizziness: 1-10% (CPS, PDR)
      Vertigo: >1% (CPS, PDR)
  Outer/Middle Ear:
      Earache/ear pain: >1% (CPS, PDR)

Risk assessment: Class 2

Notes:

  [1] *Twinrix* is a combination of **Hepatitis A** and **Hepatitis B** vaccines. (See the generic drug **Hepatitis A vaccine** for its specific ototoxic properties.)

Herceptin   (see **Trastuzumab**)

Hexadimethrine

Pronunciation guide: hex-ah-DIE-meth-reen

Drug classification: Anti-viral drugs (see section 7.17 in Table 14-1)

Brand names: *Polybrene*

Ototoxic effects:
  Unspecified/General Ear Conditions:
      Ototoxicity: [234]

Risk assessment: Not enough information to rate

Hexadrol   (see **Dexamethasone**)

Hexalen   (see **Altretamine**)

Hexamine   (see **Methenamine**)

Hibiclens   (see **Chlorhexidine**)

Hibistat   (see **Chlorhexidine**)

Hiprex   (see **Methenamine**)

Histase   (see **Methapyrilene**)

Histrelin

Pronunciation guide: HISS-trah-lyn

Drug classification: PITUITARY HORMONES (see section 40.44 in Table 14-1)

Brand names: *Supprelin*

Ototoxic effects:
    Cochlear:
        Hearing loss: 1-3% (PDR, USP)
    Vestibular:
        Dizziness: 1-3% (PDR, USP)
    Outer/Middle Ear:
        Earache/ear pain: 1-3% (PDR, USP)

Risk assessment: Class 2

Hivid (see **Zalcitabine**)

Homatropine

Pronunciation guide: hoe-MAH-troe-peen

Drug classification: ANTI-CHOLINERGIC DRUGS (see section 17.1 in Table 14-1)

Brand names: *Isopto Homatropine, Mimims Homatropine*

Ototoxic effects:
    Cochlear:
        Tinnitus: (San, She)
    Vestibular:
        Dizziness: [235]
    Unspecified/General Ear Conditions:
        Ototoxicity: (San)

Risk assessment: Class 2

Hp-PAC (see **Lansoprazole**)

Humatin (see **Paromomycin**)

Humatrope (see **Somatropin**)

Humira (see **Adalimumab**)

Hycanthone

Pronunciation guide: hye-KAN-thone

Drug classification: ANTHELMINTIC DRUGS (see section 7.1 in Table 14-1)

Brand names: —

Ototoxic effects:
    Vestibular:
        Dizziness: (NTP)
        Vertigo: (NTP)

Risk assessment: Class 1

Hycodan   (see **Hydrocodone**)

Hydeltrasol   (see **Prednisolone**)

Hydeltra-TBA   (see **Prednisolone**)

Hydrochlorothiazide (HCTZ)

Pronunciation guide: hye-droe-klor-oh-THYE-ah-zide

Drug classification: DIURETICS—THIAZIDE-RELATED (see section 30.5.12 in Table 14-1)

Brand names: *Aldoril*[1], *Apo-Hydro*, *Apresazide*[2], *Esidrix*, *Esimil*[3], *HydroDIURIL*,

    Hydropres[4], *Microzide*, *Oretic*

Ototoxic effects:
    Cochlear:
        Tinnitus: [5,6]
    Vestibular:
        Dizziness: 8% [5.6% above placebo results] (CPS, PDR)
        Vertigo: (CPS, PDR)

Risk assessment: Class 1

Notes:

[1] *Aldoril* is a combination of **Hydrochlorothiazide** and **Methyldopa**. (See the generic drug **Methyldopa** for its specific ototoxic properties.)

[2] *Apresazide* is a combination of **Hydrochlorothiazide** and Hydralazine. (**Hydrochlorothiazide** is the ototoxic agent.)

[3] *Esimil* is a combination of **Hydrochlorothiazide** and Guanethidine. (**Hydrochlorothiazide** is the ototoxic agent.)

[4] *Hydropres* is a combination of **Hydrochlorothiazide** and **Reserpine**. (See the generic drug **Reserpine** for its specific ototoxic properties.)

[5] I have an anecdotal report in my files of a lady whose tinnitus gets louder when she takes **Hydrochlorothiazide**.

[6] I have another anecdotal report in my files of a lady who also reveals, "I currently take **Hydrochlorothiazide** which causes my ears to ring worse".

Hydrocodone

Pronunciation guide: hye-droe-KOE-doan

Drug classification: OPIATE AGONIST DRUGS (see section 1.4.1 in Table 14-1)

Brand names: *Hycodan*[1], *Lortab*[2], *Norco*[2], *Tussend*[3], *Vicodin*[2], *Zydone*[2]

Ototoxic effects:
    Cochlear:
        Hearing loss: [4] (PDR)
        Tinnitus: (Med)
    Vestibular:
        Dizziness: (CPS, PDR)

Risk assessment: normally Class 1, but Class 5 if taking high doses and/or for a long time
    (see warning below)

Notes:

Hydrocodone is one of the ingredients in a number of compound drugs too numerous to list here. As always, check the labels and then look up each drug listed to see its ototoxic properties.

[1] *Hycodan* is a combination of **Hydrocodone** and **Homatropine**. (See the generic drug **Homatropine** for its specific ototoxic properties.)

[2] *Lortab*, *Norco*, *Vicodin* and *Zydone* are combinations of **Acetaminophen** and **Hydrocodone**. (See the drug **Acetaminophen** for its specific ototoxic properties.)

[3] *Tussend* is a combination of **Hydrocodone**, **Pseudoephedrine** and **Chlorpheniramine**. (See the generic drugs **Chlorpheniramine** and **Pseudoephedrine** for their specific ototoxic properties.)

[4] Although earlier reports have implicated **Hydrocodone** as the culprit in hearing loss, current experiments in cochlear cultures show that the death of both the inner and outer hair cells occurs with high doses of **Acetaminophen**, but not with even the highest doses of **Hydrocodone**.[236] However, when taken in combination with **Acetaminophen**, **Hydrocodone** has a somewhat synergistic effect and makes the resulting hearing loss even worse that it would have been by taking **Acetaminophen** alone.[237]

Warning: House Ear physicians reported a previously unknown and devastating side effect of *Vicodin*—rapid, profound, bilateral, irreversible hearing loss after overuse of this drug.[238] Apparently, hearing loss has not been reported when taking *Vicodin* at recommended dosages.

After this report was published, two audiologists called the Journal that published this study to report that each of them had had a patient who experienced sudden and significant hearing loss after taking *Vicodin*.

According to Dr. John W. House, "Some patients have retained some hearing if they stop using the painkillers immediately, but for most, the damage is already done. Once the process starts, it seems irreversible".[239]

Although *Vicodin* has been on the market since 1982, hearing loss attributed to *Vicodin* did not begin showing up until 11 years later, in 1993.[240] This was likely because no one was looking for a link between sudden hearing loss and *Vicodin*.

One man was taking 20 to 30 *Vicodin* pills a day for pain. One day he noticed his ears were ringing. From the time he first noticed his ears ringing until he was completely deaf was only 4 weeks.[241]

Dr. John House of the House Ear Institute wrote, "My colleagues and I [at the House Clinic] have seen a significant number of patients who have become addicted to *Vicodin* and have gone completely deaf. They have been taking 15 to 75 tablets per day and in a short period of time have developed a rapidly progressive hearing loss, which leads to permanent total deafness".

He went on to say, "*Vicodin* and other **Hydrocodone/Acetaminophen** prescription painkillers affect people differently. One person may take *Vicodin* for years and not suffer any hearing loss. Another person may take large doses for only six months and suffer profound permanent hearing loss".

For example, "Shannon was taking 40 to 50 *Vicodin* a day" for more than a year. The *Vicodin* "permanently killed the sensorineural hair cells in her inner ears, leaving her completely deaf".[242]

In my files I have anecdotal reports of two women who took *Vicodin* for several months. During that time both definitely noticed a drop in their hearing.

I have another anecdotal report of a woman that now has "profound hearing loss as a result of *Vicodin* abuse".

Also, I have correspondence in my files with a woman who totally lost her hearing from taking *Vicodin*. Here is her story.

Jodi had back surgery, and her doctor put her on *Vicodin* for the pain. She built up a tolerance to it, and consequently had to take more and more to kill the pain. The pain persisted, and she ended up taking high doses of *Vicodin* for several years. Then one day she noticed her ears were ringing, and she couldn't hear things she used to hear. In a matter of months, her hearing dropped from normal to so bad that even hearing aids couldn't help her. Now she has a cochlear implant to help her hear.

Vicodin is typically prescribed for short-term use of two to three weeks at most. The typical dose is one pill every six hours. Trouble to your ears develops when you take much higher doses such as 20 or more pills a day for two months or longer.[243]

Here are two things you should know. First, *Vicodin* was the number one prescription drug in the United States in 2000.[244] Second, it is addictive and thus subject to abuse. Put these two facts together, and you can readily see the staggering potential for severe hearing loss when used wrongly.

The following warning was first included in the 2002 edition of the PDR under *Vicodin*. "Very rare cases of hearing loss have been reported in patients predominantly receiving very high doses of **Hydrocodone/Acetaminophen** for long periods of time" (PDR). In the 2010 edition of the PDR it is reported as, "Cases of hearing impairment or permanent loss have been reported predominantly in patients with chronic overdose".

See Chapter 2 "Ototoxic Drugs—What Are They?", and also the section entitled "The Story of Vicodin)" in Chapter 5 for further information on **Acetaminophen/Hydrocodone**.

Hydrocortisone

Pronunciation guide: hye-droe-KOR-tih-sone

Drug classification: GLUCOCORTICOIDS (see section 40.1.4 in Table 14-1)

Brand names: *Colocort, Cortef, Cortenema, Hydrocortone, Solu-Cortef*

Ototoxic effects:
  Vestibular:
      Vertigo: (CPS, PDR)

Risk assessment: Class 1

Hydrocortone   (see **Hydrocortisone**)

HydroDIURIL   (see **Hydrochlorothiazide**)

Hydroflumethiazide

Pronunciation guide: hye-droe-floo-meth-EYE-ah-zide

Drug classification: DIURETICS—THIAZIDE-RELATED (see section 30.5.12 in Table 14-1)

Brand names: *Diucardin*

Ototoxic effects:
  Vestibular:
      Dizziness: (PDR)
      Vertigo: (PDR)

Risk assessment: Class 1

Hydromorph Contin   (see **Hydromorphone**)

Hydromorphone

Pronunciation guide: hye-droe-MOR-fone

Drug classification: OPIATE AGONIST DRUGS (see section 1.4.1 in Table 14-1)

Brand names: *Dilaudid, Dilaudid-HP, Hydromorph Contin*

Ototoxic effects:
  Cochlear:
      Hyperacusis: <1% (DFC)
      Tinnitus: >1% (DFC)

Vestibular:
    Ataxia: (CPS, PDR)
    Dizziness: (CPS, PDR)
    Nystagmus: <1% (CPS, PDR)
    Vertigo: (BNF)
    Vestibular disorder: (CP2, CPS)

Risk assessment: Class 2

Hydromox   (see **Quinethazone**)

Hydropres   (see **Hydrochlorothiazide**)

Hydroxychloroquine

Pronunciation guide: hye-drox-ee-KLOR-oh-kwin

Drug classification: ANTI-MALARIAL DRUGS (see section 7.14.8 in Table 14-1)

Brand names: *Plaquenil*

Ototoxic effects:
    Cochlear:
        Hearing loss: (CPS, PDR) [1]
        Tinnitus: (CPS, PDR)
    Vestibular:
        Ataxia: (NDH, PDR)
        Dizziness: (NDH, PDR)
        Nystagmus: (NDH, PDR) [2]
        Vertigo: (CPS, PDR)

Risk assessment: Class 3

Notes:

[1] Hearing loss is often temporary, but may be permanent (CPS).

[2] Nystagmus is typically irreversible (NDH).

See Chapter 7, "We 'Hear' With Our Eyes" for further information on this drug.

Hydroxyzine

Pronunciation guide: hye-DROX-ih-zeen

Drug classification: PIPERAZINE DERIVATIVES (see section 10.8.1 in Table 14-1)

Brand names: *Atarax, Vistaril*

Ototoxic effects:
    Vestibular:
        Ataxia: >1% (CPS, AHF)
        Dizziness: >1% (CPS, AHF)

Risk assessment: Class 1

Hygromix 2.4 (see **Hygromycin B**)

Hygromycin B

Pronunciation guide: hye-groe-MY-sin BEE

Drug classification: AMINOGLYCOSIDES (see section 7.4.1 in Table 14-1)

Brand names: *Antihelmycin, Hygromix 2.4*

Ototoxic effects:
Cochlear:
Hearing loss: (NTP)

Risk assessment: Class 5

Notes:

Hygromycin B is an AMINOGLYCOSIDE antibiotic that is not used on humans in North America. Therefore, all the ear-related side effects are unknown, but in animals, it can cause deafness.

See Chapter 9, "Aminoglycoside Antibiotics are the Ototoxic 'Bad boys'" for further information on this drug.

Hygroton (see **Chlorthalidone**)

Hyoscyamine

Pronunciation guide: hye-AH-skah-meen

Drug classification: ANTI-CHOLINERGIC DRUGS (see section 17.1 in Table 14-1)

Brand names: *Levbid, Levsin, Levsinex, NuLev*

Ototoxic effects:
Vestibular:
Ataxia: (CPS, PDR)
Dizziness: (CPS, PDR)

Risk assessment: Class 1

Hyperstat (see **Diazoxide**)

Hytrin (see **Terazosin**)

Hyzaar (see **Losartan**)

Ibandronate (Ibandronic acid)

Pronunciation guide: eh-BAN-drow-nate

Drug classification: BISPHOSPHONATES (see section 50.1.1 in Table 14-1)

Brand names: *Boniva*

Ototoxic effects:
Cochlear:
Tinnitus: [1]
Vestibular:
Ataxia: [1]
Dizziness: 1.0-3.7% [<1.1% above placebo results] (AHF, PDR)
Vertigo: 3.5% [0.5% above placebo results] (AHF, PDR)
Unspecified/General Ear Conditions:
Ear disorder: [1]

Risk assessment: Class 2

[1] Adverse event reports for **Ibandronate** include tinnitus, gait disturbance (ataxia), dizziness and ear disorder.[245, 246]

IBU   (see **Ibuprofen**)

Ibuprofen

Pronunciation guide: eye-byoo-PROE-fen

Drug classification: PROPIONIC ACIDS (see section 1.1.13 in Table 14-1)

Brand names: *Advil, Advil Cold & Sinus*[1], *Dristan Sinus*[1], *IBU, Motrin, Nuprin, Sudafed Sinus Advance*[1], *Vicoprofen*[2]

Ototoxic effects:
Cochlear:
Hearing loss: <1% (CPS, PDR)
Tinnitus: 1-3% (CPS, PDR)
Vestibular:
Dizziness: 3-14% (CPS, PDR)
Nystagmus: (AHF, CPS)
Vertigo: <1% (CPS, PDR)

Risk assessment: Class 3

Notes:

[1] *Advil Cold & Sinus, Dristan Sinus* and *Sudafed Sinus Advance* are combinations of **Ibuprofen** and **Pseudoephedrine.** (See the generic drug **Pseudoephedrine** for its specific ototoxic properties.)

[2] *Vicoprofen* is a combination of **Ibuprofen** and **Hydrocodone.** (See the generic drug **Hydrocodone** for its specific ototoxic properties.)

Using **Ibuprofen** regularly over time can increase your risk of hearing loss. For example, in one study of 26,917 men between the ages of 40 and 75 at the beginning of the study, men that used **Ibuprofen** at least twice a week had a 33% increased risk of hearing loss over men who were not regular users of **Ibuprofen**. However, when only men under the age of 50 were considered, the risk factor for hearing loss jumped to 61%.[247]

Taking **Ibuprofen** inhibits cyclooxygenase and decreases prostaglandin activity, potentially reducing cochlear blood flow.[248] Symptoms of **Ibuprofen** overdose include dizziness, nystagmus and tinnitus (CPS, PDR).

I have an anecdotal report in my files of a man who took **Ibuprofen** and has had permanent tinnitus ever since. He wrote, "I have taken **Ibuprofen** three times in the last nine years—and after the instant tinnitus problem caused by the first occasion, I only took the drug twice more (in error, thinking it was [**Acetaminophen**]). My tinnitus has remained from the first occasion to today, and increased in intensity on the second and third occasions".

I have another anecdotal report in my files of a man who took large doses of **Ibuprofen** to relieve a severe tooth ache. He reported, "Within two days my tinnitus started, and has persisted for the last two years. I have not taken any more **Ibuprofen** since the original dose". This shows that tinnitus from **Ibuprofen** can be permanent.

In another anecdotal report in my files, a woman wrote, "I used **Ibuprofen** 800 mg. for several nights in a row for shoulder pain. I have had a high-pitched ringing sound ever since—for the past month or so now. It's very loud and wakes me up at night. I have moments of panic at the idea that this will never end".

In still another anecdotal report in my files, a man had much the same experience as above. He wrote, "I've had the same thing happen to me and it hasn't gone away. It's been two days of this [tinnitus] and I can't handle living like this. I wish I had have never taken the *Advil* to begin with".

In another anecdotal report in my files a lady reported that she took *Advil* for a few weeks and got tinnitus. In another anecdotal report a lady wrote, "I got tinnitus through **Ibuprofen**," while another lady stated, "I have been taking **Ibuprofen** and my ears have started ringing". And still another lady wrote, "I am in my 50s and took *Advil* for a few weeks last year and started getting tinnitus".

A man reported in another anecdotal report in my files, "I took **Ibuprofen** for 3 weeks, and now my ears are ringing constantly. I've been off the **Ibuprofen** for 4 days, but if anything, my tinnitus seems even louder," while another man reported, "I took *Advil* for back pain about 6 months ago that resulted in the rather loud tinnitus I am still suffering from today".

I have yet another anecdotal report in my files of a man who had been taking **Ibuprofen** for his headaches and other pains for some time. Some months ago he noticed he had a hearing loss in one ear. He explained, "I could barely hear the person speaking to me on the phone. I could hear with my left ear, but not my right". A hearing test revealed that he had a moderately-severe to mild reverse slope sensorineural hearing loss up to 1000 Hz rising to normal beyond 1000 Hz in his right ear. He then switched to another pain killer and stopped taking **Ibuprofen** completely. A few weeks later he wrote, "I went for a hearing test today and my hearing has come back. Both my ears are now hearing normally and there is no hint of tinnitus in either ear. I have continued to avoid **Ibuprofen**, which appears to have been responsible for my hearing loss".

In another anecdotal report in my files a man wrote, "I had a noticeable drop in hearing acuity after a 7-day course of **Ibuprofen** for post-surgical pain. I took 800 mg. every 6 hours for about 7 days. My hearing loss was then apparent after I stopped taking the

Ibuprofen. I have much more tinnitus and it feels like my ears are full of wax or water. Discontinuing **Ibuprofen** did not bring back my hearing. I had hearing loss before I took **Ibuprofen**, and this makes it so much worse".

In yet another anecdotal report in my files, a man wrote, "My doctor recently prescribed 800 mg. of **Ibuprofen** three times a day for ten days. On the tenth day I noticed sudden hearing loss in my left ear, and tremendous roaring and ringing too. It is now two weeks later and my doctor is very pessimistic regarding my regaining my hearing back".

In still another anecdotal report in my files, a man wrote, "I had an injury to my foot and took **Ibuprofen** for the pain. Shortly thereafter, the ringing in my ears started. I had no idea this could happen, and would never have taken the **Ibuprofen** if I had known this would happen. I have been off of it about a week, but the ringing continues".

In another anecdotal report in my files, a lady wrote, "I have been using **Ibuprofen** for 6 months. I now have loud, constant ringing in my ears that started about 3 weeks ago".

I have a couple of anecdotal reports in my files of **Ibuprofen** apparently affecting the hearing of people with cochlear implants. A man wrote, "I have experienced a decline in the clarity of my hearing when taking medications that are NSAIDs. (**Aspirin**, **Ibuprofen**, **Nabumetone**, **Naproxen**, etc.) I've had recurring back problems for over a year now and take NSAIDS to get it under control. I've noticed from time to time that the sound from my cochlear implant seems a little fuzzy or muddy and now realize that it may be during times when I'm taking those drugs that it happens". A lady with a cochlear implant also wrote, "I have been taking **Ibuprofen** (*Advil*) for the past ten days. In that time I have not been able to understand on the phone as well as I usually do. It might be the *Advil*". Four days after stopping the **Ibuprofen**, she exclaimed, "Today I can hear fine on the phone. I never associated my hearing loss with taking *Advil*".

See Chapter 4 "Are You at Risk?" and Chapter 12, "Potpourri" for some further important information on this drug.

Idarac (see **Floctafenine**)

Idursulfase

Pronunciation guide: eye-dur-SUL-fase

Drug classification: ENZYMES (see section 32.1 in Table 14-1)

Brand names: *Elaprase*

Ototoxic effects:
  Vestibular:
    Dizziness: 6.3% [same as placebo] (CPS)
    Vertigo: (CPS)
  Unspecified/General Ear Conditions:
    Ear disorder: 9.4% [placebo 0] (CPS)

Risk assessment: Class 2

Ifex (see **Ifosfamide**)

Ifosfamide

Pronunciation guide: eye-FOSS-fah-mide

Drug classification: ALKYLATING DRUGS (see section 14.1 in Table 14-1)

Brand names: *Ifex*

Ototoxic effects:
    Cochlear:
        Auditory hallucinations: (AHF)
    Vestibular:
        Dizziness: (AHF, DFC)

Risk assessment: Class 1

Ilaris   (see **Canakinumab**)

Iloperidone

Pronunciation guide: eye-loe-PEER-ih-dohn

Drug classification: ANTIPSYCHOTIC DRUGS (see section 60.8 in Table 14-1)

Brand names: *Fanapt*, *Fanapta*, *Zomaril*

Ototoxic effects:
    Cochlear:
        Tinnitus: 0.1-1% (PDR)
    Vestibular:
        Dizziness: 10-20% [3-13% above placebo results] (PDR)
        Vertigo: 0.1-1% (PDR)

Risk assessment: Class 2

Ilosone   (see **Erythromycin**)

Ilotycin   (see **Erythromycin**)

Imatinib

Pronunciation guide: ih-MAT-ih-nib

Drug classification: TYROSINE KINASE INHIBITORS (see section 14.40 in Table 14-1)

Brand names: *Gleevec*

Ototoxic effects:
    Cochlear:
        Hearing loss: 0.1-1% (CPS, PDR)
        Tinnitus: 0.1-1% (CPS, PDR)

Vestibular:
> Dizziness: 0.9-19.4% (NDH, PDR)
> Vertigo: 0.1-1% (CPS, PDR)

Risk assessment: Class 2

Imdur (see **Isosorbide**)

Imidapril

Pronunciation guide: ih-MID-ah-pril

Drug classification: Angiotensin-converting enzyme (ACE) inhibitors (see section 20.8.8 in Table 14-1)

Brand names: *Tanatril*

Ototoxic effects:
> Cochlear:
>> Tinnitus: (BNF)
> Vestibular:
>> Dizziness: (BNF)

Risk assessment: Class 1

Imidourea (see **Guanidine**)

Imipenem—Cilastatin

Pronunciation guide: im-ih-PEN-em sye-lah-STAT-in

Drug classification: Carbapenems (see section 7.4.12.1 in Table 14-1)

Brand names: *Primaxin*

Ototoxic effects:
> Cochlear:
>> Hearing loss: <0.1% (CPS, PDR)
>> Tinnitus: <0.1% (CPS, PDR)
> Vestibular:
>> Ataxia: (PDR)
>> Dizziness: 0.3% (CPS, PDR)
>> Vertigo: 0.1% (CPS, PDR)

Risk assessment: Class 2

Notes:

> Hearing loss may be temporary (CPS).

> Ataxia is a sign of **Imipenem—Cilastatin** overdose (PDR).

Imipramine

Pronunciation guide: im-IP-rah-meen

Drug classification: Tricyclic anti-depressants (see section 60.1.8 in Table 14-1)

Brand names: *Tofranil*

Ototoxic effects:
    Cochlear:
        Tinnitus: 0.01-1% (CPS, PDR)
    Vestibular:
        Ataxia: 0.01-1% (CPS, PDR)
        Dizziness: 1-10% (CPS, PDR)

Risk assessment: Class 2

Notes:

In my files I have an anecdotal report of a woman who got tinnitus when she began taking **Imipramine**.

Caution: Eating grapefruit or drinking grapefruit juice during the time you are taking this drug may make the listed side effects worse than shown here.

See Chapter 11, "Grapefruit Juice and Ototoxic Drugs" for further information on this drug.

Imitrex   (see **Sumatriptan**)

Immune globulin

Pronunciation guide: ih-MUNE GLOB-yoo-lin

Drug classification: Serums (see section 70.1 in Table 14-1)

Brand names: *Gammagard, Gamunex*

Ototoxic effects:
    Vestibular:
        Dizziness: 0.4-9.8% (CPS, PDR)
        Vertigo: 0.5% (CPS)
    Outer/Middle Ear:
        Earache/ear pain: 14-18% (PDR)

Risk assessment: Class 2

Imovane   (see **Zopiclone**)

Imovax   (see **Rabies vaccine**)

Implanon   (see **Etonogestrel**)

Increlex   (see **Mecasermin**)

Indacrinone

Pronunciation guide: in-dah-KRIN-own

Drug classification: DIURETICS—LOOP (see section 30.5.4 in Table 14-1)

Brand names: —

Ototoxic effects:
    Unspecified/General Ear Conditions:
        Ototoxicity: [249]

Risk assessment: Not enough information to rate

Indapamide

Pronunciation guide: in-DAP-ah-mide

Drug classification: DIURETICS—THIAZIDE-RELATED (see section 30.5.12 in Table 14-1)

Brand names: *Apo-Indapamide, Lozide, Lozol*

Ototoxic effects:
    Cochlear:
        Tinnitus: <1% (CPS)
    Vestibular:
        Ataxia: (CPS)
        Dizziness: 1.9-7% (CPS, PDR)
        Vertigo: 2.2% (CPS, PDR)
    Outer/Middle Ear:
        Earache/ear pain: <1% (CPS)
        Otitis: <1% (CPS)
    Unspecified/General Ear Conditions:
        Ear disorder: (CPS)

Risk assessment: Class 2

Inderal   (see **Propranolol**)

Inderal-LA   (see **Propranolol**)

Inderide   (see **Propranolol**)

Indinavir

Pronunciation guide: in-DIN-ah-ver

Drug classification: ANTI-RETROVIRAL PROTEASE INHIBITORS (see section 7.17.1.1 in Table 14-1)

Brand names: *Crixivan*

Ototoxic effects:

    Vestibular:

        Dizziness: <3.9% (AHF, PDR)

        Vertigo: <2% (CPS, PDR)

Risk assessment: Class 1

Notes:

    Caution: Eating grapefruit or drinking grapefruit juice during the time you are taking this drug may make the listed side effects worse than shown here.

    See Chapter 11, "Grapefruit Juice and Ototoxic Drugs" for further information on this drug.

Indocid   (see **Indomethacin**)

Indocin   (see **Indomethacin**)

Indomethacin

Pronunciation guide: in-doe-METH-ah-sin

Drug classification: ACETIC ACIDS (see section 1.1.1 in Table 14-1)

Brand names: *Indocid, Indocin, Indotec, Rhodacine*

Ototoxic effects:

    Cochlear:

        Hearing disorder: 1-3% (AHF, PDR)

        Hearing loss: 1-3% (CPS, PDR)

        Tinnitus: 1-3% (CPS, PDR)

    Vestibular:

        Ataxia: (AHF)

        Dizziness: 3-9% (CPS, PDR)

        Vertigo: 1-3% (CPS, PDR)

Risk assessment: Class 3

Notes:

    See Chapter 4 "Are You at Risk?" and Chapter 7, "We 'Hear' With Our Eyes" for further information on this drug.

Indoprofen

Pronunciation guide: IN-doe-proe-fen

Drug classification: PROPIONIC ACIDS (see section 1.1.13 in Table 14-1)

Brand names: *Fosint*

Ototoxic effects:

    Cochlear:

        Tinnitus: (San, She)

Unspecified/General Ear Conditions:
Ototoxicity: (San)

Risk assessment: Class 2

Indotec   (see **Indomethacin**)

Infanrix   (see **Tetanus vaccine**)

Infergen   (see **Interferon alfacon-1**)

Infliximab

Pronunciation guide: in-FLICKS-ih-mab

Drug classification: MONOCLONAL ANTIBODIES (see section 7.17.8 in Table 14-1)

Brand names: *Remicade*

Ototoxic effects:
Vestibular:
Ataxia: (CPS)
Dizziness: 4-11% [0-6% above placebo results] (CPS, PDR)
Vertigo: 1-5% [0-1% above placebo results] (CPS, PDR)
Outer/Middle Ear
Earache/ear pain: 2% (CPS)
Increased ear wax: <2% (CPS, PDR)
Otitis: 1-2% [<2% above placebo results] (CPS)
Otitis externa: (CPS)
Otitis media: 2% (CPS)

Risk assessment: Class 2

Influenza vaccine

Pronunciation guide: in-flue-EN-zah VAK-seen

Drug classification: VACCINES (see section 70.8 in Table 14-1)

Brand names: *Fluarix, Flulaval, FluShield, Fluviral S/F, Fluzone, Vaxigrip*

Ototoxic effects:
Cochlear:
Hearing loss: [1]
Vestibular:
Dizziness: (PDR)
Labyrinthitis: (CPS, PDR)
Vertigo: (PDR)

Risk assessment: Class 2

Notes:

[1] Flu shots contain mercury (**Thimerosal**). **Thimerosal** is known to cause hearing loss (see the generic drug **Thimerosal** for its specific ototoxic properties.)

I have an anecdotal report in my files of a boy that lost "a significant amount of his hearing, and experienced dizziness after getting a flu shot".

In another anecdotal report in my files, a mother wrote, "My daughter's hearing dropped significantly—30 dB at every frequency—one week to the day after receiving her flu shot last year".

In another anecdotal report in my files, a man reported a "major hearing drop the day after I took a seasonal flu shot".

I have an anecdotal report of a man who got the N1H1 (swine flu) shot and within a week suffered severe sudden hearing loss in his right ear.

I have another anecdotal report in my files of a man who also got the N1H1 (swine flu) shot and 15 days later suddenly lost all hearing in his left ear. Only a minimal amount has since returned in spite of treatment.

In yet another anecdotal report in my files a man wrote, "My wife suddenly lost hearing in her right ear one week after the H1N1 (swine flu) injection. Two days later she saw her ear specialist who injected **Prednisone** in her ear. It has been 9 days, and her hearing has not returned".

INH   (see **Isoniazid**)

Inhibace   (see **Cilazapril**)

Innopran XL   (see **Propranolol**)

Insulin aspart

Pronunciation guide: IN-suh-lin ASS-part

Drug classification: INSULINS (see section 40.8.4 in Table 14-1)

Brand names: *NovoMix*

Ototoxic effects:
    Vestibular:
        Dizziness: 2-3% (CPS)
        Vertigo: <1-2% (CPS)

Risk assessment: Class 1

Insulin detemir

Pronunciation guide: IN-suh-lin DEH-teh-meer

Drug classification: INSULINS (see section 40.8.4 in Table 14-1)

Brand names: *Levemir*

Ototoxic effects:
    Vestibular:
        Dizziness: 1.8% (CPS)
        Vestibular disorder: <1% (CPS)
    Outer/Middle Ear
        Earache/ear pain: <1% (CPS)
    Unspecified/General Ear Conditions:
        Ear disorder: <1% (CPS)

Risk assessment: Class 1

Insulin, human

Pronunciation guide: IN-suh-lin, HEU-man

Drug classification: INSULINS (see section 40.8.4 in Table 14-1)

Brand names: *Exubera*

Ototoxic effects:
    Outer/Middle Ear
        Earache/ear pain: 3.9% (PDR)
        Otitis media: 6.5% (PDR)
    Unspecified/General Ear Conditions:
        Ear disorder: 1.3% (PDR)

Risk assessment: Class 1

Intal   (see **Cromolyn sodium**)

Intelence   (see **Etravirine**)

Interferon alfa-2a

Pronunciation guide: in-ter-FEER-on AL-fah

Drug classification: INTERFERONS (see section 7.17.4 in Table 14-1)

Brand names: *Roferon-A*

Ototoxic effects:
    Cochlear:
        Hearing disorder: <5% (CPS, PDR)
        Hearing loss: 35% [250]
        Tinnitus: 29% [251]
    Vestibular:
        Ataxia: <1% (AHF, PDR)
        Dizziness: 11-40% (CPS, PDR)
        Vertigo: <3-5% (CPS, PDR)

Outer/Middle Ear:
    Earache/ear pain: <1% (AHF, PDR)

Risk assessment: Class 4

Notes:

Hearing loss generally is overlooked because it is often mild and sub-clinical (hearing loss above 8,000 Hz). However, when it affects the frequencies below 8,000 Hz, it is readily detected by serial audiograms. Hearing loss ranges from 20-30 dB at 8,000 Hz. Both the hearing loss and tinnitus tend to occur more frequently when you take higher doses. Normally, your hearing will return and your tinnitus will go away within 7 to 14 days after stopping **Interferon** treatment.[252]

Interferon alfa-2b

Pronunciation guide: in-ter-FEER-on AL-fah

Drug classification: INTERFERONS (see section 7.17.4 in Table 14-1)

Brand names: *Intron A, Rebetron*[1]

Ototoxic effects:
    Cochlear:
        Hearing disorder: <5% (CPS, PDR)
        Hearing loss: 5-35% (CPS, PDR)
        Hyperacusis: (CPS)
        Tinnitus: 2-29% (CPS, PDR)
    Vestibular:
        Ataxia: <5% (CPS, PDR)
        Dizziness: 7-24% (CPS, PDR)
        Labyrinthine disorder: <5% (PDR)
        Nystagmus: <5% (PDR)
        Vertigo: 2-8% (CPS, PDR)
    Outer/Middle Ear:
        Earache/ear pain: 2-5% (CPS, PDR)
        Otitis media: 2-5% (CPS, PDR)

Risk assessment: Class 4

Notes:

[1] *Rebetron* is a combination of **Ribavirin** and **Interferon alfa-2b**. (See the generic drug **Ribavirin** for its specific ototoxic properties.)

Hearing loss generally is overlooked because it is often mild and sub-clinical (hearing loss above 8,000 Hz). However, when it affects the frequencies below 8,000 Hz, it is readily detected by serial audiograms. Hearing loss ranges from 20-30 dB at 8,000 Hz. Both the hearing loss and tinnitus tend to occur more frequently when you take higher doses. Normally, your hearing will return and your tinnitus will go away within 7 to 14 days after stopping **Interferon** treatment.[253]

Interferon alfacon-1

Pronunciation guide: in-ter-FEER-on AL-fah-kon

Drug classification: INTERFERONS (see section 7.17.4 in Table 14-1)

Brand names: *Infergen*

Ototoxic effects:
    Cochlear:
        Tinnitus: 2-6% (CPS, PDR)
    Vestibular:
        Dizziness: 18-25% (CPS, PDR)
    Outer/Middle Ear:
        Earache/ear pain: 5-7% (CPS, PDR)
        Otitis: 1-5% (CPS, PDR)

Risk assessment: Class 2

Interferon alfa-n3

Pronunciation guide: in-ter-FEER-on AL-fah

Drug classification: INTERFERONS (see section 7.17.4 in Table 14-1)

Brand names: *Alferon N*

Ototoxic effects:
    Cochlear:
        Tinnitus: 3% (DFC, PDR)
    Vestibular:
        Dizziness: 9% [5% above placebo results] (DFC, PDR)

Risk assessment: Class 1

Interferon beta-1a

Pronunciation guide: in-ter-FEER-on BAY-tuh

Drug classification: INTERFERONS (see section 7.17.4 in Table 14-1)

Brand names: *Avonex, Rebif*

Ototoxic effects:
    Cochlear:
        Hearing loss: 3-41% [placebo 0] (CPS, PDR)
        Hyperacusis: <1% (CPS)
        Tinnitus: 1.2-3.6% [<1.2% above placebo results] (CPS)
    Vestibular:
        Ataxia: 2-5.4% [<3% above placebo results] (CPS, PDR)
        Dizziness: 9.1-15% [1.1-8.5% above placebo results] (CPS, PDR)
        Labyrinthitis: (CPS, PDR)

Nystagmus: <1% (CPS)
Vertigo: 1.2-5.8% (CPS)
Vestibular disorder: <1% (CPS)
Outer/Middle Ear:
Earache/ear pain: 0.4-4.9% [<3.9% above placebo results] (CPS, PDR)
Otitis externa: 0.8-2.9% (CPS)
Otitis media: 0.4-6% [<1% above placebo results] (CPS, PDR)
Unspecified/General Ear Conditions:
Meniere's syndrome: <1% (CPS)

Risk assessment: Class 4

Notes:

Hearing loss generally is overlooked because it is often mild and sub-clinical (hearing loss above 8,000 Hz). However, when it affects the frequencies below 8,000 Hz, it is readily detected by serial audiograms. Hearing loss ranges from 20-30 dB at 8,000 Hz. Both the hearing loss and tinnitus tend to occur more frequently when you take higher doses. Normally, your hearing will return and your tinnitus will go away within 7 to 14 days after stopping **Interferon** treatment.[254]

I have an anecdotal report in my files of a woman that had a "considerable change in her hearing" after 4 months of taking **Interferon beta-1a**. When she noticed the hearing loss, she stopped taking this drug immediately. However, a year later, her "hearing went completely out on me". She now wears a cochlear implant. Thus it appears there are no guarantees that lost hearing will always come back.

Interferon beta-1b

Pronunciation guide: in-ter-FEER-on BAY-tuh

Drug classification: INTERFERONS (see section 7.17.4 in Table 14-1)

Brand names: *Betaseron, Extavia*

Ototoxic effects:
Cochlear:
Hearing loss: 1-41% (CPS, PDR)
Tinnitus: 1% [same as placebo] (CPS)
Vestibular:
Ataxia: 19% [2% above placebo results] (CPS, PDR)
Dizziness: 35% [7% above placebo results] (CPS, PDR)
Nystagmus: (CPS, PDR)
Outer/Middle Ear:
Earache/ear pain: (CPS, PDR)
Otitis externa: (CPS, PDR)
Otitis media: 2% [same as placebo] (CPS, PDR)
Unspecified/General Ear Conditions:
Ear disorder: 1% [same as placebo] (CPS)

Risk assessment: Class 4

Notes:

Hearing loss generally is overlooked because it is often mild and sub-clinical (hearing loss above 8,000 Hz). However, when it affects the frequencies below 8,000 Hz, it is readily detected by serial audiograms. Hearing loss ranges from 20-30 dB at 8,000 Hz. Both the hearing loss and tinnitus tend to occur more frequently when you take higher doses. Normally, your hearing will return and your tinnitus will go away within 7 to 14 days after stopping **Interferon** treatment.[255]

Interferon gamma-1b

Pronunciation guide: in-ter-FEER-on GAM-mah

Drug classification: INTERFERONS (see section 7.17.4 in Table 14-1)

Brand names: *Actimmune*

Ototoxic effects:
    Vestibular:
        Ataxia: (PDR)
        Dizziness: (PDR)

Risk assessment: Class 1

Intron A   (see **Interferon alfa-2b**)

Invanz   (see **Ertapenem**)

Invega   (see **Paliperidone**)

Invega Sustenna   (see **Paliperidone**)

Invirase   (see **Saquinavir**)

Iodixanol

Pronunciation guide: eye-oh-DIX-ah-nole

Drug classification: RADIOPAQUE DRUGS (see section 26.4 in Table 14-1)

Brand names: *Visipaque*

Ototoxic effects:
    Cochlear:
        Hearing loss: <1% (CPS)
        Tinnitus: <1% (CPS)
    Vestibular:
        Dizziness: <1% (CPS)
        Vertigo: 2.4-28.3% (CPS)
    Outer/Middle Ear:
        Earache/ear pain: <1% (CPS)

Risk assessment: Class 2, can be Class 4 [1]

Notes:

[1] The incidence of vertigo is much higher for cerebral arteriography than for other tests (CPS), hence the higher risk assessment in these cases.

Iodoquinol

Pronunciation guide: eye-oh-doe-KWIN-ole

Drug classification: AMEBICIDES (see section 7.14.1 in Table 14-1)

Brand names: *Diodoquin, Yodoxin*

Ototoxic effects:
Vestibular:
Ataxia: (AHF)
Vertigo: (CPS, PDR)

Risk assessment: Class 1

Notes:

Large doses for long periods can result in Ataxia (AHF).

Iohexol

Pronunciation guide: eye-oh-HEX-ole

Drug classification: RADIOPAQUE DRUGS (see section 26.4 in Table 14-1)

Brand names: *Omnipaque*

Ototoxic effects:
Cochlear:
Hearing loss: <0.1% (CPS)
Tinnitus: <0.4% (CPS)
Vestibular:
Dizziness: <0.7-2% (CPS)
Nystagmus: <0.4% (CPS)
Vertigo: <0.7% (CPS)

Risk assessment: Class 2

Ionsys   (see **Fentanyl**)

Iopromide

Pronunciation guide: eye-oh-PROE-mide

Drug classification: RADIOPAQUE DRUGS (see section 26.4 in Table 14-1)

Brand names: *Ultravist*

Ototoxic effects:
    Cochlear:
        Hearing loss: (CPS)
    Vestibular:
        Dizziness: 0.1% (CPS)
        Vertigo: 0.1% (CPS)

Risk assessment: Class 2

Iotrolan

Pronunciation guide: eye-oh-TROE-lan

Drug classification: RADIOPAQUE DRUGS (see section 26.4 in Table 14-1)

Brand names: *Osmovist*

Ototoxic effects:
    Cochlear:
        Tinnitus: 1.1% (CPS)
    Vestibular:
        Dizziness: 1.9% (CPS)
        Nystagmus: <1% (CPS)
    Outer/Middle Ear:
        Earache/ear pain: <1% (CPS)

Risk assessment: Class 2

Ioversol

Pronunciation guide: eye-oh-VER-sole

Drug classification: RADIOPAQUE DRUGS (see section 26.4 in Table 14-1)

Brand names: *Optiray*

Ototoxic effects:
    Cochlear:
        Tinnitus: (CPS)
    Vestibular:
        Nystagmus: (CPS)
        Vertigo: <1% (CPS)

Risk assessment: Class 1

Ipratropium

Pronunciation guide: ih-prah-TROE-pee-um

Drug classification: BRONCHODILATORS—BETA ADRENERGIC AGONISTS (see section 63.4 in Table 14-1)

Brand names: *Atrovent, Combivent* [1]

Ototoxic effects:
> Cochlear:
>> Tinnitus: <1% (AHF, PDR)
> Vestibular:
>> Ataxia: (CPS, PDR)
>> Dizziness: 2.4% (CPS, PDR)
>> Equilibrium disorder: (AHF)
>> Vertigo: <2% (CPS)

Risk assessment: Class 2

Notes:

> [1] *Combivent* is a combination of **Ipratropium** and **Salbutamol (Albuterol)**. (See the generic drug **Albuterol** for its specific ototoxic properties.)

Irbesartan

Pronunciation guide: er-beh-SAR-tan

Drug classification: ANGIOTENSIN-2-RECEPTOR ANTAGONISTS (see section 20.8.4 in Table 14-1)

Brand names: *Avalide* [1], *Avapro*

Ototoxic effects:
> Cochlear:
>> Hearing disorder: 0.3-1% (CPS, PDR)
>> Tinnitus: [2] (BNF)
> Vestibular:
>> Dizziness: 4.9-6% [2-4% above placebo results] (CPS, PDR)
>> Vertigo: <1% [same as placebo] (CPS, PDR)
> Outer/Middle Ear:
>> Earache/ear pain: 0.3-1% (DFC, PDR)
>> Otitis: 0.3-1% (DFC, PDR)
> Unspecified/General Ear Conditions:
>> Ear disorder: 0.3-1% (DFC, PDR)

Risk assessment: Class 2

Notes:

> [1] *Avalide* is a combination of **Irbesartan** and **Hydrochlorothiazide**. (See the generic drug **Hydrochlorothiazide** for its specific ototoxic properties.)

> [2] I have an anecdotal report in my files of a woman whose existing tinnitus became noticeably louder when she was put on a higher dose of **Irbesartan**. When she complained to her doctor, he reduced the dose and her tinnitus returned to its previous level.

Irinotecan

Pronunciation guide: eh-rin-OH-teh-kan

Drug classification: NATURAL ANTI-NEOPLASTICS (see section14.20 in Table 14-1)

Brand names: *Camptosar*

Ototoxic effects:
    Vestibular:
        Dizziness: 15-23.1% (CPS, PDR)
        Vertigo: (PDR)

Risk assessment: Class 1

Iron sucrose

Pronunciation guide: EYE-urn SOO-krose

Drug classification: MINERALS (see section 75.8 in Table 14-1)

Brand names: *Venofer*

Ototoxic effects:
    Vestibular:
        Dizziness: 2.8-6.7% (DFC)
    Outer/Middle Ear:
        Earache/ear pain: 0.7-2.2% (DHC)

Risk assessment: Class 1

Isentress   (see **Raltegravir**)

Isepacin   (see **Isepamicin**)

Isepamicin

Pronunciation guide: eye-sep-ah-MY-sin

Drug classification: AMINOGLYCOSIDES (see section 7.4.1 in Table 14-1)

Brand names: *Isepacin*

Ototoxic effects:
    Cochlear:
        Tinnitus: (She)
    Unspecified/General Ear Conditions:
        Ototoxicity: [1]

Risk assessment: Class 5 [1]

Notes:

[1] **Isepamicin** is a **Gentamicin** derivative with a chemical structure similar to **Amikacin**[256] so you could logically expect it to have much the same ototoxic properties as both **Gentamicin** and **Amikacin**. (See the generic drugs **Amikacin** and **Gentamicin** for their specific ototoxic properties.) I can't find a good description of its ototoxic properties in English so I don't know exactly how ototoxic it is. Until I learn otherwise, I am assuming it is similar in ototoxicity to **Gentamicin**.

Isepamicin is a relatively new drug that is used in the Far East.

See Chapter 9, "Aminoglycoside Antibiotics are the Ototoxic 'Bad boys'" for further information on this drug.

Ismo   (see **Isosorbide**)

Isocarboxazid

Pronunciation guide: eye-soh-kar-BOX-ah-zid

Drug classification: Monoamine oxidase inhibitors (MAO) (see section 60.1.1 in Table 14-1)

Brand names: *Marplan*

Ototoxic effects:
Vestibular:
Ataxia: (PDR)
Dizziness: 15-29% [1-15% above placebo results] (PDR)

Risk assessment: Class 2

Notes:

See Chapter 7, "We 'Hear' With Our Eyes" for further information on this drug.

Isoniazid (INH)

Pronunciation guide: eye-soh-NYE-ah-zid

Drug classification: Anti-tuberculosis drugs (see section 7.7.1 in Table 14-1)

Brand names: *Isotamine*

Ototoxic effects:
Cochlear:
Hearing Loss: (NTP)
Tinnitus: (AHF, CPS)
Vestibular:
Ataxia: (AHF, CPS)
Dizziness: (CPS, NTP)
Vertigo: (BNF, NTP)

Risk assessment: Class 2

Notes:

I have an anecdotal report in my files of an woman who developed tinnitus and hearing loss after taking **Isoniazid**.

See Chapter 7, "We 'Hear' With Our Eyes" for further information on this drug.

Isoproterenol

Pronunciation guide: eye-soe-proe-TER-eh-nole

Drug classification: BRONCHODILATORS—BETA ADRENERGIC AGONISTS (see section 63.4 in Table 14-1)

Brand names: *Isuprel*

Ototoxic effects:
Cochlear:
Tinnitus: (AHF)
Vestibular:
Dizziness: (AHF)

Risk assessment: Class 1

Isoptin   (see **Verapamil**)

Isopto Homatropine   (see **Homatropine**)

Isosorbide

Pronunciation guide: eye-soe-SORE-bide

Drug classification: CORONARY VASODILATORS (see section 20.8.40.1 in Table 14-1)

Brand names: *Imdur*, *Ismo*, *Monoket*

Ototoxic effects:
Cochlear:
Tinnitus: <1% (CPS, PDR)
Vestibular:
Dizziness: 3-11% [2-7% above placebo results] (CPS, PDR)
Vertigo: 1-3% (CPS, PDR)
Outer/Middle Ear:
Earache/ear pain: <1% (CPS, PDR)
Perforated eardrum: <1% (CPS, PDR)

Risk assessment: Class 2

Notes:

See Chapter 7, "We 'Hear' With Our Eyes" for further information on this drug.

Isotamine   (see **Isoniazid**)

Isotretinoin

Pronunciation guide: eye-soh-TRET-ih-noyn

Drug classification: VITAMIN A ANALOGS (see section 23.4 in Table 14-1)

Brand names: *Accutane*, *Clarus*

Ototoxic effects:
    Cochlear:
        Hearing loss: (CPS, PDR)
        Tinnitus: <1% (CPS, PDR)
    Vestibular:
        Ataxia: (CPS, PDR)
        Dizziness: (CPS, PDR)

Risk assessment: Class 3

Notes:

Warning: There is an extremely high risk that you will have a deformed child if you take **Isotretinoin** while you are pregnant. Your baby might be born with no external ears, tiny external ears, tiny ear canals or no ear canals at all (PDR).

Taking **Isotretinoin** can result in either temporary or permanent hearing loss. If you experience either tinnitus or hearing loss you should discontinue **Isotretinoin** treatment and seek specialized medical care (PDR).

Isoxicam

Pronunciation guide: eye-SOX-ih-kam

Drug classification: Oxicams (see section 1.1.10 in Table 14-1)

Brand names: *Floxicam, Maxicam, Pacyl, Vectren*

Ototoxic effects:
    Cochlear:
        Tinnitus: (Ka8)

Risk assessment: Class 1

Isradipine

Pronunciation guide: is-RAH-dih-peen

Drug classification: Calcium-channel-blocking drugs (Calcium Blockers) (see section 20.8.16 in Table 14-1)

Brand names: *DynaCirc*

Ototoxic effects:
    Vestibular:
        Dizziness: (RXL)
    Unspecified/General Ear Conditions:
        Ototoxicity: (San)

Risk assessment: Not enough information to rate

Isuprel   (see **Isoproterenol**)

Itraconazole

Pronunciation guide: eye-trah-KON-ah-zole

Drug classification: ANTI-FUNGAL ANTIBIOTICS (see section 7.10 in Table 14-1)

Brand names: *Sporanox*

Ototoxic effects:
  Cochlear:
    Hearing loss: CPS)
    Tinnitus: <2% (PDR)
  Vestibular:
    Dizziness: 0.5-4.4% (CPS, PDR)
    Vertigo: 1% (CPS, PDR)

Risk assessment: Class 2

Notes:

Hearing loss may be temporary or permanent (CPS).

Caution: Eating grapefruit or drinking grapefruit juice during the time you are taking this drug may make the listed side effects worse than shown here.

See Chapter 11, "Grapefruit Juice and Ototoxic Drugs" for further information on this drug.

Ivermectin

Pronunciation guide: eye-ver-MEK-tin

Drug classification: ANTHELMINTIC DRUGS (see section 7.1 in Table 14-1)

Brand names: *Stromectol*

Ototoxic effects:
  Vestibular:
    Ataxia: (PDR)
    Dizziness: 2.8% (DFC, PDR)
    Vertigo: 0.9% (DFC, PDR)

Risk assessment: Class 1

Notes:

Ataxia is a sign of **Ivermectin** overdose (PDR).

Kadian   (see **Morphine**)

Kaletra   (see **Ritonavir**)

Kanamycin

Pronunciation guide: kan-ah-MY-sin

Drug classification: AMINOGLYCOSIDES (see section 7.4.1 in Table 14-1)

Brand names: *Kantrex*

Ototoxic effects:
    Cochlear:
        Hearing loss: (DFC, RXL)
        Tinnitus: (RXL)
    Vestibular:
        Dizziness: (RXL)
        Nystagmus: (RXL)
        Loss of balance: [1] (DFC)
        Vertigo: (CP2, RXL)
    Unspecified/General Ear Conditions:
        Ototoxicity: (CP2, Med)

Risk assessment: Class 4

Notes:

Hearing loss and loss of balance may be partially reversible or permanent, and may occur in both ears (DFC).

Kanamycin mostly affects the cochlea and can cause profound cochlear hair cell damage. This often results in bilateral (often permanent) high-frequency hearing loss and even complete deafness.[257] Less commonly, it can cause tinnitus. **Kanamycin** sometimes affects the vestibular system, and can result in dizziness, nystagmus and vertigo (RXL).

Hearing loss in the high frequencies usually occurs before you notice any clinical symptoms. As a result, you may not have any clinical symptoms to warn you of developing cochlear damage (RXL).

The more **Kanamycin** you take, the more your risk of hearing loss increases. Your hearing loss can still continue to get worse even after you stop taking **Kanamycin** (RXL).

You are at much greater risk of having severe ototoxic reactions to **Kanamycin** if you have kidney problems, or if you have normal kidney function but receive high doses or for a prolonged time. You are also at high risk if you are receiving other ototoxic or rapidly-acting diuretics at the same time or following **Kanamycin** therapy. Therefore, you should not take **Kanamycin** at the same time as potent diuretics such as **Ethacrynic acid**, **Furosemide** or **Mannitol** (RXL). You are also at greater risk if you are older or become dehydrated (RXL).

If you are taking **Kanamycin** and are exposed to loud noise, you could be making your hearing even worse than would otherwise be expected. A number of studies have shown that **Kanamycin** plus noise exposure has a synergistic effect on hearing loss.[258]

You should have serial audiograms (before, during and after **Kanamycin** treatment), especially if you are at high risk. You should have audiograms periodically after you have stopped taking **Kanamycin** if you have any hearing loss or vestibular symptoms, or if you are taking other potentially ototoxic drugs either at the same time or sequentially (RXL).

If you have evidence of ototoxicity (hearing loss, tinnitus, dizziness, vertigo, etc.), your doctor should strongly consider either reducing your dose or discontinuing **Kanamycin** treatment altogether (RXL).

See Chapter 8, "The Sinister Partnership Between Ototoxic Agents and Noise," Chapter 9, "Aminoglycoside Antibiotics are the Ototoxic 'Bad boys'" and Chapter 12, "Potpourri" for further information on this drug.

Kantrex   (see **Kanamycin**)

Kapidex   (see **Dexlansoprazole**)

Keflex   (see **Cephalexin**)

Kefurox   (see **Cefuroxime**)

Kenacomb   (see **Neomycin**)

Kenalog   (see **Triamcinolone**)

Keppra   (see **Levetiracetam**)

Keral   (see **Dexketoprofen**)

Kerlone   (see **Betaxolol**)

Ketek   (see **Telithromycin**)

Ketoconazole

Pronunciation guide: kee-toe-KOE-nah-zole

Drug classification: ANTI-FUNGAL ANTIBIOTICS (see section 7.10 in Table 14-1)

Brand names: *Nizoral*

Ototoxic effects:
    Cochlear:
        Tinnitus: <1% (AHF, She)
    Vestibular:
        Dizziness: <1% (AHF, CPS)

Risk assessment: Class 1

Notes:

Caution: Eating grapefruit or drinking grapefruit juice during the time you are taking this drug may make the listed side effects worse than shown here.

See Chapter 11, "Grapefruit Juice and Ototoxic Drugs" for further information on this drug.

Ketoprofen

Pronunciation guide: kee-toe-PROE-fen

Drug classification: PROPIONIC ACIDS (see section 1.1.13 in Table 14-1)

Brand names: *Apo-Keto, Orafen, Orudis, Oruvail, Rhodis, Rhovail*

Ototoxic effects:
    Cochlear:
        Hearing loss: <1% (CPS, PDR)
        Tinnitus: >1% (CPS, PDR)
    Vestibular:
        Dizziness: >1% (CPS, PDR)
        Vertigo: <1% (CPS, PDR)

Risk assessment: Class 2

Notes:

Tinnitus has occurred in about 1-3%, and hearing loss in less than 1% of **Ketoprofen**-treated patients (AHF).

Ketorolac

Pronunciation guide: KEE-toe-role-ack

Drug classification: ACETIC ACIDS (see section 1.1.1 in Table 14-1)

Brand names: *Apo-Ketorolac, Toradol*

Ototoxic effects:
    Cochlear:
        Hearing loss: <1% (CPS, PDR)
        Tinnitus: <1% (CPS, PDR)
    Vestibular:
        Dizziness: 2-7% (CPS, PDR)
        Vertigo: <1% (PDR)
    Outer/Middle Ear:
        Earache/ear pain: <1% (CPS)

Risk assessment: Class 2

Klonopin   (see **Clonazepam**)

Kogenate   (see **Antihemophilic factor**)

Kytril   (see **Granisetron**)

Labetalol

Pronunciation guide: lah-BET-ah-lawl

Drugclassification:BETA-ADRENERGIC-BLOCKINGDRUGS(BETA-BLOCKERS)(seesection20.8.12 in Table 14-1)

Brand names: *Normodyne, Trandate*

Ototoxic effects:
>   Vestibular:
>>   Dizziness: 1-16% [<8% above placebo results] (CPS, PDR)
>>   Vertigo: 2% [1% above placebo results] (CPS, PDR)

Risk assessment: Class 1

Lacidipine

Pronunciation guide: lah-SID-dih-peen

Drug classification: CALCIUM-CHANNEL-BLOCKING DRUGS (CALCIUM BLOCKERS) (see section 20.8.16 in Table 14-1)

Brand names: *Caldine*

Ototoxic effects:
>   Vestibular:
>>   Dizziness: [259]
>   Unspecified/General Ear Conditions:
>>   Ototoxicity: (San)

Risk assessment: Class 1

Lacosamide

Pronunciation guide: lah-KOE-sah-mide

Drug classification: ANTI-CONVULSANT DRUGS (see section 53.12 in Table 14-1)

Brand names: *Vimpat*

Ototoxic effects:
>   Cochlear:
>>   Tinnitus: (PDR)
>   Vestibular:
>>   Ataxia: 4-15% [2-13% above placebo results] (PDR)
>>   Dizziness: 16-53% [8-45% above placebo results] (PDR)
>>   Equilibrium disorder: 1-6% [placebo 0] (PDR)
>>   Vertigo: 3-5% [2-4% above placebo results] (PDR)

Risk assessment: Class 2

Lactisal   (see **Salicylic acid**)

Lamictal   (see **Lamotrigine**)

Lamivudine

Pronunciation guide: lah-MEH-vyoo-deen

Drug classification: ANTI-RETROVIRAL REVERSE TRANSCRIPTASE INHIBITORS (see section 7.17.1.4 in Table 14-1)

Brand names: *3TC, Epivir, Trizivir* [1]

Ototoxic effects:
   Vestibular:
       Dizziness: 10% [6% above placebo results] (CPS, PDR)
   Outer/Middle Ear:
       Otitis: 25% [4% above placebo results] (PDR)
   Unspecified/General Ear Conditions:
       Ear disorder: [2] 7% (CPS)

Risk assessment: Class 1

Notes:

   [1] *Trizivir* is a combination of Abacavir, **Lamivudine** and **Zidovudine**. (See the drug **Zidovudine** for its specific ototoxic properties.)

   [2] Includes ear pain, discharge from ear, erythema (redness) or swelling of an ear (CPS).

Lamotrigine

Pronunciation guide: lah-MAW-trih-geen

Drug classification: ANTI-CONVULSANT DRUGS (see section 53.12 in Table 14-1)

Brand names: *Lamictal*

Ototoxic effects:
   Cochlear:
       Hearing loss: <0.1% (AHF, PDR)
       Tinnitus: 0.1-1% (AHF, PDR)
   Vestibular:
       Ataxia: 2-28% [<18% above placebo results] (CPS, PDR)
       Dizziness: 14-54% [<27% above placebo results] (CPS, PDR)
       Nystagmus: 2% [placebo 0] (CPS, PDR)
       Oscillopsia: 0.1-1% (DFC, PDR)
       Vertigo: 2-4% [1-4% above placebo results] (CPS, PDR)
   Outer/Middle Ear:
       Earache/ear pain: 1% [placebo 0] (CPS, PDR)
   Unspecified/General Ear Conditions:
       Ear disorder: 2% [1% above placebo results] (AHF, PDR)

Risk assessment: Class 3

Lanicor   (see **Digoxin**)

Lanoxicaps   (see **Digoxin**)

Lanoxin   (see **Digoxin**)

Lansoprazole

Pronunciation guide: lanz-AH-pray-zol

Drug classification: PROTON PUMP INHIBITORS (see section 34.8.4 in Table 14-1)

Brand names: *Hp-PAC*[1], *Prevacid*, *PREVPAC*[1]

Ototoxic effects:
> Cochlear:
>> Hearing loss: <1% (CPS, PDR)
>> Tinnitus: <1% (CPS, PDR)
> Vestibular:
>> Dizziness: 1.0-2.8% [0.2-2.4% above placebo results] (CPS, PDR)
>> Vertigo: <1% (CPS, PDR)
> Outer/Middle Ear:
>> Otitis media: <1% (CPS, PDR)
> Unspecified/General Ear Conditions:
>> Ear disorder: <1% (CPS, PDR)

Risk assessment: Class 2

Notes:

> [1] *Hp-Pac* and *PREVPAC* are combinations of **Lansoprazole**, Amoxicillin and **Clarithromycin**. (See the generic drug **Clarithromycin** for its specific ototoxic properties.)

> I have an anecdotal report in my files of a woman who lost more hearing each time her doctor prescribed **Lansoprazole** for her.

Lanthanum

Pronunciation guide: LAN-thah-num

Drug classification: MISCELLANEOUS DRUGS (see section 46 in Table 14-1)

Brand names: *Fosrenol*

Ototoxic effects:
> Vestibular:
>> Dizziness: >0.1% (CPS)
>> Vertigo: <0.1% (CPS)

Risk assessment: Class 1

Lariam　(see **Mefloquine**)

Larodopa　(see **Levodopa**)

Lasix　(see **Furosemide**)

l-Deprenyl   (see **Selegiline**)

Lederfen   (see **Fenbufen**)

Leflunomide

Pronunciation guide: leh-FLEW-noh-mide

Drug classification: Musculoskeletal drugs (see section 50 in Table 14-1)

Brand names: *Arava*

Ototoxic effects:
  Vestibular:
    Dizziness: 5% [2% above placebo results] (CPS, PDR)
    Vertigo: 1-3% (CPS, PDR)

Risk assessment: Class 1

Legatrin   (see **Quinine**)

Lenalidomide

Pronunciation guide: leh-nah-LIH-doe-mide

Drug classification: Tumor necrosis factor modifiers (see section 14.36 in Table 14-1)

Brand names: *Revlimid*

Ototoxic effects:
  Vestibular:
    Dizziness: 19.6-20.8% (DFC)
    Vertigo: (DFC)

Risk assessment: Class 1

Lercanidipine

Pronunciation guide: ler-kah-NIH-dih-peen

Drug classification: Dihydropyridine Calcium-Channel Blockers (see section 20.8.16.1 in Table 14-1)

Brand names: *Zanidip*

Ototoxic effects:
  Vestibular:
    Dizziness: 1% [0.4% above placebo results] [260]
    Loss of balance: [261]
    Vertigo: 0.1-1% [262]

Risk assessment: Class 1

Notes:

Caution: Eating grapefruit or drinking grapefruit juice during the time you are taking this drug may make the listed side effects worse than shown here.

See Chapter 11, "Grapefruit Juice and Ototoxic Drugs" for further information on these kind of drugs.

Lescol   (see **Fluvastatin**)

Letrozole

Pronunciation guide: LEH-troh-zol

Drug classification: Non-steroidal aromatase inhibitors (see section 14.24 in Table 14-1)

Brand names: *Femara*

Ototoxic effects:
Vestibular:
Dizziness: 3-5% (CPS, PDR)
Vertigo: <5% (AHF, PDR)

Risk assessment: Class 1

Leukeran   (see **Chlorambucil**)

Leuprolide

Pronunciation guide: loo-PROE-lide

Drug classification: Gonadotropins (see section 40.24 in Table 14-1)

Brand names: *Eligard, Lupron, Lupron Depot*

Ototoxic effects:
Cochlear:
Hearing disorder: (CPS, PDR)
Tinnitus: <5% (CPS, PDR)
Vestibular:
Dizziness/vertigo: 3.1-16% [placebo 0] (CPS, PDR)
Vertigo: <2% (CPS, PDR)
Outer/Middle Ear:
Earache/ear pain: <5% (CPS, PDR)

Risk assessment: Class 2

Levalbuterol

Pronunciation guide: lev-al-BYOO-ter-all

Drug classification: Bronchodilators—beta adrenergic agonists (see section 63.4 in Table 14-1)

Brand names: *Xopenex, Xopenex HFA*

Ototoxic effects:
Vestibular:
Dizziness: 1.4-2.7% [0.1-1.4% above placebo results] (PDR)
Vertigo: (PDR)
Outer/Middle Ear:
Earache/ear pain: <2% (PDR)

Risk assessment: Class 1

Levamisole

Pronunciation guide: lee-VAM-ih-sole

Drug classification: ANTI-NEOPLASTICS (ANTI-CANCER DRUGS) (see section 14 in Table 14-1)

Brand names: *Ergamisol*

Ototoxic effects:
Vestibular:
Ataxia: 2-3% (CPS, PDR)
Dizziness: (CPS)
Dizziness/vertigo: 1-4% (CPS, PDR)
Nystagmus: (PDR)

Risk assessment: Class 1

Levaquin   (see **Levofloxacin**)

Levbid   (see **Hyoscyamine**)

Levemir   (see **Insulin detemir**)

Levetiracetam

Pronunciation guide: lee-vah-tih-RACE-ah-tam

Drug classification: ANTI-CONVULSANT DRUGS (see section 53.12 in Table 14-1)

Brand names: *Keppra*

Ototoxic effects:
Vestibular:
Ataxia: 3% [2% above placebo results] (NDH, PDR)
Dizziness: >10% [5% above placebo results] (NDH, PDR)
Vertigo: 3-5% [2% above placebo results] (NDH, PDR)
Outer/Middle Ear:
Earache/ear pain: 2% [placebo 0] (DFC, PDR)
Otitis media: >1% (CPS, PDR)

Risk assessment: Class 2

Levitra (see **Vardenafil**)

Levobetaxolol

Pronunciation guide: lee-voe-beh-TAX-oh-lole

Drug classification: BETA-ADRENERGIC-BLOCKING DRUGS (BETA-BLOCKERS) (see section 20.8.12 in Table 14-1)

Brand names: *Betaxon*

Ototoxic effects:
    Cochlear:
        Tinnitus: <2% (DFC, PDR)
    Vestibular:
        Dizziness: <2% (DFC, PDR)
        Vertigo: <2% (DFC, PDR)
    Outer/Middle Ear:
        Earache/ear pain: <2% (DFC, PDR)
        Otitis media: <2% (DFC, PDR)

Risk assessment: Class 2

Levobunolol

Pronunciation guide: lee-voe-BYOO-noe-lole

Drug classification: BETA-ADRENERGIC-BLOCKING DRUGS (BETA-BLOCKERS) (see section 20.8.12 in Table 14-1)

Brand names: *Betagan*

Ototoxic effects:
    Vestibular:
        Ataxia, transient: (CPS, PDR)
        Dizziness: (CPS, PDR)

Risk assessment: Class 1

Levobupivacaine

Pronunciation guide: lee-voe-byoo-PIV-ah-kane

Drug classification: LOCAL ANESTHETICS (see section 4.10 in Table 14-1)

Brand names: *Chirocaine*

Ototoxic effects:
    Cochlear:
        Tinnitus: <1% (CP2, PDR)
    Vestibular:
        Dizziness: 5.1-6% (CP2, PDR)

Risk assessment: Class 1

Levocabastine

Pronunciation guide: lee-voe-KAB-as-teen

Drug classification: ANTIHISTAMINES (see section 10 in Table 14-1)

Brand names: *Livostin*

Ototoxic effects:
    Cochlear:
        Hearing loss: <1% [placebo 0] (CPS)
    Vestibular:
        Dizziness: <1% [same as placebo] (CPS)
    Outer/Middle Ear:
        Otitis externa: <1% [placebo 0] (CPS)

Risk assessment: Class 2

Levocarnitine

Pronunciation guide: lee-voe-KAR-nih-teen

Drug classification: AMINO ACIDS (see section 75.1 in Table 14-1)

Brand names: *Carnitor*

Ototoxic effects:
    Vestibular:
        Dizziness: 10-18% [<5% above placebo results] (CPS, PDR)
        Vertigo: 2-6% (CPS, PDR)

Risk assessment: Class 2

Levocetirizine

Pronunciation guide: LEE-voe-seh-TIR-ah-zeen

Drug classification: PIPERAZINE DERIVATIVES (see section 10.8.1 in Table 14-1)

Brand names: *Xyzal*

Ototoxic effects:
    Outer/Middle Ear:
        Otitis media: 3% [placebo 0] (PDR)

Risk assessment: Class 1

Notes:

    Levocetirizine is a purified form of **Cetirizine**. It basically replaced **Cetirizine** in the USA in 2007 when the patent on **Cetirizine** ran out. Since it is a purified form of **Cetirizine**, **Levocetirizine** likely has the same ototoxic properties as **Cetirizine** although none of these side effects have been listed so far. (See the drug **Cetirizine** for its specific ototoxic properties.)

Levodopa

Pronunciation guide: lee-voe-DOE-pah

Drug classification: ANTI-PARKINSONIAN DRUGS (see section 53.16 in Table 14-1)

Brand names: *Larodopa, Lodosyn* [1], *Prolopa* [2], *Sinemet* [3], *Stalevo* [4]

Ototoxic effects:
    Vestibular:
        Ataxia: 1.2% [0.7% above placebo results] (CPS, PDR)
        Dizziness: 2.3-7.5% [1.5% above placebo results] (CPS, PDR)

Risk assessment: Class 1

Notes:

[1] *Lodosyn* is a brand name for the generic drug **Carbidopa** (kar-bih-DOE-pah). **Carbidopa** does not seem to be ototoxic by itself, but when used in combination with **Levodopa** (the normal situation), together they can cause ataxia and dizziness (PDR). Like **Levodopa**, **Carbidopa** is an ANTI-PARKINSONIAN DRUG (see section 53.16 in Table 14-1).

[2] *Prolopa* is a combination of **Levodopa** and Benserazide. (**Levodopa** is the ototoxic agent).

[3] *Sinemet* is a combination of **Levodopa** and **Carbidopa**. (**Levodopa** is the more ototoxic agent.) (PDR).

[4] *Stalevo* is a combination of **Levodopa**, **Carbidopa** and **Entacapone**. (See the generic drug **Entacapone** for its specific ototoxic properties).

See Chapter 7, "We 'Hear' With Our Eyes" for further information on this drug.

Levofloxacin

Pronunciation guide: leev-oh-FLOX-ah-sin

Drug classification: QUINOLONES (see section 7.4.48 in Table 14-1)

Brand names: *Levaquin*

Ototoxic effects:
    Cochlear:
        Auditory hallucinations: [1]
        Hearing disorder: (BNF)
        Hearing loss: (CPS, PDR)
        Hyperacusis: [2]
        Tinnitus: 0.3-0.5% (CPS, PDR)
    Vestibular:
        Ataxia: (CPS, PDR)
        Dizziness: 0.4-2.9% (CPS, PDR)
        Vertigo: <0.3% (CPS, PDR)

Outer/Middle Ear:
> Earache/ear pain: (CPS)

Unspecified/General Ear Conditions:
> Ear disorder: 0.5-1% (CPS, PDR)

Risk assessment: Class 3

Notes:

[1] I have an anecdotal report of a lady that was put on a high dose of **Levofloxacin** for 5 days. On the second day, she began hearing phantom music. This phantom music has persisted for over 3 months. Although not listed as causing hallucinations, her psychiatrist said he was not at all surprised it caused them, as it is a very strong drug.

[2] In another anecdotal report in my files, a woman, after taking just two doses of **Levofloxacin** had severe dizziness, ringing in her ears and "sensitivity to loud noises" (hyperacusis).

I have an anecdotal report in my files of a lady that took **Levofloxacin** for 3 weeks. One result is that she now has permanent hearing loss in both ears.

I also have an anecdotal report in my files of a lady that took **Levofloxacin** for 10 days. The result is that she now suffers from tinnitus.

I have an anecdotal report in my files of a man that took **Levofloxacin** which resulted in tinnitus.

In another anecdotal report in my files, a lady who took **Levofloxacin** for 10 days reported that "the ringing in my head is maddening!"

Levonorgestrel

Pronunciation guide: lee-voe-nor-JES-trel

Drug classification: PROGESTINS (see section 40.32 in Table 14-1)

Brand names: *Mirena, Plan B*

Ototoxic effects:
Vestibular:
> Dizziness: 1-13.3% (CPS)
> Vertigo: <1% (CPS)

Outer/Middle Ear:
> Otitis: (CPS)

Risk assessment: Class 1

Levonorgestrel—Ethinyl estradiol (see **Ethinyl estradiol**)

Levsin (see **Hyoscyamine**)

Levsinex (see **Hyoscyamine**)

Lexapro (see **Escitalopram**)

Lexxel   (see **Enalapril**)

Lialda   (see **Mesalamine**)

Librium   (see **Chlordiazepoxide**)

Lidocaine

Pronunciation guide: LYE-doe-kane

Drug classification: AMIDES (see section 4.1 in Table 14-1)

Brand names: *Depo-Medrol with Lidocaine* [1], *ELA-Max, Emla, Lidoderm, Xylocaine, Xylocard*

Ototoxic effects:
Cochlear:
     Hyperacusis: 0.1-1% (CPS)
     Tinnitus: >10% (NDH, PDR)
Vestibular:
     Dizziness: 1-10% (CPS, PDR)

Risk assessment: Class 2

Notes:

[1] *Depo-Medrol with Lidocaine* is a combination of **Methylprednisolone** and **Lidocaine**. (See the generic drug **Methylprednisolone** for its specific ototoxic properties.)

I have an anecdotal report in my files of a woman who finds that when her dentist gives her **Lidocaine** her tinnitus becomes temporarily worse.

Although **Lidocaine** can cause tinnitus, a recent study suggests that **Lidocaine** injections actually can help control tinnitus.

Dr. John Shea of the Shea Ear Clinic in Memphis, Tennessee presented a paper at a recent American Otological Society meeting. He reported that injections of **Lidocaine**, both into the ear and intravenously, repeated on three consecutive days, had resulted in partial or complete tinnitus relief.

This treatment works for people with tinnitus deriving from conditions involving disturbed hair cells such as Meniere's disease, positional vertigo and *Aspirin*, as well as those with hearing loss. So far, there are no reports of hearing loss or other side effects from this treatment.

Treating tinnitus with **Lidocaine** seems to be quite effective. According to Shea, "almost all patients get immediate relief". What is even more impressive is that a month after the treatment, 70% of the patients still report either complete or partial relief from their tinnitus.[263] Unfortunately, the tinnitus eventually returns, and thus the treatment has to be repeated every month or so. This limits its usefulness as a permanent solution to tinnitus.

Lidoderm   (see **Lidocaine**)

Lidone   (see **Molindone**)

Limbitrol   (see **Amitriptyline**)

Lincocin   (see **Lincomycin**)

Lincomycin

Pronunciation guide: lin-koe-MY-sin

Drug classification: LINCOMYCINS (see section 7.4.24 in Table 14-1)

Brand names: *Lincocin, Lincorex*

Ototoxic effects:
    Cochlear:
        Tinnitus: (DFC, She)
    Vestibular:
        Dizziness: (Med)
        Vertigo: (DFC, Med)
    Unspecified/General Ear Conditions:
        Ototoxicity: (San)

Risk assessment: Class 1

Lincorex   (see **Lincomycin**)

Linessa 28   (see **Ethinyl estradiol**)

Linezolid

Pronunciation guide: lih-NEH-zoe-lid

Drug classification: OXAZOLINIDONES (see section 7.4.36 in Table 14-1)

Brand names: *Zyvox, Zyvoxam*

Ototoxic effects:
    Cochlear:
        Tinnitus: 0.1-1% (BNF, CPS)
    Vestibular:
        Ataxia: (CPS)
        Dizziness: 0.1-2% [0.1% above placebo results] (CPS, PDR)
        Vertigo: 1.2% (AHF, PDR)

Risk assessment: Class 1

Lioresal   (see **Baclofen**)

Lipidil   (see **Fenofibrate**)

Lipitor   (see **Atorvastatin**)

Liposomal daunorubicin   (see **Daunorubicin**)

Liposomal doxorubicin   (see **Doxorubicin**)

Lisinopril

Pronunciation guide: lye-SIN-oh-pril

Drug classification: ANGIOTENSIN-CONVERTING ENZYME (ACE) INHIBITORS (see section 20.8.8 in Table 14-1)

Brand names: *Apo-Lisinopril, Prinivil, Prinzide* [1]*, Zestoretic* [1]*, Zestril*

Ototoxic effects:
    Cochlear:
        Tinnitus: 0.3-1% (PDR)
    Vestibular:
        Ataxia: 0.3-1% (PDR)
        Dizziness: 4.4-18.9% [3.5-9.5% above placebo results] (CPS, PDR)
        Vertigo: 0.2-1.1% [placebo 0] (CPS, PDR)
    Outer/Middle Ear:
        Earache/ear pain: 0.3-1% (PDR)

Risk assessment: Class 2

Notes:

[1] *Prinzide* and *Zestoretic* are both combinations of **Lisinopril** and **Hydrochlorothiazide**. (See the generic drug **Hydrochlorothiazide** for its specific ototoxic properties.)

Lithane   (see **Lithium**)

Lithium

Pronunciation guide: LITH-ee-um

Drug classification: ANTI-MANICS (see section 60.4 in Table 14-1)

Brand names: *Carbolith, Duralith, Eskalith, Lithane, Lithobid, PMS-Lithium Carbonate*

Ototoxic effects:
    Cochlear:
        Tinnitus: (CPS, PDR)
    Vestibular:
        Ataxia: (CPS, PDR)
        Dizziness: (CPS, PDR)
        Nystagmus: (CPS, PDR)
        Vertigo: 15% (AHF, PDR)

Risk assessment: Class 2

Notes:

The toxic levels for **Lithium** are close to the therapeutic levels. Therefore it is important to watch for the early symptoms of drug overdose such as ataxia, nystagmus and tinnitus (CPS).

Lithobid   (see **Lithium**)

Livostin   (see **Levocabastine**)

Lodine   (see **Etodolac**)

Lodosyn   (see **Levodopa**)

Loestrin   (see **Ethinyl estradiol**)

Lomefloxacin

Pronunciation guide: low-me-FLOX-ah-sin

Drug classification: QUINOLONES (see section 7.4.48 in Table 14-1)

Brand names: *Maxaquin*

Ototoxic effects:
    Cochlear:
        Tinnitus: <1% (DFC, PDR)
    Vestibular:
        Ataxia: (PDR)
        Dizziness: 2.1-2.3% (DFC, PDR)
        Nystagmus: (PDR)
        Vertigo: <1% (DFC, PDR)
    Outer/Middle Ear:
        Earache/ear pain: <1% (DFC, PDR)

Risk assessment: Class 2

Lomustine (CCNU)

Pronunciation guide: loe-MUSS-teen

Drug classification: ALKYLATING DRUGS (see section 14.1 in Table 14-1)

Brand names: *CeeNU*

Ototoxic effects:
    Vestibular:
        Ataxia: (CPS, PDR)

Risk assessment: Class 1

Lonidamine

Pronunciation guide: law-NIH-dah-meen

Drug classification: ANTI-NEOPLASTICS (ANTI-CANCER DRUGS) (see section 14 in Table 14-1)

Brand names: —

Ototoxic effects:
    Unspecified/General Ear Conditions:
        Ototoxicity: (San)

Risk assessment: Not enough information to rate

Lopid   (see **Gemfibrozil**)

Lopinavir   (see **Ritonavir**)

Loprazolam

Pronunciation guide: loe-PRAH-zoe-lam

Drug classification: BENZODIAZEPINES (see section 60.12.8 in Table 14-1)

Brand names: *Dormonoct*

Ototoxic effects:
    Vestibular:
        Ataxia: (BNF)
        Vertigo: (BNF)

Risk assessment: Class 1

Notes:
    See Chapter 10 "Beware of Benzodiazepines—Don't Let This Nasty Time-Bomb Ambush You and Your Ears" for further information on this drug.

Lopresor   (see **Metoprolol**)

Lopressor   (see **Metoprolol**)

Lopressor HCT   (see **Metoprolol**)

Loratadine

Pronunciation guide: lore-AT-ah-deen

Drug classification: H_1 RECEPTOR ANTAGONISTS (see section 10.1 in Table 14-1)

Brand names: *Apo-Loratadine, Chlor-Tripolon N.D.[1], Claritin, Claritin-D[1], Claritin Extra[1], Claritin Liberator*

Ototoxic effects:
    Cochlear:
        Tinnitus: (CPS, PDR)
    Vestibular:
        Dizziness: 1-4% [<2% above placebo results] (CPS, PDR)
        Vertigo: (CPS, PDR)
    Outer/Middle Ear:
        Earache/ear pain: 2-3% (AHF, PDR)
        Otitis: (PDR)

Risk assessment: Class 2

Notes:

[1] *Chlor-Tripolon, Claritin-D* and *Claritin Extra* are combinations of **Loratadine** and **Pseudoephedrine**. (See the generic drug **Pseudoephedrine** for its specific ototoxic properties.)

Caution: Eating grapefruit or drinking grapefruit juice during the time you are taking this drug may make the listed side effects worse than shown here.

See Chapter 11, "Grapefruit Juice and Ototoxic Drugs" for further information on this drug.

Lorazepam

Pronunciation guide: lore-AZ-eh-pam

Drug classification: BENZODIAZEPINES (see section 60.12.8 in Table 14-1)

Brand names: *Ativan*

Ototoxic effects:
    Cochlear:
        Hearing loss: (PDR)
        Tinnitus: (She)
    Vestibular:
        Ataxia: 0.1-1% (CPS, PDR)
        Dizziness: 6.9% (CPS, PDR)
        Vertigo: (BNF, CPS)

Risk assessment: Class 2

Notes:

Depressed hearing was infrequently reported during the peak-effect period (PDR).

I have an anecdotal report in my files of a woman who took four doses of **Lorazepam** within 3 hours. The result was "awful tinnitus" and dizziness.

I have an anecdotal report in my files of a man that was feeling particularly anxious, so his doctor prescribed **Lorazepam**. After a while, he noticed that his constant "hissing" tinnitus oftentimes became a pulsating hiss. He asked his pharmacist if she had ever heard of *Ativan* causing a pulsating sound. She said that it didn't show up in the literature that she had, but that more than one of her patients had told her they had had pulsating tinnitus from taking *Ativan*.

See Chapter 4 "Are You at Risk?" and Chapter 10 "Beware of Benzodiazepines—Don't Let This Nasty Time-Bomb Ambush You and Your Ears" for further information on this drug.

Lorelco   (see **Probucol**)

Lormetazepam

Pronunciation guide: lore-meh-TAZ-ee-pam

Drug classification: BENZODIAZEPINES (see section 60.12.8 in Table 14-1)

Brand names: *Noctamide*, *Octonox*

Ototoxic effects:
    Vestibular:
        Ataxia: (BNF)
        Vertigo: (BNF)

Risk assessment: Class 1

Notes:

See Chapter 10 "Beware of Benzodiazepines—Don't Let This Nasty Time-Bomb Ambush You and Your Ears" for further information on this drug.

Lornoxicam

Pronunciation guide: lore-NOX-ih-kam

Drug classification: OXICAMS (see section 1.1.10 in Table 14-1)

Brand names: *Xefo*

Ototoxic effects:
    Cochlear:
        Tinnitus: (BNF)
    Vestibular:
        Dizziness: (BNF)
        Vertigo: (BNF)

Risk assessment: Class 1

Lortab   (see **Hydrocodone**)

Losartan

Pronunciation guide: LOW-sar-tan

Drug classification: ANGIOTENSIN-2-RECEPTOR ANTAGONISTS (see section 20.8.4 in Table 14-1)

Brand names: *Cozaar*, *Hyzaar* [1]

Ototoxic effects:
    Cochlear:
        Tinnitus: <1% (CPS, PDR)

Vestibular:
    Ataxia: <1% (DFC, PDR)
    Dizziness: 3.5-5.7% [1.4-2.8% above placebo results] (CPS, PDR)
    Vertigo: <1% (CPS, PDR)

Risk assessment: Class 2

Notes:

[1] *Hyzaar* is a combination of **Losartan** and **Hydrochlorothiazide**. (See the generic drug **Hydrochlorothiazide** for its specific ototoxic properties.)

I have an anecdotal report in my files of a man that began taking **Losartan** and within two days his existing tinnitus became much worse. He stopped the **Losartan** after one week. Two months later his tinnitus had decreased a bit, but it was still a lot louder than it was before he began the **Losartan**. His increased tinnitus appears to be permanent.

Caution: Eating grapefruit or drinking grapefruit juice during the time you are taking this drug may make the listed side effects worse than shown here.

See Chapter 11, "Grapefruit Juice and Ototoxic Drugs" for further information on this drug.

Losec   (see **Omeprazole**)

Lotemax   (see **Loteprednol**)

Lotensin   (see **Benazepril**)

Lotensin HCT   (see **Benazepril**)

Loteprednol

Pronunciation guide: law-tee-PRED-nol

Drug classification: CORTICOSTEROIDS (see section 40.1.2 in Table 14-1)

Brand names: *Lotemax*

Ototoxic effects:
    Cochlear:
        Hearing disorder: [1]
        Tinnitus: [264]
    Unspecified/General Ear Conditions:
        Ear disorder: [2]

Risk assessment: Class 2

Notes:

Lotemax is a combination of **Loteprednol** and **Benzalkonium**. (See the generic drug **Benzalkonium** for its specific ototoxic properties.) It is unknown whether the side effects listed here are the result of the **Loteprednol** or the **Benzalkonium** (or the combination of these two drugs).

[1] I have an anecdotal report in my files of a man who began using *Lotemax* one day. The following day he noticed pressure in his ears, and sounds were distorted (as strange "wobbling" quality).

I have another anecdotal report in my files of a boy who took **Loteprednol** and had the same above problems.

[2] After being treated with *Lotemax*, a woman experienced an unspecified ear disorder.[265]

Lotrel   (see **Amlodipine**)

Lotrisone   (see **Betamethasone**)

Lotronex   (see **Alosetron**)

Lovastatin

Pronunciation guide: loe-vah-STA-tin

Drug classification: HMG-CoA REDUCTASE INHIBITORS (see section 20.12.8 in Table 14-1)

Brand names: *Advicor* [1], *Altocor, Apo-Lovastatin, Mevacor*

Ototoxic effects:
Vestibular:
Dizziness: 0.5-7% [<0.8% above placebo results] (CPS, PDR)
Vertigo: (CPS, PDR)

Risk assessment: Class 1

Notes:

[1] *Advicor* is a combination of Niacin and **Lovastatin**. (**Lovastatin** is the ototoxic agent.)

Caution: Eating grapefruit or drinking grapefruit juice during the time you are taking this drug may make the listed side effects worse than shown here. In fact, taking **Lovastatin** with grapefruit juice can increase the potency of **Lovastatin** by as much as 1,500%!

See Chapter 11, "Grapefruit Juice and Ototoxic Drugs" for further information on this drug.

Lovaza   (see **Omega-3-acid ethyl esters**)

Loxapac   (see **Loxapine**)

Loxapine

Pronunciation guide: LOX-ah-peen

Drug classification: ANTIPSYCHOTIC DRUGS (see section 60.8 in Table 14-1)

Brand names: *Loxapac, Loxitane*

Ototoxic effects:
Cochlear:
Tinnitus: (AHF)

Vestibular:
    Ataxia: (CPS, PDR)
    Dizziness: (CPS, PDR)

Risk assessment: Class 1

Loxitane   (see **Loxapine**)

Lozide   (see **Indapamide**)

Lozol   (see **Indapamide**)

Lubiprostone

Pronunciation guide: loo-bee-PRAHS-tohn

Drug classification: CHLORIDE CHANNEL ACTIVATORS (see section 34.12 in Table 14-1)

Brand names: *Amitiza*

Ototoxic effects:
    Vestibular:
        Dizziness: 3.4-4.0% [>2.1% above placebo results] (NDH, PDR)
        Vertigo: >0.2% (DFC, PDR)

Risk assessment: Class 1

Lucentis   (see **Ranibizumab**)

Ludiomil   (see **Maprotiline**)

Lumefantrine   (see **Artemether/Lumefantrine**)

Lunesta   (see **Eszopiclone**)

Lupron   (see **Leuprolide**)

Lupron Depot   (see **Leuprolide**)

Luvox   (see **Fluvoxamine**)

Lyrica   (see **Pregabalin**)

Lysocline   (see **Methacycline**)

Lysodren   (see **Mitotane**)

Maalox Total Stomach Relief   (see **Bismuth subsalicylate**)

MabCampath   (see **Alemtuzumab**)

MacroBID　(see **Nitrofurantoin**)

Macrodantin　(see **Nitrofurantoin**)

Macugen　(see **Pegaptanib**)

Magnesium salicylate

Pronunciation guide: mag-NEE-zee-um sah-LIH-sih-late

Drug classification: SALICYLATES (see section 1.1.16 in Table 14-1)

Brand names: *Backache Caplets, Doan's Analgesic Caplets, Momentum Backache Relief*

Ototoxic effects:
　　Cochlear:
　　　　Hearing loss: (PDR, PDR-N)
　　　　Tinnitus: (PDR, PDR-N)

Risk assessment: Class 2

Magnevist　(see **Gadopentetate**)

Malarone　(see **Atovaquone/Proguanil**)

Mandelamine　(see **Methenamine**)

Manerix　(see **Moclobemide**)

Mannitol

Pronunciation guide: MAN-ih-tall

Drug classification: HEXITOL IRRIGANTS (see section 30.10.1 in Table 14-1)

Brand names: *Osmitrol*

Ototoxic effects:
　　Vestibular:
　　　　Dizziness: (AHF, NDH)
　　　　Vertigo: (DFC)
　　Unspecified/General Ear Conditions:
　　　　Ototoxicity: [266]

Risk assessment: Class 1

Notes:

　　May cause hearing loss when used in combination with **Kanamycin**.[267]

　　See Chapter 9, "Aminoglycoside Antibiotics are the Ototoxic 'Bad boys'" for further information on this drug.

Maprotiline

Pronunciation guide: mah-PROE-tih-leen

Drug classification: TETRACYCLIC ANTI-DEPRESSANTS (see section 60.1.12 in Table 14-1)

Brand names: *Ludiomil*

Ototoxic effects:
  Cochlear:
      Tinnitus: <0.01-1% (CPS, PDR)
  Vestibular:
      Ataxia: <0.01% (CPS, PDR)
      Dizziness: 8% (CPS, PDR)
      Vertigo: >10% (CPS)

Risk assessment: Class 2

Maraviroc

Pronunciation guide: mahr-AY-vih-rock

Drug classification: ANTI-RETROVIRAL CC CHEMOKINE RECEPTOR 5 (CCR5) ANTAGONISTS (see section 7.17.1.8 in Table 14-1)

Brand names: *Celsentri*

Ototoxic effects:
  Cochlear:
      Auditory hallucinations: <2% (CPS)
      Hearing loss: <2% (CPS)
  Vestibular:
      Dizziness: 8.7% [0.5% above placebo results] (CPS)
  Outer/Middle Ear:
      Otitis media: 2.1% [1.6% above placebo results] (CPS)

Risk assessment: Class 2

Marax   (see **Ephedrine**)

Marcaine   (see **Bupivacaine**)

Marinol   (see **Dronabinol**)

Marplan   (see **Isocarboxazid**)

Marvelon   (see **Ethinyl estradiol**)

Marzine   (see **Cyclizine**)

Matulane   (see **Procarbazine**)

Mavik   (see **Trandolapril**)

Maxalt   (see **Rizatriptan**)

Maxaquin   (see **Lomefloxacin**)

Maxicam   (see **Isoxicam**)

Maxzide   (see **Triamterene**)

Measles vaccine

Pronunciation guide: MEE-zills VAK-seen

Drug classification: VACCINES (see section 70.8 in Table 14-1)

Brand names: *Attenuvax*

Ototoxic effects:
    Cochlear:
        Hearing loss: (DFC, PDR)
    Vestibular:
        Ataxia: (DFC, PDR)
        Dizziness: (PDR)
    Outer/Middle Ear:
        Otitis media: (DFC, PDR)

Risk assessment: Class 2

Measles, mumps & rubella vaccine

Pronunciation guide: MEE-zills, mumps, rue-BELL-a VAK-seen

Drug classification: VACCINES (see section 70.8 in Table 14-1)

Brand names: *M-M-R II*, *Priorix*, *Proquad* [1]

Ototoxic effects:
    Cochlear:
        Hearing loss: (CPS, PDR)
    Vestibular:
        Ataxia: (CPS, PDR)
        Dizziness: (CPS, PDR)
    Outer/Middle Ear:
        Earache/ear pain: 0.3-1.1% (CPS, PDR)
        Otitis media: 0.3-12.5% (CPS, PDR)

Risk assessment: Class 2

Notes:

[1] *Proquad* is a combination of **Measles**, **Mumps**, **Rubella** and **Varicella** vaccines. (See the vaccine **Varicella** for its specific ototoxic properties.)

Although the risk is low, hearing loss can happen and the results may be severe. I have an anecdotal report in my files of a lawsuit filed November, 1998 in England against a certain vaccine manufacturer claiming that a 14 year old boy became deaf as a result of being vaccinated.

Measles, rubella vaccine

Pronunciation guide: MEE-zills, rue-BELL-a VAK-seen

Drug classification: VACCINES (see section 70.8 in Table 14-1)

Brand names: *MoRu-Viraten Berna*, *M-R-VAX II*

Ototoxic effects:
    Cochlear:
        Hearing loss: (CPS)
    Vestibular:
        Ataxia: (Med, PDR)
        Dizziness: (CP2, PDR)
    Outer/Middle Ear:
        Otitis media: (Med)

Risk assessment: Class 2

Mebaral   (see **Mephobarbital**)

Mebendazole

Pronunciation guide: meh-BEN-dah-zole

Drug classification: ANTHELMINTIC DRUGS (see section 7.1 in Table 14-1)

Brand names: *Amoebriz* [1], *Exbenzol*

Ototoxic effects:
    Cochlear:
        Tinnitus: (AHF)
    Vestibular:
        Dizziness: (AHF)

Risk assessment: Class 1

Notes:

[1] *Amoebriz* is a combination of **Mebendazole** and Quinfamide. (**Mebendazole** is the ototoxic agent.)

Mecasermin

Pronunciation guide: meh-KAH-ser-min

Drug classification: GROWTH FACTORS (see section 40.28 in Table 14-1)

Brand names: *Increlex*

Ototoxic effects:
    Cochlear:
        Hearing loss: >5% (DFC, PDR)
    Vestibular:
        Dizziness: >5% (NDH, PDR)
    Outer/Middle Ear:
        Earache/ear pain: >5% (DFC, PDR)
        Otitis media: [1] >5% (NDH, PDR)

Risk assessment: Class 3

Notes:

[1] Including serous otitis media, fluid in the middle ear and abnormal tympanometry (PDR).

Mechlorethamine (Nitrogen mustard)

Pronunciation guide: me-klor-ETH-ah-meen (NIE-troe-jen MUS-tard)

Drug classification: ALKYLATING DRUGS (see section 14.1 in Table 14-1)

Brand names: *Mustargen*

Ototoxic effects:
    Cochlear:
        Hearing loss: (CPS, PDR)
        Tinnitus: (CPS, PDR)
    Vestibular:
        Vertigo: (CPS, PDR)

Risk assessment: Class 3

Notes:

Nitrogen mustard is a general name for several drugs including **Mechlorethamine** (described here), **Chlorambucil** (described elsewhere), **Estramustine** (ESS-truh-muss-TEEN), **Melphalan** (mel-FAL-an), **Mustine** (MUSS-teen), and **Uracil mustard** (YOO-rah-sill MUS-tard). All these drugs are ototoxic to some degree.[268] I do not have specific information on the ototoxicity of **Estramustine**, **Melphalan**, **Mustine** and **Uracil mustard**.

Nitrogen mustard can cause permanent hearing loss and tinnitus[269], especially in high doses (NDH).

Meclan   (see **Tetracycline**)

Meclizine

Pronunciation guide: MEK-lih-zeen

Drug classification: PIPERAZINES (see section 10.8 in Table 14-1)

Brand names: *Antivert, Bonamine, Bonine*

Ototoxic effects:
    Cochlear:
        Auditory hallucinations: (DFC, NDH)
        Tinnitus: (DFC, NDH)
    Vestibular:
        Vertigo: (DFC)

Risk assessment: Class 1

Notes:
    See Chapter 4 "Are You at Risk?" for further information on this drug.

Meclocycline   (see **Tetracycline**)

Meclofenamate

Pronunciation guide: MEK-low-fen-ah-mate

Drug classification: FENAMATES (see section 1.1.7 in Table 14-1)

Brand names: *Meclomen*

Ototoxic effects:
    Cochlear:
        Tinnitus: 1-3% (AHF, RXL)
    Vestibular:
        Dizziness: 3-9% (AHF, RXL)
        Vertigo: (AHF, Med)

Risk assessment: Class 2

Meclomen   (see **Meclofenamate**)

Medrol   (see **Methylprednisolone**)

Medrone   (see **Medroxyprogesterone**)

Medroxyprogesterone

Pronunciation guide: meh-DROX-ee-proe-JESS-teh-rone

Drug classification: PROGESTINS (see section 40.32 in Table 14-1)

Brand names: *Amen, Cycrin, Depo-Provera, Farlutal, Medrone, Premique, Premplus* [1],

Prempro, Proclim, Provera

Ototoxic effects:
    Cochlear:
        Hearing loss: (CPS)
        Tinnitus: <2% (CPS)

Vestibular:
    Ataxia: (CPS)
    Dizziness: 2-6% (CPS, PDR)
    Vertigo: <2% (CPS)
Unspecified/General Ear Conditions:
    Ototoxicity: [270]

Risk assessment: Class 2

Notes:

[1] *Premplus* is a combination of **Medroxyprogesterone** and conjugated estrogens. (**Medroxyprogesterone** is the ototoxic agent.)

PROGESTINS (such as **Medroxyprogesterone**, **Megestrol** and **Progesterone**) can cause hearing loss in women. PROGESTINS are typically used in hormone replacement therapy (HRT). One study found women who take the most common form of HRT had a hearing loss of 10% to 30% greater than women who have not taken HRT.[271] That's a loss equivalent to aging another 10 years or so. This hearing loss is particularly noticeable when trying to understand someone in a noisy environment.[272] The results showed that women who had received progestin had problems both in their cochleas and in the auditory circuits in their brains.

Progesterone (and synthetic **Progesterone** such as **Medroxyprogesterone**) are the likely culprits in this kind of hearing loss. There is some anecdotal evidence that women prescribed supplemental **Progesterone** to help maintain a pregnancy often complain their hearing gets noticeably worse while they're on **Progesterone**. In fact, a few studies have also shown that young women don't hear as well during the latter part of their monthly periods when **Progesterone** is the highest.[273]

In an anecdotal report in my files, one lady who lost most of her hearing to HRT summed up her situation as, "[in retrospect] my life would have been much easier if I'd just withstood the hot flashes and not medicated them away!"

Mefenamic acid

Pronunciation guide: MEF-en-ah-mik ASS-id

Drug classification: FENAMATES (see section 1.1.7 in Table 14-1)

Brand names: *Apo-Mefenamic, Ponstan, Ponstel*

Ototoxic effects:
    Cochlear:
        Hearing loss: <1% (CPS, PDR)
        Tinnitus: 1-10% (AHF, PDR)
    Vestibular:
        Dizziness: 1-10% (CPS, PDR)
        Vertigo: (AHF, PDR)
    Outer/Middle Ear:
        Earache/ear pain: (CPS, PDR)

Risk assessment: Class 2

Notes:

See Chapter 7, "We 'Hear' With Our Eyes" for further information on this drug.

Mefloquine

Pronunciation guide: MEH-flow-kwin

Drug classification: ANTI-MALARIAL DRUGS (see section 7.14.8 in Table 14-1)

Brand names: *Lariam*

Ototoxic effects:
    Cochlear:
        Auditory hallucinations: [1]
        Hearing loss: (CPS, PDR)
        Hyperacusis: [2]
        Tinnitus: >1% (CPS, PDR)
    Vestibular:
        Ataxia: (CPS, PDR)
        Dizziness: >1% (CPS, PDR)
        Loss of balance: (CPS, PDR)
        Vertigo: >1% (CPS, PDR)
        Vestibular disorder: (CPS, PDR)
    Outer/Middle Ear:
        Earache/ear pain: [2]

Risk assessment: Class 3

Notes:

The side effects of **Mefloquine** can "persist for years after the end of dosing".[274]

[1] Auditory hallucinations can persist for months after the last dose.[275]

[2] I have an anecdotal report in my files of a woman who began having balance and other ear problems just two days after taking her first **Mefloquine** pill. She experienced "a dull earache and extreme dizziness," as well as tinnitus. In addition, she began experiencing hyperacusis (where normal sounds are now much too loud). In her case, she couldn't stand the sound of people clapping. She had to cover her ears. Three years later the hyperacusis is still there but it is more tolerable, and the dizziness is much better.

I have another anecdotal report in my files of a woman who took **Mefloquine** as a precautionary measure when visiting Senegal in Africa. The result is that she now has a 50 dB hearing loss at 6,000 Hz and annoying tinnitus—both a high-pitched hissing sound, and also a low-pitched rumbling sound. This tinnitus has continued unabated for 9 years now.

Mefloquine given to a Navy Commander while he was serving in Iraq resulted in severe permanent balance problems. "A year after he stopped taking the drug, he still suffers from severe balance problems". [276]

Three people taking **Mefloquine** as a precautionary measure to protect against malaria had resulting high-frequency hearing loss and tinnitus. Of the three, only one had some of his hearing return. In the other two, the hearing loss was permanent. Furthermore, all three were left with permanent tinnitus.[277]

Mefloquine has so many harmful side effects (both ototoxic and otherwise) that there is an entire website dedicated to exposing the dangers of taking this drug (http://www. lariaminfo.org).

Megace (see **Megestrol**)

Megestrol

Pronunciation guide: meh-JESS-trole

Drug classification: PROGESTINS (see section 40.32 in Table 14-1)

Brand names: *Megace*

Ototoxic effects:
  Cochlear:
      Hearing loss: (CPS)
  Vestibular:
      Dizziness: (CP2)

Risk assessment: Class 2

Notes:

PROGESTINS (such as **Medroxyprogesterone**, **Megestrol** and **Progesterone**) can cause hearing loss in women. PROGESTINS are typically used in hormone replacement therapy (HRT). One study found women who take the most common form of HRT had a hearing loss of 10% to 30% greater than women who have not taken HRT.[278] That's a loss equivalent to aging another 10 years or so. This hearing loss is particularly noticeable when trying to understand someone in a noisy environment.[279] The results showed that women who had received progestin had problems both in their cochleas and in the auditory circuits in their brains.

Melitracen

Pronunciation guide: meh-lih-TRAY-sen

Drug classification: TRICYCLIC ANTI-DEPRESSANTS (see section 60.1.8 in Table 14-1)

Brand names: *Deanxit*[1], *Dixeran*

Ototoxic effects:
  Cochlear:
      Tinnitus: (Ka7, She)

Risk assessment: Class 1

Notes:

[1] *Deanxit* is a combination of **Melitracen** and Flupentixol. (**Melitracen** is the ototoxic agent.)

Mellaril (see **Thioridazine**)

Meloxicam

Pronunciation guide: mel-OX-ih-kam

Drug classification: OXICAMS (see section 1.1.10 in Table 14-1)

Brand names: *Mobic*, *Mobicox*

Ototoxic effects:
    Cochlear:
        Tinnitus: <2% (CPS, PDR)
    Vestibular:
        Dizziness: 1.1-3.8% [<0.6% above placebo results] (CPS, PDR)
        Vertigo: <2% (CPS, PDR)

Risk assessment: Class 2

Notes:

I have an anecdotal report in my files of a woman who gets loud tinnitus and her dizziness gets worse whenever she takes **Meloxicam** for her fibromyalgia.

I have another anecdotal report in my files of a woman who has pain from arthritis in her back. She took **Meloxicam**—15 mg. daily for 12 days. The result was horrible tinnitus—likely permanent as it has been two months since she stopped taking the **Meloxicam**. She lamented, "The back pain is awful, but the tinnitus is worse!"

Melphalan (see **Mechlorethamine**)

Memantine

Pronunciation guide: meh-MAN-teen

Drug classification: NMDA RECEPTOR ANTAGONIST (see section 53.4.4 in Table 14-1)

Brand names: *Ebixa*, *Namenda*

Ototoxic effects:
    Cochlear:
        Auditory hallucinations: 3% [1% above placebo results] (PDR)
        Hearing loss: 0.1-1% (CPS, PDR)
        Tinnitus: 0.1-1% (CPS, PDR)
    Vestibular:
        Ataxia: >1% (NDH, PDR)
        Dizziness: 7% [2% above placebo results] (NDH, PDR)
        Vertigo: >1% (CPS, PDR)
    Outer/Middle Ear:
        Earache/ear pain: 0.1-1% (CPS)
        Otitis media: [280] (CPS)

Unspecified/General Ear Conditions:
Ear disorder: 0.1-1% (CPS)

Risk assessment: Class 3

Meningitec   (see **Meningococcal serogroup C vaccine**)

Meningococcal serogroup C conjugate vaccine

Pronunciation guide: meh-nin-goe-KAW-kal SEER-oh-group C CON-joo-gate VAK-seen

Drug classification: VACCINES (see section 70.8 in Table 14-1)

Brand names: *Meningitec*

Ototoxic effects:
Vestibular:
Dizziness: < 0.01% (CPS)
Outer/Middle Ear:
Otitis media: 2% (CPS)

Risk assessment: Class 1

Menopur   (see **Menotropins**)

Menotropins

Pronunciation guide: meh-noe-TROP-inz

Drug classification: GONADOTROPINS (see section 40.24 in Table 14-1)

Brand names: *Menopur*

Ototoxic effects:
Vestibular:
Dizziness: 2.6-13% (CPS)
Vertigo: <1% (CPS)
Outer/Middle Ear:
Earache/ear pain: <1% (CPS)

Risk assessment: Class 1

Mepacrine   (see **Quinacrine**)

Mepergan   (see **Meperidine**)

Meperidine

Pronunciation guide: meh-PER-ih-deen

Drug classification: OPIATE AGONIST DRUGS (see section 1.4.1 in Table 14-1)

Brand names: *Demerol, Mepergan* [1]

Ototoxic effects:
    Vestibular:
        Ataxia: (CPS, PDR)
        Dizziness: >10% (NDH, PDR)

Risk assessment: Class 1

Notes:

    [1] *Mepergan* is a combination of **Meperidine** and **Promethazine**. (See **Promethazine** for its specific ototoxic properties.)

Mephentermine

Pronunciation guide: meh-FEN-ter-meen

Drug classification: SYMPATHOMIMETIC DRUGS (see section 17.16 in Table 14-1)

Brand names: *Wyamine*

Ototoxic effects:
    Cochlear:
        Tinnitus: (San, She)
    Unspecified/General Ear Conditions:
        Ototoxicity: (San)

Risk assessment: Not enough information to rate

Mephobarbital

Pronunciation guide: meh-foe-BAR-bih-tal

Drug classification: BARBITURATES (see section 60.12.4 in Table 14-1)

Brand names: *Mebaral*

Ototoxic effects:
    Vestibular:
        Ataxia: <1% (PDR)
        Dizziness: <1% (Med, PDR)
        Nystagmus: (PDR)

Risk assessment: Class 1

Notes:

These [above] adverse reactions were compiled from observing thousands of hospitalized patients. Because such patients may be less aware of adverse effects, the incidence of these adverse reactions may be somewhat higher in people that are normally up and walking around (PDR).

Mepivacaine

Pronunciation guide: meh-PIV-ah-kane

Drug classification: AMIDES (see section 4.1 in Table 14-1)

Brand names: *Carbocaine, Polocaine, Scandonest*

Ototoxic effects:
Cochlear:
    Hyperacusis: (CPS)
    Tinnitus: (CPS, PDR)
Vestibular:
    Dizziness: (CPS, PDR)

Risk assessment: Class 1

Meprobamate

Pronunciation guide: meh-proe-BAH-mate

Drug classification: ANXIOLYTICS (see section 60.12.1 in Table 14-1)

Brand names: *Miltown, PMB* [1]

Ototoxic effects:
Vestibular:
    Ataxia: (DFC, PDR)
    Dizziness: (DFC, PDR)
    Vertigo: (DFC, PDR)

Risk assessment: Class 1

Notes:

[1] *PMB* is a combination of **Meprobamate** and conjugated estrogens. (**Meprobamate** is the ototoxic agent.)

Mepron　(see **Atovaquone/Proguanil**)

Mercurio Cromo　(see **Thimerosal**)

Meridia　(see **Sibutramine**)

Mersyndol with Codeine　(see **Doxylamine**)

Meruvax II　(see **Rubella vaccine**)

Mervan....(see **Alclofenac**)

Mesalamine (5-ASA)

Pronunciation guide: meh-SAL-ah-meen

Drug classification: SALICYLATES (see section 1.1.16 in Table 14-1)

Brand names: *Apriso, Asacol, Colazal, Lialda, Mezavant, Pentasa, Rowasa, Salofalk*

Ototoxic effects:
  Cochlear:
    Hearing loss: 2% [placebo 0] (CPS, Med+)
    Tinnitus: <5% (CPS, PDR)
  Vestibular:
    Ataxia: (PDR)
    Dizziness: 2-8% [1% above placebo results] (AHF, PDR)
    Vertigo: <5% (CPS, PDR)
  Outer/Middle Ear:
    Earache/ear pain: >2% (AHF, PDR)
    Ears feel "plugged up": (AHF, PDR)
    Otitis: (PDR)
  Unspecified/General Ear Conditions:
    Ear disorder: >2% (CPS, PDR)

Risk assessment: Class 2

Notes:

Other names for **Mesalamine** include **Aminosalicylic acid** (technically **5-Aminosalicylic acid**) (ah-mee-noe-sal-ih-SIKE-lik ASS-id), **Balsalazide** (bal-SAL-ah-zide) and **Mesalazine** (meh-SAL-ah-zeen).

Colazal is a brand name of **Balsalazide. Balsalazide** is a prodrug that is converted by the enzymes in your colon into **Mesalamine** (PDR).

Mesalazine (see **Mesalamine**)

M-Eslon   (see **Morphine**)

Mesoridazine

Pronunciation guide: mez-oh-RID-ah-zeen

Drug classification: PHENOTHIAZINES (see section 60.8.1 in Table 14-1)

Brand names: *Serentil*

Ototoxic effects:
  Vestibular:
    Ataxia: (PDR)
    Dizziness: (PDR)

Risk assessment: Class 1

Notes:

See Chapter 7, "We 'Hear' With Our Eyes" for further information on this drug.

Metacycline   (see **Methacycline**)

Metformin

Pronunciation guide: met-FORE-min

Drug classification: BIGUANIDE ANTI-DIABETIC DRUGS (see section 40.8.1 in Table 14-1)

Brand names: *Glumetza*

Ototoxic effects:
    Vestibular:
        Dizziness: 1-5% (CPS, DFC)
    Outer/Middle Ear:
        Earache/ear pain: 1-5% (CPS, DFC)

Risk assessment: Class 1

Methacycline (Metacycline)

Pronunciation guide: meth-ah-SYE-kleen (met-ah-SYE-kleen)

Drug classification: TETRACYCLINES (see section 7.4.60 in Table 14-1)

Brand names: *Lysocline, Rondomycin*

Ototoxic effects:
    Unspecified/General Ear Conditions:
        Ototoxicity: (San)

Risk assessment: Not enough information to rate

Methapyrilene

Pronunciation guide: meth-ah-PYE-ril-een

Drug classification: ANTIHISTAMINES (see section 10 in Table 14-1)

Brand names: *Histase*

Ototoxic effects:
    Cochlear:
        Tinnitus: (NTP)
    Vestibular:
        Dizziness: (NTP)
        Nystagmus: (NTP)

Risk assessment: Class 1

Methazolamide

Pronunciation guide: meth-ah-ZOLE-ah-mide

Drug classification: DIURETICS—CARBONIC ANHYDRASE INHIBITORS (see section 30.5.1 in Table 14-1)

Brand names: *Apo-Methazolamide, Neptazane*

Ototoxic effects:
  Cochlear:
      Hearing disorder: (PDR)
      Tinnitus: (CPS, PDR)
  Vestibular:
      Ataxia: (CPS)
      Dizziness: (CPS, PDR)
      Vertigo: (CPS)

Risk assessment: Class 2

Methdilazine

Pronunciation guide: meth-DILL-ah-zeen

Drug classification: H$_1$ RECEPTOR ANTAGONISTS (see section 10.1 in Table 14-1)

Brand names: *Tacaryl*

Ototoxic effects:
  Cochlear:
      Tinnitus: (Med, NTP)
  Vestibular:
      Dizziness: (CP2, NTP)

Risk assessment: Class 1

Methenamine (Hexamine)

Pronunciation guide: meth-EN-ah-meen (HEX-ah-meen)

Drug classification: URINARY ANTI-INFECTIVES (see section 7.20 in Table 14-1)

Brand names: *Dehydral, Hiprex, Mandelamine, Prosed* [1], *Urasal, Urex, Urised* [1]

Ototoxic effects:
  Cochlear:
      Tinnitus: (CPS, Med)
  Vestibular:
      Dizziness: (PDR)
  Unspecified/General Ear Conditions:
      Ototoxicity: [281]

Risk assessment: Class 1

Notes:

[1] *Prosed* and *Urised* are combinations of **Methenamine**, Phenyl salicylate, Methylene blue, Benzoic acid, **Atropine** and **Hyoscyamine**. (See the generic drugs **Atropine** and **Hyoscyamine** for their specific ototoxic properties.)

Methergine   (see **Methylergonovine**)

425

Methimazole

Pronunciation guide: meth-IM-ah-zole

Drug classification: ANTI-THYROID DRUGS (see section 40.42.1 in Table 14-1)

Brand names: *Tapazole*

Ototoxic effects:
　　Vestibular:
　　　　Dizziness: <1% (CPS, Med)
　　　　Vertigo: (CPS, PDR)

Risk assessment: Class 1

Methocarbamol

Pronunciation guide: meth-oh-KAR-bah-mole

Drug classification: SKELETAL MUSCLE RELAXANTS (see section 53.36 in Table 14-1)

Brand names: *Robax Platinum* [1], *Robaxacet* [2], *Robaxin*

Ototoxic effects:
　　Vestibular:
　　　　Dizziness: (CPS, PDR)
　　　　Nystagmus: (AHF, PDR)
　　　　Vertigo: (AHF, PDR)

Risk assessment: Class 1

Notes:

[1] *Robax Platinum* is a combination of **Methocarbamol** and **Ibuprofen**. (See the generic drug **Ibuprofen** for its specific ototoxic properties.)

[2] *Robaxacet* is a combination of **Methocarbamol** and **Acetaminophen**. (See the generic drug **Acetaminophen** for its specific ototoxic properties.)

See Chapter 7, "We 'Hear' With Our Eyes" for further information on this drug.

Methotrexate

Pronunciation guide: meth-oh-TREX-ate

Drug classification: ANTI-METABOLITE DRUGS (see section 14.8 in Table 14-1)

Brand names: *Rheumatrex*

Ototoxic effects:
　　Cochlear:
　　　　Hearing loss: [1]
　　　　Tinnitus: <1% (CPS, PDR)
　　Vestibular:
　　　　Ataxia: (AHF, NTP)
　　　　Dizziness: 1-3% (CPS, PDR)

Risk assessment: Class 2

Notes:

[1] A recent study determined the effectiveness of using low doses of **Methotrexate** in treating 18 people with longstanding immune-mediated Meniere's disease in both ears.

Here are the results. Vertigo went away in 78%, was controlled in 17% and remained unchanged in 6%. Hearing improved for 28%, worsened in 22% and stabilized in 39%. In 12% the hearing improved in one ear and worsened in the other. Tinnitus went away in 6%, was reduced in 59%, remained unchanged in 29% and got worse in 6%. The feeling of fullness in the ears went away in 43%, improved in 50% and worsened in 7%.[282]

Since other treatments had not worked, this is good news for certain Meniere's sufferers! However, a word of warning. Notice that hearing loss actually **increased** in about 1 in 4 people so for some people **Methotrexate** may be quite ototoxic. (However, since this wasn't a controlled study, there is no way to determine if this hearing loss was due to the continued effects of Meniere's disease instead.)

I have an anecdotal report in my files of a lady that takes 15 mg. of **Methotrexate** weekly. She writes, "Those days are particularly hard on my tinnitus. It is almost unbearable!"

Methrazone   (see **Feprazone**)

Methsuximide

Pronunciation guide: meth-SUX-ih-mide

Drug classification: ANTI-CONVULSANT DRUGS (see section 53.12 in Table 14-1)

Brand names: *Celontin*

Ototoxic effects:
  Cochlear:
      Auditory hallucinations: (CPS, PDR)
  Vestibular:
      Ataxia: (CPS, PDR)
      Dizziness: (CPS, PDR)

Risk assessment: Class 1

Notes:

See Chapter 7, "We 'Hear' With Our Eyes" for further information on this drug.

Methyclothiazide

Pronunciation guide: meth-ee-kloe-THYE-ah-zide

Drug classification: DIURETICS—THIAZIDE-RELATED (see section 30.5.12 in Table 14-1)

Brand names: *Enduron*

Ototoxic effects:
    Cochlear:
        Tinnitus: (Eps)
    Vestibular:
        Dizziness: (DFC, PDR)
        Vertigo: (DFC, PDR)

Risk assessment: Class 1

Methyl salicylate (Oil of Wintergreen)

Pronunciation guide: METH-il sah-LISS-ih-late

Drug classification: SALICYLATES (see section 1.1.16 in Table 14-1)

Brand names: *BenGay*

Ototoxic effects:
    Cochlear:
        Hearing loss: (NTP)
        Tinnitus: (NTP)
    Vestibular:
        Dizziness: (NTP)

Risk assessment: Class 2

Notes:

    Methyl salicylates are often found in liniments.

Methyldopa

Pronunciation guide: meth-ill-DOE-pah

Drug classification: CENTRALLY ACTING ANTIADRENERGIC DRUGS (see section 20.8.20 in Table 14-1)

Brand names: *Presinol*

Ototoxic effects:
    Vestibular:
        Dizziness: (AHF)
        Vertigo: (CPS, AHF)

Risk assessment: Class 1

Methylergonovine

Pronunciation guide: meth-ill-er-goe-NOE-veen

Drug classification: ERGOT ALKALOIDS (see section 17.4 in Table 14-1)

Brand names: *Methergine*

Ototoxic effects:
 Cochlear:
  Tinnitus: (DFC, PDR)
 Vestibular:
  Dizziness: (DFC, PDR)

Risk assessment: Class 1

Methylnaltrexone

Pronunciation guide: meth-ill-NAL-trek-zone

Drug classification: NARCOTIC ANTAGONIST DRUGS (see section 1.7 in Table 14-1)

Brand names: *Relistor*

Ototoxic effects:
 Cochlear:
  Tinnitus: 1.8% (CPS)
 Vestibular:
  Dizziness: 4.2-9.1% [<9.1% above placebo results] (CPS)

Risk assessment: Class 1

Methylphenidate

Pronunciation guide: meth-ill-FEN-ih-date

Drug classification: ANXIOLYTICS, SEDATIVES & HYPNOTICS (see section 60.12 in Table 14-1)

Brand names: *Biphentin, Concerta*

Ototoxic effects:
 Cochlear:
  Auditory hallucinations: (PDR)
 Vestibular:
  Dizziness: 1.5-10% [1.5-3% above placebo results] (CPS, PDR)
  Vertigo: 1.7-2.5% [placebo 0] (CPS, PDR)
 Outer/Middle Ear:
  Earache/ear pain: <1% (CPS)
  Otitis media: 5-10% (CPS)
 Unspecified/General Ear Conditions:
  Ear disorder: 2.0% (CPS)

Risk assessment: Class 2

Methylprednisolone

Pronunciation guide: meth-ill-pred-NISS-oh-lone

Drug classification: GLUCOCORTICOIDS (see section 40.1.4 in Table 14-1)

Brand names: *Depo-Medrol, Medrol, Solu-Medrol*

Ototoxic effects:
> Vestibular:
>> Vertigo: (CPS, PDR)

Risk assessment: Class 1

Methysergide

Pronunciation guide: meth-ih-SIR-jide

Drug classification: ERGOT ALKALOIDS (see section 17.4 in Table 14-1)

Brand names: *Sansert*

Ototoxic effects:
> Vestibular:
>> Ataxia: (CPS, PDR)
>> Dizziness: (CPS, PDR)
>> Vertigo: (AHF)

Risk assessment: Class 1

Notes:
> See Chapter 7, "We 'Hear' With Our Eyes" for further information on this drug.

Metoclopramide

Pronunciation guide: met-oh-KLOE-prah-mide

Drug classification: PROKINETIC DRUGS (see section 34.24 in Table 14-1)

Brand names: *Reglan*

Ototoxic effects:
> Vestibular:
>> Ataxia: (AHF)
>> Dizziness: (AHF)
>> Vertigo: (AHF)

Risk assessment: Class 1

Notes:
> Ataxia and vertigo can occur following an overdose of **Metoclopramide** (AHF).

Metolazone

Pronunciation guide: meh-TOLE-ah-zone

Drug classification: DIURETICS—THIAZIDE-RELATED (see section 30.5.12 in Table 14-1)

Brand names: *Mykrox, Zaroxolyn*

Ototoxic effects:
    Cochlear:
        Tinnitus: <2% (PDR)
    Vestibular:
        Dizziness: 10.2% [2.8% above placebo results] (CPS, PDR)
        Vertigo: (CPS, PDR)

Risk assessment: Class 2

Metoprolol

Pronunciation guide: meh-TOH-pruh-lawl

Drug classification: BETA-ADRENERGIC-BLOCKING DRUGS (BETA-BLOCKERS) (see section 20.8.12 in Table 14-1)

Brand names: *Betaloc*, *Lopresor*, *Lopressor*, *Lopressor HCT*[1], *Toprol-XL*

Ototoxic effects:
    Cochlear:
        Hearing loss: (CPS)
        Tinnitus: 1% (CPS, PDR)
    Vestibular:
        Dizziness: 10% (CPS, PDR)
        Dizziness/Vertigo: 1.8% [0.8% above placebo results] (PDR)
        Vertigo: (CPS, PDR)
    Outer/Middle Ear:
        Earache/ear pain: 1% (PDR)
        Feeling of fullness in ears: [2]

Risk assessment: Class 3

Notes:

[1] *Lopressor HCT* is a combination of **Metoprolol** and **Hydrochlorothiazide**. (See the generic drug **Hydrochlorothiazide** for its specific ototoxic properties.)

Hearing difficulties (hearing loss) can result when the dose exceeds the recommended dose (CPS).

I have an anecdotal report in my files of a woman who got a bad case of tinnitus when she began taking **Metoprolol**. Her tinnitus went away when her doctor prescribed a different medication.

[2] I have another anecdotal report in my files of a woman who explained, "I started taking *Lopressor* 25 mg. about 5 months ago. Although my blood pressure is now under control, I have had a couple of experiences of "fullness" along with tinnitus and not being able to hear hardly anything out of one ear at times. Fortunately, the feeling of fullness and hearing loss eventually passes".

In yet another anecdotal report in my files a lady wrote, "I've been on **Metoprolol** intermittently for several months. During this time, I've been experiencing increasingly-loud tinnitus".

I have still another anecdotal report in my files of a woman who wrote, "Three months after I was put on *Lopressor,* I woke up with tinnitus, and it's never gone away these past 5 years". Perhaps it is because this lady is still taking **Metoprolol ER**.

A Doctor of Pharmacy explained: "An MD had a patient with worsening hearing loss over the previous year. She was totally deaf when he asked me to figure out which drug might be causing it. I told him to discontinue the **Metoprolol ER** 50 mg. a day she was taking. A week later this lady could hear normally. It happens more often in people with atherosclerosis. MDs don't understand the effect drugs have on the cochlear artery".

Metreton   (see **Prednisone**)

Metrogel-Vaginal   (see **Metronidazole**)

Metronidazole

Pronunciation guide: meh-troe-NIH-dah-zole

Drug classification: AMEBICIDES (see section 7.14.1 in Table 14-1)

Brand names: *Flagyl, Florazole, Metrogel-Vaginal, NidaGel, Protostat*

Ototoxic effects:
    Cochlear:
        Hearing loss: [1]
        Tinnitus: (She)
    Vestibular:
        Ataxia: (CPS, PDR)
        Dizziness: 1-4% (CPS, PDR)
        Nystagmus: (CPS)
        Vertigo: (CPS, PDR)

Risk assessment: Class 2

Notes:

[1] Two people experienced bilateral moderate to severe sensorineural hearing loss after taking **Metronidazole**. Their hearing gradually recovered over a period of 4 to 6 weeks after stopping the drug.[283] In another case, a person received **Metronidazole** for 14 days. This resulted in temporary hearing loss, tinnitus and ataxia.[284]

Mevacor   (see **Lovastatin**)

Mexiletine

Pronunciation guide: mex-ILL-eh-teen

Drug classification: ANTI-ARRHYTHMICS (HEART RHYTHM REGULATORS) (see section 20.4 in Table 14-1)

Brand names: *Mexitil*

Ototoxic effects:
    Cochlear:
        Tinnitus: 0.1-2.4% (CPS, PDR)
    Vestibular:
        Ataxia: >10% (AHF, NDH)
        Dizziness: 18.9-26.4% [12.1% above placebo results] (NDH, PDR)
        Nystagmus: (AHF, CPS)

Risk assessment: Class 2

Mexitil   (see **Mexiletine**)

Mezavant   (see **Mesalamine**)

Miacalcin   (see **Calcitonin**)

Micardis   (see **Telmisartan**)

Micardis HCT   (see **Telmisartan**)

Micardis Plus   (see **Telmisartan**)

Micronomicin

Pronunciation guide: my-kron-oh-MY-sin

Drug classification: AMINOGLYCOSIDES (see section 7.4.1 in Table 14-1)

Brand names: *Sagamicin*

Ototoxic effects:
    Cochlear:
        Hearing loss: 0.1% [1]
        Tinnitus: 0.1% [1]
    Vestibular:
        Vertigo: 0.1% [1]
        Vestibular disorder: [1]
    Outer/Middle Ear:
        Earache/ear pain: 0.1% [1]
        Feeling of fullness in ears: [1]

Risk assessment: Class 4

Notes:

[1] Reported by the manufacturer, Kyowa Hakko Kogyo Co, Ltd. in Japan.[285]

Micronomicin is a fairly new drug and is used in Japan and the Far East.

You should not take **Micronomicin** if you have had previous ear damage from taking any AMINOGLYCOSIDE antibiotics, or if you already have a hearing loss. If you are taking **Micronomicin**, you should have your hearing tested. AMINOGLYCOSIDE-induced hearing loss normally begins at the very high frequencies and works its way down to the speech frequencies.[286]

See Chapter 9, "Aminoglycoside Antibiotics are the Ototoxic 'Bad boys'" for further information on this drug.

Microzide   (see **Hydrochlorothiazide**)

Midamor   (see **Amiloride**)

Midazolam

Pronunciation guide: mid-AY-zoh-lam

Drug classification: BENZODIAZEPINES (see section 60.12.8 in Table 14-1)

Brand names: *Apo-Midazolam, Versed*

Ototoxic effects:
    Cochlear:
        Tinnitus: (Eps)
    Vestibular:
        Ataxia: <1% (CPS, PDR)
        Dizziness: 0.2-1.2% (CPS, PDR)
        Loss of balance: <1% (CPS, PDR)
        Nystagmus: 1.1% (CPS, PDR)
        Vertigo: <1% (AHF, PDR)
    Outer/Middle Ear:
        Ears feel "plugged up": <1% (CPS, PDR)

Risk assessment: Class 2

Notes:

Caution: Eating grapefruit or drinking grapefruit juice during the time you are taking this drug may make the listed side effects worse than shown here. In fact, taking **Midazolam** with grapefruit juice can increase the potency of **Midazolam** by as much as 240%.

See Chapter 10 "Beware of Benzodiazepines—Don't Let This Nasty Time-Bomb Ambush You and Your Ears" and Chapter 11, "Grapefruit Juice and Ototoxic Drugs" for further information on this drug.

Midol Extra Strength   (see **Pyrilamine**)

Miglustat

Pronunciation guide: MIG-loo-stat

Drug classification: ENZYME INHIBITORS (see section 32.4 in Table 14-1)

Brand names: *Zavesca*

Ototoxic effects:
    Vestibular:
        Dizziness: 8-11% (CPS, DFC)
        Vertigo: 3% (CPS)

Risk assessment: Class 1

Migranal   (see **Dihydroergotamine**)

Milnacipran

Pronunciation guide: mil-NAH-sih-pran

Drug classification: SELECTIVE SEROTONIN & NOREPINEPHRINE REUPTAKE INHIBITORS (see section 60.1.28 in Table 14-1)

Brand names: *Savella*

Ototoxic effects:
    Cochlear:
        Tinnitus: (DIO)
    Vestibular:
        Ataxia: (DIO)
        Dizziness: 10-17% [<11% above placebo results] (DIO, PDR)
        Vertigo: (DFC)

Risk assessment: Class 1

Milophene   (see **Clomiphene**)

Miltown   (see **Meprobamate**)

Mimims Homatropine   (see **Homatropine**)

Minestrin   (see **Ethinyl estradiol**)

Minipress   (see **Prazosin**)

Minitran   (see **Nitroglycerin**)

Minizide   (see **Prazosin**)

Minocin   (see **Minocycline**)

Minocycline

Pronunciation guide: mih-noe-SYE-kleen

Drug classification: TETRACYCLINES (see section 7.4.60 in Table 14-1)

Brand names: *Arestin, Dynacin, Minocin, Novo-Minocycline, Solodyn, Vectrin*

Ototoxic effects:
    Cochlear:
        Hearing loss: (AHF, PDR)
        Tinnitus: 2% [1% above placebo results] (CPS, PDR)
    Vestibular:
        Ataxia: (AHF, CPS)
        Dizziness: 9% [4% above placebo results] (CPS, PDR)
        Vertigo: (CPS, PDR)

Risk assessment: Class 2

Notes:

> **Minocycline** causes temporary vestibular damage in 30 to 90% of those treated with the usual dosages (AHF).[287] Vestibular symptoms appear to be dose-related (AHF).

> You can develop symptoms of ototoxicity after only one or two doses. These symptoms normally disappear a day or two after you stop taking this drug.[288]

> Dizziness, tinnitus and vertigo are more common in women than in men (AHF, BNF).

Minoxidil

Pronunciation guide: mih-NOX-ih-dill

Drug classification: VASODILATORS (see section 20.8.40 in Table 14-1)

Brand names: *Rogaine, Rogaine for Men Extra Strength, Rogaine for Women*

Ototoxic effects:
    Vestibular:
        Dizziness: 1-2% (CPS, DFC)
        Vertigo: 1.2% [same as placebo] (AHF,DFC)
    Outer/Middle Ear:
        Otitis externa:[1] 0.1-1% (AHF, CPS)

Risk assessment: Class 1

Notes:

  [1] Includes ear infections and ear inflammation (CPS).

Mintezol   (see **Thiabendazole**)

Mirapex   (see **Pramipexole**)

Mircette   (see **Ethinyl estradiol**)

Mirena   (see **Levonorgestrel**)

Mirtazapine

Pronunciation guide: mer-TAH-zah-peen

Drug classification: TETRACYCLIC ANTI-DEPRESSANTS (see section 60.1.12 in Table 14-1)

Brand names: *Remeron, Remeron RD, Remeron SolTab*

Ototoxic effects:
  Cochlear:
    Hearing loss: 0.1-1% (CPS, PDR)
    Hyperacusis: 0.1%-1% (CPS, PDR)
    Tinnitus: [same as placebo] (CPS, PDR)
  Vestibular:
    Ataxia: 0.1-1% (CPS, PDR)
    Dizziness: 7% [4% above placebo results] (CPS, PDR)
    Nystagmus: <0.1% (CPS, PDR)
    Vertigo: >1% (CPS, PDR)
  Outer/Middle Ear:
    Earache/ear pain: 0.1%-1% (CPS, PDR)
    Otitis media: <0.1% (CPS, PDR)

Risk assessment: Class 3

Notes:

Hearing loss may be temporary (PDR).

I have an anecdotal report in my files of a man who experienced hyperacusis as a result of taking **Mirtazapine**. He also wrote, "I've read of many other folks (on message boards) having hyperacusis made worse" from **Mirtazapine**.

I have an anecdotal report in my files of a woman who suffered mild hearing loss as a result of taking **Mirtazapine**. The good news is that when she started tapering off the **Mirtazapine**, she felt her hearing was improving.

Misonidazole

Pronunciation guide: mis-on-nih-DAH-zole

Drug classification: ANTI-NEOPLASTICS (ANTI-CANCER DRUGS) (see section 14 in Table 14-1)

Brand names: —

Ototoxic effects:
  Cochlear:
    Auditory disorder: [1]
    Tinnitus: [289]

Risk assessment: Not enough information to rate

Notes:

[1] This drug is toxic to the cochlea.[290]

Misoprostol

Pronunciation guide: mye-soe-PROST-ole

Drug classification: GASTRIC MUCOSAL DRUGS (see section 34.8.1 in Table 14-1)

Brand names: *Apo-Misoprostol*, *Cytotec*

Ototoxic effects:
Cochlear:
Hearing loss: (AHF, PDR)
Tinnitus: (AHF, PDR)
Vestibular:
Dizziness: (AHF, PDR)
Vertigo: (AHF)
Outer/Middle Ear:
Earache/ear pain: (AHF, PDR)

Risk assessment: Class 2

Mitomycin

Pronunciation guide: mye-toe-MYE-sin

Drug classification: ANTI-NEOPLASTICS (ANTI-CANCER DRUGS) (see section 14 in Table 14-1)

Brand names: *Mutamycin*

Ototoxic effects:
Vestibular:
Ataxia: (CPS)
Nystagmus: (NTP)
Vertigo (NTP)

Risk assessment: Class 1

Mitotane

Pronunciation guide: MYE-toe-tane

Drug classification: ADRENAL DRUGS (see section 40.1 in Table 14-1)

Brand names: *Lysodren*

Ototoxic effects:
Cochlear:
Hearing loss: (AHF)
Vestibular:
Ataxia: (AHF)
Dizziness/vertigo: 15% (CPS, PDR)

Risk assessment: Class 2

M-M-R II   (see **Measles, mumps & rubella vaccine**)

Moban   (see **Molindone**)

Mobic   (see **Meloxicam**)

Mobicox   (see **Meloxicam**)

Mobiflex   (see **Tenoxicam**)

Moclobemide

Pronunciation guide: moe-KLOE-beh-mide

Drug classification: MONOAMINE OXIDASE INHIBITORS (see section 60.1.1 in Table 14-1)

Brand names: *Apo-Moclobemide, Manerix, Novo-Moclobemide*

Ototoxic effects:
  Cochlear:
      Tinnitus: <1% (CPS)
  Vestibular:
      Dizziness: 5.1% (CPS)

Risk assessment: Class 1

Modafinil

Pronunciation guide: moe-DAF-ih-nil

Drug classification: PSYCHOSTIMULANTS (see section 60.20 in Table 14-1)

Brand names: *Alertec, Provigil*

Ototoxic effects:
  Cochlear:
      Auditory hallucinations: (AHF)
      Hearing loss: 0.3% (CPS)
      Hyperacusis: 0.3% (CPS)
  Vestibular:
      Ataxia: 0.3-1% [placebo 0] (CPS, PDR)
      Dizziness: 0.8-8.8% [<7.7% above placebo results] (CPS, PDR)
      Vertigo: 0.7-1% (placebo 0] (CPS, PDR)
  Outer/Middle Ear:
      Earache/ear pain: >1% [same as placebo] (CPS, PDR)
  Unspecified/General Ear Conditions:
      Ear disorder: >1% [same as placebo] (PDR)

Risk assessment: Class 2

Modalim   (see **Ciprofibrate**)

Moderil   (see **Rescinnamine**)

Modulon   (see **Trimebutine**)

Moduret   (see **Amiloride**)

Moduretic   (see **Amiloride**)

Moexipril

Pronunciation guide: moe-EKS-ih-pril

Drug classification: ANGIOTENSIN-CONVERTING ENZYME (ACE) INHIBITORS (see section 20.8.8 in Table 14-1)

Brand names: *Uniretic* [1], *Univasc*

Ototoxic effects:
    Cochlear:
        Hearing loss: <1% (PDR)
        Tinnitus: <1% (DFC, PDR)
    Vestibular:
        Ataxia: <1% (PDR)
        Dizziness: 1.4-4.3% [0.4-2.1% above placebo results] (AHF, PDR)
        Vertigo: >1% (PDR)
    Outer/Middle Ear:
        Earache/ear pain: <1% (PDR)
        Otitis media: <1% (PDR)

Risk assessment: Class 2

Notes:

    [1] *Uniretic* is a combination of **Moexipril** and **Hydrochlorothiazide**. (See the generic drug **Hydrochlorothiazide** for its specific ototoxic properties.)

Mogadon   (see **Nitrazepam**)

Molindone

Pronunciation guide: moe-LIN-doan

Drug classification: ANTIPSYCHOTIC DRUGS (see section 60.8 in Table 14-1)

Brand names: *Lidone*, *Moban*

Ototoxic effects:
    Cochlear:
        Tinnitus: (AHF, Ka8)
    Vestibular:
        Dizziness: (AHF, Med+)
        Loss of balance: (Med+)

Risk assessment: Class 1

Momentum Backache Relief   (see **Magnesium salicylate**)

Mometasone

Pronunciation guide: moe-MEH-tah-zone

Drug classification: GLUCOCORTICOIDS (see section 40.1.4 in Table 14-1)

Brand names: *Asmanex, Elocon, Nasonex*

Ototoxic effects:
    Outer/Middle Ear:
        Earache/ear pain: 2-5% (DFC, PDR)
        Otitis media: 2-5% (DFC, PDR)

Risk assessment: Class 1

Monitan   (see **Acebutolol**)

Monocor   (see **Bisoprolol**)

Mono-Gesic   (see **Salsalate**)

Monoket   (see **Isosorbide**)

Monopril   (see **Fosinopril**)

Monopril HCT   (see **Fosinopril**)

Montelukast

Pronunciation guide: mon-tell-OO-kast

Drug classification: RESPIRATORY ANTI-INFLAMMATORY DRUGS (see section 63.8 in Table 14-1)

Brand names: *Singulair*

Ototoxic effects:
    Vestibular:
        Dizziness: 1.9% [0.5% above placebo results] (CPS, PDR)
    Outer/Middle Ear:
        Earache/ear pain: >2% (AHF, PDR)
        Otitis: >2% (AHF, PDR)
        Otitis media: >2% (AHF, PDR)

Risk assessment: Class 1

Notes:

Caution: Eating grapefruit or drinking grapefruit juice during the time you are taking this drug may make the listed side effects worse than shown here.

See Chapter 11, "Grapefruit Juice and Ototoxic Drugs" for further information on this drug.

Monurol   (see **Fosfomycin**)

Moricizine

Pronunciation guide: mor-IH-sih-zeen

Drug classification: ANTI-ARRHYTHMICS (HEART RHYTHM REGULATORS) (see section 20.4 in Table 14-1)

Brand names: *Ethmozine*

Ototoxic effects:
Cochlear:
Tinnitus: <2% (DFC, PDR)
Vestibular:
Ataxia: <2% (DFC, PDR)
Dizziness: 11.3% [6% above placebo results] (DFC, PDR)
Nystagmus: <2% (DFC, PDR)
Vertigo: <2% (DFC, PDR)

Risk assessment: Class 2

Morphine

Pronunciation guide: MOR-feen

Drug classification: OPIATE AGONIST DRUGS (see section 1.4.1 in Table 14-1)

Brand names: *Avinza, Embeda [1], Kadian, M-Eslon, MS Contin, MS-IR, Oramorph, RMS, Roxanol*

Ototoxic effects:
Vestibular:
Ataxia: <5% (CPS, PDR)
Dizziness: 6% (CPS, PDR)
Nystagmus: <3% (CPS, PDR)
Vertigo: <5% (CPS, PDR)

Risk assessment: Class 2

Notes:

[1] *Embeda* is a combination of **Morphine** and **Naltrexone**. (See the generic drug **Naltrexone** for its specific ototoxic properties.)

See Chapter 7, "We 'Hear' With Our Eyes" for further information on this drug.

MoRu-Viraten Berna   (see **Measles, rubella vaccine**)

Motrin   (see **Ibuprofen**)

Moxifloxacin

Pronunciation guide: mocks-ih-FLOX-ah-sin

Drug classification: QUINOLONES (see section 7.4.48 in Table 14-1)

Brand names: *Avelox, Vigamox*

Ototoxic effects:
    Cochlear:
        Hearing loss: <0.1% (CPS)
        Hyperacusis: <0.1% (CPS)
        Tinnitus: 0.05-1% (CPS, PDR)
    Vestibular:
        Ataxia: <0.1% (CPS)
        Dizziness: 3% (CPS, PDR)
        Vertigo: 0.1-3% (CPS, PDR)
        Vestibular disorder: <0.1% (CPS)
    Outer/Middle Ear:
        Earache/ear pain: <0.1% (CPS)
        Otitis media: 1-4% (AHF, PDR)

Risk assessment: Class 2

Notes:

Hearing loss may be permanent (CPS).

I have an anecdotal report in my files of a girl that applied *Vigamox* eye drops 3 times to a supposedly infected eye. The next morning she had an 85 dB sensorineural hearing loss in her ear on the same side. In the month following, her hearing partially came back, but she is left with roughly a 50 dB hearing loss.

M-R-VAX II   (see **Measles, rubella vaccine**)

MS Contin   (see **Morphine**)

MSD Enteric coated ASA   (see **Acetylsalicylic acid**)

MS-IR   (see **Morphine**)

Mucomyst   (see **Acetylcysteine**)

Multitol   (see **Sorbitol**)

Mumps vaccine

Pronunciation guide: MUMPS VAK-seen

Drug classification: VACCINES (see section 70.8 in Table 14-1)

Brand names: *Mumpsvax*

Ototoxic effects:
    Cochlear:
        Hearing loss: (CPS, PDR)

Vestibular:
Ataxia: (CPS)
Outer/Middle Ear:
Otitis media: (DFC, PDR)

Risk assessment: Class 2

Notes:

Sensorineural hearing loss rarely occurs. Also, rarely there are reports of hearing loss in just one ear, that occurs within 30 days of the vaccination (AHF, Med).

Mumpsvax   (see **Mumps vaccine**)

Mupirocin

Pronunciation guide: myoo-PEER-oh-sin

Drug classification: ANTI-BACTERIAL DRUGS (see section 7.4 in Table 14-1)

Brand names: *Bactroban*

Ototoxic effects:
Vestibular:
Dizziness: <1% (AHF, PDR)
Outer/Middle Ear:
Earache/ear pain: <1% (DFC, PDR)

Risk assessment: Class 1

Muromonab-CD3

Pronunciation guide: myoo-roe-MOH-nab

Drug classification: MONOCLONAL ANTIBODIES (see section 7.17.8 in Table 14-1)

Brand names: *Orthoclone OKT3*

Ototoxic effects:
Cochlear:
Auditory hallucinations: (CPS, PDR)
Hearing loss: <1% (CPS, PDR)
Tinnitus: 1% (CPS, PDR)
Vestibular:
Dizziness: 6% (CPS, PDR)
Vertigo: (CPS, PDR)
Outer/Middle Ear:
Ears feel "plugged up": (CPS, PDR)
Otitis media: (CPS, PDR)

Risk assessment: Class 2

Mustargen   (see **Mechlorethamine**)

Mustine   (see **Mechlorethamine**)

Mutamycin   (see **Mitomycin**)

Mycifradin   (see **Neomycin**)

Mycophenolate

Pronunciation guide: mye-koe-FIN-oh-late

Drug classification: IMMUNOSUPPRESSANT DRUGS (see section 43 in Table 14-1)

Brand names: *CellCept*

Ototoxic effects:
    Cochlear:
        Hearing loss: >3% (CPS, PDR)
        Tinnitus: >3% (CPS, PDR)
    Vestibular:
        Dizziness: 5.7-28.7% (CPS, PDR)
        Vertigo: >3% (CPS, PDR)
    Outer/Middle Ear: [1]
        Earache/ear pain: >3% (CPS, PDR)
    Unspecified/General Ear Conditions:
        Ear disorder: >3% (CPS, PDR)

Risk assessment: Class 4

Notes:

[1] If you take **Mycophenolate** when you are pregnant, you increase the risk of your child being born with congenitally deformed outer ears.[291]

Mykrox   (see **Metolazone**)

Mylan-Nifedipine Extended Release   (see **Nifedipine**)

Myleran   (see **Busulfan**)

Myobloc   (see **Botulinum Toxin Type B**)

Myocet   (see **Doxorubicin**)

Myoflex   (see **Triethanolamine**)

Myozyme   (see **Alglucosidase alfa**)

Mysoline   (see **Primidone**)

Nabilone

Pronunciation guide: NAB-ih-lone

Drug classification: ANTI-VERTIGO (see section 53.20 in Table 14-1)

Brand names: *Cesamet*

Ototoxic effects:
    Cochlear:
        Tinnitus: (DFC)
    Vestibular:
        Ataxia: 12.8-14% [placebo 0] (CPS, DFC)
        Dizziness: (AHF, CPS)
        Equilibrium disorder: (DFC)
        Vertigo: 52-58.8% [49% above placebo results] (CPS, DFC)

Risk assessment: Class 2

Nabumetone

Pronunciation guide: nah-BYOO-meh-tone

Drug classification: NON-STEROIDAL ANTI-INFLAMMATORY DRUGS (NSAIDs) (see section 1.1 in Table 14-1)

Brand names: *Apo-Nabumetone, Relafen*

Ototoxic effects:
    Cochlear:
        Hearing loss: [1]
        Tinnitus: 4% (CPS, PDR)
    Vestibular:
        Dizziness: 6% (CPS, PDR)
        Vertigo: 0.9% (CPS, PDR)

Risk assessment: Class 2

Notes:

[1] In my files I have an anecdotal report of a lady that took **Nabumetone** for 6 days. The result was mild to moderate hearing loss and severe (high-pitched whine) tinnitus in both ears. The results are permanent as it is now 13 years later.

In my files I have a letter from Dr. Stephen Nagler advising that taking **Nabumetone** can result in permanent, severe tinnitus.

Nadolol

Pronunciation guide: NAY-doe-lole

Drug classification: BETA-ADRENERGIC-BLOCKING DRUGS (BETA-BLOCKERS) (see section 20.8.12 in Table 14-1)

Brand names: *Corgard*

Ototoxic effects:
    Cochlear:
        Tinnitus: 0.1-0.5% (CPS, PDR)
    Vestibular:
        Dizziness: 2-3% (CPS, PDR)

Risk assessment: Class 1

Nafarelin

Pronunciation guide: NAF-ah-reh-lynn

Drug classification: PITUITARY HORMONES (see section 40.44 in Table 14-1)

Brand names: *Synarel*

Ototoxic effects:
    Vestibular:
        Dizziness: 1% (CPS)
        Vertigo: 1% (CPS)
    Outer/Middle Ear:
        Earache/ear pain: 0.5% (CPS)

Risk assessment: Class 1

Nafidimide   (see **Amonafide**)

Naganol   (see **Suramin**)

Naglazyme   (see **Galsulfase**)

Nalbuphine

Pronunciation guide: NAL-byoo-feen

Drug classification: OPIATE AGONIST/ANTAGONIST DRUGS (see section 1.4.4 in Table 14-1)

Brand names: *Nubain*

Ototoxic effects:
    Vestibular:
        Dizziness/vertigo: 5% (CPS, PDR)
        Vertigo: (AHF, NDH)

Risk assessment: Class 1

Nalfon   (see **Fenoprofen**)

Nalidixic acid

Pronunciation guide: nal-ih-DIX-ik ASS-id

Drug classification: QUINOLONES (see section 7.4.48 in Table 14-1)

Brand names: *NegGram*

Ototoxic effects:
    Cochlear:
        Hearing disorder: (BNF)
    Vestibular:
        Dizziness: (CPS, PDR)
        Vertigo: (CPS, PDR)

Risk assessment: Class 2

Notes:
    See Chapter 7, "We 'Hear' With Our Eyes" for further information on this drug.

Naltrexone

Pronunciation guide: nal-TREX-own

Drug classification: NARCOTIC ANTAGONIST DRUGS (see section 1.7 in Table 14-1)

Brand names: *ReVia*

Ototoxic effects:
    Cochlear:
        Tinnitus: <1% (CPS, PDR)
    Vestibular:
        Dizziness: 3-13% (AHF, PDR)
    Outer/Middle Ear:
        Ears feel "plugged up": <1% (CPS, PDR)
        Earache/ear pain: <1% (CPS, PDR)

Risk assessment: Class 2

Namenda   (see **Memantine**)

Naprelan   (see **Naproxen**)

Naprosyn   (see **Naproxen**)

Naproxen

Pronunciation guide: nah-PROX-en

Drug classification: PROPIONIC ACIDS (see section 1.1.13 in Table 14-1)

Brand names: *Aleve, Anaprox, EC-Naprosyn, Naprelan, Naprosyn*

Ototoxic effects:
>   Cochlear:
>>   Hearing disorder: 1-3% (CPS, PDR)
>>   Hearing loss: <1% (CPS, PDR)
>>   Tinnitus: 3-9% (CPS, PDR)
>   Vestibular:
>>   Dizziness: 1-9% (CPS, PDR)
>>   Vertigo: 1-3% (CPS, PDR)
>   Outer/Middle Ear:
>>   Otitis media: <1% (CPS, PDR)
>   Unspecified/General Ear Conditions:
>>   Ear disorder: <1% (PDR)

Risk assessment: Class 4

Notes:

Hearing loss may be temporary or permanent. For example, in one study five people suffered hearing loss as the result of taking **Naproxen**. Of these, only two recovered their hearing when they stopped taking **Naproxen**. The other three were left with permanent hearing loss.[292]

I have an anecdotal report in my files of a woman who is experiencing hearing loss after being on **Naproxen** for 3 or 4 years. She is also experiencing dizziness and tinnitus.

I have another anecdotal report in my files of a man who had been taking **Naproxen** on and off for several years, sometimes in high doses, with never a ototoxic side effect. He now reports that when he takes **Naproxen**, he gets tinnitus for about 10 hours or so, then it goes away.

I have an anecdotal report in my files of a woman who took **Naproxen** for 1 month and now has a feeling of fullness in her ears and tinnitus. She explains, "I have a lot of clicking when I swallow. It is horrid. Everything sounds odd, even my own voice. I had no idea that anti-inflammatories could do this".

I also have an anecdotal report in my files of a woman who was prescribed **Naproxen** for a neck injury. She was instructed to take a 220 mg. tablet in the evening for 7 days. She stopped after the second day because "my ear was ringing very loudly, and I feel a significant loss in my hearing on my left side. It has been one week since I stopped the medicine, and the increased tinnitus and hearing loss has persisted".

I have yet another anecdotal report in my files of a woman who explained, "My tinnitus simply started 3 months ago while I was sitting. It is a constant tone at about 1,000 Hz in my right ear. A week later the sounds started in my left ear. Two months later I began to hear high pitched screeching sounds in both ears when moving my head left or right, or up or down. The only drug I take is Naproxen".

See Chapter 4 "Are You at Risk?" and Chapter 12, "Potpourri" for further information on this drug.

Naquasone   (see **Trichlormethiazide**)

Naratriptan

Pronunciation guide: nar-ah-TRIP-tan

Drug classification: SEROTONIN-RECEPTOR AGONISTS (see section 53.32 in Table 14-1)

Brand names: *Amerge*

Ototoxic effects:
    Cochlear:
        Hearing loss: <0.1% (CPS, PDR)
        Phonophobia: 0.1-1% (DFC)
        Tinnitus: 0.1-1% (CPS, PDR)
    Vestibular:
        Dizziness: 1-5% [<1% above placebo results] (CPS, PDR)
        Labyrinthitis: <0.1% (CPS, PDR)
        Vertigo: >1% (CPS, PDR)
    Outer/Middle Ear:
        Otorrhea: <0.1% (CPS)
        Otitis media: >1% (CPS, PDR)

Risk assessment: Class 2

Nardil   (see **Phenelzine**)

Naropin   (see **Ropivacaine**)

Nasacort   (see **Triamcinolone**)

Nasarel   (see **Flunisolide**)

Nascobal   (see **Cyanocobalamin**)

Nasonex   (see **Mometasone**)

Natalizumab

Pronunciation guide: nah-tah-LIZ-yoo-mab

Drug classification: MONOCLONAL ANTIBODIES (see section 7.17.8 in Table 14-1)

Brand names: *Tysabri*

Ototoxic effects:
    Vestibular:
        Dizziness: <10% (DIO)
        Vertigo: 6% [1% above placebo results] (DIO, NDH)

Risk assessment: Class 1

Navane   (see **Thiothixene**)

Navelbine   (see **Vinorelbine**)

Nebcin   (see **Tobramycin**)

Nebivolol

Pronunciation guide: neh-BIH-voh-lawl

Drug classification: BETA-ADRENERGIC-BLOCKING DRUGS (BETA-BLOCKERS) (see section 20.8.12 in Table 14-1)

Brand names: *Bystolic*

Ototoxic effects:
    Vestibular:
        Dizziness: 2-4% [<2% above placebo results] (AHF, PDR)
        Vertigo: (PDR)

Risk assessment: Class 1

Necon 1/35   (see **Ethinyl estradiol**)

Nefazodone

Pronunciation guide: neh-FAZ-oh-doan

Drug classification: ANTI-DEPRESSANT DRUGS (see section 60.1 in Table 14-1)

Brand names: *Serzone*

Ototoxic effects:
    Cochlear:
        Hearing loss: 0.1-1% (CPS, PDR)
        Hyperacusis: 0.1-1% (CPS, PDR)
        Tinnitus: 1.2-3% [0.1-2% above placebo results] (CPS, PDR)
    Vestibular:
        Ataxia: 2% [placebo 0] (CPS, PDR)
        Dizziness: 10-22% [5.2-18% above placebo results] (CPS, PDR)
        Vertigo: 0.1-1% (CPS, PDR)
        Vestibular disorder: <0.1% (CPS)
    Outer/Middle Ear:
        Earache/ear pain: 0.1-1% (CPS, PDR)
        Otitis media: <0.1% (CPS)

Risk assessment: Class 3

Notes:

    Banned from Canada in 2003, and in the USA in 2004.

NegGram   (see **Nalidixic acid**)

Nelarabine

Pronunciation guide: neh-LAR-uh-been

Drug classification: ANTI-NEOPLASTIC DRUGS (ANTI-CANCER DRUGS) (see section 14 in Table 14-1)

Brand names: *Arranon*, *Atriance*

Ototoxic effects:
    Vestibular:
        Ataxia: 0-9% (NDH, PDR)
        Dizziness: 0-21% (NDH, PDR)
        Nystagmus: 0-2%(PDR)
        Vestibular disorder: 0-2% (PDR)

Risk assessment: Class 2

Nembutal   (see **Pentobarbital**)

Neomycin (Fradiomycin)

Pronunciation guide: nee-oh-MYE-sin

Drug classification: AMINOGLYCOSIDES (see section 7.4.1 in Table 14-1)

Brand names: *Cicatrin*[1], *Cortisporin*[2], *Kenacomb*[3], *Mycifradin*, *Neosporin*[4], *Pediotic*[2],

Triacomb[3]

Ototoxic effects:
    Cochlear:
        Hearing loss: (CPS)
        Tinnitus: (CPS)
    Vestibular:
        Vestibular disorder: (CPS)
    Outer/Middle Ear:
        Burning/stinging: (CPS, PDR)
    Unspecified/General Ear Conditions:
        Ototoxicity: (CPS, PDR)

Risk assessment: Class 5

Notes:

[1] *Cicatrin* is a combination of **Bacitracin**, **Neomycin** and amino acids. (See the generic drug **Bacitracin** for its specific ototoxic properties.)

[2] *Cortisporin* and *Pediotic* are combinations of **Neomycin**, **Polymyxin B** and **Hydrocortisone**. Some formulations also include **Bacitracin**. (See the generic drugs **Bacitracin**, **Hydrocortisone** and **Polymyxin B** for their specific ototoxic properties.)

[3] *Kenacomb* and *Triacomb* are combinations of **Neomycin** and **Triamcinolone**, Nystatin and **Gramicidin**. (See the generic drugs **Gramicidin** and **Triamcinolone** for their specific ototoxic properties.)

Note that corticosteroids (like **Triamcinolone**) can damage the collagen that constitutes the middle layer of your tympanic membrane (eardrum) when you use drugs like these (CPS, PDR).

[4] *Neosporin* has several formulations. It may be a combination of **Neomycin** and **Polymyxin B**; a combination of **Neomycin**, **Polymyxin B** and **Gramicidin**; or a combination of **Neomycin**, **Polymyxin B** and **Bacitracin** (CPS, PDR). (See the generic drugs **Gramicidin** and **Polymyxin B** for their specific ototoxic properties.)

Neomycin is a neurotoxin and can destroy the tiny nerve fibers (hair cells) in your cochlea. The result is permanent sensorineural hearing loss in both ears (CPS, PDR). In fact, **Neomycin** is the most damaging to the cochlea of all the AMINOGLYCOSIDE antibiotics.[293]

Hearing loss often does not appear right away. This is because **Neomycin** is one of the slowest of the AMINOGLYCOSIDE antibiotics to clear from the inner ear fluids (endolymph and perilymph).[294] Therefore, while you are taking **Neomycin** you may not have any obvious symptoms to warn you that you are damaging your hearing. The result is that you may end up with partial or total hearing loss long after you have stopped taking **Neomycin** (CPS).

Therefore, if you take **Neomycin**, you should have serial vestibular (balance) and audiometric (hearing) tests—before, during and after treatment (CPS).

You are particularly at risk to **Neomycin** ototoxicity if you have kidney problems or if you have normal kidney function, but take **Neomycin** at higher doses, or for longer periods than recommended (CPS), if you are dehydrated, are an infant or are elderly (PDR). However, you can still end up with hearing loss, even if you only take **Neomycin** at the recommended dose (CPS).

Do not use **Neomycin** in your external ear canals if your eardrums are perforated (PDR). Also, be cautious when using the otic solution if you have longstanding chronic otitis media because of the possibility of ototoxicity. Note that **Neomycin** can cause stinging and burning if it gets into your middle ears (CPS, PDR).

Neomycin is quickly and almost totally absorbed from body surfaces (except the urinary bladder). As a result, you may end up with permanent hearing loss following topical application of minute amounts of **Neomycin** to both small and large surgical sites (CPS). Therefore, avoid prolonged use. Also, do not use large amounts in the treatment of skin infections following burns, trophic ulceration and other conditions where **Neomycin** might be absorbed (CPS). The same applies to open wounds and granulating surfaces. In these cases, serum concentrations are comparable to, and are often higher than those attained following oral and parenteral (injections and intravenous) therapy (PDR).

I have an anecdotal report in my files of a lady that took **Neomycin** for a leg infection. She lost almost all her hearing as a result. She explained, "I have an autoimmune disorder called Pyoderma gangrenosum. The doctor had me using *Neosporin* on the sores I had on my legs. When I questioned him about my hearing, he always had an excuse. Within 6 months, my hearing had dropped to 10% in my right ear. I can't even hear my own voice without my hearing aid".

Note that the ototoxic side effects are additive when **Neomycin** and **Polymyxin B** are taken together (*Cortisporin*, *Neosporin*) (CPS, PDR).

See Chapter 9, "Aminoglycoside Antibiotics are the Ototoxic 'Bad boys'" and Chapter 12, "Potpourri" for further information on this drug.

Neoral   (see **Cyclosporine**)

Neosar   (see **Cyclophosphamide**)

Neosporin   (see **Neomycin**)

Neptazane   (see **Methazolamide**)

Nesacaine   (see **Chloroprocaine**)

Netilmicin

Pronunciation guide: neh-till-MYE-sin

Drug classification: AMINOGLYCOSIDES (see section 7.4.1 in Table 14-1)

Brand names: *Netromycin*

Ototoxic effects:
    Cochlear:
        Hearing loss: (CPS, PDR)
        Tinnitus: (CPS, PDR)
    Vestibular:
        Dizziness: (CPS, PDR)
        Nystagmus: (PDR)
        Vertigo: (PDR)
        Vestibular disorder: (CPS)
    Unspecified/General Ear Conditions:
        Ototoxicity: (CPS)

Risk assessment: Class 5

Notes:

Netilmicin can cause balance problems and hearing loss. You are at greater risk if you have kidney problems, if you have been previously treated with ototoxic drugs, if you have been receiving higher doses than recommended, or if you are dehydrated (CPS, PDR).

About 4% of people taking **Netilmicin** show audiometric changes in the high frequencies while about 0.4% have a noticeable hearing loss (PDR). Ototoxicity can occur in 2.4% to 10% of the people taking **Netilmicin**.[295] Another source reports that **Netilmicin** has a 2% incidence rate of ototoxicity in newly-born babies.[296] Vestibular problems such as vertigo, dizziness and nystagmus occur about 0.7% of the time (PDR)

To avoid greater risk of ototoxic reactions, you should only take **Netilmicin** for 7 to 14 days.[297]

In order to have a chance at reversing developing ototoxicity, you must recognize the signs and symptoms of ototoxicity such as tinnitus, dizziness and hearing loss (CPS).

Netilmicin ototoxicity is usually permanent (PDR). Also, the ototoxic side effects of **Netilmicin** such as hearing loss may not appear until **after** you have finished taking a course of **Netilmicin** (PDR).

If you have kidney problems or hearing loss, you should have audiograms done both before and during treatment with **Netilmicin**. If you experience tinnitus or hearing loss, you should stop taking **Netilmicin** (CPS).

Do not take **Netilmicin** at the same time as Loop Diuretics such as **Furosemide** or **Ethacrynic acid** as they increase your chances of ototoxicity (CPS, PDR).

Also, you should not take **Netilmicin** at the same time, nor before or after taking other drugs that are ototoxic or nephrotoxic (damaging to your kidneys). Some such drugs include: **Acyclovir, Amikacin, Amphotericin B, Bacitracin, Cisplatin,** Cephaloridine, **Colistin, Gentamicin, Kanamycin, Neomycin, Paromomycin, Polymyxin B, Sisomicin, Streptomycin, Tobramycin, Vancomycin** and **Viomycin** (CPS, PDR).

See Chapter 9, "Aminoglycoside Antibiotics are the Ototoxic 'Bad boys'" for further information on this drug.

Netromycin   (see **Netilmicin**)

Neupro   (see **Rotigotine**)

Neurontin   (see **Gabapentin**)

Nevirapine

Pronunciation guide: neh-VEER-ah-pine

Drug classification: Anti-retroviral reverse transcriptase inhibitors (see section 7.17.1.4 in Table 14-1)

Brand names: *Viramune*

Ototoxic effects:
    Vestibular:
        Dizziness: 1-10% (CPS)
        Vertigo: (CPS, PDR)

Risk assessment: Class 1

Notes:

   Nevirapine overdose can cause vertigo (PDR).

Nexavar   (see **Sorafenib**)

Nexium   (see **Esomeprazole**)

Niacin (Vitamin B$_3$)

Pronunciation guide: NIE-ah-sin

Drug classification: VITAMINS (see section 75.4 in Table 14-1)

Brand names: *Niaspan*

Ototoxic effects:
    Cochlear:
        Tinnitus: 2% [1% above placebo results] (CPS)
    Vestibular:
        Dizziness: <2% (CPS)
        Vertigo: <2% (CPS)

Risk assessment: Class 1

Notes:

Niacin is used to treat certain kinds of tinnitus, however, it seems that in some cases, **Niacin** can actually make existing tinnitus worse.

I have an anecdotal report in my files of a person who took just one 50 mg. tablet of **Niacin** and reported, "The hissing in my ears became excruciating. This lasted for several hours, and then went. Since my tinnitus symptoms vary so much during the day and evening, I couldn't tell if this was a coincidence. I took a 2nd **Niacin** and again had dramatically worse hissing tinnitus".

I have another anecdotal report in my files of a man who found his tinnitus increased as he steadily increased his dose of **Niacin** from 100 mg. a day to 1,000 mg. a day.

It appears that **Niacin's** effect on tinnitus is temporary, so if you find you have increased tinnitus from taking **Niacin**, consider stopping taking it altogether, or take a reduced dose that doesn't affect your tinnitus.

Niaspan   (see **Niacin**)

Nicardipine

Pronunciation guide: nye-KAR-deh-peen

Drug classification: CALCIUM-CHANNEL-BLOCKING DRUGS (CALCIUM BLOCKERS) (see section 20.8.16 in Table 14-1)

Brand names: *Cardene*

Ototoxic effects:
    Cochlear:
        Tinnitus: <1% (CPS, PDR)
    Vestibular:
        Ataxia: <1% (CPS)
        Dizziness: 1.4-11% [0.9-6.9% above placebo results] (CPS, PDR)
        Vertigo: <1% (AHF, CPS)
    Unspecified/General Ear Conditions:
        Ear disorder: (AHF, PDR)

Risk assessment: Class 2

Nicoderm   (see **Nicotine**)

Nicorette   (see **Nicotine**)

Nicotine

Pronunciation guide: NIK-oh-teen

Drug classification: CHOLINERGIC AGONIST DRUGS (see section 17.12.1 in Table 14-1)

Brand names: *Habitrol, Nicoderm, Nicorette, Nicotrol*

Ototoxic effects:
    Cochlear:
        Hearing disorder: (CPS, PDR)
        Tinnitus: (CPS)
    Vestibular:
        Dizziness: 2.1-19% (CPS, PDR)
        Vertigo: 3.1% [2.3% above placebo results] (CPS)
    Outer/Middle Ear:
        Earache/ear pain: 1-2% (CPS, PDR)
        Otitis media: 0.4-1.1% [<0.7% above placebo results] (CPS)
    Unspecified/General Ear Conditions:
        Ear disorder: <1% (CPS)

Risk assessment: Class 2

Notes:

    See Chapter 8, "The Sinister Partnership Between Ototoxic Agents and Noise" for further information on this drug.

Nicotrol   (see **Nicotine**)

NidaGel   (see **Metronidazole**)

Nifedipine

Pronunciation guide: nye-FED-ih-peen

Drug classification: CALCIUM-CHANNEL-BLOCKING DRUGS (CALCIUM BLOCKERS) (see section 20.8.16 in Table 14-1)

Brand names: *Adalat, Mylan-Nifedipine Extended Release, Procardia*

Ototoxic effects:
    Cochlear:
        Hearing loss: [1]
        Tinnitus: <1% (CPS, PDR)

Vestibular:

Ataxia: <1% (CPS, PDR)

Dizziness: 2.3-27% [2-12% above placebo results] (CPS, PDR)

Loss of Balance: <2% (PDR)

Vertigo: <3% (CPS, PDR)

Risk assessment: Class 2

Notes:

[1] I have an anecdotal report in my files of a woman who now has permanent hearing loss thought to be the result of taking **Nifedipine**.

Caution: Eating grapefruit or drinking grapefruit juice during the time you are taking this drug may make the listed side effects worse than shown here. In fact, the latest report from the FDA warns that taking **Nifedipine** with grapefruit juice can increase the potency of **Nifedipine** by 200%.[298]

See Chapter 11, "Grapefruit Juice and Ototoxic Drugs" for further information on this drug.

Nilotinib

Pronunciation guide: nye-low-TIH-nib

Drug classification: TYROSINE KINASE INHIBITORS (see section 14.40 in Table 14-1)

Brand names: *Tasigna*

Ototoxic effects:

Cochlear:

Hearing loss: (CPS, PDR)

Vestibular:

Dizziness: 1-10% (NDH, PDR)

Vertigo: 1-10% (NDH, PDR)

Outer/Middle Ear:

Earache/ear pain: (CPS, PDR)

Risk assessment: Class 2

Nilvadipine

Pronunciation guide: nil-VAH-dih-peen

Drug classification: CALCIUM-CHANNEL-BLOCKING DRUGS (CALCIUM BLOCKERS) (see section 20.8.16 in Table 14-1)

Brand names: *Nivadil*

Ototoxic effects:

Cochlear:

Tinnitus: <0.1% (San, She)

Vestibular:

Dizziness: 0.1-5%

Unspecified/General Ear Conditions:
Ototoxicity: (San)

Risk assessment: Class 2

Notes:

Adverse reactions include dizziness and tinnitus.[299]

Nimodipine

Pronunciation guide: nye-MOE-dih-peen

Drug classification: CALCIUM-CHANNEL-BLOCKING DRUGS (CALCIUM BLOCKERS) (see section 20.8.16 in Table 14-1)

Brand names: *Nimotop*

Ototoxic effects:
Cochlear:
Tinnitus: (San, She)
Vestibular:
Dizziness: <1% (AHF, RXL)
Unspecified/General Ear Conditions:
Ototoxicity: (San)

Risk assessment: Class 2

Notes:

Caution: Eating grapefruit or drinking grapefruit juice during the time you are taking this drug may make the listed side effects worse than shown here.

See Chapter 11, "Grapefruit Juice and Ototoxic Drugs" for further information on this drug.

Nimotop   (see **Nimodipine**)

Nipent   (see **Pentostatin**)

Nisoldipine

Pronunciation guide: nih-SAWL-dih-peen

Drug classification: CALCIUM-CHANNEL-BLOCKING DRUGS (CALCIUM BLOCKERS) (see section 20.8.16 in Table 14-1)

Brand names: *Sular*

Ototoxic effects:
Tinnitus: <1% (DFC, PDR)
Vestibular:
Ataxia: <1% (PDR)
Dizziness: 5-10% [1-6% above placebo results] (NDH, PDR)
Vertigo: <1% (DFC, PDR)

Outer/Middle Ear:
    Earache/ear pain: <1% (DFC, PDR)
    Otitis media: <1% (DFC, PDR)

Risk assessment: Class 2

Notes:

Caution: Eating grapefruit or drinking grapefruit juice during the time you are taking this drug may make the listed side effects worse than shown here. In fact, taking **Nisoldipine** with grapefruit juice can increase the potency of **Nisoldipine** by as much as 900%!

See Chapter 11, "Grapefruit Juice and Ototoxic Drugs" for further information on this drug.

Nitazoxanide

Pronunciation guide: nye-tah-ZOX-ah-nide

Drug classification: ANTI-PROTOZOALS (see section 7.14 in Table 14-1)

Brand names: *Alinia*

Ototoxic effects:
    Vestibular:
        Dizziness: <1% (DFC, RXL)
    Outer/Middle Ear:
        Earache/ear pain: <1% (DFC, RXL)

Risk assessment: Class 1

Nitisinone

Pronunciation guide: nih-TIS-ih-known

Drug classification: ENZYME INHIBITORS (see section 32.4 in Table 14-1)

Brand names: *Orfadin*

Ototoxic effects:
    Outer/Middle Ear:
        Otitis: <1% (DFC)

Risk assessment: Class 1

Nitrazadon   (see **Nitrazepam**)

Nitrazepam

Pronunciation guide: nie-TRA-zeh-pam

Drug classification: BENZODIAZEPINES (see section 60.12.8 in Table 14-1)

Brand names: *Mogadon, Nitrazadon*

Ototoxic effects:
>   Vestibular:
>>   Ataxia: (BNF, CPS)
>>   Dizziness: (CPS)
>>   Vertigo: (BNF)
>   Unspecified/General Ear Conditions:
>>   Ototoxicity: (San)

Risk assessment: Class 2

Notes:

>   Common ototoxic side effects include ataxia and dizziness[300] and vertigo.[301]

>   See Chapter 10 "Beware of Benzodiazepines—Don't Let This Nasty Time-Bomb Ambush You and Your Ears" for further information on this drug.

Nitrendipine

Pronunciation guide: nie-TREN-dih-peen

Drug classification: CALCIUM-CHANNEL-BLOCKING DRUGS (CALCIUM BLOCKERS) (see section 20.8.16 in Table 14-1)

Brand names: *Cardif, Nitrepin*

Ototoxic effects:
>   Cochlear:
>>   Tinnitus: (San, She)
>   Unspecified/General Ear Conditions:
>>   Ototoxicity: (San)

Risk assessment: Class 2

Nitrepin   (see **Nitrendipine**)

Nitro-Bid   (see **Nitroglycerin**)

Nitro-Dur   (see **Nitroglycerin**)

Nitrofurantoin

Pronunciation guide: nye-troe-fyoor-AN-toy-in

Drug classification: URINARY ANTI-INFECTIVES (see section 7.20 in Table 14-1)

Brand names: *Furadantin, MacroBID, Macrodantin*

Ototoxic effects:
>   Vestibular:
>>   Ataxia: (NTP)
>>   Dizziness: <1% (CPS, PDR)
>>   Nystagmus: (CPS, PDR)
>>   Vertigo: (CPS, PDR)

Risk assessment: Class 1

Notes:

See Chapter 7, "We 'Hear' With Our Eyes" for further information on this drug.

Nitrogen mustard   (see **Mechlorethamine**)

Nitroglycerin

Pronunciation guide: nye-troe-GLIH-ser-in

Drug classification: CORONARY VASODILATORS (see section 20.8.40.1 in Table 14-1)

Brand names: *Minitran, Nitro-Bid, Nitro-Dur, Nitrostat, Transderm-Nitro, Trinipatch*

Ototoxic effects:
Vestibular:
Dizziness: (CPS, PDR)
Vertigo: (CPS, PDR)

Risk assessment: Class 1

Notes:

See Chapter 7, "We 'Hear' With Our Eyes" for further information on this drug.

Nitrostat   (see **Nitroglycerin**)

Nivadil   (see **Nilvadipine**)

Nizoral   (see **Ketoconazole**)

Noctamide   (see **Lormetazepam**)

Nolvadex   (see **Tamoxifen**)

Norco   (see **Hydrocodone**)

Norditropin   (see **Somatropin**)

Norelgestromin

Pronunciation guide: nor-ell-JESS-troe-min

Drug classification: PROGESTINS (see section 40.32 in Table 14-1)

Brand names: *Evra* [1]

Ototoxic effects:
Cochlear:
Hearing loss: [2]
Tinnitus: (CPS)

Vestibular:
    Dizziness: 3% (CPS)
    Vertigo: (CPS)
    Vestibular disorder: (CPS)
Outer/Middle Ear:
    Earache/ear pain: (CPS)
    Otosclerosis: (CPS)
Unspecified/General Ear Conditions:
    Ear disorder: (CPS)

Risk assessment: Class 2

Notes:

[1] *Evra* is a combination of **Norelgestromin** and **Ethinyl estradiol**. (See the generic drug **Ethinyl estradiol** for its specific ototoxic properties.)

[2] PROGESTINS (such as **Norelgestromin**) can cause hearing loss in women. PROGESTINS are typically used in hormone replacement therapy (HRT) although **Norelgestromin** is used in CONTRACEPTIVES. One study found women who take the most common form of HRT had a hearing loss of 10% to 30% greater than women who have not taken HRT.[302] That's a loss equivalent to aging another 10 years or so. This hearing loss is particularly noticeable when trying to understand someone in a noisy environment.[303] The results showed that women who had received progestin had problems both in their cochleas and in the auditory circuits in their brains.

The CPS lists otosclerosis as a side effect of taking **Norelgestromin** in some women. Since otosclerosis is exacerbated by hormonal changes in women at puberty, pregnancy and menopause, women taking CONTRACEPTIVES containing **Norelgestromin** and who are also prone to otosclerosis could expect similar results.

Norethindrone

Pronunciation guide: nor-eth-IN-drone

Drug classification: CONTRACEPTIVES (see section 40.12 in Table 14-1)

Brand names: *Activelle, Norinyl*[1], *Ortho-Novum*[1]

Ototoxic effects:
Cochlear:
    Auditory disorder: (CPS)
Vestibular:
    Dizziness: (CPS, PDR)
Unspecified/General Ear Conditions:
    Ear disorder: 1.1% [placebo 0] (CPS)

Risk assessment: Class 1

Notes:

[1] *Norinyl* and *Ortho-Novum* are combinations of **Norethindrone** and Mestranol. (**Norethindrone** is the ototoxic agent.)

See the drug **Medroxyprogesterone** for more information on auditory disorder (hearing loss) as **Norethindrone** is a PROGESTIN class of drug and likely causes similar hearing loss as other drugs in this class.

Norethindrone—Ethinyl estradiol   (see **Ethinyl estradiol**)

Norethindrone—Mestranol   (see **Norethindrone**)

Norflex   (see **Orphenadrine**)

Norfloxacin

Pronunciation guide: nor-FLOX-ah-sin

Drug classification: QUINOLONES (see section 7.4.48 in Table 14-1)

Brand names: *Apo-Norflox, Chibroxin, Noroxin, Novo-Norfloxacin*

Ototoxic effects:
  Cochlear:
    Hearing disorder: (BNF)
    Hearing loss: (CPS, PDR)
    Tinnitus: (CPS, PDR)
  Vestibular:
    Ataxia: (CPS, PDR)
    Dizziness: 1.2-2.6% (CPS, PDR)
    Nystagmus: (CPS, PDR)
    Vertigo: (CPS)

Risk assessment: Class 2

Notes:

Hearing loss is transient and occurs rarely (CPS, PDR).

See Chapter 7, "We 'Hear' With Our Eyes" for further information on this drug.

Norgesic   (see **Acetylsalicylic acid**)

Norgestimate—Ethinyl estradiol   (see **Ethinyl estradiol**)

Norinyl   (see **Norethindrone**)

Normodyne   (see **Labetalol**)

Noroxin   (see **Norfloxacin**)

Norpramin   (see **Desipramine**)

Nortriptyline

Pronunciation guide: nor-TRIP-tih-leen

Drug classification: TRICYCLIC ANTI-DEPRESSANTS (see section 60.1.8 in Table 14-1)

Brand names: *Apo-Nortriptyline*, *Aventyl*, *Pamelor*

Ototoxic effects:
    Cochlear:
        Tinnitus: (CPS, PDR)
    Vestibular:
        Ataxia: (CPS, PDR)
        Dizziness: >10% (NDH, PDR)

Risk assessment: Class 2

Norvasc   (see **Amlodipine**)

Norvir   (see **Ritonavir**)

Novo-Amiodarone   (see **Amiodarone**)

Novo-AZT   (see **Zidovudine**)

Novobiocin

Pronunciation guide: noe-voe-BIE-oh-sin

Drug classification: ANTI-BACTERIAL DRUGS (see section 7.4 in Table 14-1)

Brand names: *Albamycin-T*, *Panalba* [1]

Ototoxic effects:
    Cochlear:
        Hearing loss: [2]

Risk assessment: Not enough information to rate

Notes:

[1] *Panalba* is a combination of **Novobiocin** and **Tetracycline**. (See the generic drug **Tetracycline** for its specific ototoxic properties.)

Panalba was introduced in 1957, but the FDA yanked it off the market in the USA in 1970 because of its many dangerous side effects. It is apparently still sold in 33 other countries under the brand name *Albamycin-T*.[304]

[2] I have an anecdotal report in my files of a man who took *Panalba* around 1960 that cost him his hearing. He wrote, "It was discontinued as being extremely ototoxic".

It appears that the combination of **Novobiocin** and **Tetracycline** caused the ototoxicity. So far, I have not seen hard evidence that **Novobiocin** by itself is ototoxic.

This drug combination has not been sold in the USA for over 33 years, so ototoxic information on it is hard to find.

Novo-Butazone   (see **Phenylbutazone**)

Novocain   (see **Procaine**)

Novo-Clopate   (see **Clorazepate**)

Novo-Cycloprine   (see **Cyclobenzaprine**)

Novo-Difenac   (see **Diclofenac**)

Novo-Diltazem   (see **Diltiazem**)

Novo-Divalproex   (see **Divalproex**)

Novo-Famotidine   (see **Famotidine**)

Novo-Fluoxetine   (see **Fluoxetine**)

Novo-Fluvoxamine   (see **Fluvoxamine**)

Novo-Gabapentin   (see **Gabapentin**)

Novo-Minocycline   (see **Minocycline**)

NovoMix   (see **Insulin aspart**)

Novo-Moclobemide   (see **Moclobemide**)

Novo-Norfloxacin   (see **Norfloxacin**)

Novo-Selegiline   (see **Selegiline**)

Novo-Sucralate   (see **Sucralfate**)

Novo-Veramil   (see **Verapamil**)

Nplate   (see **Romiplostim**)

Nubain   (see **Nalbuphine**)

Nucynta   (see **Tapentadol**)

NuLev   (see **Hyoscyamine**)

Nuprin   (see **Ibuprofen**)

NuvaRing   (see **Ethinyl estradiol**)

Nytol   (see **Diphenhydramine**)

Occlusal   (see **Salicylic acid**)

Octonox   (see **Lormetazepam**)

Octreotide

Pronunciation guide: ock-TREE-oh-tide

Drug classification: SOMATOSTATIC DRUGS (see section 40.48 in Table 14-1)

Brand names: *Sandostatin, Sandostatin LAR*

Ototoxic effects:
    Cochlear:
        Hearing loss: 1-2% (CPS, PDR)
        Tinnitus: 1-4% (CPS, PDR)
    Vestibular:
        Ataxia: 1-4% (PDR)
        Dizziness: 1.5-20% [<4% above placebo results] (CPS, PDR)
        Vertigo: 1.6-3.5% (CPS, PDR)
    Outer/Middle Ear:
        Earache/ear pain: 5-15% (DFC, PDR)
        Otitis: 1-2% (CPS, PDR)
        Otitis media: 1.8-15% (CPS, PDR)
        Otorrhea: 1-2% (CPS)
    Unspecified/General Ear Conditions:
        Ear disorder: 2.3% (CPS)

Risk assessment: Class 4

Ofloxacin

Pronunciation guide: oh-FLOX-ah-sin

Drug classification: QUINOLONES (see section 7.4.48 in Table 14-1)

Brand names: *Floxin*

Ototoxic effects:
    Cochlear:
        Hearing disorder: (AHF, CPS)
        Hearing loss: <1% (CPS, PDR)
        Tinnitus: 0.3-1% (CPS, PDR)
    Vestibular:
        Ataxia: (CPS, PDR)
        Dizziness: 1-5% (CPS, PDR)
        Nystagmus: (CPS, PDR)
        Vertigo: 0.5-1% (CPS, PDR)
        Vestibular disorder: (CPS)

Outer/Middle Ear:
    Earache/ear pain: 1% (AHF, PDR)
    Otitis externa: (AHF, PDR)
    Otitis media: (AHF)
    Otorrhagia: 0.6% (AHF, PDR)

Risk assessment: Class 3

Notes:

Hearing loss is usually reversible after discontinuing drug treatment (CPS, PDR).

Oil of Wintergreen (see **Methyl salicylate**)

Olanzapine

Pronunciation guide: oh-LAN-zah-peen

Drug classification: SALICYLATES (see section 1.1.16 in Table 14-1)

Brand names: *Symbyax* [1], *Zyprexa*

Ototoxic effects:
    Cochlear:
        Hearing loss: 0.1-1% (AHF, PDR)
        Tinnitus: >1% (AHF, PDR)
    Vestibular:
        Ataxia: 6% [5% above placebo results] (AHF, PDR)
        Dizziness: 4-18% [2-12% above placebo results] (CPS, PDR)
        Nystagmus: <0.1% (AHF, PDR)
        Vertigo: 0.1-1% (AHF, PDR)
    Outer/Middle Ear:
        Earache/ear pain: 0.1-1% (AHF, PDR)
        Otitis media: 2% [placebo 0] (PDR)

Risk assessment: Class 3

Notes:

[1] *Symbyax* is a combination of **Olanzapine** and **Fluoxetine**. (See the generic drug **Fluoxetine** for its specific ototoxic properties.)

Olmesartan

Pronunciation guide: all-mah-SAR-tan

Drug classification: ANGIOTENSIN-2-RECEPTOR ANTAGONISTS (see section 20.8.4 in Table 14-1)

Brand names: *Benicar, Olmetec, Olmetec Plus* [1]

Ototoxic effects:
    Vestibular:
        Dizziness: 3% (2% above placebo results] (AHF, PDR)
        Vertigo: 0.5-1% (CPS, PDR)

Risk assessment: Class 1

Notes:

[1] *Olmetec Plus* is a combination of **Olmesartan** and **Hydrochlorothiazide**. (See the generic drug **Hydrochlorothiazide** for its specific ototoxic properties.)

I have an anecdotal report in my files of a man that after taking **Olmesartan** for two weeks reported: "I began to notice that I was running into walls and felt like I was unbalanced all the time. Sometimes even sitting down I would feel a sensation as if I was being pushed or rocked. [Note: although vertigo is normally a spinning sensation, it can also be a rocking sensation such as this man experienced.] I also felt a distinct pressure in both my ears that I've never experienced before. I stopped the *Benicar* after about two months, but I've had the balance problems ever since. When I stopped the *Benicar*, the ear pressure went away after about 2 weeks, and when I resumed the *Benicar* one time after that, the ear pressure came back! I also experienced a drop in hearing in the ear that I had hearing in".

Olmetec   (see **Olmesartan**)

Olmetec Plus   (see **Olmesartan**)

Olsalazine

Pronunciation guide: all-SAL-uh-zeen

Drug classification: SALICYLATES (see section 1.1.16 in Table 14-1)

Brand names: *Dipentum*

Ototoxic effects:
    Cochlear:
        Tinnitus: <1% (DFC, PDR)
    Vestibular:
        Dizziness: 1% [placebo 0] (CPS, PDR)
        Dizziness/vertigo: 1% [placebo 0] (CPS, PDR)
        Vertigo: (DFC, NDH)

Risk assessment: Class 1

Omalizumab

Pronunciation guide: oh-mah-LIZ-uh-mab

Drug classification: MONOCLONAL ANTIBODIES (see section 7.17.8 in Table 14-1)

Brand names: *Xolair*

Ototoxic effects:
    Vestibular:
        Dizziness: 3% [1% above placebo results] (DFC, PDR)

Outer/Middle Ear:
Earache/ear pain: 2% [1% above placebo results] (DFC, PDR)

Risk assessment: Class 1

Omega-3-acid ethyl esters

Pronunciation guide: oh-MAY-gah three ASS-id ETH-el ESS-ters

Drug classification: ANTI-LIPEMICS (see section 20.12 in Table 14-1)

Brand names: *Lovaza*

Ototoxic effects:
Vestibular:
Dizziness: (PDR)
Vertigo: (PDR)

Risk assessment: Class 1

Omeprazole

Pronunciation guide: oh-ME-pray-zole

Drug classification: PROTON PUMP INHIBITORS (see section 34.8.4 in Table 14-1)

Brand names: *Losec, Prilosec, Zegerid*

Ototoxic effects:
Cochlear:
Hearing loss: [1]
Tinnitus: <1% (AHF, PDR)
Vestibular:
Dizziness: 1.5% [placebo 0] (CPS, PDR)
Vertigo: <1% (CPS, PDR)
Outer/Middle Ear:
Earache/ear pain: [1]
Otitis media: 23% (AHF)
Unspecified/General Ear Conditions:
Ototoxicity: [1]

Risk assessment: Class 3

Notes:

[1] In a report by the FDA on **Omeprazole** (*Prilosec*) dated August 14, 2000, ototoxic side effects reported to the FDA at that time included 68 cases of tinnitus, 21 cases of vertigo, 17 incidents of hearing loss, 14 episodes of dizziness, 10 cases of ear pain and 2 cases of "ototoxicity". Of the hearing loss cases, 35% proved to be permanent. The remaining 65% of the cases was split between hearing returning to "normal" or showing some degree of improvement.[305]

A 42-year-old man with no known allergies was placed on **Omeprazole** 20 mg. daily for the treatment of GERD. Seven days later this man experienced hearing loss in one ear. He stopped taking the **Omeprazole** at that time, but his hearing loss only improved slightly.[306]

Omnaris   (see **Ciclesonide**)

Omnipaque   (see **Iohexol**)

Omniscan   (see **Gadodiamide**)

Oncovin   (see **Vincristine**)

Ondansetron

Pronunciation guide: on-DAN-seh-tron

Drug classification: Serotonin-receptor antagonists (see section 34.1.4 in Table 14-1)

Brand names: *Zofran*

Ototoxic effects:
    Vestibular:
        Ataxia: (AHF)
        Dizziness: 4-12% (AHF)

Risk assessment: Class 1

Ony-clear   (see **Benzalkonium**)

OptiMARK   (see **Gadoversetamide**)

Optimine   (see **Azatadine**)

Optiray   (see **Ioversol**)

Orafen   (see **Ketoprofen**)

Oraflex   (see **Benoxaprofen**)

Oramorph   (see **Morphine**)

Orap   (see **Pimozide**)

Orapred   (see **Prednisolone**)

Orencia   (see **Abatacept**)

Oretic   (see **Hydrochlorothiazide**)

Oreticyl   (see **Deserpidine**)

Orfadin   (see **Nitisinone**)

Orinase   (see **Tolbutamide**)

Orlistat

Pronunciation guide: ORE-lih-stat

Drug classification: LIPASE INHIBITORS (see section 34.20 in Table 14-1)

Brand names: *Xenical*

Ototoxic effects:
  Vestibular:
    Dizziness: 5.2% [0.2% above placebo results] (CPS, PDR)
  Outer/Middle Ear:
    Otitis: 2.9-4.3% [0.4-0.9% above placebo results] (CPS, PDR)

Risk assessment: Class 1

Ornade Spansule   (see **Phenylpropanolamine**)

Orphenadrine

Pronunciation guide: ore-FEN-ah-dreen

Drug classification: H_1 RECEPTOR ANTAGONISTS (see section 10.1 in Table 14-1)

Brand names: *Norflex*

Ototoxic effects:
  Cochlear:
    Tinnitus: (NTP)
  Vestibular:
    Ataxia: (NTP)
    Dizziness: (CPS, PDR)
    Nystagmus: (NTP)
    Vertigo: (NTP)

Risk assessment: Class 1

Notes:
  See Chapter 7, "We 'Hear' With Our Eyes" for further information on this drug.

Ortho   (see **Ethinyl estradiol**)

Ortho 7/7/7   (see **Ethinyl estradiol**)

Ortho-Cept   (see **Ethinyl estradiol**)

Orthoclone OKT3   (see **Muromonab-CD3**)

Ortho-Novum   (see **Norethindrone**)

Orudis   (see **Ketoprofen**)

Oruvail   (see **Ketoprofen**)

Oseltamivir

Pronunciation guide: oz-el-TAM-ih-veer

Drug classification: ANTI-RETROVIRAL PROTEASE INHIBITORS (see section 7.17.1.1 in Table 14-1)

Brand names: *Tamiflu*

Ototoxic effects:
    Vestibular:
        Dizziness: 2.1% [same as placebo] (CPS, PDR)
        Vertigo: 1% [0.6% above placebo results] (CPS, PDR)
    Unspecified/General Ear Conditions:
        Ear disorder: 2% [1% above placebo results] (AHF, PDR)

Risk assessment: Class 1

Osmitrol   (see **Mannitol**)

Osmovist   (see **Iotrolan**)

Ostoforte   (see **Ergocalciferal**)

Oxaliplatin

Pronunciation guide: ox-ah-lih-PLAH-tin

Drug classification: ALKYLATING DRUGS (see section 14.1 in Table 14-1)

Brand names: *Eloxatin*

Ototoxic effects:
    Cochlear:
        Hearing loss: (DFC, PDR)
    Vestibular:
        Ataxia: 2-5% (CPS, PDR)
        Dizziness 7-15% (NDH, PDR)
        Vertigo: 2-5% (CPS, PDR)
    Unspecified/General Ear Conditions:
        Ototoxicity: (BNF)

Risk assessment: Class 3

Oxaprozin

Pronunciation guide: OK-ah-proe-zin

Drug classification: PROPIONIC ACIDS (see section 1.1.13 in Table 14-1)

Brand names: *Apo-Oxaprozin, Daypro*

Ototoxic effects:
    Cochlear:
        Hearing loss: <1% (CPS, PDR)
        Tinnitus: 1-3% (CPS, PDR)

Risk assessment: Class 2

Notes:

I have an anecdotal report in my files of a woman who took **Oxaprozin**. After a few months on it, her hearing, which had been slowly dropping, took a nosedive.

Oxazepam

Pronunciation guide: ox-AZ-eh-pam

Drug classification: BENZODIAZEPINES (see section 60.12.8 in Table 14-1)

Brand names: *Serax*

Ototoxic effects:
    Cochlear:
        Tinnitus: (She)
    Vestibular:
        Ataxia: (NTP, PDR)
        Dizziness: (CPS, PDR)
        Nystagmus: (NTP)
        Vertigo: (CPS, PDR)

Risk assessment: Class 2

Notes:

See Chapter 10 "Beware of Benzodiazepines—Don't Let This Nasty Time-Bomb Ambush You and Your Ears" for further information on this drug.

Oxcarbazepine

Pronunciation guide: ox-kar-BAZ-eh-peen

Drug classification: ANTI-CONVULSANT DRUGS (see section 53.12 in Table 14-1)

Brand names: *Trileptal*

Ototoxic effects:
    Cochlear:
        Tinnitus: (CPS, PDR)

Vestibular:
Ataxia: 1-31% [<26% above placebo results] (CPS, PDR)
Dizziness: 1.3-49% [<36% above placebo results] (CPS, PDR)
Nystagmus: 1.1-26% [<21% above placebo results] (CPS, PDR)
Vertigo: 2-15% [<13% above placebo results] (CPS, PDR)
Outer/Middle Ear:
Earache/ear pain: 1-2% (CPS, PDR)
Otitis: 2% (CPS, PDR)
Otitis externa: (CPS, PDR)

Risk assessment: Class 4

Oxprenolol

Pronunciation guide: ox-PREN-oh-lole

Drug classification: BETA-ADRENERGIC-BLOCKING DRUGS (BETA-BLOCKERS) (see section 20.8.12 in Table 14-1)

Brand names: *Slow-Trasicor*, *Trasicor*

Ototoxic effects:
Cochlear:
Tinnitus: (CPS)
Vestibular:
Dizziness: (CPS)
Vertigo: (CPS)

Risk assessment: Class 1

Oxy IR   (see **Oxycodone**)

Oxybutynin

Pronunciation guide: ox-ih-BYOO-tih-nin

Drug classification: MUSCARINIC RECEPTOR ANTAGONISTS (see section 17.1.1 in Table 14-1)

Brand names: *Uromax*

Ototoxic effects:
Cochlear:
Tinnitus: <1% (CPS)
Vestibular:
Dizziness: 6.4-15.3% (CPS)

Risk assessment: Class 1

Oxycodone

Pronunciation guide: ox-ih-KOE-done

Drug classification: Opiate agonist drugs (see section 1.4.1 in Table 14-1)

Brand names: *OxyContin, Oxy IR, Percocet* [1], *Percodan* [2], *Roxicet* [1], *Supeudol*

Ototoxic effects:
    Cochlear:
        Hearing loss: (PDR)
        Tinnitus: <1% (CPS, PDR)
    Vestibular:
        Ataxia: <1% (CPS, PDR)
        Dizziness: 13-16% [4-7% above placebo results] (CPS, PDR)
        Vertigo: <1% (CPS, PDR)

Risk assessment: Class 2

Notes:

[1] *Percocet* and *Roxicet* are combinations of **Oxycodone** and **APAP** (**Acetaminophen**). (See the generic drug **Acetaminophen** for its specific ototoxic properties.)

[2] *Percodan* is a combination of **Oxycodone** and *Aspirin* (**Acetylsalicylic acid**). (See the generic drug **Acetylsalicylic acid** for its specific ototoxic properties.)

Hearing loss is likely due to the **Acetaminophen** in *Percocet* and *Roxicet*, rather than due to the ototoxicity of **Oxycodone** itself. (See the generic drug **Acetaminophen** for more on its specific ototoxic properties.) Likewise, in *Percodan*, hearing loss may be due to the **Acetylsalicylic acid** (*Aspirin*), rather than the **Oxycodone**. (See the generic drug **Acetylsalicylic acid** for more on its specific ototoxic properties.)

OxyContin   (see **Oxycodone**)

Ozolinone

Pronunciation guide: oh-ZOE-lih-noan

Drug classification: Diuretics—loop (see section 30.5.4 in Table 14-1)

Brand names: —

Ototoxic effects:
    Unspecified/General Ear Conditions:
        Ototoxicity: [307]

Risk assessment: Not enough information to rate

Pabalate   (see **Sodium salicylate**)

Pacerone   (see **Amiodarone**)

Paclitaxel

Pronunciation guide: pak-lih-TAX-ell

Drug classification: ANTI-NEOPLASTICS (ANTI-CANCER DRUGS) (see section 14 in Table 14-1)

Brand names: *Taxol*

Ototoxic effects:
    Cochlear:
        Hearing loss: (DFC, PDR)
        Tinnitus: (DFC, PDR)
    Vestibular:
        Ataxia: <1% (AHF, PDR)

Risk assessment: Class 2

Pacyl   (see **Isoxicam**)

Paliperidone

Pronunciation guide: pahl-ee-PEER-ih-dohn

Drug classification: ANTIPSYCHOTIC DRUGS (see section 60.8 in Table 14-1)

Brand names: *Invega, Invega Sustenna*

Ototoxic effects:
    Vestibular:
        Dizziness: 1-6% [<2% above placebo results] (AHF, PDR)
        Vertigo: (PDR)

Risk assessment: Class 1

Palivizumab

Pronunciation guide: pal-ih-VIH-zuh-mab

Drug classification: MONOCLONAL ANTIBODIES (see section 7.17.8 in Table 14-1)

Brand names: *Synagis*

Ototoxic effects:
    Outer/Middle Ear:
        Otitis media: 36.4-41.9% [1.8-1.9% above placebo results] (CPS, PDR)
    Unspecified/General Ear Conditions:
        Ear disorder: >1% (CPS)

Risk assessment: Class 1

Palonosetron

Pronunciation guide: pal-on-OSS-eh-tron

Drug classification: Serotonin 5-HT$_3$ RECEPTOR ANTAGONISTS (see section 17.8.1 in Table 14-1)

Brand names: *Aloxi*

Ototoxic effects:
    Cochlear:
        Tinnitus: <1% (DFC, PDR)
    Vestibular:
        Dizziness: 1% (DFC, PDR)

Risk assessment: Class 1

Pamelor   (see **Nortriptyline**)

Panalba   (see **Novobiocin**)

Panectyl   (see **Trimeprazine**)

Panimycin   (see **Dibekacin**)

Panitumumab

Pronunciation guide: pan-eh-TOO-moo-mab

Drug classification: MONOCLONAL ANTIBODIES (see section 7.17.8 in Table 14-1)

Brand names: *Vectibix*

Ototoxic effects:
    Vestibular:
        Dizziness: 1-2% (CPS)
        Vertigo: 1-2% (CPS)

Risk assessment: Class 1

Pan-Streptomycin   (see **Streptomycin**)

Panto   (see **Pantoprazole**)

Panto IV   (see **Pantoprazole**)

Pantoloc   (see **Pantoprazole**)

Pantoprazole

Pronunciation guide: pan-TOE-pra-zol

Drug classification: PROTON PUMP INHIBITORS (see section 34.8.4 in Table 14-1)

Brand names: *Panto, Panto IV, Pantoloc, Protonix, Tecta*

Ototoxic effects:
    Cochlear:
        Hearing loss: <1% (DFC, PDR)
        Tinnitus: <1% (CPS, PDR)
    Vestibular:
        Ataxia: (PDR)
        Dizziness: 0.7-1.4% (CPS, PDR)
        Vertigo: 0.1-1% (CPS, PDR)
    Outer/Middle Ear:
        Earache/ear pain: <1% (DFC, PDR)
        Otitis externa: <1% (DFC, PDR)

Risk assessment: Class 2

Notes:

> The PDR also notes an absence of ear reflex, presumably indicating severe to profound hearing loss.

Papaverine

Pronunciation guide: pah-PAV-er-een

Drug classification: VASODILATORS (see section 20.8.40 in Table 14-1)

Brand names: *Pavabid*

Ototoxic effects:
    Vestibular:
        Dizziness: (AHF)
        Vertigo: (AHF, PDR)

Risk assessment: Class 1

Notes:

> **Papaverine** is a vasodilator. Some people have good results when their doctors prescribe it to stop certain types of hearing losses. I have an anecdotal report of a woman who regained "quite a bit" of her lost hearing after just three weeks on **Papaverine**.

Paracetamol   (see **Acetaminophen**)

Parafon Forte   (see **Acetaminophen**)

Paraplatin   (see **Carboplatin**)

Parecoxib

Pronunciation guide: PAH-reh-kox-ib

Drug classification: COX-2 INHIBITORS (see section 1.1.4 in Table 14-1)

Brand names: *Dynastat*

Ototoxic effects:
    Cochlear:
        Tinnitus: (BNF)
    Vestibular:
        Dizziness: (BNF)
        Vertigo: (BNF)

Risk assessment: Class 1

Paricalcitol

Pronunciation guide: par-rih-KAL-sih-tol

Drug classification: VITAMINS (see section 75.4 in Table 14-1)

Brand names: *Zemplar*

Ototoxic effects:
    Vestibular:
        Dizziness: 5% [1% above placebo results] (PDR)
        Vertigo: 5% [placebo 0] (PDR)

Risk assessment: Class 1

Notes:

    Paricalcitol is a synthetic form of Vitamin D. (See also **Ergocalciferal**.)

Pariet   (see **Rabeprazole**)

Parlodel   (see **Bromocriptine**)

Parnate   (see **Tranylcypromine**)

Paromomycin (Aminosidine)

Pronunciation guide: par-oh-moe-MY-sin (ah-MEEN-oh-sid-deen)

Drug classification: AMINOGLYCOSIDES (see section 7.4.1 in Table 14-1)

Brand names: *Humatin*

Ototoxic effects:
    Cochlear:
        Hearing loss: [1]
        Tinnitus: [1]
    Vestibular:
        Dizziness: [1]
        Vertigo: <1% (AHF, Med)

Risk assessment: Class 4

Notes:

[1] Hearing loss, tinnitus and dizziness are all ototoxic side effects of this drug.[308] Hearing loss may be temporary (AHF).

See the drug listings for **Amikacin**, **Kanamycin** and **Neomycin** for a more complete understanding of the severity and kinds of side effects you could expect from taking **Paromomycin**.

See Chapter 9, "Aminoglycoside Antibiotics are the Ototoxic 'Bad boys'" for further information on this drug.

Paroxetine

Pronunciation guide: pah-ROX-eh-teen

Drug classification: SELECTIVE SEROTONIN REUPTAKE INHIBITORS (see section 60.1.32 in Table 14-1)

Brand names: *Paxil, Paxil CR*

Ototoxic effects:
> Cochlear:
>> Hearing loss: <0.1% (CPS, PDR)
>> Hyperacusis: <0.1% (CPS, PDR)
>> Tinnitus: >1% (CPS, PDR)
> Vestibular:
>> Ataxia: 0.1-1% (CPS, PDR)
>> Dizziness: 1.4-14.1% [<11.7% above placebo results] (CPS, PDR)
>> Nystagmus: 0.1-1% (CPS, PDR)
>> Vertigo: 2-3.3% [0-1% above placebo results] (CPS, PDR)
> Outer/Middle Ear:
>> Earache/ear pain: 0.1-1% (CPS, PDR)
>> Otitis externa: <0.1% (CPS, PDR)
>> Otitis media: 0.1-1% (CPS, PDR)

Risk assessment: Class 3

Parsitan   (see **Ethopropazine**)

Pavabid   (see **Papaverine**)

Paxil   (see **Paroxetine**)

Paxil CR   (see **Paroxetine**)

PBZ   (see **Tripelennamine**)

PCE   (see **Erythromycin**)

Pediapred   (see **Prednisolone**)

Pediazole   (see **Erythromycin**)

Pediotic   (see **Neomycin**)

PedvaxHIB   (see **Haemophilus vaccine**)

Peganone   (see **Ethotoin**)

Pegaptanib

Pronunciation guide: peh-GAP-tah-nib

Drug classification: MACULAR DEGENERATION THERAPY ADJUNCT (see section 56.1.1 in Table 14-1)

Brand names: *Macugen*

Ototoxic effects:
    Cochlear:
        Hearing loss: 1-5% (DFC)
        Tinnitus: >1% (CPS)
    Vestibular:
        Dizziness: 6-10% (CPS, DFC)
        Vertigo: 1-5% (CPS, DFC)

Risk assessment: Class 2

Pegasys   (see **Peginterferon alfa-2a**)

Pegasys RBV   (see **Peginterferon alfa-2a**)

Pegetron   (see **Peginterferon alfa-2b**)

Peginterferon alfa-2a

Pronunciation guide: peg-in-ter-FEER-on AL-fah

Drug classification: INTERFERONS (see section 7.17.4 in Table 14-1)

Brand names: *Pegasys, Pegasys RBV* [1]

Ototoxic effects:
    Cochlear:
        Hearing loss: <1% (CPS)
        Tinnitus: 2-5% (CPS)
    Vestibular:
        Dizziness: 2-15% (CPS)
        Vertigo: 2-5% (CPS)
    Outer/Middle Ear:
        Earache/ear pain: 2-5% (CPS)
        Otitis externa: <1% (CPS)

Risk assessment: Class 2

Notes:

> [1] *Pegasys RBV* is a combination of **Ribavirin** and **Peginterferon alfa-2a**. (See the generic drug **Ribavirin** for its specific ototoxic properties.)

Peginterferon alfa-2b

Pronunciation guide: peg-in-ter-FEER-on AL-fah

Drug classification: INTERFERONS (see section 7.17.4 in Table 14-1)

Brand names: *Pegetron*[1], *PEG-Intron, Unitron PEG*

Ototoxic effects:
    Cochlear:
        Hearing loss: 0.1-5% (CPS, PDR)
        Tinnitus: 2-5% (CPS)
    Vestibular:
        Dizziness: 8-21% (CPS, NDH)
        Vertigo: 2-5% (CPS, PDR)
    Outer/Middle Ear:
        Otitis media: 2-5% (CPS)

Risk assessment: Class 3

Notes:

> [1] *Pegetron* is a combination of **Ribavirin** and **Peginterferon alfa-2b**. (See the generic drug **Ribavirin** for its specific ototoxic properties.)

PEG-Intron　(see **Peginterferon alfa-2b**)

Pelidorm　(see **Carbromal**)

Pemoline

Pronunciation guide: PEM-oh-leen

Drug classification: PSYCHOSTIMULANTS (see section 60.20 in Table 14-1)

Brand names: *Cylert*

Ototoxic effects:
    Vestibular:
        Dizziness: (CPS, PDR)
        Nystagmus: (CPS, PDR)

Risk assessment: Class 1

Penetrex　(see **Enoxacin**)

Penglobe　(see **Bacampicillin**)

Penicillamine

Pronunciation guide: pen-ih-SILL-ah-meen

Drug classification: Heavy metal antagonists/chelating agents (see section 66.4 in Table 14-1)

Brand names: *Cuprimine*, *Depen*

Ototoxic effects:
    Cochlear:
        Tinnitus: (CPS, PDR)

Risk assessment: Class 1

Notes:
    See Chapter 7, "We 'Hear' With Our Eyes" for further information on this drug.

Penicillin G   (see **Penicillin**)

Penicillin/Penicillin G

Pronunciation guide: pen-ih-SILL-in

Drug classification: Penicillins (see section 7.4.40 in Table 14-1)

Brand names: *Bicillin*, *Veetids*

Ototoxic effects:
    Cochlear:
        Auditory hallucinations: (PDR)
        Tinnitus: (PDR)
    Vestibular:
        Dizziness: (NDH, PDR)

Risk assessment: Class 1

Notes:

    The above side effects can occur when taking **Penicillin G** either intravenously or by injection. These effects are temporary (PDR).

Pennsaid   (see **Diclofenac**)

Pentacarinat   (see **Pentamidine**)

Pentamidine

Pronunciation guide: pen-TAH-mih-deen

Drug classification: Anti-protozoals (see section 7.14 in Table 14-1)

Brand names: *Pentacarinat*

Ototoxic effects:
    Cochlear:
        Hearing loss: <1% (DFC)
        Tinnitus: <1% (CPS)
    Vestibular:
        Ataxia: <1% (AHF, CPS)
        Dizziness: 10-23% (BNF, CPS)
        Vertigo: <1% (AHF, CPS)

Risk assessment: Class 2

Pentamycetin   (see **Chloramphenicol**)

Pentasa   (see **Mesalamine**)

Pentazocine

Pronunciation guide: pen-TAZ-oh-seen

Drug classification: OPIATE AGONIST/ANTAGONIST DRUGS (see section 1.4.4 in Table 14-1)

Brand names: *Talacen*[1]*, Talwin, Talwin Compound*[2]*, Talwin Nx*[3]

Ototoxic effects:
    Cochlear:
        Tinnitus: (CPS, PDR)
    Vestibular:
        Dizziness: >10% (NDH, PDR)
        Nystagmus: (CPS, PDR)
        Vertigo: (BNF, CPS)

Risk assessment: Class 2

Notes:

[1] *Talacen* is a combination of **Pentazocine** and **Acetaminophen**. (See the generic drug **Acetaminophen** for its specific ototoxic properties.)

[2] *Talwin Compound* is a combination of **Pentazocine** and **Acetylsalicylic acid**. (See the generic drug **Acetylsalicylic acid** for its specific ototoxic properties.)

[3] *Talwin Nx* is a combination of **Pentazocine** and Naloxone. (**Pentazocine** is the ototoxic agent.)

See Chapter 7, "We 'Hear' With Our Eyes" for further information on this drug.

Pentobarbital

Pronunciation guide: pen-toe-BAR-bih-tal

Drug classification: BARBITURATES (see section 60.12.4 in Table 14-1)

Brand names: *Nembutal*

Ototoxic effects:
Vestibular:
Ataxia: <1% (PDR)
Dizziness: <1% (PDR)
Nystagmus: (PDR)

Risk assessment: Class 1

Notes:

Ataxia and nystagmus are two symptoms of **Pentobarbital** overdose. Withdrawal can cause dizziness (PDR).

Pentosan

Pronunciation guide: PEN-toe-san

Drug classification: ANTI-CLOTTING DRUGS (see section 36.1 in Table 14-1)

Brand names: *Elmiron*

Ototoxic effects:
Cochlear:
Tinnitus: <1% (PDR, USP)
Vestibular:
Dizziness: 1% (CPS, PDR)
Nystagmus: 1% [same as placebo] (DFC, PDR)

Risk assessment: Class 1

Pentostam   (see **Sodium stibogluconate**)

Pentostatin

Pronunciation guide: pen-toe-STA-tin

Drug classification: ANTI-METABOLITE DRUGS (see section 14.8 in Table 14-1)

Brand names: *Nipent*

Ototoxic effects:
Cochlear:
Hearing loss: <3% (AHF, PDR)
Tinnitus: <3% (AHF, PDR)
Vestibular:
Ataxia: <3% (AHF, PDR)
Dizziness: 3-10% (AHF, PDR)
Labyrinthitis: <3% (AHF, PDR)
Vertigo: <3% (AHF, PDR)
Outer/Middle Ear:
Earache/ear pain: 3-10% (AHF, PDR)
Otitis media: <3% (AHF)

Risk assessment: Class 3

Pentoxifylline

Pronunciation guide: pen-tox-IH-fih-leen

Drug classification: BLOOD-FLOW DRUGS (see section 36.12 in Table 14-1)

Brand names: *Albert Pentoxifylline, ratio-Pentoxifylline, Trental*

Ototoxic effects:
    Cochlear:
        Auditory hallucinations: [1]
    Vestibular:
        Dizziness: 1.9-11.9% [<7.4% above placebo results] (CPS, PDR)
    Outer/Middle Ear:
        Earache/ear pain: <1% (AHF, PDR)

Risk assessment: Class 1

Notes:

[1] I have a report in my files of a woman who had musical auditory hallucinations every time she was on **Pentoxifylline**. When she would go off, the hallucinations would go away.[309]

Pepcid   (see **Famotidine**)

Pepcid AC   (see **Famotidine**)

Pepto-Bismol Original   (see **Bismuth subsalicylate**)

Percocet   (see **Oxycodone**)

Percodan   (see **Oxycodone**)

Perflutren

Pronunciation guide: per-FLOO-tren

Drug classification: ULTRASOUND CONTRAST AGENTS (see section 26.8 in Table 14-1)

Brand names: *Definity*

Ototoxic effects:
    Cochlear:
        Hearing loss: <0.5% (CPS)
        Tinnitus: 0.6-1.2% [placebo 0] (CPS, DFC)
    Vestibular:
        Dizziness: 1.1-2% (CPS)
        Vertigo: 0.6-1.2% [placebo 0] (CPS)

Risk assessment: Class 2

Pergolide

Pronunciation guide: PER-go-lide

Drug classification: ERGOT ALKALOIDS (see section 17.4 in Table 14-1)

Brand names: *Permax*

Ototoxic effects:
    Cochlear:
        Hearing loss: 0.1-1% (CPS, PDR)
        Tinnitus: 0.1-1% (CPS, PDR)
    Vestibular:
        Ataxia: 0.1-1% (CPS, PDR)
        Dizziness: 19.1% [5.2% above placebo results] (CPS, PDR)
        Vertigo: 0.1-1% (CPS, PDR)
    Outer/Middle Ear:
        Earache/ear pain: 0.1-1% (CPS, PDR)
        Otitis media: 0.1-1% (CPS, PDR)

Risk assessment: Class 3

Periactin   (see **Cyproheptadine**)

Perindopril

Pronunciation guide: per-IN-doe-pril

Drug classification: ANGIOTENSIN-CONVERTING ENZYME (ACE) INHIBITORS (see section 20.8.8 in Table 14-1)

Brand names: *Aceon, Coversyl, Coversyl Plus* [1]

Ototoxic effects:
    Cochlear:
        Tinnitus: 1.5% (CPS, PDR)
    Vestibular:
        Dizziness: 1.4-8.6% (CPS, PDR)
        Vertigo: 0.3-1% (CPS, PDR)
    Outer/Middle Ear:
        Earache/ear pain: 0.3-1% (CPS, PDR)
        Otitis: 1.3% [placebo 0] (NDH, PDR)
        Otitis media: <1% (CPS)

Risk assessment: Class 2

Notes:

    [1] *Coversyl Plus* is a combination of **Perindopril** and **Indapamide**. (See the generic drug **Indapamide** for its specific ototoxic properties.)

Permax   (see **Pergolide**)

Perphenazine

Pronunciation guide: per-FEN-ah-zeen

Drug classification: ANTIPSYCHOTIC DRUGS (see section 60.8 in Table 14-1)

Brand names: *Trilafon*

Ototoxic effects:
Vestibular:
Ataxia: (CPS, PDR)
Dizziness: (CPS, PDR)

Risk assessment: Class 1

Notes:

See Chapter 7, "We 'Hear' With Our Eyes" for further information on this drug.

Persantine   (see **Dipyridamole**)

Pertofrane   (see **Desipramine**)

Phenaphen with Codeine   (see **Phenobarbital**)

Phenelzine

Pronunciation guide: FEN-el-zeen

Drug classification: MONOAMINE OXIDASE INHIBITORS (see section 60.1.1 in Table 14-1)

Brand names: *Nardil*

Ototoxic effects:
Cochlear:
Tinnitus: (Ka7)
Vestibular:
Ataxia: (CPS, PDR)
Dizziness: (CPS, PDR)
Nystagmus: (CPS, PDR)

Risk assessment: Class 1

Phenergan   (see **Promethazine**)

Pheniramine

Pronunciation guide: fen-EER-ah-meen

Drug classification: H_1 RECEPTOR ANTAGONISTS (see section 10.1 in Table 14-1)

Brand names: [1]

Ototoxic effects:
    Cochlear:
        Tinnitus: (CPS)
    Vestibular:
        Dizziness: (CPS)

Risk assessment: Class 1

Notes:

[1] There are a number of drug preparations that use **Pheniramine** as one of their compounds. They are too numerous to mention here. As always, check the labels and then look up each drug listed to see its ototoxic properties.

Phenobarbital

Pronunciation guide: fee-noe-BAR-bih-tall

Drug classification: BARBITURATES (see section 60.12.4 in Table 14-1)

Brand names: *Phenaphen with Codeine* [1]

Ototoxic effects:
    Vestibular:
        Ataxia: <1% (BNF, PDR)
        Dizziness: <1% (CPS, PDR)
        Nystagmus: (NTP)
        Vertigo: (CPS, PDR)

Risk assessment: Class 1

Notes:

[1] *Phenaphen with Codeine* is a combination of **Phenobarbital, Acetylsalicylic acid** and **Codeine**. (See the generic drugs **Acetylsalicylic acid** and **Codeine** for their specific ototoxic properties.)

Phenopropazine   (see **Ethopropazine**)

Phentermine

Pronunciation guide: FEN-ter-meen

Drug classification: SYMPATHOMIMETIC DRUGS (see section 17.16 in Table 14-1)

Brand name: *Adipex-P*

Ototoxic effects:
    Cochlear:
        Tinnitus: [1]
    Vestibular:
        Dizziness: (NDH, PDR)

Risk assessment: Class 1

Notes:

[1] I have an anecdotal report in my files of a lady that took "very little" **Phentermine**. She reported, "I have had loud ringing in my ears ever since. It's been at least 3 weeks since I stopped taking the drug".

Although **Phentermine** is not listed as causing tinnitus, most of the drugs in its class can cause tinnitus, so it would be surprising if **Phentermine** didn't also cause tinnitus in some people.

Phenylbutazone

Pronunciation guide: fen-ill-BYOO-tah-zone

Drug classification: NON-STEROIDAL ANTI-INFLAMMATORY DRUGS (NSAIDs) (see section 1.1 in Table 14-1)

Brand names: *Apo-Phenylbutazone, Novo-Butazone*

Ototoxic effects:
Cochlear:
Hearing loss: (Med, NTP)
Tinnitus: (Med, NTP)
Vestibular:
Dizziness: (Med, NTP)
Vertigo: (BNF, NTP)

Risk assessment: Class 2

Notes:

See Chapter 7, "We 'Hear' With Our Eyes" for further information on this drug.

Phenylephrine

Pronunciation guide: fen-ill-EFF-rin

Drug classification: SYMPATHOMIMETIC DRUGS (see section 17.16 in Table 14-1)

Brand names: [1]

Ototoxic effects:
Vestibular:
Dizziness: (NDH, PDR)

Risk assessment: Class 1

Notes:

[1] There are many drug preparations that use **Phenylephrine** as one of their compounds. They are too numerous to mention here. As always, check the labels and then look up each drug listed to see its ototoxic properties.

Phenylpropanolamine

Pronunciation guide: fen-ill-proe-pah-NOLE-ah-meen

Drug classification: SYMPATHOMIMETIC DRUGS (see section 17.16 in Table 14-1)

Brand names: *Alumadrine* [1], *Atrohist Plus* [2], *Coricidin D* [3], *Ornade Spansule* [4]

Ototoxic effects:
  Cochlear:
    Tinnitus: (PDR)
  Vestibular:
    Dizziness: (CPS, PDR)
    Labyrinthitis, acute: (PDR)
    Vertigo: (PDR)

Risk assessment: Class 1

Notes:

[1] *Alumadrine* is a combination of **Acetaminophen**, **Phenylpropanolamine**, and **Chlorpheniramine**. (See the generic drugs **Acetaminophen** and **Chlorpheniramine** for their specific ototoxic properties.)

[2] *Atrohist Plus* is a combination of **Phenylpropanolamine**, **Phenylephrine**, **Scopolamine** and **Hyoscyamine**. See the generic drugs **Phenylephrine**, **Scopolamine** and **Hyoscyamine** for their specific ototoxic properties.)

[3] *Coricidin D* is a combination of **Phenylpropanolamine**, **Acetaminophen** and **Chlorpheniramine**. (See the generic drugs **Acetaminophen** and **Chlorpheniramine** for their specific ototoxic properties.)

[4] *Ornade Spansule* is a combination of **Phenylpropanolamine** and **Chlorpheniramine**. (See the generic drug **Chlorpheniramine** for its specific ototoxic properties.)

In November 2000, the FDA began taking steps to remove **Phenylpropanolamine** from the American market because of health hazards.[310] **Phenylpropanolamine** is an ingredient in more than 300 drug products.

Phenytek   (see **Phenytoin**)

Phenytoin (Diphenylhydantoin)

Pronunciation guide: FEN-ih-toe-in (die-fen-ill-hie-dan-TOY-in)

Drug classification: ANTI-CONVULSANT DRUGS (see section 53.12 in Table 14-1)

Brand names: *Dilantin, Phenytek*

Ototoxic effects:
  Vestibular:
    Ataxia: >10% (NDH, PDR)
    Dizziness: (CPS, PDR)

Nystagmus: >10% (NDH, PDR)
Oscillopsia: (NTP)
Vertigo: (NTP)

Risk assessment: Class 2

Notes:

The initial symptoms of **Phenytoin** overdose include ataxia, nystagmus and dizziness (PDR). Nystagmus generally appears at about 20 mg/L and ataxia at around 30 mg/L (PDR).

See Chapter 7, "We 'Hear' With Our Eyes" for further information on this drug.

Phrenilin   (see **Butalbital**)

Phrenilin Forte   (see **Butalbital**)

Phrenilin with Caffeine and Codeine   (see **Butalbital**)

Pilocarpine

Pronunciation guide: pie-low-KAR-peen

Drug classification: CHOLINERGIC AGONIST DRUGS (see section 17.12.1 in Table 14-1)

Brand names: *Salagen*

Ototoxic effects:
    Cochlear:
        Hearing loss: <1% (DFC, PDR)
        Tinnitus: 1-2% (CPS, PDR)
    Vestibular:
        Dizziness: 5-12% [1-8% above placebo results] (CPS, PDR)
    Outer/Middle Ear:
        Earache/ear pain: <1% (DFC, PDR)
    Unspecified/General Ear Conditions:
        Ear disorder: <1% (DFC, PDR)

Risk assessment: Class 2

Notes:

See Chapter 7, "We 'Hear' With Our Eyes" for further information on this drug.

Pimecrolimus

Pronunciation guide: pie-meck-roh-LYE-mus

Drug classification: IMMUNOSUPPRESSANT DRUGS (see section 43 in Table 14-1)

Brand names: *Elidel*

Ototoxic effects:
    Outer/Middle Ear:
        Earache/ear pain: 0.7-2.9% [0.2% above placebo results] (DFC, PDR)
        Otitis: 2.2-5.7% [<2.4% above placebo results] (DFC, PDR)
        Otitis media: 2.2-3% [<1.5% above placebo results] (DFC, PDR)

Risk assessment: Class 1

Pimozide

Pronunciation guide: PIM-oh-zide

Drug classification: ANTIPSYCHOTIC DRUGS (see section 60.8 in Table 14-1)

Brand names: *Apo-Pimozide, Orap*

Ototoxic effects:
    Vestibular:
        Dizziness: (AHF, CPS)
        Vertigo: (CPS)

Risk assessment: Class 1

Notes:

    Caution: Eating grapefruit or drinking grapefruit juice during the time you are taking this drug may make the listed side effects worse than shown here.

    See Chapter 11, "Grapefruit Juice and Ototoxic Drugs" for further information on this drug.

Pinaverium

Pronunciation guide: pin-ah-VEER-ee-um

Drug classification: ANTI-CHOLINERGIC DRUGS (see section 17.1 in Table 14-1)

Brand names: *Dicetel*

Ototoxic effects:
    Vestibular:
        Vertigo: 0.2% (CPS)

Risk assessment: Class 1

Pindolol

Pronunciation guide: PIN-doe-lole

Drug classification: BETA-ADRENERGIC-BLOCKING DRUGS (BETA-BLOCKERS) (see section 20.8.12 in Table 14-1)

Brand names: *Viskazide* [1], *Visken*

Ototoxic effects:
    Cochlear:
        Tinnitus: (CPS)
    Vestibular:
        Dizziness: (CPS)
        Vertigo: (CPS)
        Vestibular disorder: (CPS)

Risk assessment: Class 1

Notes:

[1] *Viskazide* is a combination of **Pindolol** and **Hydrochlorothiazide**. (See the generic drug **Hydrochlorothiazide** for its specific ototoxic properties.)

Piperacillin–Tazobactam

Pronunciation guide: pie-PER-ah-SILL-in—taz-oh-BAK-tem

Drug classification: PENICILLINS (see section 7.4.40 in Table 14-1)

Brand names: *Pipracil*[1], *Tazocin*, *Zosyn*

Ototoxic effects:
    Cochlear:
        Hearing loss: <1% (PDR)
        Tinnitus: <1% (CPS, PDR)
    Vestibular:
        Dizziness: 1.4% (CPS, PDR)
        Vertigo: <1% (CPS, PDR)
    Outer/Middle Ear:
        Earache/ear pain: <1% (PDR)

Risk assessment: Class 2

Notes:

[1] *Pipracil* is just the drug **Piperacillin** by itself (CPS).

Piperazine

Pronunciation guide: PIH-per-ah-zeen

Drug classification: PIPERAZINES (see section 10.8 in Table 14-1)

Brand names: *Entacyl*

Ototoxic effects:
    Vestibular:
        Ataxia: (CPS)
        Dizziness: (BNF)
        Vertigo: (CPS)

Risk assessment: Class 1

Pipracil   (see **Piperacillin—Tazobactam**)

Piretanide

Pronunciation guide: pie-REH-tah-nide

Drug classification: DIURETICS—LOOP (see section 30.5.4 in Table 14-1)

Brand names: *Arelix*

Ototoxic effects:
Vestibular:
Dizziness: [311]
Unspecified/General Ear Conditions:
Ototoxicity: [312] (San)

Risk assessment: Not enough information to rate

Piroxicam

Pronunciation guide: peer-OX-ih-kam

Drug classification: OXICAMS (see section 1.1.10 in Table 14-1)

Brand names: *Brexidol, Feldene*

Ototoxic effects:
Cochlear:
Auditory disturbances: (NDH)
Hearing loss: (CPS, PDR)
Tinnitus: 1-10% (CPS, PDR)
Vestibular:
Dizziness: 1-10% (CPS, PDR)
Vertigo: 1-3% (CPS, PDR)

Risk assessment: Class 2

Pirprofen

Pronunciation guide: peer-PROE-fen

Drug classification: PROPIONIC ACIDS (see section 1.1.13 in Table 14-1)

Brand names: *Rengasil*

Ototoxic effects:
Cochlear:
Tinnitus: (San, She)
Unspecified/General Ear Conditions:
Ototoxicity: (San)

Risk assessment: Not enough information to rate

Pizotifen

Pronunciation guide: pih-ZOT-ih-fen

Drug classification: SEROTONIN ANTAGONISTS (see section 60.1.36 in Table 14-1)

Brand names: *Sandomigran*

Ototoxic effects:
    Vestibular:
        Ataxia: (CPS)
        Dizziness: (BNF, CPS)

Risk assessment: Class 1

Plan B   (see **Levonorgestrel**)

Plaquenil   (see **Hydroxychloroquine**)

Platinol   (see **Cisplatin**)

Plavix   (see **Clopidogrel**)

Plendil   (see **Felodipine**)

Pletal   (see **Cilostazol**)

PMB   (see **Meprobamate**)

PMS-Lithium Carbonate   (see **Lithium**)

Pneumococcal vaccine

Pronunciation guide: NEW-moe-KOK-al VAK-seen

Drug classification: VACCINES (see section 70.8 in Table 14-1)

Brand names: *Prevnar*

Ototoxic effects:
    Outer/Middle Ear:
        Otitis media: (PDR)

Risk assessment: Class 1

Polaramine   (see **Chlorpheniramine**)

Polocaine   (see **Mepivacaine**)

Polybrene   (see **Hexadimethrine**)

Polymyxin B

Pronunciation guide: pol-ee-MIX-in

Drug classification: POLYPEPTIDES (see section 7.4.44 in Table 14-1)

Brand names: *Aerosporin*

Ototoxic effects:
Vestibular:
Ataxia: (AHF, DFC)
Dizziness: (AHF, DFC)
Nystagmus: (AHF, Med)
Unspecified/General Ear Conditions:
Ototoxicity: [1]

Risk assessment: Class 2

Notes:

[1] "**Polymyxin B** is highly ototoxic when administered topically. However, no ototoxicity has been reported with systemic administration of this drug".[313]

Polymyxin E   (see **Colistin**)

Polythiazide

Pronunciation guide: pol-ee-THYE-ah-zide

Drug classification: DIURETICS—THIAZIDE-RELATED (see section 30.5.12 in Table 14-1)

Brand names: *Renese*

Ototoxic effects:
Vestibular:
Dizziness: (PDR)
Vertigo: (PDR)

Risk assessment: Class 1

Ponstan   (see **Mefenamic acid**)

Ponstel   (see **Mefenamic acid**)

Pontocaine   (see **Tetracaine**)

Posaconazole

Pronunciation guide: pahs-ah-KON-ah-zall

Drug classification: ANTI-FUNGAL ANTIBIOTICS (see section 7.10 in Table 14-1)

Brand names: *Posanol*

Ototoxic effects:
    Cochlear:
        Hearing loss: <2% (CPS)
        Tinnitus: <2% (CPS)
    Vestibular:
        Ataxia: <2% (CPS)
        Dizziness: 1-3% (CPS)
        Vertigo: <2% (CPS)
        Vestibular disorder: <2% (CPS)
    Outer/Middle Ear:
        Earache/ear pain: <2% (CPS)

Risk assessment: Class 2

Posanol   (see **Posaconazole**)

Potassium gluconate

Pronunciation guide: poe-TAS-see-um GLUE-koh-nate

Drug classification: MINERALS (see section 75.8 in Table 14-1)

Brand names: *Gluco-K*

Ototoxic effects:
    Cochlear:
        Hearing loss: [1]
        Tinnitus: [1]
    Vestibular:
        Vertigo: [2]

Risk assessment: Class 3 in higher doses

Notes:

[1] "ringing in your ears, or sudden hearing loss" "**Potassium gluconate** can decrease blood flow to the optic nerve of the eye, causing sudden vision loss".[314] By the same token, it seems that it can do the same to the tiny arteries in the inner ear causing the hair cells to be starved for oxygen. The result can be tinnitus and a mostly-temporary sudden hearing loss, as well as balance problems such as vertigo when taking **Potassium gluconate** in higher doses.

[2] I have an anecdotal report in my files of a woman who took daily 550 mg. doses of **Potassium gluconate**. She explained, "Almost as soon as I started on it, my tinnitus started to roar and I was hearing very little. I experienced slight to severe vertigo at least two out of every three days during that time. When I stopped taking the **Potassium gluconate**, I noticed an improvement in my tinnitus after only one day. After 2-3 days it was back to its familiar hiss. The vertigo stopped completely the first day, and has not come back in the week I have been off the potassium. My hearing rebounded almost back to normal in the week I have been off the potassium, but an audiogram confirmed I have lost a bit more hearing". This same lady, a few weeks later, wrote, "I recently decided (again) that it was time to lose weight, and though I'd use SlimFast to get a jump start

on it. I immediately experienced extreme tinnitus and hearing loss. When I checked the label, I found that it is high in potassium—in fact it contains 550 mg.—the same amount I was taking in the supplement that caused me trouble before. I stopped the SlimFast and the problems decreased again. I have not gotten back to where I was before the 30 days on potassium, but at least it's no longer getting worse".

Pramipexole

Pronunciation guide: pram-ih-PEX-ole

Drug classification: DOPAMINE RECEPTOR AGONISTS (see section 53.16.1 in Table 14-1)

Brand names: *Mirapex*

Ototoxic effects:
> Cochlear:
>> Tinnitus: [same as placebo] (CPS, PDR)
> Vestibular:
>> Ataxia: 7% [2% above placebo results] (CPS, PDR)
>> Dizziness: 25-26% [1% above placebo results] (CPS, PDR)
>> Equilibrium disorder: (CPS)
>> Vertigo: [same as placebo] (CPS, PDR)
> Outer/Middle Ear:
>> Otitis media: (CPS)
> Unspecified/General Ear Conditions:
>> Ear disorder: (CPS)

Risk assessment: Class 2

Pravachol   (see **Pravastatin**)

Pravastatin

Pronunciation guide: prah-vah-STA-tin

Drug classification: HMG-CoA REDUCTASE INHIBITORS (see section 20.12.8 in Table 14-1)

Brand names: *Pravachol*

Ototoxic effects:
> Cochlear:
>> Hearing loss: 0.6% [0.1% above placebo results] (CPS)
>> Tinnitus: 0.6% [0.1% above placebo results] (CPS)
> Vestibular:
>> Dizziness: 1-3.3% [0.1-0.5% above placebo results] (CPS, PDR)
>> Vertigo: <1% (CPS, PDR)

Risk assessment: Class 2

Notes:

> Caution: Eating grapefruit or drinking grapefruit juice during the time you are taking this drug may make the listed side effects worse than shown here.

See Chapter 11, "Grapefruit Juice and Ototoxic Drugs" for further information on this drug.

Praziquantel

Pronunciation guide: pray-zih-KWON-tel

Drug classification: ANTHELMINTIC DRUGS (see section 7.1 in Table 14-1)

Brand names: *Biltricide*

Ototoxic effects:
Vestibular:
Dizziness: (CPS, PDR)
Vertigo: (AHF, CPS)

Risk assessment: Class 1

Prazosin

Pronunciation guide: PRAH-zoh-sin

Drug classification: ALPHA ADRENERGIC BLOCKING DRUGS (see section 20.8.1 in Table 14-1)

Brand names: *Apo-Prazo, Minipress, Minizide* [1]

Ototoxic effects:
Cochlear:
Tinnitus: <1% (CPS, PDR)
Vestibular:
Dizziness: 10.3% (CPS, PDR)
Vertigo: 1-4% (CPS, PDR)

Risk assessment: Class 2

Notes:

[1] *Minizide* is a combination of **Prazosin** and **Polythiazide**. (See the generic drug **Polythiazide** for its specific ototoxic properties.)

Prednisolone

Pronunciation guide: pred-NISS-oh-lone

Drug classification: GLUCOCORTICOIDS (see section 40.1.4 in Table 14-1)

Brand names: *Hydeltrasol, Hydeltra-TBA, Orapred, Pediapred, Prelone, Solupred*

Ototoxic effects:
Cochlear:
Tinnitus: (Ka7)
Vestibular:
Vertigo: (CPS, PDR)

Risk assessment: Class 1

Prednisone

Pronunciation guide: PRED-nih-sone

Drug classification: GLUCOCORTICOIDS (see section 40.1.4 in Table 14-1)

Brand names: *Deltasone, Metreton* [1]

Ototoxic effects:
Cochlear:
Hearing loss: [2]
Hyperacusis: [3]
Tinnitus: [4]
Vestibular:
Vertigo: (CP2, CPS)

Risk assessment: Class 2

Notes:

[1] *Metreton* is a combination of **Prednisone**, **Chlorpheniramine** and Ascorbic acid. (See the generic drug **Chlorpheniramine** for its specific ototoxic properties.)

[2] I have an anecdotal report in my files of a man that had hearing loss while taking **Prednisone**. Also, hearing loss is listed in a comprehensive list of **Prednisone** side effects, compiled from various sources, that I have in my files.

[3] I have an anecdotal report in my files of a woman who got hyperacusis while taking **Prednisone**.

[4] Tinnitus is listed in a comprehensive list of **Prednisone** side effects, compiled from various sources, that I have in my files. I also have an anecdotal report in my files of a man who was put on **Prednisone** and the very first dose of 40 mg. caused a "tremendous increase in the whooshing noise in both ears" (his kind of tinnitus).

Prednisone is commonly used to treat sudden hearing loss caused by autoimmune disorders and suchlike. Sometimes hearing returns (or partially returns) and sometimes it doesn't. Left untreated, basically you get the same results—sometimes hearing returns and sometimes it doesn't. Taking **Prednisone** is currently a popular treatment, but be aware of **all** the adverse side effects that can mess up your body. I have several reports in my files of people who call it a "wretched" drug.

See Chapter 7, "We 'Hear' With Our Eyes" for further information on this drug.

Pregabalin

Pronunciation guide: pray-GAB-ah-lin

Drug classification: ANTI-CONVULSANT DRUGS (see section 53.12 in Table 14-1)

Brand names: *Lyrica*

Ototoxic effects:

    Cochlear:

        Hearing loss: <2% (CPS)

        Hyperacusis: 0.1-1% (DFC, PDR)

        Tinnitus: 2.9% [placebo 0] (CPS, PDR)

    Vestibular:

        Ataxia: 1-20% [<19% above placebo results] (PDR, RXL)

        Dizziness: 8-45% [3-36% above placebo results] (DFC, PDR)

        Equilibrium disorder: 2-9% [placebo 0] (DFC, PDR)

        Nystagmus: >1% (DFC, PDR)

        Vertigo: 1-4% [<3% above placebo results] (DFC, PDR)

    Outer/Middle Ear:

        Otitis externa: <2% (CPS)

        Otitis media: <2% (CPS, PDR)

    Unspecified/General Ear Conditions:

        Ear disorder: <2% (CPS)

Risk assessment: Class 4

Notes:

Received FDA approval in December, 2004. Replacing **Gabapentin**.

I have an anecdotal report in my files of a man that noticed a "huge increase" in his tinnitus after he started taking **Pregabalin**.

See Chapter 7, "We 'Hear' With Our Eyes" for further information on this drug.

Prelone   (see **Prednisolone**)

Premarin   (see **Estradiol**)

Premique   (see **Medroxyprogesterone**)

Premplus   (see **Medroxyprogesterone**)

Prempro   (see **Medroxyprogesterone**)

Prepulsid   (see **Cisapride**)

Preservex   (see **Aceclofenac**)

Presinol   (see **Methyldopa**)

Pressyn   (see **Vasopressin**)

Pressyn AR   (see **Vasopressin**)

Prevacid   (see **Lansoprazole**)

Prevnar (see **Pneumococcal vaccine**)

PREVPAC (see **Lansoprazole**)

Prezista (see **Darunavir**)

Prialt (see **Ziconotide**)

Prilocaine

Pronunciation guide: PRIL-oh-kane

Drug classification: AMIDES (see section 4.1 in Table 14-1)

Brand names: *Citanest*

Ototoxic effects:
    Cochlear:
        Hyperacusis: (CPS)
        Tinnitus: (CPS)
    Vestibular:
        Dizziness: (CP2, CPS)

Risk assessment: Class 1

Prilosec (see **Omeprazole**)

Primaxin (see **Imipenem—Cilastatin**)

Primidone

Pronunciation guide: PRIH-mih-done

Drug classification: ANTI-CONVULSANT DRUGS (see section 53.12 in Table 14-1)

Brand names: *Mysoline*

Ototoxic effects:
    Vestibular:
        Ataxia: >10% (NDH, PDR)
        Dizziness: (Med, NTP)
        Nystagmus: (NDH, PDR)
        Vertigo: <1% (NDH, PDR)

Risk assessment: Class 2

Notes:
    See Chapter 7, "We 'Hear' With Our Eyes" for further information on this drug.

Prinivil (see **Lisinopril**)

Prinzide (see **Lisinopril**)

Priorix   (see **Measles, mumps & rubella vaccine**)

Pristiq   (see **Desvenlafaxine**)

ProAir HFA   (see **Albuterol**)

Probucol

Pronunciation guide: PROE-byoo-kole

Drug classification: ANTI-LIPEMICS (see section 20.12 in Table 14-1)

Brand names: *Lorelco*

Ototoxic effects:
    Cochlear:
        Tinnitus: (CP2)
    Vestibular:
        Dizziness: (CP2, Med)

Risk assessment: Class 1

Procainamide

Pronunciation guide: proe-KANE-ah-mide

Drug classification: ANTI-ARRHYTHMICS (HEART RHYTHM REGULATORS) (see section 20.4 in Table 14-1)

Brand names: *Procan, Procanbid, Pronestyl*

Ototoxic effects:
    Cochlear:
        Tinnitus: (Ka8)
    Vestibular:
        Dizziness: >10% (AHF, NDH)

Risk assessment: Class 1

Procaine

Pronunciation guide: PROE-kane

Drug classification: AMIDES (see section 4.1 in Table 14-1)

Brand names: *Novocain*

Ototoxic effects: [315]
    Cochlear:
        Tinnitus:
    Vestibular:
        Dizziness:

Risk assessment: Class 1

Procan   (see **Procainamide**)

Procanbid   (see **Procainamide**)

Procarbazine

Pronunciation guide: proe-KAR-bah-zeen

Drug classification: ANTI-METABOLITE DRUGS (see section 14.8 in Table 14-1)

Brand names: *Matulane*

Ototoxic effects:
    Cochlear:
        Hearing disorder: (CPS)
        Hearing loss: (CPS, PDR)
    Vestibular:
        Ataxia: (CPS, PDR)
        Dizziness: (CPS, PDR)
        Nystagmus: (CPS, PDR)

Risk assessment: Class 2

Notes:

    Procarbazine rarely causes altered hearing (CPS).

Procardia   (see **Nifedipine**)

Proclim   (see **Medroxyprogesterone**)

Procytox   (see **Cyclophosphamide**)

Pro-Diaban   (see **Glisoxepide**)

Progesterone

Pronunciation guide: proe-JES-ter-own

Drug classification: PROGESTINS (see section 40.32 in Table 14-1)

Brand names: *Prometrium*

Ototoxic effects:
    Cochlear:
        Hearing loss: [1]
        Tinnitus: (PDR)
    Vestibular:
        Ataxia: (PDR)
        Dizziness: 15-24% [6-20% above placebo results] (CPS, PDR)
        Vertigo: <1% (CPS, PDR)

Outer/Middle Ear:
   Earache/ear pain: <5% (PDR)

Risk assessment: Class 2

Notes:

[1] PROGESTINS (such as **Medroxyprogesterone**, **Megestrol** and **Progesterone**) can cause hearing loss in women. PROGESTINS are typically used in hormone replacement therapy (HRT). One study found women who take the most common form of HRT had a hearing loss of 10% to 30% greater than women who have not taken HRT.[316] That's a loss equivalent to aging another 10 years or so. This hearing loss is particularly noticeable when trying to understand someone in a noisy environment.[317] The results showed that women who had received progestin had problems both in their cochleas and in the auditory circuits in their brains.

Progesterone is the likely culprit in this kind of hearing loss. There is some anecdotal evidence from women prescribed supplemental **Progesterone** to help maintain a pregnancy that often complain that their hearing gets noticeably worse while they're on **Progesterone**. In fact, a few studies have also shown that young women don't hear as well during the latter part of their monthly periods when **Progesterone** is the highest.[318]

In an anecdotal report in my files, one lady who lost most of her hearing to HRT summed up her situation as, "[in retrospect] my life would have been much easier if I'd just withstood the hot flashes and not medicated them away!"

Proglumetacin

Pronunciation guide: proe-glue-MEH-tah-sin

Drug classification: ACETIC ACIDS (see section 1.1.1 in Table 14-1)

Brand names: *Afloxan, Protaxon Forte*

Ototoxic effects:
   Cochlear:
      Tinnitus: (Ka7)

Risk assessment: Class 1

Prograf   (see **Tacrolimus**)

Proguanil   (see **Atovaquone**)

ProHance   (see **Gadoteridol**)

Proleukin   (see **Aldesleukin**)

Prolopa   (see **Levodopa**)

Proloprim   (see **Trimethoprim**)

Promethazine

Pronunciation guide: proe-METH-ah-zeen

Drug classification: H$_1$ RECEPTOR ANTAGONISTS (see section 10.1 in Table 14-1)

Brand names: *Phenergan*

Ototoxic effects:
    Cochlear:
        Tinnitus: (AHF, PDR)
    Vestibular:
        Ataxia: (NTP, PDR)
        Dizziness: (CPS, PDR)

Risk assessment: Class 1

Notes:

Ataxia may be a sign of **Promethazine** overdose (PDR).

See Chapter 4, "Are You at Risk?" and Chapter 7, "We 'Hear' With Our Eyes" for further information on this drug.

Prometrium   (see **Progesterone**)

Pronestyl   (see **Procainamide**)

Propafenone

Pronunciation guide: proe-PAF-eh-none

Drug classification: ANTI-ARRHYTHMICS (HEART RHYTHM REGULATORS) (see section 20.4 in Table 14-1)

Brand names: *Rythmol*

Ototoxic effects:
    Cochlear:
        Hearing loss: (PDR)
        Tinnitus: 1.9% (CPS, PDR)
    Vestibular:
        Ataxia: 0.3-2% (CPS, PDR)
        Dizziness: 3.6-23% [1.2-9% above placebo results] (CPS, PDR)
        Loss of balance: 1.2% [placebo 0] (DFC, PDR)
        Vertigo: <1% (CPS, PDR)

Risk assessment: Class 2

Notes:

Caution: Eating grapefruit or drinking grapefruit juice during the time you are taking this drug may make the listed side effects worse than shown here.

See Chapter 11, "Grapefruit Juice and Ototoxic Drugs" for further information on this drug.

Propofol

Pronunciation guide: PROE-poe-fol

Drug classification: General anesthetics (see section 4.8 in Table 14-1)

Brand names: *Diprivan*

Ototoxic effects:
    Cochlear:
        Tinnitus: <1% (CPS, PDR)
    Vestibular:
        Dizziness: <1.7% (CPS, PDR)
        Nystagmus: <1% (CPS, PDR)
    Outer/Middle Ear:
        Earache/ear pain: <1% (CPS, PDR)

Risk assessment: Class 2

Propoxyphene

Pronunciation guide: proe-POX-ih-feen

Drug classification: Opiate agonist drugs (see section 1.4.1 in Table 14-1)

Brand names: *Darvon, Darvon-N* [1]

Ototoxic effects:
    Cochlear:
        Tinnitus: (Med, She)
    Vestibular:
        Dizziness: (AHF, CPS)

Risk assessment: Class 1

Notes:

[1] *Darvon-N* is a combination of **Propoxyphene** and **Acetaminophen**. (See the generic drug **Acetaminophen** for its specific ototoxic properties.)

Propranolol

Pronunciation guide: proe-PRAN-oh-lawl

Drug classification: Beta-adrenergic-blocking drugs (Beta-Blockers) (see section 20.8.12 in Table 14-1)

Brand names: *Inderal, Inderal-LA, Inderide* [1], *Innopran XL*

Ototoxic effects:
    Cochlear:
        Auditory Hallucinations: [319]
        Hearing loss: (AHF, CPS)
        Tinnitus: (CPS)

Vestibular:
  Ataxia: (AHF)
  Dizziness: 4-7% [2-5% above placebo results] (CPS, NDH)
  Vertigo: (CPS)

Risk assessment: Class 2

Notes:

[1] *Inderide* is a combination of **Propranolol** and **Hydrochlorothiazide**. (See the generic drug **Hydrochlorothiazide** for its specific ototoxic properties.)

See Chapter 7, "We 'Hear' With Our Eyes" for further information on this drug.

Propulsid (see **Cisapride**)

Propylene glycol

Pronunciation guide: PRAH-puh-leen GLY-call

Drug classification: CERUMENOLYTIC DRUGS (EAR-WAX REMOVERS) (see section 56.4.1 in Table 14-1)

Brand names: *Rhinaris, Salinol, Secaris*

Ototoxic effects:
  Vestibular:
    Ataxia: (NTP)
  Outer/Middle Ear:
    Cholesteatoma: [1]
  Unspecified/General Ear Conditions:
    Ototoxicity: [320]

Risk assessment: Class 2

Notes:

[1] Many oto-topical preparations contain **Propylene glycol**, a solvent and penetrance enhancer. **Propylene glycol** has been associated with extensive middle ear adhesions and cholesteatomas in experimental animals—so caution is warranted in humans.[321]

In light of the above findings, you might want to watch out for your pets. For example, one brand of pet ear wax remover, called *Ear Clear*, says on the front of the bottle that it is "nontoxic" yet it lists two potentially ototoxic substances in the ingredients—**Propylene glycol** and **Salicylic acid**. (See the generic drug **Salicylic acid** for its specific ototoxic properties.)

Propylthiouracil (PTU)

Pronunciation guide: proe-pill-thye-oh-YOOR-ah-sill

Drug classification: ANTI-THYROID DRUGS (see section 40.42.1 in Table 14-1)

Brand names: *Propyl-Thyracil*

Ototoxic effects:
  Cochlear:
    Hearing loss: (CPS) [1]
  Vestibular:
    Dizziness: (CPS, Med)
    Vertigo: (AHF, NDH)

Risk assessment: Class 2

Notes:

  [1] Unilateral sensorineural hearing loss (CPS).

Propyl-Thyracil   (see **Propylthiouracil**)

Proquad   (see **Measles, mumps & rubella vaccine**)

Proquazone

Pronunciation guide: proe-KWA-zon

Drug classification: NON-STEROIDAL ANTI-INFLAMMATORY DRUGS (NSAIDs) (see section 1.1 in Table 14-1)

Brand names: *Biarison*

Ototoxic effects:
  Cochlear:
    Tinnitus: (Ka7)

Risk assessment: Class 1

Prosed   (see **Methenamine**)

ProSom   (see **Estazolam**)

Prostin E2   (see **Dinoprostone**)

Protaxon Forte   (see **Proglumetacin**)

Prothiaden   (see **Dothiepin**)

Protonix   (see **Pantoprazole**)

Protopic   (see **Tacrolimus**)

Protostat   (see **Metronidazole**)

Protriptyline

Pronunciation guide: pro-TRIP-tih-leen

Drug classification: Tricyclic anti-depressants (see section 60.1.8 in Table 14-1)

Brand names: *Triptil*, *Vivactil*

Ototoxic effects:
    Cochlear:
        Tinnitus: (CPS, PDR)
    Vestibular:
        Ataxia: (CPS, PDR)
        Dizziness: (CPS, PDR)

Risk assessment: Class 1

Proventil   (see **Albuterol**)

Provera   (see **Medroxyprogesterone**)

Provigil   (see **Modafinil**)

Prozac   (see **Fluoxetine**)

Prozepam

Pronunciation guide: PROE-zeh-pam

Drug classification: Benzodiazepines (see section 60.12.8 in Table 14-1)

Brand names: *Centrax*

Ototoxic effects:
    Cochlear:
        Tinnitus: (Ka8)

Risk assessment: Class 1

Notes:

See Chapter 10 "Beware of Benzodiazepines—Don't Let This Nasty Time-Bomb Ambush You and Your Ears" for further information on this drug.

Pseudoephedrine

Pronunciation guide: soo-doe-eh-FED-rin

Drug classification: Sympathomimetic drugs (see section 17.16 in Table 14-1)

Brand names: [1] *Actifed, Co-Actifed* [2], *Sudafed*

Ototoxic effects:
    Cochlear:
        Tinnitus: (CPS)
    Vestibular:
        Ataxia: (CPS)
        Dizziness: (CPS, PDR)

Risk assessment: Class 1

Notes:

[1] **Pseudoephedrine** is used in combination with other drugs (both prescription and non-prescription) in formulations too numerous to mention here.

[2] *Co-Actifed* is a combination of Triprolidine, **Pseudoephedrine** and **Codeine**. (See the generic drug **Codeine** for its specific ototoxic properties.)

PTU   (see **Propylthiouracil**)

Pulmicort   (see **Budesonide**)

Pyrantel

Pronunciation guide: PYE-ran-tel

Drug classification: ANTHELMINTIC DRUGS (see section 7.1 in Table 14-1)

Brand names: *Ascarel, Reese's Pinworm Medicine*

Ototoxic effects:
Vestibular:
Dizziness: (AHF)
Unspecified/General Ear Conditions:
Ototoxicity: [1] (AHF)

Risk assessment: Class 1

Notes:

[1] Reported rarely (AHF).

Pyribenzamine   (see **Tripelennamine**)

Pyridostigmine

Pronunciation guide: peer-id-oh-STIG-meen

Drug classification: CHOLINESTERASE INHIBITORS (see section 17.12.4 in Table 14-1)

Brand names: *Regonol*

Ototoxic effects:
Vestibular:
Ataxia: (CPS)
Nystagmus: (BNF)
Vertigo: (AHF, CPS)

Risk assessment: Class 1

B6   (see **Pyridoxine**)

Pyridoxine (Vitamin B$_6$)

Pronunciation guide: peer-ih-DOX-een

Drug classification: VITAMINS (see section 75.4 in Table 14-1)

Brand names: *B6*

Ototoxic effects:
   Vestibular:
      Ataxia: (DFC)

Risk assessment: Class 1

Pyrilamine

Pronunciation guide: pye-RIL-ah-meen

Drug classification: H$_1$ RECEPTOR ANTAGONISTS (see section 10.1 in Table 14-1)

Brand names: [1] *Atrohist* [2], *Midol Extra Strength* [3]

Ototoxic effects:
   Cochlear:
      Tinnitus: (NTP)
   Vestibular:
      Nystagmus: (NTP)
      Vertigo: (NTP)

Risk assessment: Class 1

Notes:

[1] There are many drug preparations that use **Pyrilamine** as one of their compounds. I have only listed two here. As always, check the labels and then look up each drug listed to see its ototoxic properties.

[2] *Atrohist* is a combination of **Phenylephrine, Chlorpheniramine** and **Pyrilamine**. (See the generic drugs **Phenylephrine** and **Chlorpheniramine** for their specific ototoxic properties.)

[3] *Midol Extra Strength* is a combination of **Pyrilamine, Acetaminophen** and **Caffeine**. (See the generic drugs **Acetaminophen** and **Caffeine** for their specific ototoxic properties.)

Pyrimethamine   (see **Sulfadoxine**)

Quadracel   (see **Tetanus vaccine**)

Quazepam

Pronunciation guide: KWA-zee-pam

Drug classification: BENZODIAZEPINES (see section 60.12.8 in Table 14-1)

Brand names: *Doral*

Ototoxic effects:
  Cochlear:
    Tinnitus: (Eps)
  Vestibular:
    Ataxia: (Med, PDR)
    Dizziness: 1.5% [0.5% above placebo results] (Med, PDR)

Risk assessment: Class 1

Notes:

  See Chapter 10 "Beware of Benzodiazepines—Don't Let This Nasty Time-Bomb Ambush You and Your Ears" for further information on this drug.

Questran   (see **Cholestyramine**)

Quetiapine

Pronunciation guide: kweh-TIE-ah-peen

Drug classification: ANTIPSYCHOTIC DRUGS (see section 60.8 in Table 14-1)

Brand names: *Seroquel*

Ototoxic effects:
  Cochlear:
    Hearing loss: <0.1% (PDR)
    Tinnitus: 0.1-1% (DFC, PDR)
  Vestibular:
    Ataxia: 0.1-1% (PDR)
    Dizziness: 10-18% [6-11% above placebo results] (CPS, PDR)
    Vertigo: 0.1-1% (DFC, PDR)
  Outer/Middle Ear:
    Earache/ear pain: 1% [placebo 0] (CPS, PDR)

Risk assessment: Class 2

Notes:

  Caution: Eating grapefruit or drinking grapefruit juice during the time you are taking this drug may make the listed side effects worse than shown here.

  See Chapter 11, "Grapefruit Juice and Ototoxic Drugs" for further information on this drug.

Quinacrine (Mepacrine)

Pronunciation guide: QWIN-ah-kreen (MEP-ah-kreen)

Drug classification: ANTHELMINTIC DRUGS (see section 7.1 in Table 14-1)

Brand names: *Atabrine*

Ototoxic effects:
  Cochlear:
      Hearing loss: [322] (Ka8)
  Vestibular:
      Dizziness: [323] (BNF)

Risk assessment: Class 2

Notes:

  In Britain, **Quinacrine** is known as **Mepacrine**.

  See Chapter 7, "We 'Hear' With Our Eyes" for further information on this drug.

Quinaglute   (see **Quinidine**)

Quinamed....(see **Amonafide**)

Quinapril

Pronunciation guide: KWIN-ah-pril

Drug classification: ANGIOTENSIN-CONVERTING ENZYME (ACE) INHIBITORS (see section 20.8.8 in Table 14-1)

Brand names: *Accupril, Accuretic* [1]

Ototoxic effects:
  Cochlear:
      Tinnitus: <0.5% (CPS)
  Vestibular:
      Ataxia: (PDR)
      Dizziness: 2.7-11.2% [1.3-2.6% above placebo results] (CPS, PDR)
      Vertigo: 0.3-1% (CPS, PDR)

Risk assessment: Class 2

Notes:

  [1] *Accuretic* is a combination of **Quinapril** and **Hydrochlorothiazide**. (See the generic drug **Hydrochlorothiazide** for its specific ototoxic properties.)

Quinate   (see **Quinidine**)

Quinethazone

Pronunciation guide: kwin-ETH-ah-zone

Drug classification: DIURETICS—THIAZIDE-RELATED (see section 30.5.12 in Table 14-1)

Brand names: *Hydromox*

Ototoxic effects:
  Vestibular:
      Vertigo: (NTP)

Risk assessment: Class 1

Quinidex   (see **Quinidine**)

Quinidine

Pronunciation guide: KWIN-ih-deen

Drug classification: ANTI-ARRHYTHMICS (HEART RHYTHM REGULATORS) (see section 20.4 in Table 14-1)

Brand names: *Biquin, Cardioquin, Quinaglute, Quinate, Quinidex*

Ototoxic effects:
    Cochlear:
        Hearing disorder: (CPS, DFC)
        Hearing loss: (CPS, PDR)
        Tinnitus: >10% (NDH, PDR)
    Vestibular:
        Ataxia: (CPS, PDR)
        Dizziness: 3% (CPS, PDR)
        Vertigo: >10% (NDH, PDR)

Risk assessment: Class 3

Notes:

The above ototoxic symptoms may occur after just a single moderate dose in sensitive people (PDR).

Taking too much **Quinidine** can cause a toxic syndrome called cinchonism. Cinchonism symptoms may include temporary or permanent hearing loss, deafness, headaches, nausea, tinnitus, vertigo and visual loss (PDR).[324]

Hearing loss typically occurs as a temporary high-frequency loss, but can result in permanent deafness (PDR). I have an anecdotal report in my files of a woman who noticed she lost her hearing after taking **Quinidine**.

See Chapter 7, "We 'Hear' With Our Eyes" for further information on this drug.

Quinine

Pronunciation guide: KWYE-nine

Drug classification: ANTI-MALARIAL DRUGS (see section 7.14.8 in Table 14-1)

Brand names: *Legatrin, Q-Vel*

Ototoxic effects:
    Cochlear:
        Hearing disorder: (CPS)
        Hearing loss: (AHF, CPS)
        Tinnitus: (AHF, CPS)

Vestibular:
    Ataxia: (AHF)
    Dizziness: (AHF)
    Vertigo: (AHF, CPS)

Risk assessment: Class 4

Notes:

Quinine (and its derivatives) can produce temporary or permanent sensorineural hearing loss with tinnitus as the major symptom.[325] In fact, some **Quinine** derivatives cause significant and long-lasting tinnitus.[326] As a result, you should not take **Quinine** if you already have tinnitus (CPS).

I have an anecdotal report in my files of a woman who had had tinnitus for many years. Her doctor prescribed **Quinine** for her leg cramps. She took one **Quinine** sulfate pill (325 mg.), and woke up the next morning with severe tinnitus. This severe tinnitus has continued unabated for several months now. She only ever took the one **Quinine** pill.

Transient hearing loss is usually the first symptom of **Quinine** ototoxicity. You have a 20% chance of suffering a hearing loss if you take **Quinine** for a long time such as is the case in the treatment for malaria.[327] Audiometric testing often reveals a characteristic sensorineural notch at 4000 Hz.[328]

Taking too much **Quinine** can cause a toxic syndrome called cinchonism. Cinchonism symptoms may include temporary or permanent hearing loss, deafness, headaches, nausea, tinnitus, vertigo and visual loss (PDR).[329]

Quinine is currently popular for treating nocturnal leg cramps. If you are taking **Quinine** for leg cramps, you should be aware of the risk to your hearing.[330]

Taking **Quinine** during pregnancy is a no no. It can result in severe inner ear abnormalities to your unborn baby.[331] If you are pregnant when you take **Quinine**, it can have devastating effects on your unborn child including damaging both his auditory and vestibular systems resulting in permanent deafness and/or balance problems. Your unborn baby is particularly vulnerable during the first trimester, especially between weeks 6 and 8.[332]

Quinine has another (illegal) use. It is sometimes used to "cut" heroin.[333] Therefore, some heroin addicts could have hearing problems from this cause.

Apparently, in the heyday of the Indian "Rajas," the British old-timers who returned to England were frequently deaf from all the tonic water they drank while in India. Tonic water contains **Quinine**. In addition, drinking tonic water can cause significant vestibular (balance) problems.[334] The United States Army found that 75% of the people drinking 1.6 L of tonic water daily for two weeks had significant vestibular (balance) dysfunction.[335] "During World War II, thousands of veterans were treated with **Quinine** for malaria and suffered the misery of partial or total loss of hearing".[336]

See Chapter 2, "Ototoxic Drugs—What Are They," Chapter 3, "Ototoxic Side Effects and Your Ears," Chapter 4, "Are You at Risk?" and Chapter 7, "We 'Hear' With Our Eyes" for further information on this drug.

Q-Vel (see **Quinine**)

RabAvert   (see **Rabies vaccine**)

Rabeprazole

Pronunciation guide: rah-BEH-pray-zol

Drug classification: PROTON PUMP INHIBITORS (see section 34.8.4 in Table 14-1)

Brand names: *Aciphex*, *Pariet*

Ototoxic effects:
    Cochlear:
        Hearing loss: <0.1% (CPS, PDR)
        Tinnitus: <1% (CPS, PDR)
    Vestibular:
        Dizziness: <1% (CPS, PDR)
        Vertigo: <1% (CPS, PDR)
        Vestibular disorder: (CPS)
    Outer/Middle Ear:
        Earache/ear pain: <1% (CPS)
        Otitis externa: <1% (CPS)
        Otitis media: <1% (CPS, PDR)
    Unspecified/General Ear Conditions:
        Ear disorder: <1% (CPS)

Risk assessment: Class 2

Rabies vaccine

Pronunciation guide: RAY-beez VAK-seen

Drug classification: VACCINES (see section 70.8 in Table 14-1)

Brand names: *Imovax*, *RabAvert*

Ototoxic effects:
    Vestibular:
        Dizziness: 9.7% (CPS, DFC)
        Vertigo: <0.1% (CPS, DFC)
    Outer/Middle Ear:
        Earache/ear pain: 3.2% (CPS)

Risk assessment: Class 1

Ralivia   (see **Tramadol**)

Raloxifene

Pronunciation guide: rah-LOX-ih-feen

Drug classification: ESTROGEN AGONIST—ANTAGONISTS (see section 40.16 in Table 14-1)

Brand names: *Evista*

Ototoxic effects:
  Vestibular:
    Vertigo: 4.1% [0.4% above placebo results] (CPS, PDR)

Risk assessment: Class 1

Raltegravir

Pronunciation guide: rahl-TEH-grah-veer

Drug classification: ANTI-RETROVIRAL INTEGRASE INHIBITORS (see section 7.17.1.16 in Table 14-1)

Brand names: *Isentress*

Ototoxic effects:
  Vestibular:
    Dizziness: 4.9% [2.8% above placebo results] (CPS)
    Labyrinthine disorder: 3% [0.9% above placebo results] (CPS)
    Vertigo: <2% (CPS)

Risk assessment: Class 1

Ramipril

Pronunciation guide: rah-MIH-pril

Drug classification: ANGIOTENSIN-CONVERTING ENZYME (ACE) INHIBITORS (see section 20.8.8 in Table 14-1)

Brand names: *Altace, Topril*

Ototoxic effects:
  Cochlear:
    Hearing loss: <1% (CPS, PDR)
    Tinnitus: <1% (CPS, PDR)
  Vestibular:
    Dizziness: 3.7-5.6% [0.9-1.7% above placebo results] (CPS, PDR)
    Equilibrium disorder: <1% (CPS)
    Vertigo: 1.5% [0.8% above placebo results] (CPS, PDR)
  Outer/Middle Ear:
    Feeling of fullness in ears: [1]

Risk assessment: Class 2

Notes:

[1] I have an anecdotal report in my files of a man who gets high-frequency hearing loss, tinnitus (loud buzzing sound) and has a feeling of fullness in his ears as long as he is on **Ramipril**. When he goes off this drug, within a few days of stopping it, the tinnitus and feeling of fullness go away, and 3 weeks or so later his hearing comes back. This

happens every time he goes on it and later comes off it, indicating that for him at least, the ototoxic effects are temporary while on this drug.

Ranexa   (see **Ranolazine**)

Ranibizumab

Pronunciation guide: rah-nih-BIZZ-yoo-mab

Drug classification: MONOCLONAL ANTIBODIES (see section 7.17.8 in Table 14-1)

Brand names: *Lucentis*

Ototoxic effects:
> Vestibular:
>> Dizziness: 4.6-7.9% (CPS)
>> Equilibrium disorder: 0.2-1.1% [<0.8% above placebo results] (CPS)
>> Vertigo: 1.4-6.6% [2.5-5% above placebo results] (CPS)
> Outer/Middle Ear:
>> Earache/ear pain: <1% (CPS)

Risk assessment: Class 2

Ranitidine

Pronunciation guide: rah-NYE-teh-deen

Drug classification: H_2 RECEPTOR ANTAGONISTS (see section 10.4 in Table 14-1)

Brand names: *Zantac*

Ototoxic effects:
> Vestibular:
>> Dizziness: (CPS, PDR)
>> Vertigo: (CPS, PDR)

Risk assessment: Class 1

Ranolazine

Pronunciation guide: ran-OH-lah-zeen

Drug classification: ANTI-ANGINALS (see section 20.1 in Table 14-1)

Brand names: *Ranexa*

Ototoxic effects:
> Cochlear:
>> Tinnitus: 0.5-2.0% (NDH, PDR)
> Vestibular:
>> Dizziness: 1.3-6.2% [<4% above placebo results](NDH, PDR)
>> Vertigo: 0.5-2.0% (NDH, PDR

Risk assessment: Class 2

Rantudil Retard   (see **Acemetacin**)

Rapacuronium

Pronunciation guide: rah-pah-koo-ROE-nee-um

Drug classification: Skeletal muscle relaxants (see section 53.36 in Table 14-1)

Brand names: *Raplon*

Ototoxic effects:
    Cochlear:
        Hearing loss: <0.1% (PDR)

Risk assessment: Class 2

Rapamune   (see **Sirolimus**)

Raplon   (see **Rapacuronium**)

Rasagiline

Pronunciation guide: reh-SAH-jih-leen

Drug classification: Monoamine oxidase inhibitors (see section 60.1.1 in Table 14-1)

Brand names: *Azilect*

Ototoxic effects:
    Cochlear:
        Hearing loss: 0.1-1% (DFC, PDR)
    Vestibular:
        Ataxia: 3-6% [2-5% greater than placebo results] (AHF, PDR)
        Dizziness: >10% (NDH, PDR)
        Vertigo: 2-6% [<5% greater than placebo results] (NDH, PDR)
        Vestibular disorder: <0.1% (DFC, PDR)

Risk assessment: Class 2

Rasilez   (see **Aliskiren**)

ratio-Fentanyl   (see **Fentanyl**)

ratio-Glyburide   (see **Glyburide**)

ratio-Pentoxifylline   (see **Pentoxifylline**)

Raxar   (see **Grepafloxacin**)

Reactine   (see **Cetirizine**)

Rebetol　(see **Ribavirin**)

Rebetron　(see **Interferon alfa-2b**)

Rebif　(see **Interferon beta-1a**)

Reboxetine

Pronunciation guide: ree-BOX-eh-teen

Drug classification: Selective noradrenaline reuptake inhibitors (see section 60.1.20 in Table 14-1)

Brand names: *Edronax*

Ototoxic effects:
　Vestibular:
　　Dizziness: (BNF)
　　Vertigo: (BNF)

Risk assessment: Class 1

Reclast　(see **Zoledronic acid**)

Recombivax HB　(see **Hepatitis B vaccine**)

Redux　(see **Dexfenfluramine**)

Reese's Pinworm Medicine　(see **Pyrantel**)

Reglan　(see **Metoclopramide**)

Regonol　(see **Pyridostigmine**)

Relafen　(see **Nabumetone**)

Relenza　(see **Zanamivir**)

Relistor　(see **Methylnaltrexone**)

Relpax　(see **Eletriptan**)

Remeron　(see **Mirtazapine**)

Remeron RD　(see **Mirtazapine**)

Remeron SolTab　(see **Mirtazapine**)

Remicade　(see **Infliximab**)

Reminyl   (see **Galantamine**)

Renedil   (see **Felodipine**)

Renese   (see **Polythiazide**)

Rengasil   (see **Pirprofen**)

Repetabs   (see **Betamethasone**)

Replagal   (see **Agalsidase alfa**)

ReQuip   (see **Ropinirole**)

Rescinnamine

Pronunciation guide: res-SIN-nah-meen

Drug classification: ANTI-HYPERTENSIVE DRUGS (see section 20.8 in Table 14-1)

Brand names: *Moderil*

Ototoxic effects:
    Cochlear:
        Hearing loss: (PDR)
    Vestibular:
        Dizziness: (CP2, PDR)

Risk assessment: Class 2

Rescriptor   (see **Delavirdine**)

Resdan Dandruff Treatment   (see **Cetrimide**)

Reserpine

Pronunciation guide: re-SER-peen

Drug classification: RAUWOLFIA ALKALOIDS (see section 20.8.32 in Table 14-1)

Brand names: *Diupres*[1], *SER-AP-ES*[2], *Serpasil*

Ototoxic effects:
    Cochlear:
        Hearing loss: (CPS, PDR)
    Vestibular:
        Dizziness: (CPS, PDR)
        Vertigo: (NTP)

Risk assessment: Class 2

Notes:

[1] *Diupres* is a combination of **Reserpine** and **Chlorothiazide**. (See the generic drug **Chlorothiazide** for its specific ototoxic properties.)

[2] *SER-AP-ES* is a combination of **Reserpine**, Hydralazine and **Hydrochlorothiazide**. (See the generic drug **Hydrochlorothiazide** for its specific ototoxic properties.)

See Chapter 7, "We 'Hear' With Our Eyes" for further information on this drug.

Restasis (see **Cyclosporine**)

Restoril (see **Temazepam**)

Retrovir (see **Zidovudine**)

Revatio (see **Sildenafil**)

ReVia (see **Naltrexone**)

Revlimid (see **Lenalidomide**)

Rexolate (see **Sodium thiosalicylate**)

Rheumatrex (see **Methotrexate**)

Rheumox (see **Azapropazone**)

Rhinaris (see **Propylene glycol**)

Rhinocort (see **Budesonide**)

Rhodacine (see **Indomethacin**)

Rhodis (see **Ketoprofen**)

Rhotral (see **Acebutolol**)

Rhotrimine (see **Trimipramine**)

Rhovail (see **Ketoprofen**)

Ribavirin

Pronunciation guide: rye-bah-VYE-rin

Drug classification: ANTI-VIRAL DRUGS (see section 7.17 in Table 14-1)

Brand names: *Rebetol, Virazole*

Ototoxic effects:
    Cochlear:
        Tinnitus: (BNF)
    Vestibular:
        Dizziness: (BNF)

Risk assessment: Class 1

Ribostamycin

Pronunciation guide: rih-boss-tah-MY-sin

Drug classification: AMINOGLYCOSIDES (see section 7.4.1 in Table 14-1)

Brand names: *Ribostat*

Ototoxic effects:
    Unspecified/General Ear Conditions:
        Ototoxicity: [337]

Risk assessment: Not enough information to rate

Notes:
    See Chapter 9, "Aminoglycoside Antibiotics are the Ototoxic 'Bad boys'" for further information on this drug.

Ribostat   (see **Ribostamycin**)

Ridaura   (see **Auranofin**)

Rifadin   (see **Rifampin**)

Rifamate   (see **Rifampin**)

Rifampin

Pronunciation guide: RIF-am-pin

Drug classification: RIFAMYCINS (see section 7.4.52 in Table 14-1)

Brand names: *Rifadin, Rifamate* [1], *Rifater* [2], *Rimactane, Rofact*

Ototoxic effects:
    Cochlear:
        Hearing loss: [338]
        Tinnitus: (PDR)
    Vestibular:
        Ataxia: (CPS, PDR)
        Dizziness: (CPS, PDR)
        Equilibrium disorder: (PDR)
        Vertigo: (PDR)

Risk assessment: Class 2

Notes:

[1] *Rifamate* is a combination of **Rifampin** and **Isoniazid**. (See the generic drug **Isoniazid** for its specific ototoxic properties.)

[2] *Rifater* is a combination of **Rifampin**, **Isoniazid** and Pyrazinamide. (See the generic drug **Isoniazid** for its specific ototoxic properties.)

When the three drugs in *Rifater* were taken in the one tablet, the incidence of tinnitus and vertigo was 2%. However, when these three drugs were taken separately, the incidence of tinnitus and vertigo rose to 5% (PDR).

Rifater   (see **Rifampin**)

Rifaximin

Pronunciation guide: rih-FAX-ih-min

Drug classification: RIFAMYCINS (see section 7.4.52 in Table 14-1)

Brand names: *Xifaxan*

Ototoxic effects:
Cochlear:
Tinnitus: <2% (DFC, PDR)
Vestibular:
Dizziness: <2% (DFC, PDR)
Outer/Middle Ear:
Earache/ear pain: <2% (DFC, PDR)

Risk assessment: Class 2

Rilutek   (see **Riluzole**)

Riluzole

Pronunciation guide: RILL-you-zole

Drug classification: ANTI-AMYOTROPHIC LATERAL SCLEROSIS DRUGS (see section 53.8 in Table 14-1)

Brand names: *Rilutek*

Ototoxic effects:
Cochlear:
Hearing loss: <0.1% (CPS, PDR)
Hyperacusis: <0.1% (CPS, PDR)
Vestibular:
Ataxia: 0.1-1% (CPS, PDR)
Dizziness: 3.8-12.7% [1.3-10.2% above placebo results] (CPS, PDR)
Vertigo: 1.9-4.5% [1-3.6 above placebo results] (CPS, PDR)
Vestibular disorder: <0.1% (CPS, PDR)

Outer/Middle Ear:
Earache/ear pain: <0.1% (CPS, PDR)

Risk assessment: Class 2

Rimactane   (see **Rifampin**)

Rimadyl   (see **Carprofen**)

Rimantadine

Pronunciation guide: rih-MAN-tah-deen

Drug classification: ANTI-VIRAL DRUGS (see section 7.17 in Table 14-1)

Brand names: *Flumadine*

Ototoxic effects:
Cochlear:
Tinnitus: 0.3-1% (AHF, PDR)
Vestibular:
Ataxia: 0.3-1% (AHF, PDR)
Dizziness: 0.7-1.9% [0.7-0.8% above placebo results] (AHF, PDR)

Risk assessment: Class 2

Risedronate

Pronunciation guide: rih-SED-roe-nate

Drug classification: BISPHOSPHONATES (see section 50.1.1 in Table 14-1)

Brand names: *Actonel*

Ototoxic effects:
Cochlear:
Hearing loss: [1]
Tinnitus: 1.6-3.3% [<1.6% above placebo results] (CPS, PDR)
Vestibular:
Dizziness: 4.9-6.7% [<1.4% above placebo results] (CPS, PDR)
Vertigo: 1.6-3.3% [0.1% above placebo results] (PDR)
Outer/Middle Ear:
Earache/ear pain: 1.6% [same as placebo] (CPS, PDR)
Otitis media: 2.5% [0.1% above placebo results] (DFC, PDR)

Risk assessment: Class 2

[1] I have an anecdotal report in my files of hearing loss from taking **Risedronate**. A woman wrote, "I was given **Risedronate** (*Actonel*) for osteoporosis. After taking the first pill I had severe chest pains and suffered profound hearing loss in one ear and some hearing loss in the other".

Risperdal   (see **Risperidone**)

Risperidone

Pronunciation guide: ris-PEER-ih-dohn

Drug classification: ANTIPSYCHOTIC DRUGS (see section 60.8 in Table 14-1)

Brand names: *Risperdal*

Ototoxic effects:
    Cochlear:
        Hearing loss: 0.1-1% (AHF, PDR)
        Hyperacusis: <0.1% (AHF, PDR)
        Tinnitus: <0.1% (AHF, PDR)
    Vestibular:
        Ataxia: 4% [placebo 0] (CPS, PDR)
        Dizziness: 3-11% [2-6% above placebo results] (CPS, PDR)
        Vertigo: 0.1-1% (AHF, PDR)
    Outer/Middle Ear:
        Earache/ear pain: <2% (CPS, PDR)
    Unspecified/General Ear Conditions:
        Ear disorder: 3% [placebo 0] (NDH, PDR)

Risk assessment: Class 2

Ritonavir

Pronunciation guide: rih-TON-ah-veer

Drug classification: ANTI-RETROVIRAL PROTEASE INHIBITORS (see section 7.17.1.1 in Table 14-1)

Brand names: *Kaletra* [1], *Norvir*

Ototoxic effects:
    Cochlear:
        Hearing loss: <2% (CPS, PDR)
        Hyperacusis: <2% (PDR)
        Tinnitus: <2% (CPS, PDR)
    Vestibular:
        Ataxia: <2% (CPS, PDR)
        Dizziness: 2.6-5.2% [1.5-2.8% above placebo results] (CPS, PDR)
        Vertigo: <2% (CPS, PDR)
        Vestibular disorder: <2% (Med, PDR)
    Outer/Middle Ear:
        Earache/ear pain: <2% (CPS, PDR)
        Increased ear wax: <2% (CPS, PDR)
        Otitis media: <2% (CPS, PDR)

Risk assessment: Class 3

Notes:

[1] *Kaletra* is a combination of **Lopinavir** and **Ritonavir**. You could expect **Lopinavir** (low-PIN-ah-veer) to have much the same ototoxic properties as **Ritonavir** since both of these drugs are in the same class (ANTI-RETROVIRAL PROTEASE INHIBITORS—section 7.17.1.1 in Table 14-1). At the very least, **Lopinavir** likely can cause ataxia, dizziness, otitis media and tinnitus (BNF, PDR).

Rituxan   (see **Rituximab**)

Rituximab

Pronunciation guide: rih-TUX-ih-mab

Drug classification: MONOCLONAL ANTIBODIES (see section 7.17.8 in Table 14-1)

Brand names: *Rituxan*

Ototoxic effects:
    Cochlear:
        Hearing loss: <1% (CPS)
        Tinnitus: 1-5% (CPS)
    Vestibular:
        Dizziness: 1-10% (CPS, PDR)
        Vertigo: 1-5% (NDH, PDR)
    Outer/Middle Ear:
        Earache/ear pain: 1-5% (CPS)
        Otitis externa: <1% (CPS)

Risk assessment: Class 3

Notes:

Hearing loss may occur up to several months after completion of **Rituximab** therapy (CPS).

Rivastigmine

Pronunciation guide: riv-ah-STIG-meen

Drug classification: CHOLINESTERASE INHIBITORS (see section 17.12.4 in Table 14-1)

Brand names: *Exelon*

Ototoxic effects:
    Cochlear:
        Hearing loss: 0.1-1% (CPS)
        Tinnitus: >1% (CPS, PDR)
    Vestibular:
        Ataxia: >1% (CPS, PDR)
        Dizziness: 2-21% [1-10% above placebo results] (CPS, PDR)
        Nystagmus: 0.1-1% (CPS, PDR)

Vertigo: >2% [1% above placebo results] (CPS, PDR)
Vestibular disorder: 0.1-1% (CPS)
Outer/Middle Ear:
Earache/ear pain: 0.1-1% (CPS)
Otitis media: 0.1-1% (CPS, PDR)
Unspecified/General Ear Conditions:
Ear disorder: 0.1-1% (CPS)
Meniere's disease: 0.1-1% (CPS, DFC)

Risk assessment: Class 3

Rivotril   (see **Clonazepam**)

Rizatriptan

Pronunciation guide: rih-zah-TRIP-tan

Drug classification: Serotonin-receptor agonists (see section 53.32 in Table 14-1)

Brand names: *Maxalt*

Ototoxic effects:
Cochlear:
Hearing loss: (PDR)
Hyperacusis: <0.1% (CPS, PDR)
Tinnitus: 0.1-1% (CPS, PDR)
Vestibular:
Ataxia: 0.1-1% (CPS, PDR)
Dizziness: 4-9% [<4% above placebo results] (CPS, PDR)
Vertigo: 0.1-1% (CPS, PDR)
Outer/Middle Ear:
Earache/ear pain: 0.1-1% (CPS, PDR)

Risk assessment: Class 2

Notes:

I have an anecdotal report in my files of a woman who has been taking **Rizatriptan** (and **Zolmitriptan**) for "some time now and gradually lost hearing in my right ear".

RMS   (see **Morphine**)

Robax Platinum   (see **Methocarbamol**)

Robaxacet   (see **Methocarbamol**)

Robaxin   (see **Methocarbamol**)

Robaxisal   (see **Acetylsalicylic acid**)

Rocephin   (see **Ceftriaxone**)

Rofact (see **Rifampin**)

Rofecoxib

Pronunciation guide: row-feh-KOK-sib

Drug classification: COX-2 INHIBITORS (see section 1.1.4 in Table 14-1)

Brand names: *Vioxx*

Ototoxic effects:
　　Cochlear:
　　　　Tinnitus: 0.1-1.9% (CPS, PDR)
　　Vestibular:
　　　　Dizziness: 3% [0.8% above placebo results] (CPS, PDR)
　　　　Vertigo: 0.1-1.9% (CPS, PDR)
　　Outer/Middle Ear:
　　　　Earache/ear pain: 0.1-1.9% (CPS, PDR)
　　　　Increased ear wax: 0.1-1.9% (CPS, PDR)
　　　　Otitis: 0.1-1.9% (CPS)
　　　　Otitis media: 0.1-1.9% (CPS, PDR)

Risk assessment: Class 2

Notes:

I have an anecdotal report in my files of a woman who got loud tinnitus whenever she took **Rofecoxib** for her fibromyalgia.

Rofecoxib was withdrawn from the USA market on September 23, 2004.

Roferon-A (see **Interferon alfa-2a**)

Rogaine (see **Minoxidil**)

Rogaine for Men Extra Strength (see **Minoxidil**)

Rogaine for Women (see **Minoxidil**)

Rohypnol (see **Flunitrazepam**)

Romazicon (see **Flumazenil**)

Romiplostim

Pronunciation guide: roe-mih-PLOE-stim

Drug classification: HEMATOPOIETIC AGENTS (see section 36.20 in Table 14-1)

Brand names: *Nplate*

Ototoxic effects:
    Cochlear:
        Tinnitus: 2.4% [placebo 0] (CPS)
    Vestibular:
        Dizziness: 12.5-16.7% [placebo 0] (CPS)
    Outer/Middle Ear:
        Earache/ear pain: 2.2% (CPS)
        Otitis: 2.4-3.7% [placebo 0] (CPS)
        Otorrhagia: 2.2-2.4% [placebo 0] (CPS)

Risk assessment: Class 2

Rondomycin (see **Methacycline**)

Ropinirole

Pronunciation guide: roe-PIN-ih-role

Drug classification: DOPAMINE RECEPTOR AGONISTS (see section 53.16.1 in Table 14-1)

Brand names: *ReQuip*

Ototoxic effects:
    Cochlear:
        Hearing loss: 0.1-1% (CPS, PDR)
        Hyperacusis: <0.1% (CPS)
        Tinnitus: 1.3% [placebo 0] (CPS, PDR)
    Vestibular:
        Ataxia: 0.1-14% (CPS, PDR)
        Dizziness: 20.1-40.1% [10.2-18.3% above placebo results] (CPS, PDR)
        Vertigo: 2-7.1% [0-2% above placebo results] (CPS, PDR)
        Vestibular disorder: 0.1-1% (CPS, PDR)
    Outer/Middle Ear:
        Earache/ear pain: 0.1-1% (CPS, PDR)
        Otitis media: 0.1-1% (CPS, PDR)
    Unspecified/General Ear Conditions:
        Ear disorder: (CPS)

Risk assessment: Class 3

Ropivacaine

Pronunciation guide: roe-PIV-ah-kane

Drug classification: AMIDES (see section 4.1 in Table 14-1)

Brand names: *Naropin*

Ototoxic effects:
    Cochlear:
        Hearing disorder: <1% (CPS, PDR)
        Tinnitus: <1% (CPS, PDR)

Vestibular:
 Dizziness: 1.1-10% (CPS, PDR)
 Vertigo: <1% (DFC, PDR)

Risk assessment: Class 2

Rosuvastatin

Pronunciation guide: row-SUE-vah-stah-tin

Drug classification: HMG-CoA REDUCTASE INHIBITORS (see section 20.12.8 in Table 14-1)

Brand names: *Crestor*

Ototoxic effects:
 Cochlear:
  Tinnitus: [1]
 Vestibular:
  Dizziness: 4% [1.2% above placebo results] (NDH, PDR)
  Vertigo: (NDH)

Risk assessment: Class 1

Notes:

[1] I have an anecdotal report in my files of a man that took **Rosuvastatin** and shortly afterwards experienced tinnitus. I also have an anecdotal report in my files of a woman that took **Rosuvastatin** and some months later developed tinnitus.

Rotashield (see **Rotavirus vaccine**)

RotaTeq (see **Rotavirus vaccine**)

Rotavirus vaccine

Pronunciation guide: ROTE-ta-vie-rus VAK-seen

Drug classification: VACCINES (see section 70.8 in Table 14-1)

Brand names: *Rotashield, RotaTeq*

Ototoxic effects:
 Outer/Middle Ear:
  Otitis media: 14.5% [1.5% above placebo results] (AHF, PDR)

Risk assessment: Class 1

Rotigotine

Pronunciation guide: roe-TIH-goh-teen

Drug classification: ANTI-PARKINSONIAN DRUGS (see section 53.16 in Table 14-1)

Brand names: *Neupro*

Ototoxic effects:
    Cochlear:
        Tinnitus: 0.1-1% (PDR)
    Vestibular:
        Ataxia: 0.1-1% (PDR)
        Dizziness: 18% [7% above placebo results] (PDR)
        Vertigo: 3% [1% above placebo results[(PDR)

Risk assessment: Class 2

Roubac   (see **Trimethoprim**)

Rowasa   (see **Mesalamine**)

Roxanol   (see **Morphine**)

Roxicet   (see **Oxycodone**)

Roxithromycin

Pronunciation guide: rocks-ith-roe-MY-sin

Drug classification: MACROLIDE ANTIBIOTICS (see section 7.4.32 in Table 14-1)

Brand names: *Cadithro, Rulid, Rulide, Surlid*

Ototoxic effects:
    Cochlear:
        Tinnitus: [1]
    Vestibular:
        Dizziness: [1,2]
        Vertigo: [2]

Risk assessment: Class 2

Notes:

    [1] Can cause ringing in the ears and dizziness.[339]

    [2] Can cause dizziness and vertigo.[340]

Royflex   (see **Triethanolamine**)

Rubella & mumps vaccine

Pronunciation guide: rue-BELL-ah, MUMPS VAK-seen

Drug classification: VACCINES (see section 70.8 in Table 14-1)

Brand names: *Bivax*

Ototoxic effects:
    Cochlear:
        Hearing loss: (PDR)
    Vestibular:
        Dizziness: (PDR)

Risk assessment: Class 2

Rubella vaccine

Pronunciation guide: rue-BELL-ah VAK-seen

Drug classification: VACCINES (see section 70.8 in Table 14-1)

Brand names: *Meruvax II*

Ototoxic effects:
    Cochlear:
        Hearing loss: (DFC, PDR)
    Vestibular:
        Dizziness: (AHF, PDR)
    Outer/Middle Ear:
        Otitis media: (DFC, PDR)

Risk assessment: Class 2

Rufinamide

Pronunciation guide: ruh-FIN-ah-mide

Drug classification: ANTI-CONVULSANT DRUGS (see section 53.12 in Table 14-1)

Brand names: *Banzel*

Ototoxic effects:
    Vestibular:
        Ataxia: 4-5.4% [<4% above placebo results] (PDR)
        Dizziness: 2.7-19% [<7% above placebo results] (PDR)
        Nystagmus: >5% (PDR)
        Vertigo: 3% [2% above placebo results] (PDR)
    Outer/Middle Ear:
        Otitis: 3% [2% above placebo results] (PDR)

Risk assessment: Class 2

Rulid   (see **Roxithromycin**)

Rulide   (see **Roxithromycin**)

Rynatan   (see **Azatadine**)

Rythmodan   (see **Disopyramide**)

Rythmol (see **Propafenone**)

Ryzolt (see **Tramadol**)

Sabril (see **Vigabatrin**)

Sagamicin (see **Micronomicin**)

Saizen (see **Somatropin**)

Salac (see **Salicylic acid**)

Salacid (see **Salicylic acid**)

Salagen (see **Pilocarpine**)

Salazopyrin (see **Sulfasalazine**)

Salbutamol (see **Albuterol**)

Salflex (see **Salsalate**)

Salicylic acid

Pronunciation guide: sal-ih-SILL-ik ASS-id

Drug classification: SALICYLATES (see section 1.1.16 in Table 14-1)

Brand names: [1] *Compound W, Diprosalic, DuoFilm, Lactisal, Occlusal, Salac, Salacid, Verukan*

Ototoxic effects:
   Cochlear:
      Hearing disorder: (CPS)
      Tinnitus:(Med)
   Vestibular:
      Dizziness: (Med)

Risk assessment: Class 2

Notes:

[1] There are over 70 brands containing **Salicylic acid**—far too many to list here—but these are a few of the more common ones.

Symptoms of **Salicylic acid** poisoning include dizziness and continuous ringing or buzzing in your ears (tinnitus).[341]

Salinol (see **Propylene glycol**)

Salmeterol

Pronunciation guide: sal-MEE-ter-all

Drug classification: BRONCHODILATORS—BETA ADRENERGIC AGONISTS (see section 63.4 in
      Table 14-1)

Brand names: *Serevent*

Ototoxic effects:
    Vestibular:
        Dizziness: 4% [<2% above placebo results] (CPS, PDR)
        Vertigo: (AHF)
    Outer/Middle Ear:
        Earache/ear pain: 1-3% (CPS, PDR)
        Otitis media: 10-19% (CPS)

Risk assessment: Class 2

Salofalk   (see **Mesalamine**)

Salsalate

Pronunciation guide: SAL-sah-late

Drug classification: SALICYLATES (see section 1.1.16 in Table 14-1)

Brand names: *Disalcid, Mono-Gesic, Salflex*

Ototoxic effects:
    Cochlear:
        Hearing loss: (PDR)
        Tinnitus: (PDR)
    Vestibular:
        Vertigo: (PDR)

Risk assessment: Class 2

Notes:

    The appearance of tinnitus and/or hearing loss is often used as a guide to therapy (PDR).
    (If either one occurs, you know you just took too much and should let your doctor know.)

    Both tinnitus and hearing loss are normally temporary and should go away after you
    complete treatment (PDR).

Sandimmune   (see **Cyclosporine**)

Sandomigran   (see **Pizotifen**)

Sandostatin   (see **Octreotide**)

Sandostatin LAR　(see **Octreotide**)

SangCya　(see **Cyclosporine**)

Sansert　(see **Methysergide**)

Saquinavir

Pronunciation guide: sah-KWIN-ah-veer

Drug classification: ANTI-RETROVIRAL PROTEASE INHIBITORS (see section 7.17.1.1 in Table 14-1)

Brand names: *Fortovase, Invirase*

Ototoxic effects:
　Cochlear:
　　　Hearing loss: <2% (CPS, PDR)
　　　Tinnitus: <2% (CPS, PDR)
　Vestibular:
　　　Ataxia: <2% (CPS, PDR)
　　　Dizziness: 1-2% (CPS, PDR)
　Outer/Middle Ear:
　　　Earache/ear pain: <2% (CPS, PDR)
　　　Middle ear pressure: <2% (CPS, PDR)
　　　Otitis: <2% (CPS, PDR)

Risk assessment: Class 2

Notes:

　Caution: Eating grapefruit or drinking grapefruit juice during the time you are taking this drug may make the listed side effects worse than shown here. In fact, taking **Saquinavir** with grapefruit juice can increase the potency of **Saquinavir** by as much as 200%.

　See Chapter 11, "Grapefruit Juice and Ototoxic Drugs" for further information on this drug.

Sarafem　(see **Fluoxetine**)

Sativex　(see **Dronabinol**)

Savella　(see **Milnacipran**)

Scandonest　(see **Mepivacaine**)

Scopolamine

Pronunciation guide: skoe-POL-ah-meen

Drug classification: ANTI-CHOLINERGIC DRUGS (see section 17.1 in Table 14-1)

Brand names: *Transderm Scop, Transderm-V*

Ototoxic effects:
    Vestibular:
        Dizziness: 12% (DFC, PDR)
        Equilibrium disturbances: (CPS, PDR)

Risk assessment: Class 1

Seasonale   (see **Ethinyl estradiol**)

Secaris   (see **Propylene glycol**)

Secbutabarbital   (see **Butabarbital**)

Secobarbital

Pronunciation guide: see-koe-BAR-bih-tall

Drug classification: BARBITURATES (see section 60.12.4 in Table 14-1)

Brand names: *Seconal*

Ototoxic effects:
    Vestibular:
        Ataxia: (PDR)
        Dizziness: (CPS, PDR)
        Vertigo: (CPS)

Risk assessment: Class 1

Seconal   (see **Secobarbital**)

Sectral   (see **Acebutolol**)

Sedapap   (see **Butalbital**)

Select   (see **Ethinyl estradiol**)

Select 1/35   (see **Ethinyl estradiol**)

Selegiline (l-Deprenyl)

Pronunciation guide: seh-LEH-jih-leen

Drug classification: MONOAMINE OXIDASE INHIBITORS (see section 60.1.1 in Table 14-1)

Brand names: *Apo-Selegiline, Carbex, Deprenyl, Eldepryl, Emsam, Novo-Selegiline*

Ototoxic effects:
    Cochlear:
        Hearing loss: (DFC)
        Tinnitus: >1% (CPS, PDR)

Vestibular:
    Ataxia: 3% [2% above placebo results] (DFC, PDR)
    Dizziness: 7-11% [3-6% above placebo results] (DFC, PDR)
    Equilibrium disorder: (PDR)
    Loss of balance: (CPS, PDR)
    Vertigo: 0.1-1% (CPS, PDR)
Outer/Middle Ear:
    Earache/ear pain: 0.1-1% (PDR)
    Otitis externa: <0.1% (DFC, PDR)
    Otitis media: 0.1-1% (PDR)

Risk assessment: Class 2

Notes:

Watch out for your pets too. Veterinarians use **Selegiline** under the brand name of *Anipryl* in treating your pooch. The literature on *Anipryl* cites studies that show 2% of dogs taking this drug end up with hearing loss.[342] If this drug can affect your dog's hearing, there is a good chance it can affect yours also.

See the section "Watch Out for Your Pet's Ears Too" in Chapter 12 for more information on this important topic.

Sensorcaine   (see **Bupivacaine**)

Septocaine   (see **Articaine**)

Septra   (see **Trimethoprim**)

Septrin   (see **Trimethoprim**)

SER-AP-ES   (see **Reserpine**)

Serax   (see **Oxazepam**)

Serentil   (see **Mesoridazine**)

Serevent   (see **Salmeterol**)

Seromycin   (see **Cycloserine**)

Serophene   (see **Clomiphene**)

Seroquel   (see **Quetiapine**)

Serostim   (see **Somatropin**)

Serpasil   (see **Reserpine**)

Sertraline

Pronunciation guide: SIR-trah-leen

Drug classification: SELECTIVE SEROTONIN REUPTAKE INHIBITORS (see section 60.1.32 in Table 14-1)

Brand names: *Zoloft*

Ototoxic effects:
Cochlear:
Hearing loss: [1]
Hyperacusis: <0.1% (AHF, PDR)
Tinnitus: 1.4-4% [0.3-1% above placebo results] (CPS, PDR)
Vestibular:
Ataxia: 0.1-1% (CPS, PDR)
Dizziness: 11-17% [4-8% above placebo results] (CPS, PDR)
Labyrinthine disorder: <0.1% (AHF, PDR)
Nystagmus: 0.1-1% (CPS, PDR)
Vertigo: 0.1-1% (CPS, PDR)
Outer/Middle Ear:
Earache/ear pain: 0.1-1% (CPS, PDR)
Otitis media: <0.1% (CPS, PDR)

Risk assessment: Class 3

Notes:

[1] I have an anecdotal report in my files of a man that began to experience hearing loss after taking **Sertraline** for 5 weeks. He continued to take **Sertraline** for 5 more weeks. Ten weeks later, he began experiencing "horrific screaming tinnitus" and severe hyperacusis such that he couldn't tolerate "the sound of two dishes slightly bumping against each other in the sink". His hearing continued to get worse and worse as time went by. In addition he experienced extreme ear pain.

Curiously, in the few months following stopping the **Sertraline**, he reported that his hyperacusis would get much better at the same time that he would occasionally lose all hearing in one ear or the other for a minute or so.

I have an anecdotal report in my files of a woman who also experienced hearing loss after she stopped taking **Sertraline**.

Serzone (see **Nefazodone**)

Sibelium (see **Flunarizine**)

Sibutramine

Pronunciation guide: sih-BUH-trah-meen

Drug classification: ANOREXIANTS (see section 60.20.1 in Table 14-1)

Brand names: *Meridia*

Ototoxic effects:
Cochlear:
Hearing loss: 0.1-1% (CPS)
Tinnitus: 0.1-1% (CPS, PDR)
Vestibular:
Ataxia: 0.1-1% (CPS, PDR)
Dizziness: 4.9-7% [1.6-3.6% above placebo results] (CPS, PDR)
Vertigo: 1.1% [0.4% above placebo results] (CPS, PDR)
Vestibular disorder: 0.1-1% (CPS)
Outer/Middle Ear:
Earache/ear pain: 1.1% [0.4% above placebo results] (CPS, PDR)
Otitis externa: 0.1-1% (CPS, PDR)
Otitis media: 0.1-1% (CPS, PDR)
Unspecified/General Ear Conditions:
Ear disorder: 1.7% [0.8 above placebo results] (DFC, PDR)

Risk assessment: Class 2

Notes:

Sibutramine with withdrawn from the USA market on October 8, 2010 due to increased heart attacks, strokes and death.[343]

Sildenafil

Pronunciation guide: sill-DEN-ah-fill

Drug classification: PHOSPHODIESTERASE TYPE 5 (PDE5) INHIBITORS (see section 20.8.28 in Table 14-1)

Brand names: *Revatio, Viagra*

Ototoxic effects:
Cochlear:
Hearing loss: <2% (CPS, PDR)
Tinnitus: <2% (CPS, PDR)
Vestibular:
Ataxia: <2% (CPS, PDR)
Dizziness: 2.2% [1% above placebo results] (CPS, PDR)
Vertigo: 1-5% [<4% above placebo results] (CPS, PDR)
Outer/Middle Ear:
Earache/ear pain: <2% (CPS, PDR)
Unspecified/General Ear Conditions:
Ear disorder: <2% (CPS)

Risk assessment: Class 4

Notes:

Sudden hearing loss (partial loss to complete loss) can occur within hours to two days of taking this drug. In the 29 cases of ear problems reported to the FDA, sudden hearing loss typically occurred in one ear. The hearing loss was sometimes accompanied by tinnitus, dizziness and/or vertigo. The hearing loss was temporary in 1/3 of the cases reported.[344]

The results in a study of 11,525 men over the age of 40 indicated that men who use **Sildenafil** (or **Tadalafil** or **Vardenafil**) were twice as likely to have hearing loss as those who did not use such drugs. The resulting hearing loss was "long term" (permanent).[345]

A 44-year-old man experienced permanent bilateral sensorineural deafness 15 days after initiating therapy with **Sildenafil** 50 mg. daily (AHF)

I have an anecdotal report in my files of a 58 year-old man who wrote, "I use *Viagra* once every 2 or 3 months. I have noticed a mild decrease in my hearing that seems to be associated with the *Viagra* use".

Caution: Eating grapefruit or drinking grapefruit juice during the time you are taking this drug may make the listed side effects worse than shown here.

See Chapter 5, "Here's How the System Works," Chapter 7, "We 'Hear' With Our Eyes" and Chapter 11, "Grapefruit Juice and Ototoxic Drugs" for further information on this drug.

Simethicone

Pronunciation guide: sih-METH-ih-kone

Drug classification: Antiflatulents (see section 34.4 in Table 14-1)

Brand names: *SonoRx*

Ototoxic effects:
Outer/Middle Ear:
Earache/ear pain: 0.5% [placebo 0] (DFC)

Risk assessment: Class 1

Simply Sleep (see **Diphenhydramine**)

Simvastatin

Pronunciation guide: sim-vah-STAH-tin

Drug classification: HMG-CoA reductase inhibitors (see section 20.12.8 in Table 14-1)

Brand names: *Vytorin* [1], *Zocor*

Ototoxic effects:
Vestibular:
Dizziness: (CPS, PDR)
Vertigo: 4.5% [0.3% above placebo results] (PDR)

Risk assessment: Class 1

Notes:

[1] *Vytorin* is a combination of Ezetimibe and **Simvastatin**. **Simvastatin** is the ototoxic drug.

Caution: Eating grapefruit or drinking grapefruit juice during the time you are taking this drug may make the listed side effects worse than shown here. In fact, taking **Simvastatin** with grapefruit juice can increase the potency of **Simvastatin** by a whopping 1,513%!

See Chapter 11, "Grapefruit Juice and Ototoxic Drugs" for further information on this drug.

Sinemet   (see **Levodopa**)

Sinequan   (see **Doxepin**)

Singulair   (see **Montelukast**)

Sirolimus

Pronunciation guide: sir-AH-lih-mus

Drug classification: IMMUNOSUPPRESSANT DRUGS (see section 43 in Table 14-1)

Brand names: *Rapamune*

Ototoxic effects:
   Cochlear:
      Hearing loss: 3-20% (NDH, PDR)
      Tinnitus: 3-20% (CPS, PDR)
   Vestibular:
      Dizziness: 3-20% [1-5% above placebo results] (CPS, PDR)
   Outer/Middle Ear:
      Earache/ear pain: 3-20% (CPS, PDR)
      Otitis media: 3-20% (NDH, PDR)

Risk assessment: Class 4

Sisomicin

Pronunciation guide: sih-soe-MY-sin

Drug classification: AMINOGLYCOSIDES (see section 7.4.1 in Table 14-1)

Brand names: *Extramycin, Sisomina*

Ototoxic effects:
   Unspecified/General Ear Conditions:
      Ototoxicity: [346]

Risk assessment: Not enough information to rate

Notes:

   See Chapter 9, "Aminoglycoside Antibiotics are the Ototoxic 'Bad boys'" for further information on this drug.

Sisomina   (see **Sisomicin**)

Sitaxsentan

Pronunciation guide: sih-TAKS-sen-tan

Drug classification: ENDOTHELIN RECEPTOR ANTAGONISTS (see section 20.8.24 in Table 14-1)

Brand names: *Thelin*

Ototoxic effects:
  Cochlear:
    Hearing loss: <1% (CPS)
    Tinnitus: <1% (CPS)
  Vestibular:
    Ataxia: <1% (CPS)
    Dizziness: <1% (CPS)
    Vertigo: <1% (CPS)
  Outer/Middle Ear:
    Earache/ear pain: <1% (CPS)
    Ears blocked: <1% (CPS)
    Otitis media: <1% (CPS)

Risk assessment: Class 2

Skelid   (see **Tiludronate**)

Slow-Trasicor   (see **Oxprenolol**)

Sodium benzoate   (see **Sodium phenylacetate**)

Sodium cromoglycate   (see **Cromolyn sodium**)

Sodium Diuril   (see **Chlorothiazide**)

Sodium ferric gluconate

Pronunciation guide: SOE-dee-um FAIR-ick GLUE-koh-nate

Drug classification: MINERALS (see section 75.8 in Table 14-1)

Brand names: *Ferrlecit*

Ototoxic effects:
  Vestibular:
    Dizziness: 13% (AHF, PDR)
  Unspecified/General Ear Conditions:
    Ear disorder: (AHF, PDR)

Risk assessment: Class 1

Sodium oxybate

Pronunciation guide: SOE-dee-um OKS-ee-bate

Drug classification: ANTI-CATAPLECTIC DRUGS (see section 53.1 in Table 14-1)

Brand names: *Xyrem*

Ototoxic effects:
    Cochlear:
        Auditory hallucinations: (DFC)
        Tinnitus: 6% [placebo 0] (CPS, PDR)
    Vestibular:
        Ataxia: >1% (CPS, PDR)
        Dizziness: 17-34% [<28% above placebo results] (AHF, PDR)
        Equilibrium disorder: >1% (DFC, PDR)
        Vertigo: >1% (DFC, PDR)
    Outer/Middle Ear:
        Earache/ear pain: >1% (DFC, PDR)
        Otitis externa: 0.1-1% (DFC)

Risk assessment: Class 2

Sodium phenylacetate

Pronunciation guide: SOE-dee-um FEN-ill-ASS-ih-tate

Drug classification: MISCELLANEOUS DRUGS (see section 46 in Table 14-1)

Brand names: *Ammonul* [1]

Ototoxic effects:
    Vestibular:
        Ataxia: <3% (DFC, RXL)

Risk assessment: Class 1

Notes:

    [1] *Ammonul* is a combination of **Sodium phenylacetate** and Sodium benzoate. (**Sodium phenylacetate** is probably the ototoxic agent.)

Sodium phenylbutyrate

Pronunciation guide: SOE-dee-um FEN-ill-BUE-tih-rate

Drug classification: MISCELLANEOUS DRUGS (see section 46 in Table 14-1)

Brand names: *Buphenyl*

Ototoxic effects:
    Cochlear:
        Hearing loss: (DFC)

Risk assessment: Class 2

Sodium salicylate

Pronunciation guide: SOE-dee-um sah-LISS-ill-ate

Drug classification: SALICYLATES (see section 1.1.16 in Table 14-1)

Brand names: *Diuretin, Dodd's Pills, Gin Pain Pills, Pabalate, Uracel*

Ototoxic effects:
    Cochlear:
        Hearing loss: (Med+)
        Tinnitus: (Med+, She)
    Vestibular:
        Dizziness: (Med+)
    Unspecified/General Ear Conditions:
        Ototoxicity: (San)

Risk assessment: Class 2

Notes:
    See Chapter 7, "We 'Hear' With Our Eyes" for further information on this drug.

Sodium stibogluconate

Pronunciation guide: SOE-dee-um stih-boe-GLUE-koe-nate

Drug classification: ANTI-PROTOZOALS (see section 7.14 in Table 14-1)

Brand names: *Pentostam*

Ototoxic effects:
    Vestibular:
        Vertigo: (BNF)

Risk assessment: Class 1

Sodium thiosalicylate

Pronunciation guide: SOE-dee-um thy-oh-sah-LISS-ill-ate

Drug classification: SALICYLATES (see section 1.1.16 in Table 14-1)

Brand names: *Rexolate, Thiocyl, Tusal*

Ototoxic effects:
    Cochlear:
        Tinnitus: (San, She)
    Unspecified/General Ear Conditions:
        Ototoxicity: (San)

Risk assessment: Class 2

Sofracort   (see **Framycetin**)

Soframycin   (see **Framycetin**)

Soliris   (see **Eculizumab**)

Solodyn   (see **Minocycline**)

Solu-Cortef   (see **Hydrocortisone**)

Solu-Medrol   (see **Methylprednisolone**)

Solupred   (see **Prednisolone**)

Soluspan   (see **Betamethasone**)

Soma   (see **Carisoprodol**)

Soma Compound   (see **Carisoprodol**)

Soma Compound with Codeine   (see **Carisoprodol**)

Somatropin

Pronunciation guide: soe-mah-TROE-pin

Drug classification: PITUITARY HORMONES (see section 40.44 in Table 14-1)

Brand names: *Genotropin, Humatrope, Norditropin, Saizen, Serostim*

Ototoxic effects:
  Cochlear:
      Hearing loss: 1% [placebo 0] (CPS, PDR)
      Tinnitus: <1% (CPS)
  Vestibular:
      Dizziness: 1-10% (CPS, PDR)
      Nystagmus: 1-10% (CPS, PDR)
      Vertigo: <1% (CPS)
  Outer/Middle Ear:
      Earache/ear pain: 1-11.6% (CPS, PDR)
      Otitis: 1.5-19% [<4.3% above placebo results] (CPS, PDR)
      Otitis media: 6.2-43% [<17% above placebo results] (CPS, PDR)
      Otorrhea: 1.3% (CPS)
  Unspecified/General Ear Conditions:
      Ear disorder: 1.5-18% [<13% above placebo results] (CPS, PDR)

Risk assessment: Class 3

Notes:

> Doctors should carefully evaluate people with Turner syndrome (see Appendix) for otitis media and other ear disorders before treating them with **Somatropin** since these people have a much higher risk of ear or hearing disorders (CPS). The results from a randomized, controlled trial versus untreated controls revealed an increase in incidence of ototoxic side effects ranging from 165% to 360%. For example, otitis media (43% vs. 26%), ear disorders (18% vs. 5%), and surgical procedures (45% vs. 27%) (CPS, PDR).

Sonata   (see **Zaleplon**)

SonoRx (see **Simethicone**)

Sorafenib

Pronunciation guide: sohr-uh-FEN-ib

Drug classification: ANTI-NEOPLASTICS (ANTI-CANCER DRUGS) (see section 14 in Table 14-1)

Brand names: *Nexavar*

Ototoxic effects:
    Cochlear:
        Tinnitus: 0.1-1% (CPS, PDR)

Risk assessment: Class 1

Sorbiline (see **Sorbitol**)

Sorbitol

Pronunciation guide: SORE-bih-tall

Drug classification: HEXITOL IRRIGANTS (see section 30.10.1 in Table 14-1)

Brand names: *Multitol, Sorbiline* [1]

Ototoxic effects:
    Vestibular:
        Vertigo: (DFC)

Risk assessment: Class 1

Notes:

    [1] *Sorbiline* is a combination of **Sorbitol** and Tricholine. (**Sorbitol** is the ototoxic agent.)

Soriatane (see **Acitretin**)

Sotacor (see **Sotalol**)

Sotalol

Pronunciation guide: SOH-tah-lawl

Drug classification: BETA-ADRENERGIC-BLOCKING DRUGS (BETA-BLOCKERS) (see section 20.8.12 in Table 14-1)

Brand names: *Apo-Sotalol, Betapace, Sotacor*

Ototoxic effects:
    Vestibular:
        Dizziness: 6-20% [0.7-3.2% above placebo results] (CPS, PDR)
        Vertigo: 0.01% (CPS, PDR)

Risk assessment: Class 1

Spanidin   (see **Gusperimus**)

Sparfloxacin

Pronunciation guide: SPAR-flox-ah-sin

Drug classification: QUINOLONES (see section 7.4.48 in Table 14-1)

Brand names: *Zagam*

Ototoxic effects:
    Cochlear:
        Tinnitus: <1% (DFC, PDR)
    Vestibular:
        Ataxia: (PDR)
        Dizziness: 2-3.8% (CP2, PDR)
        Nystagmus: (PDR)
        Vertigo: <1% (DFC, PDR)
    Outer/Middle Ear:
        Earache/ear pain: <1% (DFC, PDR)
        Otitis media: <1% (DFC, PDR)
    Unspecified/General Ear Conditions:
        Ear disorder: <1% (DFC, PDR)

Risk assessment: Class 2

Spectinomycin

Pronunciation guide: speck-tih-noe-MY-sin

Drug classification: ANTI-BACTERIAL DRUGS (see section 7.4 in Table 14-1)

Brand names: *Trobicin*

Ototoxic effects:
    Vestibular:
        Dizziness: (Med+)
    Unspecified/General Ear Conditions:
        Ototoxicity: (San)

Risk assessment: Not enough information to rate

Notes:

    See Chapter 9, "Aminoglycoside Antibiotics are the Ototoxic 'Bad boys'" for further information on this drug.

Spirbon   (see **Chlorphenoxamine**)

Spironolactone

Pronunciation guide: speer-on-oh-LAK-tone

Drug classification: DIURETICS—POTASSIUM-SPARING (see section 30.5.8 in Table 14-1)

Brand names: *Aldactazide* [1], *Aldactone*

Ototoxic effects:
    Vestibular:
        Ataxia: (CPS, PDR)
        Dizziness: (CPS, Med)

Risk assessment: Class 1

Notes:

    [1] *Aldactazide* is a combination of **Spironolactone** and **Hydrochlorothiazide**. (See the generic drug **Hydrochlorothiazide** for its specific ototoxic properties.)

    See Chapter 7, "We 'Hear' With Our Eyes" for further information on this drug.

Sporanox   (see **Itraconazole**)

Sprycel   (see **Dasatinib**)

Stadol   (see **Butorphanol**)

Stadol NS   (see **Butorphanol**)

Stalevo   (see **Levodopa**)

Starnoc   (see **Zaleplon**)

Stavudine

Pronunciation guide: stay-VYOO-deen

Drug classification: ANTI-RETROVIRAL REVERSE TRANSCRIPTASE INHIBITORS (see section 7.17.1.4 in Table 14-1)

Brand names: *Zerit*

Ototoxic effects:
    Vestibular:
        Dizziness: 11% [3% above placebo results] (BNF, CPS)
        Vertigo: 2% [1% above placebo results] (CPS)

Risk assessment: Class 1

Stilnoct   (see **Zolpidem**)

Stilnox   (see **Zolpidem**)

St. Joseph Aspirin   (see **Acetylsalicylic acid**)

Strattera   (see **Atomoxetine**)

Streptomycin

Pronunciation guide: strep-toe-MYE-sin

Drug classification: AMINOGLYCOSIDES (see section 7.4.1 in Table 14-1)

Brand names: *Pan-Streptomycin*

Ototoxic effects:
        Auditory disorder: (CPS)
        Hearing loss: (CPS, PDR)
        Tinnitus: (CPS)
    Vestibular:
        Ataxia: (CPS)
        Nystagmus: (CPS)
        Vertigo: (CPS, PDR)
        Vestibular disorder: (CPS)
    Outer/Middle Ear:
        Feeling of fullness in ears: (CPS)
    Unspecified/General Ear Conditions:
        Ototoxicity: (CPS, NDH)

Risk assessment: Class 5

Notes:

Streptomycin was first reported to be ototoxic in 1945.[347] **Streptomycin** use declined a number of years ago because of this, and also because many organisms had become resistant to it. Unfortunately, **Streptomycin** use has been climbing in recent years because it is effective in treating the increasing numbers of tuberculosis cases found today.[348]

Use **Streptomycin** with extreme caution if you already have a sensorineural hearing loss or vestibular (balance) problems (CPS). You are at sharply increased risk of damaging your ears if you have kidney problems. Your risk is also greater if you are older (CPS).

With **Streptomycin**, hearing loss is less common/severe than vestibular damage and is usually preceded by vestibular symptoms such as vertigo and other balance problems (CPS). With the closely related drug, **Dihydrostreptomycin** (die-hye-droe-strep-toe-MY-sin), hearing loss is more common/severe than vestibular problems.[349] **Dihydrostreptomycin** is also an AMINOGLYCOSIDE (see section 7.4.1 in Table 14-1).

You have a high risk of permanent vestibular (balance system) damage if you take **Streptomycin** (PDR). **Streptomycin** frequently affects the vestibular branch of the auditory nerve causing severe nausea, vomiting and vertigo. Your chance of having an ototoxic reaction to **Streptomycin** is directly proportional to the length of time you take this drug, and to the size of the dose you take. A large percentage of the people taking 1.8 to 2 g/day of **Streptomycin** will likely develop ototoxic symptoms within four weeks (CPS, PDR).

Between 4% and 15% of the people who receive 1 g/day of **Streptomycin** for more than one week develop a measurable hearing loss. This hearing loss usually appears after about 7 to 10 days and worsens if treatment is continued. Complete, permanent deafness may follow.[350] Other ototoxic side effects are often temporary. However, hearing loss, when severe, is usually permanent (CPS).

Vestibular symptoms appear early and usually can be reversed if they are detected early enough, and if **Streptomycin** therapy is stopped immediately. However, even after stopping **Streptomycin**, you may still be left with balance problems. Consequently, you may have difficulty walking in the dark or on rough terrain (CPS, PDR).

If you have to take **Streptomycin**, you should have audiometric tests done prior to, during, and following intensive **Streptomycin** therapy. This is because you usually lose your high-frequency hearing before you become aware that you even have a hearing loss. High-frequency audiometric testing can detect any sub-clinical hearing loss (hearing loss above 8,000 Hz) before it becomes noticeable (CPS). This can give your doctor a chance to stop **Streptomycin** therapy before you end up with a severe hearing loss.

If you notice tinnitus or a sense of fullness in your ears while you are taking **Streptomycin**, you need to have an audiometric examination, or stop taking **Streptomycin**, or both (CPS).

Taking **Streptomycin** (or **Dihydrostreptomycin**) while you are pregnant is a no no. AMINOGLYCOSIDES cross the placenta and there have been several reports of total permanent, bilateral, congenital deafness in children whose mothers received **Streptomycin** during pregnancy (PDR). These drugs can have devastating effects on your unborn child. For example, your child could be born with total permanent hearing loss in both ears (CPS) and/or balance problems. Your unborn baby is particularly vulnerable during the first trimester, especially between weeks 6 and 8.[351]

Also, avoid using **Streptomycin** at the same time as, or before, or after, taking Cephaloridine, **Colistin**, **Cyclosporine**, **Gentamicin**, **Kanamycin**, **Neomycin**, **Paromomycin**, **Polymyxin B**, **Tobramycin**, or **Viomycin** (CPS, PDR).

See Chapter 4, "Are You at Risk," Chapter 7, "We 'Hear' With Our Eyes," Chapter 9, "Aminoglycoside Antibiotics are the Ototoxic 'Bad boys'" and Chapter 12, "Potpourri" for further information on **Streptomycin** (**Dihydrostreptomycin**: Chapters 4 and 9 only).

Stromectol   (see **Ivermectin**)

Stugeron   (see **Cinnarizine**)

Suboxone   (see **Buprenorphine**)

Succimer

Pronunciation guide: SUX-ih-mer

Drug classification: HEAVY METAL ANTAGONISTS/CHELATING AGENTS (see section 66.4 in Table 14-1)

Brand names: *Chemet*

Ototoxic effects:
   Vestibular:
      Ataxia: (PDR)

554

Dizziness: 1-12.7% (NDH, PDR)
Outer/Middle Ear:
Ears feel "plugged up": 1-3.7% (NDH, PDR)
Otitis media: 1-3.7% (NDH, PDR)

Risk assessment: Class 1

Sucralfate

Pronunciation guide: soo-KRAL-fate

Drug classification: GASTRIC MUCOSAL DRUGS (see section 34.8.1 in Table 14-1)

Brand names: *Carafate*, *Novo-Sucralate*, *Sulcrate*

Ototoxic effects:
Vestibular:
Dizziness: <0.5% (CPS, PDR)
Vertigo: <0.5% (CPS, PDR)

Risk assessment: Class 1

Sudafed (see **Pseudoephedrine**)

Sudafed Sinus Advance (see **Ibuprofen**)

Sular (see **Nisoldipine**)

Sulcrate (see **Sucralfate**)

Sulfadiazine

Pronunciation guide: sul-fah-DYE-ah-zeen

Drug classification: SULFONAMIDES (see section 7.4.56 in Table 14-1)

Brand names: *Coptin*[1]

Ototoxic effects:
Cochlear:
Tinnitus: (BNF, CPS)
Vestibular:
Ataxia: (BNF, CPS)
Dizziness: (AHF, BNF)
Vertigo: (BNF, CPS)

Risk assessment: Class 1

Notes:

[1] *Coptin* is a combination of **Sulfadiazine** and **Trimethoprim**. (See the generic drug **Trimethoprim** for its specific ototoxic properties.)

Sulfadoxine--Pyrimethamine

Pronunciation guide: sul-fah-DOX-een—peer-ih-METH-ah-meen

Drug classification: ANTI-MALARIAL DRUGS (see section 7.14.8 in Table 14-1)

Brand names: *Fansidar*

Ototoxic effects:
    Cochlear:
        Tinnitus: 6% (CPS, PDR)
    Vestibular:
        Ataxia: (CPS, PDR)
        Dizziness: 6% (CPS)
        Vertigo: (CPS, PDR)

Risk assessment: Class 2

Sulfamethazine

Pronunciation guide: sul-fah-METH-ah-zeen

Drug classification: SULFONAMIDES (see section 7.4.56 in Table 14-1)

Brand names: *Trisulfaminic* [1]

Ototoxic effects:
    Vestibular:
        Vertigo: (NTP)

Risk assessment: Class 1

Notes:

    [1] *Trisulfaminic* is a combination of **Phenylpropanolamine**, **Pheniramine**, **Pyrilamine**, **Sulfadiazine**, Sulfamerazine and **Sulfamethazine**. (See the generic drugs **Phenylpropanolamine**, **Pheniramine**, **Pyrilamine** and **Sulfadiazine** for their specific ototoxic properties.)

Sulfamethizole

Pronunciation guide: sul-fuh-METH-ih-zole

Drug classification: SULFONAMIDES (see section 7.4.56 in Table 14-1)

Brand names: *Thiosulfil Forte*, *Urobiotic*

Ototoxic effects:
    Cochlear:
        Tinnitus: (San, She)
    Vestibular:
        Dizziness: (Med+)
    Unspecified/General Ear Conditions:
        Ototoxicity: (San)

Risk assessment: Class 2

Sulfamethoxazole

Pronunciation guide: sul-fah-meth-OX-ah-zole

Drug classification: SULFONAMIDES (see section 7.4.56 in Table 14-1)

Brand names: *Gantanol*

Ototoxic effects:
    Cochlear:
        Tinnitus: <1% (CPS, PDR)
    Vestibular:
        Ataxia: <1% (CPS, PDR)
        Dizziness: (BNF)
        Vertigo: <1% (CPS, PDR)

Risk assessment: Class 2

Notes:

    See Chapter 12, "Potpourri" for further information on this drug.

Sulfanilamide

Pronunciation guide: sul-fah-NIL-ah-mide

Drug classification: SULFONAMIDES (see section 7.4.56 in Table 14-1)

Brand names: *AVC*

Ototoxic effects:
    Vestibular:
        Ataxia: (NTP)
        Dizziness: (NTP)

Risk assessment: Class 1

Sulfasalazine

Pronunciation guide: sul-fah-SAH-lah-zeen

Drug classification: SULFONAMIDES (see section 7.4.56 in Table 14-1)

Brand names: *Azulfidine*, *Salazopyrin*

Ototoxic effects:
    Cochlear:
        Hearing loss: <0.1% (CPS, PDR)
        Tinnitus: <0.1% (CPS, PDR)
    Vestibular:
        Ataxia: <0.1% (CPS, PDR)
        Dizziness: 4% (DFC, PDR)
        Vertigo: <0.1% (CPS, PDR)

Risk assessment: Class 2

Sulfisoxazole

Pronunciation guide: sul-fih-SOZ-ah-zole

Drug classification: SULFONAMIDES (see section 7.4.56 in Table 14-1)

Brand names: *Gantrisin*

Ototoxic effects:
   Cochlear:
      Hearing loss: (PDR)
      Tinnitus: (PDR)
   Vestibular:
      Ataxia: (PDR)
      Dizziness: (NDH, PDR)
      Vertigo: (PDR)

Risk assessment: Class 2

Sulindac

Pronunciation guide: sul-IN-dak

Drug classification: ACETIC ACIDS (see section 1.1.1 in Table 14-1)

Brand names: *Clinoril*

Ototoxic effects:
   Cochlear:
      Hearing loss: <1% (CPS, PDR)
      Tinnitus: 1-3% (CPS, PDR)
   Vestibular:
      Dizziness: 4% (CPS, PDR)
      Vertigo: <1% (CPS, PDR)

Risk assessment: Class 2

Notes:
   See Chapter 12, "Potpourri" for further information on this drug.

Sultamicillin

Pronunciation guide: SUL-ta-mih-sill-in

Drug classification: ANTI-BACTERIAL DRUGS (see section 7.4 in Table 14-1)

Brand names: *Ampigen SB, Unasyn Oral*

Ototoxic effects:
   Unspecified/General Ear Conditions:
      Ototoxicity: (San)

Risk assessment: Not enough information to rate

Sumatriptan

Pronunciation guide: sue-mah-TRIP-tan

Drug classification: SEROTONIN-RECEPTOR AGONISTS (see section 53.32 in Table 14-1)

Brand names: *Imitrex, Treximet* [1]

Ototoxic effects:
    Cochlear:
        Hearing disorder: 0.1-1% (AHF, PDR)
        Hearing loss: >1% (AHF, PDR)
        Hyperacusis: 1.5-4.4% [<1.3% above placebo results] (CPS, PDR)
        Phonophobia: >1% (AHF) [352]
        Tinnitus: >1% (AHF, PDR)
    Vestibular:
        Ataxia: 0.1-1% (AHF, PDR)
        Dizziness: 3.1-7.9% [0.6-4.2% above placebo results] (CPS, PDR)
        Nystagmus: (CPS)
        Vertigo: 1-2% [0.4-1% above placebo results] (CPS, PDR)
    Outer/Middle Ear:
        Earache/ear pain: 0.1-1% (AHF, PDR)
        Feeling of fullness in ears: <0.1% (AHF, PDR)
        Otitis externa: >1% (AHF, PDR)
        Otitis media: (AHF, PDR)
    Unspecified/General Ear Conditions:
        Meniere's disease: (PDR)

Risk assessment: Class 3

Notes:

[1] *Treximet* is a combination of **Sumatriptan** and **Naproxen**. (See the drug **Naproxen** for its specific ototoxic properties.)

I have an anecdotal report in my files of a woman who noticed a significant hearing loss in just a few months while taking **Sumatriptan** for migraine headaches. Also, I have reports of two other women who suspect they lost their hearing because of this drug.

I have an anecdotal repot in my files of another lady that has had continued hearing loss and tinnitus from taking **Sumatriptan**. In addition, her hearing loss began in the low frequencies and she has exhibited some of the Meniere's disease symptoms since she began the **Sumatriptan**.

Meniere's disease has also been associated with this drug (PDR) [353].

Supeudol   (see **Oxycodone**)

Supprelin   (see **Histrelin**)

Supracaine (see **Tetracaine**)

Suprefact (see **Buserelin**)

Suprefact Depot (see **Buserelin**)

Supres (see **Chlorothiazide**)

Suramin

Pronunciation guide: SOO-rah-min

Drug classification: ANTI-PROTOZOALS (see section 7.14 in Table 14-1)

Brand names: *Antrypol, Naganol*

Ototoxic effects:
  Unspecified/General Ear Conditions:
    Ototoxicity: (San)

Risk assessment: Not enough information to rate

Surgam (see **Tiaprofenic acid**)

Surlid (see **Roxithromycin**)

Surmontil (see **Trimipramine**)

Sustiva (see **Efavirenz**)

Symbicort (see **Budesonide**)

Symbyax (see **Olanzapine**)

Symmetrel (see **Amantadine**)

Synacthen Depot (see **Cosyntropin**)

Synagis (see **Palivizumab**)

Synapause-E3 (see **Estriol**)

Synarel (see **Nafarelin**)

Synphasic (see **Ethinyl estradiol**)

Systral C (see **Chlorphenoxamine**)

Tacaryl (see **Methdilazine**)

Tacrine

Pronunciation guide: TA-kreen

Drug classification: CHOLINESTERASE INHIBITORS (see section 53.4.1 in Table 14-1)

Brand names: *Cognex*

Ototoxic effects:
    Cochlear:
        Hearing loss: 0.1-1% (DFC, PDR)
        Tinnitus: 0.1-1% (DFC, PDR)
    Vestibular:
        Ataxia: 6% [2% above placebo results] (DFC, PDR)
        Dizziness: 12% [1% above placebo results] (DFC, PDR)
        Labyrinthitis: <0.1% (DFC, PDR)
        Vertigo: >1% (DFC, PDR)
    Outer/Middle Ear:
        Earache/ear pain: 0.1-1% (DFC, PDR)
        Otitis media: 0.1-1% (DFC, PDR)

Risk assessment: Class 3

Tacrolimus

Pronunciation guide: tack-ROW-lim-us

Drug classification: IMMUNOSUPPRESSANT DRUGS (see section 43 in Table 14-1)

Brand names: *Advagraf, Prograf, Protopic*

Ototoxic effects:
    Cochlear:
        Hearing loss: (CPS, PDR) [354]
        Tinnitus: 3-15% (CPS, PDR)
    Vestibular:
        Ataxia: (AHF, PDR)
        Dizziness: 3-19% (CPS, PDR)
        Nystagmus: 0.8% (CPS)
        Vertigo: >1% (AHF, PDR)
    Outer/Middle Ear:
        Earache/ear pain: 1-15% (AHF, PDR) [355]
        Otitis externa: 0.2-1% (DFC, PDR)
        Otitis media: 3-15% (CPS, PDR)
    Unspecified/General Ear Conditions:
        Ear disorder: 0.2-1% (DFC, PDR)

Risk assessment: Class 3

Notes:

    Hearing loss includes deafness (PDR).

Caution: Eating grapefruit or drinking grapefruit juice during the time you are taking this drug may make the listed side effects worse than shown here. In fact, taking **Tacrolimus** with grapefruit juice can increase the potency of **Tacrolimus** by as much as 400%.

See Chapter 11, "Grapefruit Juice and Ototoxic Drugs" for further information on this drug.

Tadalafil

Pronunciation guide: tah-DAL-ah-fill

Drug classification: PHOSPHODIESTERASE TYPE 5 (PDE5) INHIBITORS (see section 20.8.28 in Table 14-1)

Brand names: *Adcirca, Cialis*

Ototoxic effects:
Cochlear:
Hearing loss: (NDH, PDR)
Tinnitus: (NDH, PDR)
Vestibular:
Dizziness: 2% [1% above placebo results] (NDH, PDR)
Vertigo: <2% (AHF, PDR)

Risk assessment: Class 3

Notes:

"Advise patients to seek immediate medical attention if sudden decrease or loss of hearing occurs". "These events may be accompanied by tinnitus and dizziness". (PDR)

Sudden hearing loss (partial loss to complete loss) can occur within hours to two days of taking this drug. In the 29 cases of ear problems reported to the FDA, sudden hearing loss typically occurred in one ear. The hearing loss was sometimes accompanied by tinnitus, dizziness and/or vertigo. The hearing loss was temporary in 1/3 of the cases reported.[356]

The results in a study of 11,525 men over the age of 40 indicated that men who use **Sildenafil** (or **Tadalafil** or **Vardenafil**) were twice as likely to have hearing loss as those who did not use such drugs. The resulting hearing loss was "long term" (permanent).[357]

Caution: Eating grapefruit or drinking grapefruit juice during the time you are taking this drug may make the listed side effects worse than shown here.

See Chapter 7, "We 'Hear' With Our Eyes" and Chapter 11, "Grapefruit Juice and Ototoxic Drugs" for further information on this drug.

Tafirol Flex (see **Chlorzoxazone**)

Talacen (see **Pentazocine**)

Talwin (see **Pentazocine**)

Talwin Compound (see **Pentazocine**)

Talwin Nx (see **Pentazocine**)

Tambocor   (see **Flecainide**)

Tamiflu   (see **Oseltamivir**)

Tamofen   (see **Tamoxifen**)

Tamoxifen

Pronunciation guide: tam-OX-ih-fen

Drug classification: ESTROGEN ANTAGONISTS (see section 40.16.1 in Table 14-1)

Brand names: *Nolvadex, Tamofen*

Ototoxic effects:
 Vestibular:
  Ataxia: (PDR)
  Dizziness: (CPS, PDR)

Risk assessment: Class 1

Notes:

 Overdose can cause ataxia (unsteady gait) and dizziness (PDR).

 Caution: Eating grapefruit or drinking grapefruit juice during the time you are taking this drug may make the listed side effects worse than shown here.

 See Chapter 11, "Grapefruit Juice and Ototoxic Drugs" for further information on this drug.

Tamsulosin

Pronunciation guide: tam-SOO-low-sin

Drug classification: ALPHA ADRENERGIC BLOCKING DRUGS (see section 20.8.1 in Table 14-1)

Brand names: *Flomax*

Ototoxic effects:
 Vestibular:
  Dizziness: 11.8-17.1% [2.9-7% above placebo results] (CPS, PDR)
  Vertigo: 0.6-1% [<0.4% above placebo results] (CP2, PDR)

Risk assessment: Class 1

Notes:

 Caution: Eating grapefruit or drinking grapefruit juice during the time you are taking this drug may make the listed side effects worse than shown here.

 See Chapter 11, "Grapefruit Juice and Ototoxic Drugs" for further information on this drug.

Tanatril   (see **Imidapril**)

Tapazole   (see **Methimazole**)

Tapentadol

Pronunciation guide: tah-PEN-tah-dol

Drug classification: CENTRALLY-ACTING SYNTHETIC ANALGESICS (see section 1.10 in Table 14-1)

Brand names: *Nucynta*

Ototoxic effects:
Vestibular:
Ataxia: <1% (PDR)
Dizziness: 24% [16% above placebo results] (PDR)

Risk assessment: Class 1

Targocid   (see **Teicoplanin**)

Targretin   (see **Bexarotene**)

Tarka   (see **Trandolapril**)

Taro-Carbamazepine   (see **Carbamazepine**)

Tasigna   (see **Nilotinib**)

Tasmar   (see **Tolcapone**)

Tavist   (see **Clemastine**)

Taxol   (see **Paclitaxel**)

Taxotere   (see **Docetaxel**)

Tazobactam   (see **Piperacillin—Tazobactam**)

Tazocin   (see **Piperacillin—Tazobactam**)

Td Adsorbed   (see **Tetanus vaccine**)

Td Polio Adsorbed   (see **Tetanus vaccine**)

Tecta   (see **Pantoprazole**)

Tegaserod

Pronunciation guide: teh-GAH-sir-rod

Drug classification: SEROTONIN 5-HT$_4$ RECEPTOR PARTIAL AGONISTS (see section 17.8.4 in Table 14-1)

Brand names: *Zelnorm*

Ototoxic effects:
  Vestibular:
    Dizziness: 4% [1% above placebo results] (CPS, PDR)
    Vertigo: (CPS, PDR)
  Outer/Middle Ear:
    Otitis media: 1% [0.4% above placebo results] (CPS)

Risk assessment: Class 1

Tegison   (see **Etretinate**)

Tegretol   (see **Carbamazepine**)

Teicoplanin

Pronunciation guide: TIE-koh-plan-in

Drug classification: GLYCOPEPTIDES (see section 7.4.20 in Table 14-1)

Brand names: *Targocid*

Ototoxic effects:
  Cochlear:
    Hearing loss: (BNF)
    Tinnitus: (BNF)
  Vestibular:
    Dizziness: (BNF)
    Vestibular disturbance: (BNF)
  Unspecified/General Ear Conditions:
    Ototoxicity: (San)

Risk assessment: Class 2

Notes:

  Can cause tinnitus and mild hearing loss,[358] as well as dizziness and vestibular disturbances.[359]

Telithromycin

Pronunciation guide: teh-lith-roe-MYE-sin

Drug classification: KETOLIDE ANTIBIOTICS (see section 7.4.32.1 in Table 14-1)

Brand names: *Ketek*

Ototoxic effects:
  Vestibular:
    Dizziness: 1.9-3.7% [0.4-1.3% above placebo results] (NDH, PDR)
    Vertigo: 0.2-2.0% (CPS, PDR)

Risk assessment: Class 1

Notes:

Telithromycin can cause dizziness and vertigo.[360]

Telithromycin is a strong inhibitor of the Cytochrome P450 3A4 system. Co-administration of **Telithromycin** and a drug primarily metabolized by the Cytochrome P450 3A4 enzyme system may result in increased plasma concentration of the drug co-administered with **Telithromycin** that could increase or prolong both the therapeutic and adverse side effects (PDR).[361]

See Chapter 11, "Grapefruit Juice and Ototoxic Drugs" for further information related to the Cytochrome P450 3A4 enzyme and **Telithromycin**.

Telmisartan

Pronunciation guide: tell-mah-SAR-tan

Drug classification: ANGIOTENSIN-2-RECEPTOR ANTAGONISTS (see section 20.8.4 in Table 14-1)

Brand names: *Micardis, Micardis HCT*[1], *Micardis Plus*[1]

Ototoxic effects:
Cochlear:
Tinnitus: >0.3% (CPS, PDR)
Vestibular:
Dizziness: 1.8-5% [<4% above placebo results] (CPS, PDR)
Vertigo: >0.3% (CPS, PDR)
Outer/Middle Ear:
Earache/ear pain: >0.3% (CPS, PDR)
Otitis media: >0.3% (CPS, PDR)

Risk assessment: Class 2

Notes:

[1] *Micardis HCT* and *Micardis Plus* are combinations of **Telmisartan** and **Hydrochlorothiazide**. (See the generic drug **Hydrochlorothiazide** for its specific ototoxic properties.)

Temaril　(see **Trimeprazine**)

Temazepam

Pronunciation guide: teh-MAZ-eh-pam

Drug classification: BENZODIAZEPINES (see section 60.12.8 in Table 14-1)

Brand names: *Apo-Temazepam, Restoril*

Ototoxic effects:
Cochlear:
Tinnitus: (Eps)

Vestibular:
    Ataxia: 0.5-0.9% (CPS, PDR)
    Dizziness: 4.5% [1.2% above placebo results] (CPS, PDR)
    Nystagmus: <0.5% (CPS, PDR)
    Vertigo: 1.2% [0.4% above placebo results] (CPS, PDR)

Risk assessment: Class 2

Notes:

See Chapter 10 "Beware of Benzodiazepines—Don't Let This Nasty Time-Bomb Ambush You and Your Ears" for further information on this drug.

Temgesic   (see **Buprenorphine**)

Temodal   (see **Temozolomide**)

Temodar   (see **Temozolomide**)

Temozolomide

Pronunciation guide: tem-oh-ZOHL-oh-mide

Drug classification: ALKYLATING DRUGS (see section 14.1 in Table 14-1)

Brand names: *Temodar, Temodal*

Ototoxic effects:
    Cochlear:
        Hearing loss: 1-5% (CPS)
        Hyperacusis: 1% (CPS)
        Tinnitus: 1-2% (CPS)
    Vestibular:
        Ataxia: 1-8% (CPS, PDR)
        Dizziness: 1-12% (CPS, PDR)
        Equilibrium disorder: 2-3% (CPS)
        Vertigo: 1% (CPS)
    Outer/Middle Ear:
        Earache/ear pain: 1-2% (CPS)
        Otitis media: 1% (CPS)

Risk assessment: Class 2

Tenex   (see **Guanfacine**)

Tenfortan   (see **Amezinium**)

Tenolin   (see **Atenolol**)

Tenoretic   (see **Atenolol**)

Tenormin   (see **Atenolol**)

Tenoxicam

Pronunciation guide: ten-OX-ih-kam

Drug classification: OXICAMS (see section 1.1.10 in Table 14-1)

Brand names: *Apo-Tenoxicam, Mobiflex*

Ototoxic effects:
Cochlear:
Hearing loss: <0.1% (CPS, Med)
Tinnitus: <0.1% (CPS, Med)
Vestibular:
Dizziness: 0.8-3.3% (CPS, Med)
Vertigo: 0.2-0.4% (BNF, CPS)

Risk assessment: Class 2

Tequin   (see **Gatifloxacin**)

Terazosin

Pronunciation guide: ter-AY-zoe-sin

Drug classification: ALPHA ADRENERGIC BLOCKING DRUGS (see section 20.8.1 in Table 14-1)

Brand names: *Hytrin*

Ototoxic effects:
Cochlear:
Tinnitus: >1% (CPS, PDR)
Vestibular:
Dizziness: 9.1-19.3% [4.9-11.8% above placebo results] (CPS, PDR)
Vertigo: 1.3-1.4% [1.1% above placebo results] (CPS, PDR)

Risk assessment: Class 2

Terbutaline

Pronunciation guide: ter-BYOO-tah-leen

Drug classification: BRONCHODILATORS—BETA ADRENERGIC AGONISTS (see section 63.4 in Table 14-1)

Brand names: *Brethaire, Bricanyl*

Ototoxic effects:
Cochlear:
Tinnitus: (AHF)

Vestibular:
  Dizziness: (AHF, CPS)
  Vertigo: (PDR)

Risk assessment: Class 1

Teriparatide

Pronunciation guide: ter-ih-PAR-uh-tide

Drug classification: PARATHYROID DRUGS (HUMAN PARATHYROID HORMONE) (see section 40.42.4 in Table 14-1)

Brand names: *Forteo*

Ototoxic effects:
  Vestibular:
    Dizziness: 8.0% [2.6% above placebo results] (AHF, PDR)
    Vertigo: 3.8% [1.1% above placebo results] (AHF, PDR)

Risk assessment: Class 1

Testosterone

Pronunciation guide: tess-TOSS-ter-own

Drug classification: ANDROGENS (MALE SEX HORMONES) (see section 40.4 in Table 14-1)

Brand names: *Androderm, AndroGel*

Ototoxic effects:
  Vestibular:
    Dizziness: (CPS)
    Vertigo: <1% (CPS, PDR)

Risk assessment: Class 1

Tetanus and Diphtheria Toxoids Adsorbed   (see **Tetanus vaccine**)

Tetanus vaccine

Pronunciation guide: TE-tan-us VAK-seen

Drug classification: TOXOIDS (see section 70.4 in Table 14-1)

Brand names: *Adacel* [1], *Daptacel* [1], *DTP Adsorbed* [1], *Infanrix* [1], *Quadracel* [1], *Td Adsorbed* [2], *Td Polio Adsorbed* [3], *Tetanus and Diphtheria Toxoids Adsorbed* [2], *Tetramune* [4], *Trihibit* [4], *Tripedia* [1]

Ototoxic effects:
  Cochlear:
    Cochlear lesions: [5] (CPS, PDR)

Vestibular:
    Dizziness: (CPS, PDR)
Outer/Middle Ear:
    Earache/ear pain: (DFC, PDR)
    Otitis media: (PDR)

Risk assessment: Class 1

Notes:

[1] *Adacel, Daptacel, DTP Adsorbed, Infanrix, Quadracel* and *Tripedia* are combinations of Diphtheria, **Tetanus** and Pertussis vaccines. *Quadracel* also includes Poliomyelitis vaccine. (**Tetanus** is the ototoxic agent.)

[2] *Tetanus and Diphtheria Toxoids Adsorbed* and *Td Adsorbed* are combinations of **Tetanus** and Diphtheria vaccines. (**Tetanus** is the ototoxic agent.)

[3] *Td Polio Adsorbed* is a combination of **Tetanus**, Diphtheria and Poliomyelitis vaccines. (**Tetanus** is the ototoxic agent.)

[4] *Tetramune* and *Trihibit* are combinations of Diphtheria, **Tetanus**, Pertussis and **Haemophilus b Conjugate** vaccines. (See **Haemophilus Vaccine** for its specific ototoxic properties.)

[5] A lesion is a injury or a pathologic change in the tissues. Cochlear lesions may be otosclerotic lesions in the cochlea and can result from vaccinations. Active lesions may be crumbly and bleed. Cochlear lesions also can cause partial nerve atrophy. Such damage can cause hearing loss and other auditory effects.

Tetrabenazine

Pronunciation guide: teh-trah-BEN-ah-zeen

Drug classification: MONOAMINE DEPLETER DRUGS (see section 60.1.1.1 in Table 14-1)

Brand names: *Xenazine*

Ototoxic effects:
    Vestibular:
        Ataxia: 4% (NDH, PDR)
        Dizziness: 4% (NDH, PDR)
        Loss of balance: 9% (NDH, PDR)

Risk assessment: Class 2

Tetracaine

Pronunciation guide: TET-rah-kane

Drug classification: ESTERS (see section 4.4 in Table 14-1)

Brand names: *Pontocaine, Supracaine*

Ototoxic effects:
    Cochlear:
        Tinnitus: (CPS, PDR)
    Vestibular:
        Dizziness: (CPS, PDR)
        Nystagmus: (CPS)

Risk assessment: Class 1

Tetracycline

Pronunciation guide: tet-rah-SYE-kleen

Drug classification: TETRACYCLINES (see section 7.4.60 in Table 14-1)

Brand names: *Achromycin*

Ototoxic effects:
    Cochlear:
        Hearing loss: (CPS, DFC)
        Tinnitus: (CPS, PDR)
    Vestibular:
        Ataxia: (CPS)
        Dizziness: (CPS, PDR)
        Vertigo: (CPS, DFC)

Risk assessment: Class 3

Notes:

> **Tetracycline** itself comes in several versions: **Tetracycline**, **Chlortetracycline**, **Demeclocycline** and **Meclocycline** (mek-loe-SYE-kleen) (brand name—*Meclan*). (See the generic drugs **Chlortetracycline** and **Demeclocycline** for their specific ototoxic properties.)

> I have an anecdotal report in my files of a man that had a severe ototoxic reaction to **Tetracycline** that left him with a severe/profound bilateral hearing loss.

> See Chapter 7, "We 'Hear' With Our Eyes" for further information on **Tetracycline**.

Tetramune   (see **Tetanus vaccine**)

Teveten   (see **Eprosartan**)

Teveten HCT   (see **Eprosartan**)

Thalidomide

Pronunciation guide: thah-LIH-doe-mide

Drug classification: TUMOR NECROSIS FACTOR MODIFIERS (see section 14.36 in Table 14-1)

Brand names: *Thalomid*

Ototoxic effects:
    Cochlear:
        Hearing loss: (DFC, PDR)
        Tinnitus: (DFC, PDR)
    Vestibular:
        Ataxia: (DFC, PDR)
        Dizziness: 4-25% [placebo 0] (DFC, PDR)
        Nystagmus: (Med, PDR)
        Vertigo: 8.3% [placebo 0] (DFC, PDR)

Risk assessment: Class 3

Thalitone (see **Chlorthalidone**)

Thalomid (see **Thalidomide**)

Thelin (see **Sitaxsentan**)

Theo-24 (see **Theophylline**)

Theochron (see **Theophylline**)

Theo-Dur (see **Theophylline**)

Theolair (see **Theophylline**)

Theophylline

Pronunciation guide: thee-OFF-ih-lin

Drug classification: BRONCHODILATORS—BETA ADRENERGIC AGONISTS (see section 63.4 in Table 14-1)

Brand names: *Theo-24, Theochron, Theo-Dur, Theolair, Uniphyl*

Ototoxic effects:
    Cochlear:
        Tinnitus: (AHF, CPS)
    Vestibular:
        Dizziness: (AHF, CPS)

Risk assessment: Class 1

Notes:

    Tinnitus is a common side effect of **Theophylline** overdose (CPS).

Thiabendazole

Pronunciation guide: thee-ah-BEN-dah-zole

Drug classification: ANTHELMINTIC DRUGS (see section 7.1 in Table 14-1)

Brand names: *Mintezol*

Ototoxic effects:
    Cochlear:
        Tinnitus: (CPS, PDR)
    Vestibular:
        Dizziness: (CPS, PDR)
        Vertigo: (AHF, NTP)

Risk assessment: Class 1

Thiethylperazine

Pronunciation guide: thye-eth-ill-PER-ah-zeen

Drug classification: PHENOTHIAZINES (see section 60.8.1 in Table 14-1)

Brand names: *Torecan*

Ototoxic effects:
    Cochlear:
        Tinnitus: (Med, PDR)
    Vestibular:
        Dizziness: (Med, PDR)

Risk assessment: Class 1

Thimerosal

Pronunciation guide: THIH-meh-roe-sal

Drug classification: ANTI-BACTERIAL DRUGS (see section 7.4 in Table 14-1)

Brand names: *Mercurio Cromo*

Ototoxic effects:
    Cochlear:
        Hearing loss: (NTP)
    Vestibular:
        Ataxia: (NTP)

Risk assessment: Class 2

Notes:

Thimerosal is an organomercurial compound (49.6% by weight mercury) that is used as a preservative in many products. These include antibiotic preparations, nasal preparations, ear preparations, cosmetics and vaccines.

For further information on the ototoxic side effects of **Mercury**, see the **Mercury** listing in the Ototoxic Chemicals section (Chapter 16).

Thiocyl   (see **Sodium thiosalicylate**)

Thioridazine

Pronunciation guide: thye-oh-RID-ah-zeen

Drug classification: PHENOTHIAZINES (see section 60.8.1 in Table 14-1)

Brand names: *Mellaril*

Ototoxic effects:
　　Vestibular:
　　　　Dizziness: (NDH, Med)
　　　　Vertigo: (CPS)

Risk assessment: Class 1

Notes:
　　See Chapter 7, "We 'Hear' With Our Eyes" for further information on this drug.

Thiosulfil Forte　(see **Sulfamethizole**)

Thiothixene

Pronunciation guide: thye-oh-THIX-een

Drug classification: ANTIPSYCHOTIC DRUGS (see section 60.8 in Table 14-1)

Brand names: *Navane*

Ototoxic effects:
　　Vestibular:
　　　　Ataxia: (CPS, PDR)
　　　　Dizziness: (CPS, PDR)

Risk assessment: Class 1

Notes:
　　Ataxia and dizziness are signs of **Thiothixene** overdose (PDR).

Thonzylamine

Pronunciation guide: thon-ZYLL-ah-meen

Drug classification: ANTIHISTAMINES (see section 10 in Table 14-1)

Brand names: *Tonamil*

Ototoxic effects:
　　Cochlear:
　　　　Tinnitus: (NTP)
　　Vestibular:
　　　　Ataxia: (NTP)
　　　　Vertigo: (NTP)

Risk assessment: Class 1

Thymoxamine

Pronunciation guide: thye-MOX-ah-meen

Drug classification: ALPHA ADRENERGIC BLOCKING DRUGS (see section 20.8.1 in Table 14-1)

Brand names: —

Ototoxic effects:
    Cochlear:
        Tinnitus: (San, She)
    Unspecified/General Ear Conditions:
        Ototoxicity: (San)

Risk assessment: Not enough information to rate

Tiagabine

Pronunciation guide: tye-AG-ah-been

Drug classification: ANTI-CONVULSANT DRUGS (see section 53.12 in Table 14-1)

Brand names: *Gabitril*

Ototoxic effects:
    Cochlear:
        Hearing loss: 0.1-1% (PDR)
        Hyperacusis: 0.1-1% (PDR)
        Tinnitus: >1% (DFC, PDR)
    Vestibular:
        Ataxia: 5-9% [2-6% above placebo results] (DFC, PDR)
        Dizziness: 27-31% [12-19% above placebo results] (DFC, PDR)
        Nystagmus: 2% [1% above placebo results] (DFC, PDR)
        Vertigo: >1% (DFC, PDR)
    Outer/Middle Ear:
        Earache/ear pain: >1% (DFC, PDR)
        Otitis externa: 0.1-1% (DFC, PDR)
        Otitis media: >1% (DFC, PDR)

Risk assessment: Class 3

Tiaprofenic acid

Pronunciation guide: tie-ah-pro-FEN-ik ASS-id

Drug classification: PROPIONIC ACIDS (see section 1.1.13 in Table 14-1)

Brand names: *Albert Tiafen, Surgam*

Ototoxic effects:
    Cochlear:
        Tinnitus: 0.2-0.7% (CPS, Med)

Vestibular:
Dizziness: 2.4-3.9% (CPS, Med)
Vertigo: (BNF, CPS)

Risk assessment: Class 1

Tiazac   (see **Diltiazem**)

Tiazac XC   (see **Diltiazem**)

Ticlid   (see **Ticlopidine**)

Ticlopidine

Pronunciation guide: tye-KLOH-pih-deen

Drug classification: ANTI-CLOTTING DRUGS (see section 36.1 in Table 14-1)

Brand names: *Ticlid*

Ototoxic effects:
Cochlear:
Tinnitus: 0.5-1% (DFC, PDR)
Vestibular:
Dizziness: 1.1% [placebo 0] (CPS, PDR)

Risk assessment: Class 1

Tigan   (see **Trimethobenzamide**)

Tigecycline

Pronunciation guide: tye-gah-SYE-klin

Drug classification: TETRACYCLINES (see section 7.4.60 in Table 14-1)

Brand names: *Tygacil*

Ototoxic effects:
Vestibular:
Dizziness: 0.1-1% (CPS)
Vertigo: 0.1-1% (CPS)

Risk assessment: Class 1

Tiludronate

Pronunciation guide: tih-LOO-droh-nate

Drug classification: BISPHOSPHONATES (see section 50.1.1 in Table 14-1)

Brand names: *Skelid*

Ototoxic effects:
    Cochlear:
        Tinnitus: (She)
    Vestibular:
        Dizziness: 4% [same as placebo] (Med, PDR)
        Vertigo: >1% (DFC, PDR)
    Outer/Middle Ear:
        Earache/ear pain: (USP)

Risk assessment: Class 1

Timolide   (see **Timolol**)

Timolol

Pronunciation guide: tye-MOE-lawl

Drug classification: Beta-adrenergic-blocking drugs (Beta-Blockers) (see section 20.8.12 in Table 14-1)

Brand names: *Apo-Timol, Betimol, Blocadren, Combigan*[1], *Cosopt*[2], *Timolide*[3], *Timoptic, Timoptic-XE, Timpilo*[4], *Xalacom*[5]

Ototoxic effects:
    Cochlear:
        Tinnitus: 0.6% [placebo 0] (CPS, PDR)
    Vestibular:
        Dizziness: 1.2-6% [1.1-2% above placebo results] (CPS, PDR)
        Vertigo: 0.6% [placebo 0] (CPS, PDR)
        Vestibular disorder: (CPS)
    Outer/Middle Ear:
        Earache/ear pain: (PDR)

Risk assessment: Class 2

Notes:

[1] *Combigan* is a combination of **Timolol** and Brimonidine. (**Timolol** is the ototoxic agent.)

[2] *Cosopt* is a combination of **Timolol** and Dorzolamide. (**Timolol** is the ototoxic agent.)

[3] *Timolide* is a combination of **Timolol** and **Hydrochlorothiazide**. (See the generic drug **Hydrochlorothiazide** for its specific ototoxic properties.)

[4] *Timpilo* is a combination of **Timolol** and **Pilocarpine**. (See the generic drug **Pilocarpine** for its specific ototoxic properties.)

[5] *Xalacom* is a combination of **Timolol** and Latanoprost. (**Timolol** is the ototoxic agent.)

Timoptic   (see **Timolol**)

Timoptic-XE   (see **Timolol**)

Timpilo (see **Timolol**)

Tinidazole

Pronunciation guide: teh-NID-ah-zol

Drug classification: AMEBICIDES (see section 7.14.1 in Table 14-1)

Brand names: *Fasigyn*

Ototoxic effects:
  Vestibular:
    Ataxia: (BNF, DFC)
    Dizziness: 0.5-1.1% (AHF, DFC)
    Vertigo: (DFC)

Risk assessment: Class 1

Tirapazamine

Pronunciation guide: tih-rah-PAZ-ah-meen

Drug classification: ANTI-NEOPLASTICS (ANTI-CANCER DRUGS) (see section 14 in Table 14-1)

Brand names: —

Ototoxic effects:
  Cochlear:
    Hearing loss: [1]
    Tinnitus: (She)

Risk assessment: Class 2

Notes:

  [1] Hearing loss is temporary and typically lasts for about 24 hours.[362]

Tizanidine

Pronunciation guide: tis-AN-ih-deen

Drug classification: SKELETAL MUSCLE RELAXANTS (see section 53.36 in Table 14-1)

Brand names: *Zanaflex*

Ototoxic effects:
  Cochlear:
    Hearing loss: 0.1-1% (CPS, PDR)
    Tinnitus: 0.1-1% (CPS, PDR)
  Vestibular:
    Dizziness: 16-45% [12-41% above placebo results] (CPS, PDR)
    Vertigo: 0.1-1% (CPS, PDR)

Outer/Middle Ear:
Earache/ear pain: 0.1-1% (CPS, PDR)
Otitis media: 0.1-1% (CPS, PDR)

Risk assessment: Class 3

TOBI   (see **Tobramycin**)

Tobradex   (see **Tobramycin**)

Tobramycin

Pronunciation guide: toe-brah-MYE-sin

Drug classification: AMINOGLYCOSIDES (see section 7.4.1 in Table 14-1)

Brand names: *Nebcin, TOBI, Tobradex*

Ototoxic effects:
Cochlear:
Auditory disorder: (CPS, PDR)
Cochlear damage: (PDR)
Hearing loss: (CPS, PDR)
Tinnitus: 3% [placebo 0] (CPS, PDR)
Vestibular:
Ataxia: (CPS, PDR)
Dizziness: (CPS, PDR)
Nystagmus: (CPS)
Vertigo: (CPS, PDR)
Vestibular disorder: (CPS, PDR)
Outer/Middle Ear:
Otitis media: 2-5.2% (CPS)
Unspecified/General Ear Conditions:
Ototoxicity: (CPS, NDH)

Risk assessment: Class 5

Notes:

Tobramycin can affect both your cochlea and your vestibular (balance) system resulting in hearing and balance problems (CPS). Between 6.1% and 11.5% of the people taking **Tobramycin** experience ototoxic side effects.[363] Hearing loss generally occurs in both ears and is usually permanent. It may be partial (and you end up hard of hearing), or it may be total (and you end up deaf). It initially shows up as a loss of high-frequency hearing (PDR).

Tinnitus is often your first warning symptom of ear damage. Therefore, if tinnitus occurs, be very cautious in proceeding further with **Tobramycin** therapy (PDR). If you experience tinnitus, your doctor should carefully monitor you for high-frequency hearing loss (CPS, PDR) since high-frequency hearing loss occurs first, and may be detected by high-frequency audiometric testing before hearing loss can be detected by standard clinical testing (CPS).

If you experience hearing loss from taking **Tobramycin**, you will frequently also experience tinnitus (PDR). You should tell your doctor if you have ringing in your ears (tinnitus), dizziness or any change in your hearing (PDR).

Symptoms of **Tobramycin** overdose can include dizziness, tinnitus, vertigo and loss of high frequency hearing (PDR).

I have an anecdotal report in my files of a man that was treated with **Tobramycin** (as ear drops) and developed tinnitus in both his ears.

You are more at risk if you already have kidney problems, or if you have normal kidney function but take **Tobramycin** at high doses or for prolonged periods of time. In order to minimize the risks of ototoxicity, you should only take **Tobramycin** for 7 to 10 days.[364] You are also more at risk if you have a pre-existing hearing loss, are dehydrated or are advanced in age. If any of these factors apply to you, you should have serial audiograms taken before, during and after you take **Tobramycin** (CPS, PDR).

You may develop cochlear damage, but not have any symptoms while you are taking **Tobramycin** to warn you. As a result, partial or total hearing loss in both ears may continue to develop even after you stop taking **Tobramycin** (PDR). In fact, ototoxic signs and symptoms may not even begin to show up until long after you have stopped taking **Tobramycin** (PDR)!

Avoid taking **Tobramycin** and other AMINOGLYCOSIDES at the same time or following one another. Not doing so can result in severe hearing loss (CPS). Some of the AMINOGLYCOSIDES to watch out for are **Amikacin**, **Gentamicin**, **Kanamycin**, **Neomycin**, **Paromomycin** and **Streptomycin**. Also watch out for such drugs as Cephaloridine, **Cisplatin**, **Colistin**, **Polymyxin B**, **Vancomycin**, and **Viomycin** (PDR). Furthermore, do not take **Tobramycin** at the same time as you are taking potent diuretics such as **Ethacrynic acid** or **Furosemide** (CPS, PDR).

I have an anecdotal report in my files of a man that was treated with intravenous **Tobramycin** for an internal infection, and at the same time was given **Furosemide**. This combination wiped out his hearing.

I also have an anecdotal report in my files of a lady with cystic fibrosis who had taken **Tobramycin** for years. Now she notices a worsening of her symptoms. She had vertigo, but that went away. Now she has constant dizziness, trouble focusing her eyes, ear fullness and pressure, pain and tinnitus. She no longer can drive her car, or do a lot of things she once could.

In another anecdotal report in my files, a man was prescribed an ointment containing **Tobramycin** for a sty on his left eyelid. He writes, "I started using the cream on my left eyelid on Tuesday at 1 PM. At 8:30 AM Wednesday, I lost the hearing in my left ear while listening on the telephone". In his case, the **Tobramycin** apparently caused sudden hearing loss just 19 hours later—and this was just from using an ointment on his eyelid!

Here's another "eye" story from my files. A man wrote, "I went to my optometrist complaining of a swollen eyelid. (I am allergic to FLUOROQUINOLONES and **Erythromycin**.) The diagnosis was a bacterial infection in the eyelid. I was prescribed a round of Amoxicillin and **Tobramycin** ointment. On day 5 I returned to the doctor complaining of dizziness. The doctor recommended I continue with the Amoxicillin and **Tobramycin**. On day 7 I was taken to the emergency room with extreme vertigo and nausea. I could not walk unassisted and was diagnosed as 'vertigo of unknown origin' and released. Four weeks later I am experiencing ongoing oscillopsia accompanied by ataxia and nystagmus".

In yet another anecdotal report in my files, a man was prescribed **Tobramycin** ear drops for one ear. The result was that he now has "permanent, profound unilateral deafness, dizziness and tinnitus all caused by a doctor who had me use *Tobradex* drops in my ear, while assuring me they were safe, despite my questions".

In an anecdotal report in my files, a woman told about her experience with **Tobramycin** (*Tobradex*) eye drops. She wrote, "I was prescribed Augmentin and *Tobradex* for conjunctivitis—2 drops each eye twice a day. After the 6th dose, I suddenly developed tinnitus—louder in the left ear than the right. I immediately stopped taking both medications". She had her hearing checked and found she had lost significant hearing at 6,000 and 8,000 Hz. She continues, "I still have the same tinnitus and hearing loss over 2 weeks later. My worst fear is that the loss will get worse".

In another anecdotal report in my files, a woman told about her similar experience with **Tobramycin** (*Tobradex*) eye drops. She wrote, "It took only one dose of two drops in each eye. After a few hours my tinnitus was greatly worse. When I got up in the morning I leaned over and fell. I took **Prednisone** for about a month and seem to be back to normal. My eye doctor said it couldn't do that, but it did".

In still another anecdotal report in my files, a man took a few doses of **Tobramycin** eye drops and developed a tinnitus "tone" in his right ear. His tinnitus seems to be permanent as it happened "a few months ago".

In yet another anecdotal report in my files, a woman wrote, "I was damaged by a **Tobramycin** IV. My symptoms have not improved. I can walk unassisted, but stumble like a drunk person. The oscillopsia is still just as bad, however I can now raise my eyes up—I couldn't at first without throwing up. I have no concentration or short term memory whatsoever. There is this 'strange' feeling in my head—like my brain is sloshing back and forth".

See Chapter 9, "Aminoglycoside Antibiotics are the Ototoxic 'Bad boys'" and Chapter 12, "Potpourri" for further information on this drug.

Tocainide

Pronunciation guide: toe-KAY-nide

Drug classification: Anti-arrhythmics (Heart Rhythm Regulators) (see section 20.4 in Table 14-1)

Brand names: *Tonocard*

Ototoxic effects:
Cochlear:
Hearing loss/tinnitus: 0.4-1.5% (CPS, PDR)
Tinnitus: (She)

Vestibular:
> Ataxia: 0.2-10.8% (CPS, PDR)
> Dizziness/vertigo: 8-25.3% (CPS, PDR)
> Nystagmus: <1.1% (CPS, PDR)

Outer/Middle Ear:
> Earache/ear pain: <1% (CPS, PDR)

Risk assessment: Class 3

Tofranil   (see **Imipramine**)

Tolazamide

Pronunciation guide: tole-AZ-ah-mide

Drug classification: SULFONYLUREAS (see section 40.8.12 in Table 14-1)

Brand names: *Tolinase*

Ototoxic effects:
Vestibular:
> Dizziness: (AHF, Med)
> Vertigo: (AHF, Med)

Risk assessment: Class 1

Tolbutamide

Pronunciation guide: tole-BYOO-tah-mide

Drug classification: SULFONYLUREAS (see section 40.8.12 in Table 14-1)

Brand names: *Orinase*

Ototoxic effects:
Cochlear:
> Tinnitus: (BNF)

Vestibular:
> Dizziness: (CP2, Med)
> Vertigo: (CP2)

Risk assessment: Class 1

Notes:
> See Chapter 7, "We 'Hear' With Our Eyes" for further information on this drug.

Tolcapone

Pronunciation guide: toll-KAP-own

Drug classification: ANTI-PARKINSONIAN DRUGS (see section 53.16 in Table 14-1)

Brand names: *Tasmar*

Ototoxic effects:
    Cochlear:
        Tinnitus: >1% (AHF, PDR)
    Vestibular:
        Dizziness: 6-13% [<3% above placebo results] (AHF, PDR)
        Equilibrium disorder: 3% [1% above placebo results] (PDR)
        Loss of balance: 2-3% [1% above placebo results] (DFC, PDR)
        Vertigo: 1-3% (AHF, PDR)
    Outer/Middle Ear:
        Earache/ear pain: 0.1-1% (AHF, PDR)
        Otitis media: 0.1-1% (AHF, PDR)

Risk assessment: Class 2

Tolectin   (see **Tolmetin**)

Tolinase   (see **Tolazamide**)

Tolmetin

Pronunciation guide: TOLE-met-in

Drug classification: ACETIC ACIDS (see section 1.1.1 in Table 14-1)

Brand names: *Tolectin*

Ototoxic effects:
    Cochlear:
        Hearing loss: (AHF, Med)
        Tinnitus: 1-3% (CPS, PDR)
    Vestibular:
        Dizziness: 3-9% (CPS, PDR)
        Vertigo: (AHF, Med)

Risk assessment: Class 2

Notes:

    See Chapter 12, "Potpourri" for further information on this drug.

Tolterodine

Pronunciation guide: toll-TEAR-oh-deen

Drug classification: MUSCARINIC RECEPTOR ANTAGONISTS (see section 17.1.1 in Table 14-1)

Brand names: *Detrol, Unidet*

Ototoxic effects:
    Vestibular:
        Dizziness: 2.2% [1.2% above placebo results] (CPS, PDR)
        Vertigo/dizziness: 5% [2% above placebo results] (CPS, PDR)

Risk assessment: Class 1

Tonamil   (see **Thonzylamine**)

Tonocard   (see **Tocainide**)

Topamax   (see **Topiramate**)

Topiramate

Pronunciation guide: toe-PIE-rah-mate

Drug classification: ANTI-CONVULSANT DRUGS (see section 53.12 in Table 14-1)

Brand names: *Topamax*

Ototoxic effects:
  Cochlear:
     Hearing loss: 1-2% [<1% above placebo results] (CPS, PDR)
     Hyperacusis: 0.1-1% (PDR)
     Tinnitus: 1-2% [placebo 0] (DFC, PDR)
  Vestibular:
     Ataxia: 1-21.2% [<14.3% above placebo results] (CPS, PDR)
     Dizziness: 4-32.1% [1-20% above placebo results] (CPS, PDR)
     Loss of balance: (USP)
     Nystagmus: 10-15% [1.8-5.7% above placebo results] (CPS, PDR)
     Vertigo: 1-4% [1% above placebo results] (CPS, PDR)
  Outer/Middle Ear:
     Earache/ear pain: 0.1-2% (CPS, PDR)
     Otitis media: 1-7% (CPS)

Risk assessment: Class 4

Toposar   (see **Etoposide**)

Topril   (see **Ramipril**)

Toprol-XL   (see **Metoprolol**)

Toradol   (see **Ketorolac**)

Torasemide   (see **Torsemide**)

Torecan   (see **Thiethylperazine**)

Toremifene

Pronunciation guide: tore-EM-ah-feen

Drug classification: SELECTIVE ESTROGEN RECEPTOR MODIFIERS (see section 40.40 in
     Table 14-1)

Brand names: *Fareston*

Ototoxic effects:
Vestibular:
Ataxia: (PDR)
Dizziness: 7-9% (CP2, PDR)
Vertigo: (BNF, PDR)

Risk assessment: Class 1

Tornalate   (see **Bitolterol**)

Torsemide (Torasemide)

Pronunciation guide: TOR-seh-mide

Drug classification: DIURETICS—LOOP (see section 30.5.4 in Table 14-1)

Brand names: *Demadex*

Ototoxic effects:
Cochlear:
Hearing loss: (CPS, PDR)
Tinnitus: (CPS, PDR)
Vestibular:
Dizziness: 3.2% [same as placebo] (CPS, PDR)
Vertigo: <1% (CPS)

Risk assessment: Class 3

Notes:

Tinnitus and hearing loss (usually reversible) can follow rapid intravenous injection of **Torsemide** or other LOOP DIURETICS. You can also get tinnitus and/or a hearing loss just from taking oral **Torsemide**. In order to minimize the risk of ototoxicity, intravenous **Torsemide** should be injected slowly over 2 minutes, and single doses should not exceed 200 mg. Ototoxicity has also been seen in animal studies when researchers induced very high plasma levels of **Torsemide** (CPS, PDR).

See Chapter 12, "Potpourri" for further information on this drug.

Tositumomab

Pronunciation guide: toe-sih-TOO-moe-mab

Drug classification: MONOCLONAL ANTIBODIES (see section 7.17.8 in Table 14-1)

Brand names: *Bexxar*

Ototoxic effects:
Cochlear:
Tinnitus: <1% (CPS)

Vestibular:
    Ataxia: <1% (CPS)
    Dizziness: 5% (CPS)
    Vestibular disorder: (CPS)
Outer/Middle Ear:
    Earache/ear pain: <1% (CPS)
Unspecified/General Ear Conditions:
    Ear disorder: 2% (CPS)

Risk assessment: Class 2

Tracleer   (see **Bosentan**)

Tramacet   (see **Tramadol**)

Tramadol

Pronunciation guide: TRAM-ah-dohl

Drug classification: Opiate agonist drugs (see section 1.4.1 in Table 14-1)

Brand names: *Ralivia, Ryzolt, Tramacet* [1], *Tridural, Ultracet* [1], *Ultram, Zytram XL*

Ototoxic effects:
  Cochlear:
    Auditory Hallucinations: [2]
    Hearing loss: (AHF, PDR)
    Tinnitus: >1% (AHF, PDR)
  Vestibular:
    Ataxia: >1% (NDH, PDR)
    Dizziness: 7-34.6% [4-26.5% above placebo results] (CPS, PDR)
    Dizziness/vertigo: 26-33% (PDR)
    Labyrinthitis: >1% (CPS)
    Vertigo: 1-10% [<2.1% above placebo results] (CPS, PDR)
  Outer/Middle Ear:
    Earache/ear pain: >1% (CPS)
    Otitis: <1% (PDR)
    Otitis media: <1% (CPS)

Risk assessment: Class 2

Notes:

[1] *Tramacet* and *Ultracet* are combinations of **Tramadol** and **Acetaminophen**. (See the generic drug **Acetaminophen** for its specific ototoxic properties.)

[2] I have a report in my files of a man that started getting auditory hallucinations soon after he began taking **Tramadol.** His auditory hallucinations stopped two days after he stopped taking the **Tramadol.**[365]

I have an anecdotal report in my files of a man who wrote, "I took one 50 mg. **Tramadol.** Shortly afterwards, I was struck with intense dizziness and nausea which was greatly relieved by laying down. It has been almost two weeks now. My balance is bad; I get dizzy if I move too fast or when I hold my head up for too long to read. I also seem to have a permanent dull headache with a feeling of fullness and flushing in my forehead area".

I have an anecdotal report in my files of a man who has been taking **Tramadol** (200 mg. daily) for ten years. He has noticed that his hearing as "dropped off in the last couple of years" and attributes it to the **Tramadol**.

Trandate   (see **Labetalol**)

Trandolapril

Pronunciation guide: tran-DOLE-ah-pril

Drug classification: ANGIOTENSIN-CONVERTING ENZYME (ACE) INHIBITORS (see section 20.8.8 in Table 14-1)

Brand names: *Mavik, Tarka* [1]

Ototoxic effects:
Cochlear:
Tinnitus: >0.3% (CPS, PDR)
Vestibular:
Dizziness: 1.3-23% [0.9-6% above placebo results] (CPS, PDR)
Loss of balance: >0.3% (CPS, PDR)
Vertigo: 1.2% (CPS, PDR)

Risk assessment: Class 2

Notes:

[1] *Tarka* is a combination of **Trandolapril** and **Verapamil**. (See the generic drug **Verapamil** for its specific ototoxic properties.)

Transderm-Nitro   (see **Nitroglycerin**)

Transderm-Scop   (see **Scopolamine**)

Transderm-V   (see **Scopolamine**)

Tranxene   (see **Clorazepate**)

Tranylcypromine

Pronunciation guide: tran-ill-SIP-roe-meen

Drug classification: MONOAMINE OXIDASE INHIBITORS (see section 60.1.1 in Table 14-1)

Brand names: *Parnate*

Ototoxic effects:
    Cochlear:
        Tinnitus: (CPS, PDR)
    Vestibular:
        Ataxia: (PDR)
        Dizziness: (CPS, PDR)
        Nystagmus: (BNF)

Risk assessment: Class 1

Notes:

    See Chapter 7, "We 'Hear' With Our Eyes" for further information on this drug.

Trasicor (see **Oxprenolol**)

Trastuzumab

Pronunciation guide: trass-too-ZOO-mab

Drug classification: MONOCLONAL ANTIBODIES (see section 7.17.8 in Table 14-1)

Brand names: *Herceptin*

Ototoxic effects:
    Cochlear:
        Hearing loss: (CPS, PDR)
    Vestibular:
        Ataxia: (AHF, PDR)
        Dizziness: 3.6-13% (CPS, PDR)
        Vertigo: 1.5% (CPS)

Risk assessment: Class 2

Travatan (see **Travoprost**)

Travoprost

Pronunciation guide: TRAH-voe-prost

Drug classification: PROSTAGLANDIN ANALOGS (see section 40.36.1 in Table 14-1)

Brand names: *DuoTrav* [1], *Travatan*

Ototoxic effects:
    Cochlear:
        Hearing loss: (CPS)
        Tinnitus: (CPS)
    Vestibular:
        Dizziness: <1% (CPS)
    Outer/Middle Ear:
        Earache/ear pain: <1% (CPS)

Risk assessment: Class 2

Notes:

[1] *DuoTrav* is a combination of **Travoprost** and **Timolol**. (See the generic drug **Timolol** for its specific ototoxic properties.)

Trazodone

Pronunciation guide: TRAYZ-oh-dohn

Drug classification: HETEROCYCLIC ANTI-DEPRESSANTS (see section 60.1.16 in Table 14-1)

Brand names: *Desyrel*

Ototoxic effects:
    Cochlear:
        Tinnitus: 1.4% [placebo 0] (CPS, PDR)
    Vestibular:
        Ataxia: (CPS, PDR)
        Dizziness: 19.7-28% [12.8-14.4% above placebo results] (CPS, PDR)
        Vertigo: (CPS, PDR)

Risk assessment: Class 2

Trecator   (see **Ethionamide**)

Trental   (see **Pentoxifylline**)

Tretinoin

Pronunciation guide: TRET-ih-noyn

Drug classification: VITAMIN A ANALOGS (see section 23.4 in Table 14-1)

Brand names: *Vesanoid*

Ototoxic effects:
    Cochlear:
        Hearing loss: <6% (AHF, PDR)
        Tinnitus: (CPS)
    Vestibular:
        Ataxia: 3% (CPS, PDR)
        Dizziness: 20% (CPS, PDR)
    Outer/Middle Ear:
        Earache/ear pain: (CPS, PDR)
        Feeling of fullness in ears: (CPS, PDR)

Risk assessment: Class 4

Notes:

People taking **Tretinoin** consistently reported various ear disorders. Earaches or a feeling of fullness in the ears was reported by 23%. Doctors observed hearing loss and other unspecified auricular disorders in 6%. Less than 1% reported permanent hearing loss (PDR).

If you take **Tretinoin** while you are pregnant, there is a high risk that your baby will be severely deformed. Among a host of other adverse side effects, your baby's external ears may be abnormal (PDR).

Treximet (see **Sumatriptan**)

Triacomb (see **Neomycin**)

Triamcinolone

Pronunciation guide: trye-am-SIN-oh-lone

Drug classification: GLUCOCORTICOIDS (see section 40.1.4 in Table 14-1)

Brand names: *Aristocort, Kenalog, Nasacort*

Ototoxic effects:
Vestibular:
Vertigo: (CPS, NDH)
Outer/Middle Ear:
Otitis media: 4.7% [1% above placebo results] (NDH, PDR)

Risk assessment: Class 1

Notes:

Corticosteroids (like **Triamcinolone**) can damage the collagen that constitutes the middle layer of your tympanic membranes (eardrums). This warning is also listed for the brands *Kenacomb* and *Triacomb* (CPS, PDR). (See the generic drug **Neomycin** for more information on these two drugs.)

Triamterene

Pronunciation guide: trye-AM-ter-een

Drug classification: DIURETICS—POTASSIUM-SPARING (see section 30.5.8 in Table 14-1)

Brand names: *Dyazide*[1], *Dyrenium, Maxzide*[1]

Ototoxic effects:
Vestibular:
Dizziness: <0.1% (CPS, PDR)
Vertigo: <0.1% (CPS, PDR)

Risk assessment: Class 1

Notes:

[1] *Dyazide* and *Maxzide* are combinations of **Triamterene** and **Hydrochlorothiazide**. (See the generic drug **Hydrochlorothiazide** for its specific ototoxic properties.)

Triavil (see **Amitriptyline**)

Triazolam

Pronunciation guide: try-AY-zoe-lam

Drug classification: BENZODIAZEPINES (see section 60.12.8 in Table 14-1)

Brand names: *Halcion*

Ototoxic effects:
Cochlear:
Auditory Hallucinations: [366]
Hearing loss: <0.5% (CPS)
Tinnitus: <0.5% (CPS, PDR)
Vestibular:
Ataxia: 1.7-4.6% [0.5-3.8% above placebo results] (CPS, PDR)
Dizziness: 4.4-9% [3.2-4.7% above placebo results] (CPS, PDR)

Risk assessment: Class 2

Notes:

Caution: Eating grapefruit or drinking grapefruit juice during the time you are taking this drug may make the listed side effects worse than shown here. In fact, taking **Triazolam** with grapefruit juice can increase the potency of **Triazolam** by as much as 48%.

See Chapter 10 "Beware of Benzodiazepines—Don't Let This Nasty Time-Bomb Ambush You and Your Ears" and Chapter 11, "Grapefruit Juice and Ototoxic Drugs" for further information on this drug.

Trichlormethiazide

Pronunciation guide: try-klor-meh-THYE-ah-zide

Drug classification: THIAZIDE-RELATED DIURETIC (see section 30.5.12 in Table 14-1)

Brand names: *Naquasone* [1]

Ototoxic effects:
Vestibular:
Dizziness: (DFC)
Vertigo: (DFC)

Risk assessment: Class 1

Notes:

[1] *Naquasone* is a combination of **Trichlormethiazide** and **Dexamethasone**. (See the generic drug **Dexamethasone** for its specific ototoxic properties.)

Tricor   (see **Fenofibrate**)

Tri-Cyclen   (see **Ethinyl estradiol**)

Tridural   (see **Tramadol**)

Triethanolamine (Trolamine)

Pronunciation guide: try-eth-ah-NOLE-ah-meen (TROE-lah-meen)

Drug classification: CERUMENOLYTIC DRUGS (EAR-WAX REMOVERS) (see section 56.4.1 in
   Table 14-1)

Brand names: *Cerumenex*, *Myoflex*, *Royflex*

Ototoxic effects:
   Cochlear:
      Tinnitus: (San, She)
   Outer/Middle Ear:
      Earache/ear pain: (PDR)
      Otitis externa: 1% (CPS, PDR)
   Unspecified/General Ear Conditions:
      Ototoxicity: (San, Str)

Risk assessment: Class 2

Notes:

   Otitis externa reactions can range from a very mild reddening of the skin and itching of
   the external ear canal to a severe eczematoid reaction (red, crusted reaction) of the outer
   ear and surrounding tissue. Such reactions generally last from 2 to 10 days (CPS, PDR).

   Some people experience burning and pain at the application site (PDR).

Trihibit   (see **Tetanus vaccine**)

Trilafon   (see **Perphenazine**)

Trileptal   (see **Oxcarbazepine**)

Trilisate   (see **Choline magnesium trisalicylate**)

Trimazosin

Pronunciation guide: trih-mah-ZOE-sin

Drug classification: ALPHA ADRENERGIC BLOCKING DRUGS (see section 20.8.1 in Table 14-1)

Brand names: *Cardovar BD*

Ototoxic effects:
   Cochlear:
      Tinnitus: (San, She)

Risk assessment: Class 1

Trimebutine

Pronunciation guide: try-MEH-boo-teen

Drug classification: INTESTINAL MOTILITY STIMULANTS (see section 17.8 in Table 14-1)

Brand names: *Modulon*

Ototoxic effects:
Cochlear:
Hearing loss: (CPS)
Vestibular:
Dizziness: <3.3% (CPS)

Risk assessment: Class 2

Notes:

Hearing loss occurs infrequently and is usually "slight" (CPS).

Trimeprazine

Pronunciation guide: try-MEP-rah-zeen

Drug classification: H$_1$ RECEPTOR ANTAGONISTS (see section 10.1 in Table 14-1)

Brand names: *Panectyl, Temaril*

Ototoxic effects:
Cochlear:
Tinnitus: (Med, She)
Vestibular:
Dizziness: (Med)

Risk assessment: Class 1

Notes:

See Chapter 7, "We 'Hear' With Our Eyes" for further information on this drug.

Trimetazadine

Pronunciation guide: tri-meh-TAH-zah-deen

Drug classification: ANTI-ANGINALS (see section 20.1 in Table 14-1)

Brand names: *Trivedon-20, Vastarel*

Ototoxic effects:
Vestibular:
Dizziness: [367]
Vertigo: [368]

Risk assessment: Class 1

Trimethobenzamide

Pronunciation guide: trye-meth-oh-BEN-zah-mide

Drug classification: ANTI-EMETICS (see section 34.1 in Table 14-1)

Brand names: *Tigan*

Ototoxic effects:
Vestibular:
Dizziness: (AHF)
Vertigo: (AHF)

Risk assessment: Class 1

Trimethoprim

Pronunciation guide: try-METH-oh-prim

Drug classification: URINARY ANTI-INFECTIVES (see section 7.20 in Table 14-1)

Brand names: *Apo-Trimethoprim, Bactrim*[1]*, Proloprim, Roubac*[1]*, Septra*[1]*, Septrin*[2]

Ototoxic effects:
Cochlear:
Tinnitus: (CPS, PDR)
Vestibular:
Ataxia: (CPS, PDR)
Dizziness: (CPS, PDR)
Vertigo: (CPS, PDR)

Risk assessment: Class 1

Notes:

[1] *Bactrim, Roubac* and *Septra* are combinations of **Trimethoprim** and **Sulfamethoxazole**. (See the generic drug **Sulfamethoxazole** for its specific ototoxic properties.)

[2] **Co-trimoxazole** (*Septrin*) is a combination of 1 part of **Trimethoprim** and 5 parts of **Sulfamethoxazole** that work together synergistically (BNF). (See the generic drug **Sulfamethoxazole** for its specific ototoxic properties.)

See Chapter 12, "Potpourri" for further information on this drug.

Trimipramine

Pronunciation guide: try-MIP-rah-meen

Drug classification: TRICYCLIC ANTI-DEPRESSANTS (see section 60.1.8 in Table 14-1)

Brand names: *Rhotrimine, Surmontil*

Ototoxic effects:
Cochlear:
Tinnitus: (CPS, PDR)
Vestibular:
Ataxia: (CPS, PDR)
Dizziness: (CPS, PDR)
Vertigo: (CPS)

Risk assessment: Class 1

Trinalin   (see **Azatadine**)

Trinipatch   (see **Nitroglycerin**)

Tripedia   (see **Tetanus vaccine**)

Tripelennamine

Pronunciation guide: tri-pel-ENN-ah-meen

Drug classification: H_1 RECEPTOR ANTAGONISTS (see section 10.1 in Table 14-1)

Brand names: *PBZ, Pyribenzamine*

Ototoxic effects:
    Cochlear:
        Tinnitus: (PDR)
    Vestibular:
        Ataxia: (NTP)
        Dizziness: (CPS, PDR)
        Vertigo: (CPS, PDR)

Risk assessment: Class 1

Notes:

    See Chapter 7, "We 'Hear' With Our Eyes" for further information on this drug.

Triple sulfas

Pronunciation guide: TRIH-pul SUL-fas

Notes:

    The Triple Sulfas are **Sulfadiazine**, **Sulfamerazine** and **Sulfamethazine** (CPS). (See the generic drugs **Sulfadiazine** and **Sulfamethazine** for their specific ototoxic properties. **Sulfamerazine** (sul-fah-MER-ah-zeen) likely has similar ototoxic side effects as the other two Triple Sulfa drugs.)

Triptil   (see **Protriptyline**)

Triquilar 28   (see **Ethinyl estradiol**)

Trisenox   (see **Arsenic trioxide**)

Trisulfaminic   (see **Sulfamethazine**)

Trivedon-20   (see **Trimetazadine**)

Trizivir   (see **Lamivudine**)

Trobicin   (see **Spectinomycin**)

Trolamine   (see **Triethanolamine**)

Trosec   (see **Trospium**)

Trospium

Pronunciation guide: TROSE-pee-um

Drug classification: Muscarinic receptor antagonists (see section 17.1.1 in Table 14-1)

Brand names: *Trosec*

Ototoxic effects:
    Outer/Middle Ear:
        Earache/ear pain: <1% (CPS)

Risk assessment: Class 1

Trovafloxacin (Alatrofloxacin)

Pronunciation guide: TROE-vah-flox-ah-sin (ah-la-troe-FLOX-ah-sin)

Drug classification: Quinolones (see section 7.4.48 in Table 14-1)

Brand names: *Trovan*

Ototoxic effects:
    Cochlear:
        Hearing loss: <1% (CPS)
        Hyperacusis: <1% (CPS, PDR)
        Tinnitus: <1% (CPS, PDR)
    Vestibular:
        Ataxia: <1% (CPS, PDR)
        Dizziness: 2-11% (CPS, PDR)
        Vertigo: <1% (CPS, PDR)
    Outer/Middle Ear:
        Earache/ear pain: <1% (CPS)

Risk assessment: Class 2

Notes:

Alatrofloxacin is a prodrug of **Trovafloxacin**. It is rapidly and completely converted in your body to **Trovafloxacin** within 5 minutes following I.V. administration (CPS).

According to the CPS, **Trovafloxacin** therapy likely does not cause hearing loss and earache. However, disturbing news from drug trials in Nigeria suggests differently. The Africa News Service reports that a meningitis outbreak in 1996 resulted in "many deaths and hearing impairments". "Over 500 children who contracted meningitis during the 1996 trials died. About 200 others who survived the administration of **Trovafloxacin** are either deaf or dumb".[369]

Since one of the side effects of meningitis can be hearing loss, what remains unknown is how many of these meningitis survivors would have had a resulting hearing loss whether or not they were treated with **Trovafloxacin**. Therefore, until proven safe, beware of **Trovafloxacin**.

Trovan   (see **Trovafloxacin**)

Trudexa   (see **Adalimumab**)

Tusal   (see **Sodium thiosalicylate**)

Tussend   (see **Hydrocodone**)

Twinrix   (see **Hepatitis B vaccine**)

Tygacil   (see **Tigecycline**)

Tylenol   (see **Acetaminophen**)

Tylenol Aches & Strains   (see **Acetaminophen**)

Tylenol, Children's   (see **Acetaminophen**)

Tylenol Flu Medication   (see **Acetaminophen**)

Tympagesic   (see **Benzocaine**)

Tysabri   (see **Natalizumab**)

Ulone   (see **Chlophedianol**)

Uloric   (see **Febuxostat**)

Ultracaine   (see **Articaine**)

Ultracet   (see **Tramadol**)

Ultradol   (see **Etodolac**)

Ultram   (see **Tramadol**)

Ultravist   (see **Iopromide**)

Unasyn Oral   (see **Sultamicillin**)

Unidet   (see **Tolterodine**)

Uniphyl　(see **Theophylline**)

Uniretic　(see **Moexipril**)

Unitron PEG　(see **Peginterferon alfa-2b**)

Univasc　(see **Moexipril**)

Uracel　(see **Sodium salicylate**)

Uracil mustard　(see **Mechlorethamine**)

Urasal　(see **Methenamine**)

Urex　(see **Methenamine**)

Urised　(see **Methenamine**)

Urispas　(see **Flavoxate**)

Urobiotic　(see **Sulfamethizole**)

Uromax　(see **Oxybutynin**)

URSO　(see **Ursodiol**)

Ursodiol

Pronunciation guide: er-soe-DIE-all

Drug classification: CHOLELITHOLYTIC AGENTS (see section 34.16 in Table 14-1)

Brand names: *URSO*

Ototoxic effects:
    Cochlear:
        Hearing loss: <1.7% (CPS)
    Vestibular:
        Dizziness: 3.3% (CPS)
        Vertigo: 1.7% (CPS)
    Outer/Middle Ear:
        Otitis media: 1.7% (CPS)

Risk assessment: Class 2

Vagifem　(see **Estradiol-17 beta**)

Valacyclovir (Acyclovir)

Pronunciation guide: val-ah-SYE-kloe-ver (aye-SYE-kloe-ver)

Drug classification: ANTI-RETROVIRAL PROTEASE INHIBITORS (see section 7.17.1.1 in Table 14-1)

Brand names: *Valtrex*, *Zovirax*

Ototoxic effects:
    Cochlear:
        Auditory hallucinations: (CPS, PDR)
    Vestibular:
        Ataxia: (AHF, PDR)
        Dizziness: 3% [1% above placebo results] (CPS, PDR)

Risk assessment: Class 1

Notes:

    When you take **Valacyclovir**, your body rapidly changes it into **Acyclovir** (PDR).

Valcyte   (see **Valganciclovir**)

Valdecoxib

Pronunciation guide: VAL-dee-kox-ib

Drug classification: COX-2 INHIBITORS (see section 1.1.4 in Table 14-1)

Brand names: *Bextra*

Ototoxic effects:
    Cochlear:
        Tinnitus: 0.1-1.9% (PDR)
    Vestibular:
        Dizziness: 2.6-2.7% [0.5-0.6% above placebo results] (PDR)
        Vertigo: 0.1-1.9% (PDR)
    Outer/Middle Ear:
        Earache/ear pain: 0.1-1.9% (PDR)
        Otitis media: 0.1-1.9% (PDR)
    Unspecified/General Ear Conditions:
        Ear disorder (ear abnormality): 0.1-1.9% (PDR)

Risk assessment: Class 2

Valganciclovir

Pronunciation guide: val-gan-SYE-kloe-ver

Drug classification: ANTI-RETROVIRAL PROTEASE INHIBITORS (see section 7.17.1.1 in Table 14-1)

Brand names: *Valcyte*

Ototoxic effects:
   Cochlear:
      Hearing loss: (BNF, CPS)
      Tinnitus: (CPS)
   Vestibular:
      Ataxia: (BNF, CPS)
      Dizziness: 9-11% (BNF, CPS)
   Outer/Middle Ear:
      Earache/ear pain: (CPS)

Risk assessment: Class 2

Notes:

   Valganciclovir is rapidly converted in the body to **Ganciclovir** (CPS). (See the generic drug **Ganciclovir** for its specific ototoxic properties.)

Valium   (see **Diazepam**)

Valproate

Pronunciation guide: val-PROH-ate

Drug classification: ANTI-CONVULSANT DRUGS (see section 53.12 in Table 14-1)

Brand names: *Depacon*

Ototoxic effects:
   Cochlear:
      Hearing loss: 1-5% (CPS, PDR)
      Tinnitus: 1-7% [<6% above placebo results] (CPS, PDR)
   Vestibular:
      Ataxia: 8% [7% above placebo results] (CPS, PDR)
      Dizziness: 5.2-25% [<12% above placebo results] (CPS, PDR)
      Nystagmus: 1-8% [<7% above placebo results] (CPS, PDR)
      Vertigo: (CPS, PDR)
   Outer/Middle Ear:
      Earache/ear pain: (CPS, PDR)
      Otitis media: 1-5% (CPS, PDR)

Risk assessment: Class 4

Notes:

   Hearing loss may be temporary or permanent (CPS, PDR).

Valproic acid

Pronunciation guide: val-PRO-ik ASS-id

Drug classification: ANTI-CONVULSANT DRUGS (see section 53.12 in Table 14-1)

Brand names: *Apo-Valproic, Depakene, Deproic*

Ototoxic effects:
    Cochlear:
        Hearing loss: 1-5% (CPS, PDR)
        Tinnitus: 7-16% [6% above placebo results] (AHF, PDR)
    Vestibular:
        Ataxia: 8% [7% above placebo results] (CPS, PDR)
        Dizziness: 18-25% [5-12% above placebo results] (CPS, PDR)
        Nystagmus: 7-8% [6-7% above placebo results] (CPS, PDR)
        Vertigo: >1% (CPS, PDR)
    Outer/Middle Ear:
        Earache/ear pain: (CPS, PDR)
        Otitis media: 1-5% (CPS, PDR)

Risk assessment: Class 4

Notes:

    Hearing loss may be temporary or permanent (CPS, PDR).

Valsartan

Pronunciation guide: val-SAR-tan

Drug classification: ANGIOTENSIN-2-RECEPTOR ANTAGONISTS (see section 20.8.4 in Table 14-1)

Brand names: *Diovan, Diovan HCT*[1], *Valturna*[2]

Ototoxic effects:
    Cochlear:
        Tinnitus: 0.2-1% (CPS, PDR)
    Vestibular:
        Dizziness: 2.8-9% [<2% above placebo results] (CPS, PDR)
        Vertigo: 0.2-1.1% [<0.8% above placebo results] (CPS, PDR)
    Outer/Middle Ear:
        Earache/ear pain: (CPS)

Risk assessment: Class 2

Notes:

    [1] *Diovan HCT* is a combination of **Valsartan** and **Hydrochlorothiazide**. (See the generic drug **Hydrochlorothiazide** for its specific ototoxic properties.)

    [2] *Valturna* is a combination of **Valsartan** and **Aliskiren**. (See the generic drug **Aliskiren** for its specific ototoxic properties.)

Valtrex   (see **Valacyclovir**)

Valturna   (see **Valsartan**)

Vancenase   (see **Beclomethasone**)

Vanceril (see **Beclomethasone**)

Vancocin (see **Vancomycin**)

Vancomycin

Pronunciation guide: van-koe-MYE-sin

Drug classification: GLYCOPEPTIDES (see section 7.4.20 in Table 14-1)

Brand names: *Vancocin*

Ototoxic effects:
Cochlear:
    Hearing loss: (CPS, PDR)
    Tinnitus: (CPS, PDR)
Vestibular:
    Dizziness: (CPS, PDR)
    Vertigo: (CPS, PDR)
Unspecified/General Ear Conditions:
    Ototoxicity: (CPS, PDR)

Risk assessment: Class 4

Notes:

Vancomycin was introduced in the 1950s. Due to early reports of ototoxicity, it was largely replaced by other antibiotics around 1958.[370]

Vancomycin can cause significant hearing loss that is frequently permanent[371] but may be temporary (PDR). Sometimes hearing loss is preceded by tinnitus (CPS). This gives you a warning that the **Vancomycin** is damaging your ears. You should stop taking **Vancomycin** if tinnitus occurs (AHF, BNF). The hearing loss may be progressive, and may continue to get worse even after you have stopped taking **Vancomycin** (AHF, CPS). If you already have a hearing loss you should avoid taking **Vancomycin** if possible (CPS).

Ototoxic side effects have occurred with **Vancomycin** blood concentrations as low as 25 mcg/ml, although more commonly, they occur at concentrations between 80 and 100 mcg/ml (AHF).

Having serial audiograms before, during and after taking **Vancomycin** may help your doctor minimize the risk of any hearing loss (CPS).

There are several dozens of cases of hearing loss reported associated with intravenously administered **Vancomycin** (DFC). You are more at risk to have a hearing loss resulting from taking **Vancomycin** if you are elderly, if you already have a hearing loss, if you have kidney problems, if you take high doses of **Vancomycin**, if you take **Vancomycin** for long periods (AHF), or if you take **Vancomycin** at the same time as other nephrotoxic (AHF), or ototoxic drugs such as the AMINOGLYCOSIDE antibiotics (CPS, PDR).

Taking **Vancomycin** in combination with AMINOGLYCOSIDE antibiotics can result in significant ototoxicity.[372]

I have an anecdotal report in my files of a man that lost almost all his hearing from an allergic reaction to taking **Vancomycin**. Shortly after his emergency surgery he came down with a surgically-caused infection. He was treated with **Vancomycin**. He explains, "While still in the hospital I began to observe for the first time a sudden and significant hearing loss. It was soon discovered that I was having a severe allergic reaction to the antibiotic, **Vancomycin**, that was being administered intravenously in very large dosages by the Hospital Staff, and later for a month by the home care nurses. The hearing loss was immediate, and continued to worsen with each passing day. Today, I have severe and permanent hearing loss, and I must now seriously consider cochlear implant surgery".

See Chapter 4, "Are You at Risk?" for further information on this drug.

Vaniqa (see **Eflornithine**)

Vanquish Extra Strength Pain Reliever (see **Acetylsalicylic acid**)

Vantin (see **Cefpodoxime**)

Vaqta (see **Hepatitis A vaccine**)

Vardenafil

Pronunciation guide: var-DEN-ah-fill

Drug classification: PHOSPHODIESTERASE TYPE 5 (PDE5) INHIBITORS (see section 20.8.28 in Table 14-1)

Brand names: *Levitra*

Ototoxic effects:
　　Cochlear:
　　　　Hearing loss: (CPS, PDR)
　　　　Tinnitus: <2% (NDH, PDR)
　　Vestibular:
　　　　Dizziness: 1.6% [1.3% above placebo results] (CPS, PDR)
　　　　Vertigo: <2% (AHF, PDR)

Risk assessment: Class 3

Notes:

Sudden hearing loss (partial loss to complete loss) can occur within hours to two days of taking this drug. In the 29 cases of ear problems reported to the FDA, sudden hearing loss typically occurred in one ear. The hearing loss was sometimes accompanied by tinnitus, dizziness and/or vertigo. The hearing loss was temporary in 1/3 of the cases reported.[373]

The results in a study of 11,525 men over the age of 40 indicated that men who use **Sildenafil** (or **Tadalafil** or **Vardenafil**) were twice as likely to have hearing loss as those who did not use such drugs. The resulting hearing loss was "long term" (permanent).[374]

"Sudden loss or decrease in hearing, sometimes with ringing in the ears and dizziness, has been rarely reported in people taking Levitra". (PDR)

Caution: Eating grapefruit or drinking grapefruit juice during the time you are taking this drug may make the listed side effects worse than shown here.

See Chapter 7, "We 'Hear' With Our Eyes" and Chapter 11, "Grapefruit Juice and Ototoxic Drugs" for further information on this drug.

Varenicline

Pronunciation guide: var-eh-NIK-leen

Drug classification: DOPAMINE REUPTAKE INHIBITORS (see section 53.24 in Table 14-1)

Brand names: *Champix*, *Chantix*

Ototoxic effects:
    Cochlear:
        Hearing loss: <0.1% (CPS, PDR)
        Tinnitus: 0.1-1% (CPS, PDR)
    Vestibular:
        Dizziness: >1% (NDH, PDR)
        Equilibrium disorder: <0.1% (CPS, PDR)
        Nystagmus: <0.1% (CPS, PDR)
        Vertigo: 0.1-1% (CPS, PDR)
    Unspecified/General Ear Conditions:
        Meniere's disease: (DFC)

Risk assessment: Class 2

Varicella vaccine

Pronunciation guide: var-ih-SELL-ah VAX-seen

Drug classification: VACCINES (see section 70.8 in Table 14-1)

Brand names: *Varivax, Varivax II, Varivax III*

Ototoxic effects:
    Vestibular:
        Ataxia: (CPS, PDR)
        Dizziness: >1% (CPS, PDR)
    Outer/Middle Ear:
        Otitis: >1% (CPS, PDR)

Risk assessment: Class 1

Notes:

It is possible that broad use of this vaccine could reveal other adverse reactions that were not observed in clinical trials (PDR).

Varivax   (see **Varicella vaccine**)

Varivax II   (see **Varicella vaccine**)

Varivax III   (see **Varicella vaccine**)

Vascor   (see **Bepridil**)

Vaseretic   (see **Enalapril**)

Vasopressin

Pronunciation guide: vay-soe-PRESS-in

Drug classification: PITUITARY HORMONES (see section 40.44 in Table 14-1)

Brand names: *Pressyn, Pressyn AR*

Ototoxic effects:
Vestibular:
Vertigo: (CPS, NDH)

Risk assessment: Class 1

Vasotec   (see **Enalapril**)

Vastarel   (see **Trimetazadine**)

Vaxigrip   (see **Influenza vaccine**)

Vectibix   (see **Panitumumab**)

Vectren   (see **Isoxicam**)

Vectrin   (see **Minocycline**)

Veetids   (see **Penicillin**)

Velban   (see **Vinblastine**)

Velbe   (see **Vinblastine**)

Velcade   (see **Bortezomib**)

Venapulse   (see **Atenolol**)

Venlafaxine

Pronunciation guide: ven-lah-FAK-seen

Drug classification: SELECTIVE SEROTONIN & NOREPINEPHRINE REUPTAKE INHIBITORS (see section 60.1.28 in Table 14-1)

Brand names: *Effexor, Effexor XR*

Ototoxic effects:
    Cochlear:
        Hearing loss: <0.1% (CPS, PDR)
        Hyperacusis: 0.1-1% (CPS, PDR)
        Tinnitus: 2-4% [2-3% above placebo results] (CPS, PDR)
    Vestibular:
        Ataxia: 0.1-1% (CPS, PDR)
        Dizziness: 3-23.9% [3-19.6% above placebo results] (CPS, PDR)
        Labyrinthitis: (CPS, PDR)
        Nystagmus: <0.1% (CPS, PDR)
        Vertigo: 2% [>1% above placebo results] (CPS, PDR)
    Outer/Middle Ear:
        Earache/ear pain: >1% (CPS, PDR)
        Otitis externa: <0.1% (CPS, PDR)
        Otitis media: 0.1-1% (CPS, PDR)

Risk assessment: Class 3

Notes:

I have an anecdotal report in my files from a hard of hearing lady that was prescribed **Venlafaxine** by one of her doctors. She wrote, "My psychiatrist said that while there was no documentation of hearing loss on *Effexor* [which is not exactly true as you can see above], he had two patients who took it for a short time. Both developed some hearing loss. At this point he took them off immediately, and decided never to prescribe this drug again. These people had not previously had hearing loss, and he felt that I was more at risk than they".

Venofer   (see **Iron sucrose**)

Ventolin   (see **Albuterol**)

VePesid   (see **Etoposide**)

Verapamil

Pronunciation guide: ver-APP-ah-mill

Drug classification: CALCIUM-CHANNEL-BLOCKING DRUGS (CALCIUM BLOCKERS) (see section 20.8.16 in Table 14-1)

Brand names: *Calan, Chronovera, Covera-HS, Isoptin, Novo-Veramil, Verelan*

Ototoxic effects:
    Cochlear:
        Tinnitus: <2% (AHF, PDR)
    Vestibular:
        Dizziness: 1.2-4.7% [<2.1 above placebo results] (CPS, PDR)
        Equilibrium disorder: <1% (CPS, PDR)
        Nystagmus: <1% (CPS, PDR)
        Vertigo: <1% (CPS, PDR)

Risk assessment: Class 2

Notes:

I have an anecdotal report in my files of a lady that was prescribed **Verapamil** by her doctor for a heart arrhythmia. She wrote, "I started taking 20 mg. of **Verapamil** three times a day. By the third day I had a high-pitched ringing/whistling sound in my right ear. I also had dizziness off and on. I stopped taking the **Verapamil** after the fifth day. It has been almost three weeks now and I feel like I am going out of my mind with the tinnitus racket. Will this ever go away?"

Caution: Eating grapefruit or drinking grapefruit juice during the time you are taking this drug may make the listed side effects worse than shown here. In fact, taking **Verapamil** with grapefruit juice can increase the potency of **Verapamil** by as much as 43%.

See Chapter 11, "Grapefruit Juice and Ototoxic Drugs" for further information on this drug.

Verelan   (see **Verapamil**)

Versed   (see **Midazolam**)

Verteporfin

Pronunciation guide: ver-teh-POR-fin

Drug classification: MACULAR DEGENERATION THERAPY ADJUNCT (see section 56.1.1 in Table 14-1)

Brand names: *Visudyne*

Ototoxic effects:
  Cochlear:
    Hearing loss: 1-10% (CPS, PDR)
  Vestibular:
    Dizziness: 4.5% [1.2% above placebo results] (CPS)
    Vertigo: 1-10% (CPS, PDR)

Risk assessment: Class 3

Verukan   (see **Salicylic acid**)

Vesanoid   (see **Tretinoin**)

Vfend   (see **Voriconazole**)

Viagra   (see **Sildenafil**)

Vibra-Tabs   (see **Doxycycline**)

Vicodin   (see **Hydrocodone**)

Vicoprofen   (see **Ibuprofen**)

Vidarabine

Pronunciation guide: vih-DARE-ah-been

Drug classification: ANTI-VIRAL DRUGS (see section 7.17 in Table 14-1)

Brand names: *Vira-A*

Ototoxic effects:
  Vestibular:
    Ataxia: (NTP)
    Dizziness: (NTP)

Risk assessment: Class 1

Videx   (see **Didanosine**)

Vigabatrin

Pronunciation guide: vih-GAB-ah-trin

Drug classification: ANTI-CONVULSANT DRUGS (see section 53.12 in Table 14-1)

Brand names: *Sabril*

Ototoxic effects:
  Cochlear:
    Hearing loss: (PDR)
    Tinnitus: 2% [1% above placebo results] (PDR)
  Vestibular:
    Ataxia: (BNF, CPS)
    Dizziness: 15-26% [5.9-9% above placebo results] (CPS, PDR)
    Nystagmus: 9-15% (CPS, PDR)
    Vertigo: 1.9-3% [1-1.8% above placebo results] (CPS, PDR)
  Outer/Middle Ear:
    Earache/ear pain: 2.3% [1.1% above placebo results] (CPS)

Risk assessment: Class 3

Vigamox   (see **Moxifloxacin**)

Viloxazine

Pronunciation guide: vih-LOX-ah-zeen

Drug classification: BICYCLIC ANTI-DEPRESSANTS (see section 60.1.4 in Table 14-1)

Brand names: *Vivalan*

Ototoxic effects:
  Vestibular:
    Ataxia: (DFC)
    Dizziness: (DFC)
    Vertigo: (WIK)

Risk assessment: Class 1

Vimpat (see **Lacosamide**)

Vinblastine

Pronunciation guide: vin-BLAS-teen

Drug classification: NATURAL ANTI-NEOPLASTICS (see section14.20 in Table 14-1)

Brand names: *Velban, Velbe*

Ototoxic effects:
    Cochlear:
        Auditory disorder: (PDR)
        Hearing loss: <1% (CPS, PDR)
        Tinnitus: (She)
    Vestibular:
        Dizziness: <1% (CPS, PDR)
        Equilibrium disorder: (PDR)
        Nystagmus: <1% (CPS, PDR)
        Vertigo: <1% (CPS, PDR)
        Vestibular disorder: (PDR)

Risk assessment: Class 3

Notes:

Both vestibular and auditory damage can result from **Vinblastine** treatment. You may end up with temporary or permanent, partial to total hearing loss, and difficulties with balance (AHF, PDR).

In order to minimize the risk of ototoxicity, you should not take **Vinblastine** at the same time as other known ototoxic drugs such as the platinum-containing anti-cancer drugs (such as **Cisplatin**) (PDR).

Caution: Eating grapefruit or drinking grapefruit juice during the time you are taking this drug may make the listed side effects worse than shown here.

See Chapter 11, "Grapefruit Juice and Ototoxic Drugs" for further information on this drug.

Vincristine

Pronunciation guide: vin-KRIS-teen

Drug classification: NATURAL ANTI-NEOPLASTICS (see section14.20 in Table 14-1)

Brand names: *Oncovin*

Ototoxic effects:
    Cochlear:
        Auditory disorder: (PDR)
        Hearing loss: (AHF, PDR)

Vestibular:
    Ataxia: (CPS, PDR)
    Dizziness: (AHF, PDR)
    Equilibrium disorder: (PDR)
    Nystagmus: (AHF, PDR)
    Vertigo: (AHF, PDR)
    Vestibular disorder: (PDR)

Risk assessment: Class 3

Notes:

Both vestibular and auditory damage can result from **Vincristine** treatment. You may end up with temporary or permanent, partial to total hearing loss, and difficulties with balance (AHF, PDR).

In order to minimize the risk of ototoxicity, you should not take **Vincristine** at the same time as other known ototoxic drugs such as the platinum-containing anti-cancer drugs (such as **Cisplatin**) (PDR).

Vinorelbine

Pronunciation guide: vih-oh-REL-been

Drug classification: NATURAL ANTI-NEOPLASTICS (see section 14.20 in Table 14-1)

Brand names: *Navelbine*

Ototoxic effects:
    Cochlear:
        Auditory disorder: (CPS, PDR)
        Hearing loss: (AHF, CPS)
    Vestibular:
        Ataxia: (CPS, PDR)
        Dizziness/vertigo: <9% (PDR)
        Vestibular disorder: (CPS, PDR)

Risk assessment: Class 2

Notes:

Vinorelbine is closely related to **Vincristine**; however, ototoxic side effects are much less common (CP2). Vestibular (balance) and auditory defects have been observed with **Vinorelbine**, usually when used in combination with **Cisplatin** (CP2, CPS). For example, hearing loss occurred in 10% of patients receiving **Vinorelbine** and **Cisplatin**, versus 1% in patients receiving **Vinorelbine** alone (AHF).

Viocin   (see **Viomycin**)

Viomycin

Pronunciation guide: vye-oh-MY-sin

Drug classification: AMINOGLYCOSIDES (see section 7.4.1 in Table 14-1)

Brand names: *Viocin*

Ototoxic effects:
    Cochlear:
        Hearing loss: [1]
    Vestibular:
        Vestibular disorder: [1]

Risk assessment: Class 4

Notes:

[1] **Viomycin** has caused both cochlear and vestibular toxicity.[375]

Viomycin is not used much anymore except to treat tuberculosis. It is not listed in current drug books like the CPS and PDR. There are several references to it in older printed works indicating it caused hearing loss and balance problems.

See Chapter 9, "Aminoglycoside Antibiotics are the Ototoxic 'Bad boys'" for further information on this drug.

Vioxx   (see **Rofecoxib**)

Vira-A   (see **Vidarabine**)

Viramune   (see **Nevirapine**)

Virazole   (see **Ribavirin**)

Visipaque   (see **Iodixanol**)

Viskazide   (see **Pindolol**)

Visken   (see **Pindolol**)

Vistaril   (see **Hydroxyzine**)

Vistide   (see **Cidofovir**)

Visudyne   (see **Verteporfin**)

Vitamin B_3 (see **Niacin**)

Vitamin B_6 (see **Pyridoxine**)

Vitamin B_{12} (see **Cyanocobalamin**)

Vitamin D_2 (see **Ergocalciferal**)

Vivactil   (see **Protriptyline**)

Vivalan   (see **Viloxazine**)

Vivelle-dot   (see **Estradiol**)

Volmax   (see **Albuterol**)

Voltaren   (see **Diclofenac**)

Voltaren Rapide   (see **Diclofenac**)

Voltaren SR   (see **Diclofenac**)

Vontrol   (see **Diphenidol**)

Voriconazole

Pronunciation guide: vor-ah-KON-ah-zole

Drug classification: ANTI-FUNGAL ANTIBIOTICS (see section 7.10 in Table 14-1)

Brand names: *Vfend*

Ototoxic effects:
    Cochlear:
        Hearing loss: <1% (CPS, PDR)
        Tinnitus: <1% (CPS, PDR)
    Vestibular:
        Ataxia: <1% (CPS, PDR)
        Dizziness: <2.6% (CPS, PDR)
        Nystagmus: <1% (DFC, PDR)
        Vertigo: <1% (CPS, PDR)
    Outer/Middle Ear:
        Earache/ear pain: <1% (CPS, PDR)
        Otitis externa: <1% (CPS, PDR)

Risk assessment: Class 2

VoSoL   (see **Benzethonium**)

Vytorin   (see **Simvastatin**)

Wellbutrin   (see **Bupropion**)

Wellbutrin SR   (see **Bupropion**)

Wellbutrin XL   (see **Bupropion**)

Welldorm   (see **Chloral hydrate**)

Wyamine   (see **Mephentermine**)

Wytensin   (see **Guanabenz**)

Xalacom   (see **Timolol**)

Xanax   (see **Alprazolam**)

Xanax TS   (see **Alprazolam**)

Xatral   (see **Alfuzosin**)

Xefo   (see **Lornoxicam**)

Xeloda   (see **Capecitabine**)

Xenazine   (see **Tetrabenazine**)

Xenical   (see **Orlistat**)

Xeomin   (see **Botulinum Toxin Type A**)

Xifaxan   (see **Rifaximin**)

Xolair   (see **Omalizumab**)

Xopenex   (see **Levalbuterol**)

Xopenex HFA   (see **Levalbuterol**)

Xylocaine   (see **Lidocaine**)

Xylocard   (see **Lidocaine**)

Xylonor   (see **Cetrimide**)

Xyrem   (see **Sodium oxybate**)

Xyzal   (see **Levocetirizine**)

Yasmin 28   (see **Ethinyl estradiol**)

Yaz   (see **Ethinyl estradiol**)

Yodoxin   (see **Iodoquinol**)

Zagam   (see **Sparfloxacin**)

Zalcitabine

Pronunciation guide: zal-SIT-ah-been

Drug classification: ANTI-RETROVIRAL REVERSE TRANSCRIPTASE INHIBITORS (see section 7.17.1.4 in Table 14-1)

Brand names: *Hivid*

Ototoxic effects:
   Cochlear:
      Hearing loss: <1% (CPS, PDR)
      Tinnitus: <1% (CPS, PDR)
   Vestibular:
      Ataxia: <1% (CPS, PDR)
      Dizziness: 1.1-3.1% (CPS, PDR)
      Equilibrium disorder: (PDR)
      Vertigo: <1% (CPS, PDR)
   Outer/Middle Ear:
      Earache/ear pain: <1% (CPS, PDR)
      Ears feel "plugged up": <0.1% (CPS, PDR)
      Otitis media: <1% (CPS, PDR)

Risk assessment: Class 2

Zaleplon

Pronunciation guide: ZAH-leh-plahn

Drug classification: PYRAZOLOPYRIMIDINES (see section 60.12.12 in Table 14-1)

Brand names: *Sonata, Starnoc*

Ototoxic effects:
   Cochlear:
      Hearing loss: <0.1% (DFC, PDR)
      Hyperacusis: 2% [>1% above placebo results] (CPS, PDR)
      Tinnitus: 0.1-1% (DFC, PDR)
   Vestibular:
      Ataxia: 0.1-1% (DFC, PDR)
      Dizziness: 7-9% [<2% above placebo results] (CPS, PDR)
      Labyrinthitis: <0.1% (DFC, PDR)
      Nystagmus: 0.1-1% (DFC, PDR)
      Vertigo: <1% (CPS, PDR)
   Outer/Middle Ear:
      Earache/ear pain: <1% [placebo 0] (CPS, PDR)

Risk assessment: Class 3

Notes:

   See Chapter 10 "Beware of Benzodiazepines—Don't Let This Nasty Time-Bomb Ambush You and Your Ears" for further information on this drug.

Zanaflex   (see **Tizanidine**)

Zanamivir

Pronunciation guide: zan-AM-ih-veer

Drug classification: NEURAMINIDASE INHIBITORS (see section 7.17.12 in Table 14-1)

Brand names: *Relenza*

Ototoxic effects:
   Vestibular:
      Dizziness: (NDH, PDR)
   Outer/Middle Ear:
      Otitis: (NDH, PDR)

Risk assessment: Class 1

Zanidip   (see **Lercanidipine**)

Zantac   (see **Ranitidine**)

Zarontin   (see **Ethosuximide**)

Zaroxolyn   (see **Metolazone**)

Zavesca   (see **Miglustat**)

Zebeta   (see **Bisoprolol**)

Zegerid   (see **Omeprazole**)

Zeldox   (see **Ziprasidone**)

Zelmid   (see **Zimeldine**)

Zelnorm   (see **Tegaserod**)

Zemplar   (see **Paricalcitol**)

Zepelin   (see **Feprazone**)

Zephiran   (see **Benzalkonium**)

Zerit   (see **Stavudine**)

Zestoretic   (see **Lisinopril**)

Zestril   (see **Lisinopril**)

Ziac   (see **Bisoprolol**)

Ziacaine   (see **Cetrimide**)

Ziconotide

Pronunciation guide: zye-KON-oh-tide

Drug classification: ANALGESIC DRUGS (PAINKILLERS) (see section 1 in Table 14-1)

Brand names: *Prialt*

Ototoxic effects:
Cochlear:
Tinnitus: (DFC)
Vestibular:
Ataxia: 16% [14% above placebo results] (DFC)
Dizziness: 47% [34% above placebo results] (DFC)
Nystagmus: 8% [placebo 0] (DFC)
Vertigo: 7% [placebo 0] (DFC)

Risk assessment: Class 3

Zidovudine

Pronunciation guide: zye-DOE-vyoo-deen

Drug classification: ANTI-RETROVIRAL REVERSE TRANSCRIPTASE INHIBITORS (see section 7.17.1.4 in Table 14-1)

Brand names: *AZT, Combivir* [1], *Novo-AZT, Retrovir*

Ototoxic effects:
Cochlear:
Hearing loss: <5% (CPS, PDR)
Tinnitus: (CPS)
Vestibular:
Ataxia: (AHF, CPS)
Dizziness: 6-20.8% [2-5.6% above placebo results] (CPS, PDR)
Vertigo: <5% (CPS, PDR)

Risk assessment: Class 2

Notes:

[1] *Combivir* is a combination of **Zidovudine** and **Lamivudine**. (See the generic drug **Lamivudine** for its specific ototoxic properties.)

Zimeldine

Pronunciation guide: zih-MEL-deen

Drug classification: SELECTIVE SEROTONIN REUPTAKE INHIBITORS (see section 60.1.32 in Table 14-1)

Brand names: *Zelmid*

Ototoxic effects:
    Cochlear:
        Tinnitus: (Ka7)

Risk assessment: Class 1

Zinacef   (see **Cefuroxime**)

Ziprasidone

Pronunciation guide: zih-PRAZ-ih-dohn

Drug classification: ANTIPSYCHOTIC DRUGS (see section 60.8 in Table 14-1)

Brand names: *Geodon, Zeldox*

Ototoxic effects:
    Cochlear:
        Tinnitus: 0.1-1% (CPS, PDR)
    Vestibular:
        Ataxia: >1% (CPS, PDR)
        Dizziness: 3-16% [2-9% above placebo results] (NDH, PDR)
        Nystagmus: <0.1% (CPS, PDR)
        Vertigo: >1% (CPS, PDR)
    Outer/Middle Ear:
        Earache/ear pain: >1% (CPS)
        Otitis externa: 0.1-1% (CPS)
        Otitis media: 0.1-1% (CPS)
    Unspecified/General Ear Conditions:
        Ear disorder: 0.1-1% (CPS)

Risk assessment: Class 2

Zithromax   (see **Azithromycin**)

Zocor   (see **Simvastatin**)

Zofran   (see **Ondansetron**)

Zoladex   (see **Goserelin**)

Zoledronic acid

Pronunciation guide: zoh-leh-DROH-nik ASS-id

Drug classification: BISPHOSPHONATES (see section 50.1.1 in Table 14-1)

Brand names: *Aclasta, Reclast*

Ototoxic effects:
> Vestibular:
>> Dizziness: 2-9% [<4.1% above placebo results] (CPS, PDR)
>> Vertigo: >1.3-4.3% [<2.6% above placebo results] (CPS, PDR)

Risk assessment: Class 1

Zoleptil   (see **Zotepine**)

Zolmitriptan

Pronunciation guide: zole-mah-TRIP-tan

Drug classification: SEROTONIN-RECEPTOR AGONISTS (see section 53.32 in Table 14-1)

Brand names: *Zomig*

Ototoxic effects:
> Cochlear:
>> Hearing loss: [1]
>> Hyperacusis: 0.1-1% (CPS, PDR)
>> Tinnitus: 0.1-1% (CPS, PDR)
> Vestibular:
>> Ataxia: 0.1-1% (CPS, PDR)
>> Dizziness: 2-10% [<6% above placebo results] (CPS, PDR)
>> Vertigo: 1.3-4.3% [<0.3% above placebo results] (CPS, PDR)
> Outer/Middle Ear:
>> Earache/ear pain: 0.1-1% (CPS, PDR)

Risk assessment: Class 2

Notes:

> [1] I have an anecdotal report in my files of a woman who has been taking **Zolmitriptan** (and **Rizatriptan**) for "some time now and gradually lost hearing in my right ear".

Zoloft   (see **Sertraline**)

Zolpidem

Pronunciation guide: ZOL-pih-dem

Drug classification: ANXIOLYTICS, SEDATIVES & HYPNOTICS (see section 60.12 in Table 14-1)

Brand names: *Ambien, Ambien CR, Edluar, Stilnoct, Stilnox*

Ototoxic effects:
> Cochlear:
>> Auditory hallucinations: <1-4% [placebo 0] (PDR)
>> Hearing loss: [1, 2]
>> Hyperacusis: [3]
>> Tinnitus: 1% [placebo 0] (AHF, PDR)

Vestibular:
    Ataxia: >1% [placebo 0] (AHF, PDR)
    Dizziness: 1-23.5% [<22% above placebo results] (AHF, PDR)
    Labyrinthitis: 1% [placebo 0] (DFC)
    Loss of balance: 2% [placebo 0] (AFH, PDR)
    Vertigo: 2% [placebo 0] (AHF, PDR)
Outer/Middle Ear:
    Earache/ear pain: [1]
    Otitis externa: 1% [placebo 0] (AHF, PDR)
    Otitis media: <0.1% (AHF, PDR)

Risk assessment: Class 3

Notes:

[1] The following ototoxic side effects have been reported for **Zolpidem**—auditory hallucinations, balance disorder, change in hearing, dizziness, ear drainage, earache, hearing loss, itching ears, loss of balance, tinnitus or other unexplained noise in the ears. [376]

[2] I have an anecdotal report in my files of a person who took **Zolpidem** for a bad case of shingles. He ended up with permanent hearing loss and permanent tinnitus.

[3] Withdrawal symptoms from **Zolpidem** (after physical dependence has been established) can include hyperacusis. [377]

Zolpidem, although not a Benzodiazepine, acts in the same way and has the same adverse effects including dependence and withdrawal reactions. [378]

See Chapter 10 "Beware of Benzodiazepines—Don't Let This Nasty Time-Bomb Ambush You and Your Ears" for further information on this drug.

Zomaril   (see **Iloperidone**)

Zomax   (see **Zomepirac**)

Zomepirac

Pronunciation guide: zoe-meh-PIR-ak

Drug classification: Acetic acids (see section 1.1.1 in Table 14-1)

Brand names: *Zomax*

Ototoxic effects:
    Cochlear:
        Tinnitus: (Ka7)

Risk assessment: Class 1

Zomig   (see **Zolmitriptan**)

Zonegran   (see **Zonisamide**)

Zonisamide

Pronunciation guide: zoh-NISS-ah-mide

Drug classification: ANTI-CONVULSANT DRUGS (see section 53.12 in Table 14-1)

Brand names: *Zonegran*

Ototoxic effects:
    Cochlear:
        Hearing loss: 0.1-1% (DFC, PDR)
        Tinnitus: >1% (NDH, PDR)
    Vestibular:
        Ataxia: 6% [5% above placebo results] (AHF, PDR)
        Dizziness: 13% [6% above placebo results] (AHF, PDR)
        Nystagmus: 4% [2% above placebo results] (AHF, PDR)
        Vertigo: 0.1-1% (DFC, PDR)

Risk assessment: Class 3

Zopiclone

Pronunciation guide: ZAW-pih-klone

Drug classification: HYPNOTIC DRUGS (see section 60.16 in Table 14-1)

Brand names: *Imovane*

Ototoxic effects:
    Vestibular:
        Ataxia: (CPS)
        Dizziness: (CPS)

Risk assessment: Class 1

Notes:

    Zopiclone, although not a BENZODIAZEPINE, acts in the same way and has the same adverse effects including dependence and withdrawal reactions.[379]

    See Chapter 10 "Beware of Benzodiazepines—Don't Let This Nasty Time-Bomb Ambush You and Your Ears" for further information on this drug.

Zosyn   (see **Piperacillin—Tazobactam**)

Zotepine

Pronunciation guide: ZOE-teh-peen

Drug classification: ANTIPSYCHOTIC DRUGS (see section 60.8 in Table 14-1)

Brand names: *Zoleptil*

Ototoxic effects:

Vestibular:
    Ataxia: (BNF)
    Dizziness: (BNF)
    Vertigo: (BNF)

Risk assessment: Class 1

Zovirax   (see **Valacyclovir**)

Zuclopenthixol

Pronunciation guide: zoo-kloe-pen-THIX-ole

Drug classification: PHENOTHIAZINES (see section 60.8.1 in Table 14-1)

Brand names: *Clopixol*

Ototoxic effects:
    Cochlear:
        Hyperacusis: <1% (CPS)
        Tinnitus: <1% (CPS)
    Vestibular:
        Ataxia: <1% (CPS)
        Dizziness: 6.8-20.6% (CPS)
        Vertigo: 1-5.2% (CPS)

Risk assessment: Class 2

Zyban   (see **Bupropion**)

Zydone   (see **Hydrocodone**)

Zyloprim   (see **Allopurinol**)

Zymar   (see **Gatifloxacin**)

Zyprexa   (see **Olanzapine**)

Zyrtec   (see **Cetirizine**)

Zytram XL   (see **Tramadol**)

Zyvox   (see **Linezolid**)

Zyvoxam   (see **Linezolid**)

---

101 *Preservex*, 1995, p. 1.
102 *Rantudil Retard*, 2002. p. 2.

103 *Rantudil Retard*, 2002. p. 2.

104 Yorgason, 2010. p. 816.

105 Yorgason, 2010. p. 814.

106 Curhan, 2010. p. 234.

107 Curhan, 2010. pp. 232, 235.

108 Kalinec, 2010. Personal communication.

109 Haybach, 1999. p. 17.

110 Stanten, 1996. p. 16.

111 *Guidelines for the Audiologic Management of Individuals Receiving Cochleotoxic Drug Therapy*, 1994. p. 4.

112 Haybach, 1999. p. 17.

113 *Disorders of the Inner Ear*. 2000. p. 10.

114 Lyos, 1992. p. 2.

115 Curhan, 2010. p. 234.

116 Curhan, 2010. p. 235.

117 Kalkanis, 2001. p. 7.

118 *Aspirin Component Prevents Antibiotic-induced Deafness*. 1999. pp. 1-2.

119 *Trudexa*. 2009. pp. 8-9.

120 *eHealth Treats—Medicine & Cure—Adalimumab*. 2009. pp. 3-4.

121 Haybach, 1999. p. 21.

122 Haybach, 1999. p. 50.

123 Rybacki, 1998. p. 76.

124 *Amonafide*, 2000. p. 1

125 Articaine, 2003. p. 2.

126 *Fortimicin for Injection*, 1998. pp. 2-3.

127 *Fortimicin for Injection*, 1998. pp. 1-2.

128 *Venapulse Tablets*, 2002. p. 2.

129 Suss, 1993. p. 215.

130 Suss, 1993. p. 214.

131 *Azapropazone (NSAID)*, 1994. p. 1.

132 Kalkanis, 2001. p. 5.

133 *Medizine: Benorylate*, 2001. p. 2.

134 Snow & Wackym, 2008. p. 277.

135 Haybach, 1999. p. 23.

136 Haybach, 1999. p. 20.

137 *Brotizolam*, 1997. p. 2.

138 Haybach, 1999. p. 19.

139 Shlafer, 2000. p. 9.

140 *Medications That Can Cause Tinnitus*, 2007. p. 1.

141 de la Cruz, 1999. p. 1.

142 Haybach, 1999. p. 20.

143 *Rimadyl Carprofen*, 2000. p. 2.

144 *Celiprolol*, 2001. p. 2.

145 Haybach, 1999. p. 22.

146 *Otology*, 1991. p. 16.

147 Snow & Wackym, 2008. p.277.

148 Carmen, 1999. p. 37.

149 Troost, 1998d. p. 5.

150 Snow & Wackym, 2008. p. 277.

151 Suss, 1993. p. 215.

152 *Guidelines for the Audiologic Management of Individuals Receiving Cochleotoxic Drug Therapy*. 1994. p. 3.

153 Fausti, 1993a. p. 661.
154 *Guidelines for the Audiologic Management of Individuals Receiving Cochleotoxic Drug Therapy*, 1994. p. 4.
155 Tange, 1985. p. 77.
156 Troost, 1998d. p. 2.
157 Haybach, 1999. p. 35.
158 Kalkanis, 2001. p. 6.
159 Kalkanis, 2001. p. 6.
160 *Audiological Aspects Of Ototoxicity*, 1996. p. 1.
161 Troost, 1998d. p. 2.
162 *Audiological Aspects Of Ototoxicity*, 1996. p. 2.
163 Kalkanis, 2001. p. 6.
164 *Audiological Aspects Of Ototoxicity*, 1996. p. 1.
165 Haybach, 1999. p. 44.
166 Kalkanis, 2001. p. 6.
167 Haybach, 1999. p. 44.
168 Fausti, 1993a. p. 661.
169 *Drug Prevents Chemotherapy-induced Hearing Loss, Study Finds*. 2004. pp. 1-2.
170 Priest, 2009. p. 2.
171 Rybacki, 1998. p. 200.
172 Roberts, 2001. p. 424.
173 Haybach, 1998. p. 7.
174 Snow & Wackym, 2008. p.277.
175 Kaufman, 1997. p. 6.
176 Kaufman, 1997. p. 6.
177 *Cosyntropin-Injectable*, 2009. p. 1.
178 Haybach, 1999. p. 20.
179 Estrada, 1997. p. 7.
180 Priuska, 1997. p. 5.
181 McIntyre, 1997. pp. 925-31.
182 *Dextromethorphan*, ~2000. p. 2.
183 Haybach, 1999. p. 20.
184 *Panimycin Injection*, 1998. pp. 2-3.
185 *Panimycin Injection*, 1998. p. 2.
186 Hain, 2001b. p. 1.
187 Troost, 1998d. p. 1.
188 Griffiths, 1999. p. 1.
189 *Dothiepin*, 2002, p. 2.
190 *Dothiepin* (tricyclic), 1994, p. 2.
191 Keeley, 2000. p.1.
192 Kalkanis, 2001. p. 4.
193 *Popular Medication Also Causes Hearing Loss*, 1991. p. 13.
194 Shlafer, 2000. p. 8.
195 Troost, 1998d. p. 3.
196 Haybach, 1999. p. 22.
197 Haybach, 1999. p. 35.
198 *Climara forte*, 2000. p. 4.
199 *Femtran*, 2000. p. 3.
200 *Climara forte*, 2000. pp. 2-4.
201 *Femtran*, 2000. p. 4.
202 *Synapause-E3*, 2003. p. 1.
203 Rickey, 2004. p. 1.

204 *Disorders of the Inner Ear*. 2000. p. 10.

205 Haybach, 1999. p. 19.

206 Haybach, 1999. p. 19.

207 Kalkanis, 2001. p. 5.

208 *Lederfen Tablets*, 1994. p. 1.

209 *Lederfen Tablets*, 1994. p. 1.

210 Haybach, 1999. p. 20.

211 *Disorders of the Inner Ear*. 2000. p. 10.

212 Haybach, 1999. p. 19.

213 Haybach, 1999. p. 19.

214 Troost, 1998d. p. 4.

215 Halmagyi, 1994. p. 1.

216 Halmagyi, 1995. p. 1.

217 Hain, 1999. p. 1.

218 Evenson, 2002. p. 1.

219 Shearer, 1991. pp. 74-75.

220 Troost, 1998a. p. 2.

221 Hain, 2001a. p. 3.

222 Troost, 1998a. p. 1.

223 Hain, 1999. p. 2.

224 Troost, 1998a. p. 2.

225 Haybach, 1999. p. 50.

226 Berner, 1996. p. 328.

227 Troost, 1998a. p. 1.

228 Hain, 2001a. p. 3.

229 Hain, 2001b, p. 3.

230 Hain, 2001a. p. 3.

231 Shea, 1994. pp. 317-324.

232 Troost, 1998c. p. 1.

233 Troost, 1998c. p. 1.

234 Hain, 2001b. p. 6.

235 *Homatropine hydrobromide*, 2000. p. 3.

236 Yorgason, 2010. p. 817.

237 Yorgason, 2010. pp. 814, 818.

238 *Consumer Warning: Medical Study Indicates Commonly Prescribed Pain Killer Abuse Can Cause Rapid, Profound Hearing Loss*, 1999. p. 1.

239 Jaeger, 2001. p. 5.

240 Jaeger, 2001. p. 4.

241 Jaeger, 2001. p. 4.

242 House, 2008. pp. 1-2.

243 Jaeger, 2001. p. 3.

244 *Top 200 Prescriptions*, 2001. p. 1.

245 *Boniva (Ibandronic Acid)—Adverse Event Reports—Other Serious Reactions—Arthralgia—Page 1*, 2009. pp. 2-6.

246 *Boniva (Ibandronic Acid)—Adverse Event Reports—Other Serious Reactions—Pain in Jaw*, 2009. pp. 1-5.

247 Curhan, 2010. p. 234.

248 Curhan, 2010. p. 235.

249 Kalkanis, 2001. p. 5.

250 Kanda, 1994. pp. 1134-5.

251 Kanda, 1994. pp. 1134-5.

252 Kanda, 1994. pp. 1134-5.

253 Kanda, 1994. pp. 1134-5.

254 Kanda, 1994. pp. 1134-5.

255 Kanda, 1994. pp. 1134-5.

256 Kafetzis, 1999. pp. 51, 54.

257 Kalkanis, 2001. p. 4.

258 Suter, 1991. p. 17.

259 *Lacidipine*, 1994. p. 1.

260 *Zanidip Product Information*, 2005. p. 8.

261 *Lercanidipine Hydrochloride*, 2004.

262 *Zanidip Product Information*, 2005. p. 8.

263 *Lidocaine Helps Relieve Ringing in the Ears*, 2000.

264 *Lotemax*, 2008. p. 5.

265 *Recent Questions and Answers about Lotemax*, 2007. p. 4.

266 Haybach, 1996. p. 2.

267 *Mannitol*, 2001. p. 2.

268 Haybach, 1999. p. 20.

269 Troost, 1998d. p. 2.

270 Haybach, 1999. p. 22.

271 *Hormone-replacement Therapy Causes Hearing Loss, Study Finds*, 2006. pp. 1-2.

272 Wingert, 2006. p. 2.

273 Wingert, 2006. pp. 2-3

274 *Lariam (Mefloquine) Info*, 2005. p. 1.

275 *Lariam (Mefloquine) Info*, 2005. p. 1.

276 Benjamin, 2004. p. 1.

277 Fusetti, 1999. p. 1.

278 *Hormone-replacement Therapy Causes Hearing Loss, Study Finds*, 2006. pp. 1-2.

279 Wingert, 2006. p. 2.

280 *Namenda Tablets*, 2003. pp. 15-17.

281 Suss, 1993. p. 216.

282 Kilpatrick, 2000. pp. 82-84.

283 Iqbal, S. M., et. al., 1999. p. 1.

284 Lawford, R & Sorrell T.C., 1994. p. 1.

285 *Sagamicin Injection 60*, 1998. pp. 2-3.

286 *Sagamicin Injection 60*, 1998. p. 1.

287 Haybach, 1999. p. 22.

288 Shlafer, 2000. p. 9.

289 *Statement of Principles concerning Tinnitus*, 1986. p. 3.

290 Troost, 1998d. p. 1.

291 *Use of CellCept (Mycophenolate mofetil) associated with increased pregnancy loss and congenital malformations*, 2007. p. 1.

292 Troost, 1998d. p. 3.

293 Kalkanis, 2001. p. 3.

294 Kalkanis, 2001. p. 3.

295 Haybach, 1999. p. 21.

296 Kalkanis, 2001. p. 4.

297 Haybach, 1999. p. 51.

298 *Procardia (Nifedipine) Capsules*, 2002. p. 1.

299 *Nivadil*, 2001. p. 2.

300 *Nitrazepam*, 2000. p. 2.

301 Fruchtengarten, 1998. p. 6.

302 *Hormone-replacement Therapy Causes Hearing Loss, Study Finds*, 2006. pp. 1-2.

303 Wingert, 2006. p. 2.

304 Mintz, 1979. pp. 1-2.

305 *Omeprazole (Prilosec) OPDA Post-marketing Safety Review*, 2000. pp. 24-25.

306 *Omeprazole (Prilosec) OPDA Post-marketing Safety Review*, 2000. p. 25.

307 Kalkanis, 2001. p. 5.

308 *Paromomycin-oral.* 2001. p. 1.

309 *"Amazing Grace"...Pentoxifylline-induced musical hallucinations*, 1993. p. 1.

310 *Phenylpropanolamine (PPA) Information Page*, 2001. p. 1.

311 *Piretanide (potassium depletion)*, 1994. p. 2.

312 Kalkanis, 2001. p. 5.

313 Snow & Wackym, 2008. p.277.

314 *Potassium gluconate*, 2009. pp. 1,3.

315 *Procain*, 2001. p. 1.

316 *Hormone-replacement Therapy Causes Hearing Loss, Study Finds*, 2006. pp. 1-2.

317 Wingert, 2006. p. 2.

318 Wingert, 2006. pp. 2-3

319 Roberts, 2001. p. 424.

320 Haybach, 1999. p. 23.

321 Estrada, 1997. p. 7.

322 Hain, 2001b. p. 5.

323 *Quinacrine hydrochloride*, 2001. p. 4.

324 Haybach, 1999. p. 18.

325 *Disorders of the Inner Ear.* 2000. p. 10.

326 Hain, 2001b. p. 5.

327 Troost, 1998d. p. 3.

328 Kalkanis, 2001. p. 7.

329 Haybach, 1999. p. 18.

330 Troost, 1998d. p. 3.

331 *Disorders of the Inner Ear*, 2000. p. 10.

332 Troost, 1998b. p. 2.

333 Haybach, 1999. p. 18.

334 Troost, 1998d. p. 3.

335 Haybach, 1999. p. 18.

336 Carmen, 1999. p. 37.

337 Haybach, 1999. p. 20.

338 Rybacki, 1998. p. 860.

339 *Side effects caused by Roxithromycin*, 2008.

340 *Roxithromycin Consumer Information*, 2008.

341 *InteliHealth*, 2001.

342 *Anipryl*, 1999. pp. 2-3.

343 FDA MedWatch - Meridia (Sibutramine), 2010. p. 1

344 *FDA Announces Revisions to Labels for Cialis, Levitra and Viagra*, 2007. p. 1.

345 *UAB Study Examines Hearing Loss, Viagra Use*, 2010. pp. 1-2.

346 Haybach, 1999. p. 20.

347 Haybach, 1999. p. 19.

348 Kalkanis, 2001. p. 3.

349 Hain, 2001b. p. 2.

350 *Inner Ear*, 2001. Section 7, Chapter 85.

351 Troost, 1998b. p. 2.

352 *Sumatriptan*, 2009, p. 19.

353 *Sumatriptan*, 2009, p. 20.

354 *Prograf*, 2002. p. 18.

355 *Prograf*, 2002. p. 18.

356 *FDA Announces Revisions to Labels for Cialis, Levitra and Viagra*, 2007. p. 1.

357 *UAB Study Examines Hearing Loss, Viagra Use*. 2010. pp. 1-2.

358 *Teicoplanin sodium*, 1997. p. 2.

359 *Teicoplanin (antibiotic)*, 1997. p. 2.

360 *Ketek*, 2004. pp. 13-14.

361 *Ketek*, 2004. p. 11.

362 *Clinical Trials of Tirapazamine Enter Final Phase*, 2001. p. 1.

363 Haybach, 1999. p. 21.

364 Haybach, 1999. p. 51.

365 Keeley, 2000. p. 1.

366 Roberts, 2001. p. 424.

367 Parikh, 2000. pp. 8-9.

368 *Trivedon-20 Tablets*, 2004. p. 2.

369 Asaju, 2001. p. 1.

370 Kalkanis, 2001. p. 4.

371 Shlafer, 2000. p. 8.

372 Snow & Wackym, 2008. p. 277.

373 *FDA Announces Revisions to Labels for Cialis, Levitra and Viagra*, 2007. p. 1.

374 *UAB Study Examines Hearing Loss, Viagra Use*, 2010. pp. 1-2.

375 *Inner Ear*, 2001. Section 7, Chapter 85.

376 *Zolpidem (Oral Route, Oromucosal Route)*, 2009. pp. 1-3.

377 *Product Information—Stilnox*, 2002. p. 4.

378 Ashton, 2002. *Introduction*. p. 1

379 Ashton, 2002. *Introduction*. p. 1

Table 14-1

Table 14-1

Ototoxic Drugs by Drug Class
(with their ototoxic side effects)

Drugs by Class	Ototoxic Side Effects (see page 659 for abbreviation key)
1 ANALGESIC DRUGS (PAINKILLERS)	
Acetaminophen	HL
Aminopyrine	D, HL, T
Antipyrine (see Benzocaine)	T
Ziconotide	A, D, N, T, V
1.1 NON-STEROIDAL ANTI-INFLAMMATORY DRUGS (NSAIDs)	
Azapropazone	D, T, V
Feprazone (Methrazone)	T
Nabumetone	D, HL, T, V
Phenylbutazone	D, HL, T, V
Proquazone	T
1.1.1 ACETIC ACIDS	
Aceclofenac	D, T, V
Acemetacin	D, HD, T, V
Alclofenac	OX, T
Amtolmetin	T
Diclofenac	D, EP, HL, T, V
Etodolac	D, EP, HL, MP, T, V
Indomethacin	A, D, HD, HL, T, V
Ketorolac	D, EP, HL, T, V
Proglumetacin	T
Sulindac	D, HL, T, V
Tolmetin	D, HL, T, V
Zomepirac	T

Table 14-1

1.1.4 Cox-2 inhibitors

Celecoxib	A, D, ED, EP, HL, L, OM, T, V
Etoricoxib	D, T, V
Parecoxib	D, T, V
Rofecoxib	C, D, EP, O, OM, T, V
Valdecoxib	D, ED, EP, OM, T, V

1.1.7 Fenamates

Floctafenine	D, T
Meclofenamate	D, T, V
Mefenamic acid	D, EP, HL, T, V

1.1.10 Oxicams

Isoxicam	T
Lornoxicam	D, T, V
Meloxicam	D, T, V
Piroxicam	D, HL, T, V
Tenoxicam	D, HL, T, V

1.1.13 Propionic acids

Benoxaprofen	T
Carprofen	A, T, VD
Dexketoprofen	D, T, V
Fenbufen	D, T, V
Fenoprofen	A, D, HL, T, V
Flurbiprofen	A, D, ED, EP, HL, T, V, VD
Ibuprofen	D, HL, N, T, V
Indoprofen	OX, T
Ketoprofen	D, HL, T, V
Naproxen	D, ED, HD, HL, OM, T, V
Oxaprozin	HL, T
Pirprofen	OX, T
Tiaprofenic acid	D, T, V

1.1.16 Salicylates

Acetylsalicylic acid (Aspirin)	D, EB, EP, HL, T, V
Benorilate (Benorylate)	D, OX, T, V
Bismuth subsalicylate	A, D, HL, T, V
Choline magnesium trisalicylate	D, HL, T
Diflunisal	D, HL, T, V
Magnesium salicylate	HL, T
Mesalamine	A, D, EB, ED, EP, HL, O, T, V
Methyl salicylate	D, HL, T
Olanzapine	A, D, EP, HL, N, OM, T, V
Olsalazine	D, T, V
Salicylic acid	D, HD, T
Salsalate	HL, T, V
Sodium salicylate	D, HL, OX, T
Sodium thiosalicylate	OX, T

1.4 NARCOTIC (OPIOID) DRUGS

    1.4.1 OPIATE AGONIST DRUGS

Buprenorphine	A, D, ED, EP, HL, OM, T, V
Codeine	D, L, N, T, V, VD
Dezocine	D, EB, T, V
Fentanyl	A, D, ED, EP, EQ, HL, T, V
Hydrocodone	D, HL, T
Hydromorphone	A, D, HY, N, T, V, VD
Meperidine	A, D
Morphine	A, D, N, V
Oxycodone	A, D, HL, T, V
Propoxyphene	D, T
Tramadol	A, AH, D, EP, HL, L, O, OM, T, V

    1.4.4 OPIATE AGONIST/ANTAGONIST DRUGS

Butorphanol	A, D, ED, EP, HL, HY, T, V
Nalbuphine	D, V
Pentazocine	D, N, T, V

1.7 NARCOTIC ANTAGONIST DRUGS

Methylnaltrexone	D, T
Naltrexone	D, EB, EP, T

1.10 CENTRALLY-ACTING SYNTHETIC ANALGESICS

Tapentadol	A, D

4 ANESTHETICS

4.1 AMIDES

Articaine	D, EP, T
Bupivacaine	D, HY, T
Etidocaine	D, T
Lidocaine	D, HY, T
Mepivacaine	D, HY, T
Prilocaine	D, HY, T
Procaine	D, T
Ropivacaine	D, HD, T, V

4.4 ESTERS

Benzocaine	BS
Chloroprocaine	D, T
Tetracaine	D, N, T

4.8 GENERAL ANESTHETICS

Propofol	D, EP, N, T

Table 14-1

Table 14-1

4.10 LOCAL ANESTHETICS

Dyclonine	D, T
Levobupivacaine	D, T

7 ANTIBIOTIC DRUGS (ANTI-INFECTIVES)

7.1 ANTHELMINTIC DRUGS

Albendazole	D, V
Hycanthone	D, V
Ivermectin	A, D, V
Mebendazole	D, T
Praziquantel	D, V
Pyrantel	D, OX
Quinacrine (Mepacrine)	D, HL
Thiabendazole	D, T, V

7.4 ANTI-BACTERIAL DRUGS

Benzalkonium	OX
Benzethonium	OX
Cetrimide (Centrimide)	OX
Chlorhexidine	HL
Gramicidin	OX
Mupirocin	D, EP
Novobiocin	HL
Spectinomycin	D, OX
Sultamicillin	OX
Thimerosal	A, HL

7.4.1 AMINOGLYCOSIDES

Amikacin	A, D, FF, HL, LB, N, OX, T, V
Astromicin	FF, HL, T, V, VD
Capreomycin	D, HL, T, V
Dibekacin	HL, OX, T, V
Dihydrostreptomycin (see Streptomycin)	HL, VD
Framycetin	OX
Gentamicin	A, D, HL, LB, OS, OX, T, V
Hygromycin B	HL
Isepamicin	OX, T
Kanamycin	D, HL, LB, N, OX, T, V
Micronomicin	EP, FF, HL, T, V, VD
Neomycin (Fradiomycin)	BS, HL, OX, T, VD
Netilmicin	D, HL, N, OX, T, V, VD
Paromomycin (Aminosidine)	D, HL, T, V
Ribostamycin	OX
Sisomicin	OX
Streptomycin	A, AD, FF, HL, N, OX, T, V, VD

Tobramycin	A, AD, CL, D, HL, N, OM, OX, T, V, VD
Viomycin	HL, VD

7.4.4 BACITRACINS

Bacitracin	OX

7.4.8 CEPHALOSPORINS

Cefaclor	D, EP, OM, V
Cefadroxil	D, V
Cefpodoxime	D, T, V
Cefprozil	D, T, VD
Ceftriaxone	A, D, T
Cefuroxime	D, HL
Cephalexin	D, HL, T, V

7.4.12 BETA-LACTAMS

7.4.12.1 CARBAPENEMS

Doripenem	D, V
Ertapenem	D, O, V
Imipenem—Cilastatin	A, D, HL, T, V

7.4.12.4 MONOBACTAMS

Aztreonam	D, HL, T, V

7.4.16 CHLORAMPHENICOLS

Chloramphenicol	HL, OX, T

7.4.20 GLYCOPEPTIDES

Teicoplanin	D, HL, OX, T, VD
Vancomycin	D, HL, OX, T, V

7.4.24 LINCOMYCINS

Clindamycin	D, T, V
Lincomycin	D, OX, T, V

7.4.28 LIPOPEPTIDES

Daptomycin	D, HL, T, V

7.4.32 MACROLIDE ANTIBIOTICS

Azithromycin	D, HL, T, V
Clarithromycin	D, ED, HD, HL, T, V
Dirithromycin	D, HL, T, V
Erythromycin	A, D, HL, HY, T, V
Roxithromycin	D, T, V

7.4.32.1 KETOLIDE ANTIBIOTICS

Telithromycin	D, V

Table 14-1

Table 14-1

7.4.36 OXAZOLINIDONES
        Linezolid   A, D, T, V

7.4.40 PENICILLINS
        Ampicillin   OX
        Bacampicillin   D, V
        Penicillin   AH, D, T
        Piperacillin—Tazobactam   D, EP, HL, T, V

7.4.44 POLYPEPTIDES
        Colistin (Colistimethate,
            Polymyxin E)   A, D, N, OX, V
        Polymyxin B   A, D, N, OX

7.4.48 QUINOLONES
        Cinoxacin   D, T
        Ciprofloxacin   A, D, EP, HD, HL, N, OE, T, V
        Enoxacin   A, D, N, T, V
        Gatifloxacin   A, D, EP, T, V
        Grepafloxacin   D, HL, T, V
        Levofloxacin   A, AH, D, ED, EP, HD, HL,
                        HY, T, V
        Lomefloxacin   A, D, EP, N, T, V
        Moxifloxacin   A, D, EP, HL, HY, OM, T, V, VD
        Nalidixic acid   D, HD, V
        Norfloxacin   A, D, HD, HL, N, T, V
        Ofloxacin   A, D, EP, HD, HL, N, OE,
                        OH, OM, T, V, VD
        Sparfloxacin   A, D, ED, EP, N, OM, T, V
        Trovafloxacin (Alatrofloxacin)   A, D, EP, HL, HY, T, V

7.4.52 RIFAMYCINS
        Rifampin   A, D, EQ, HL, T, V
        Rifaximin   D, EP, T

7.4.56 SULFONAMIDES
        Sulfadiazine   A, D, T, V
        Sulfamethazine   V
        Sulfamethizole   D, OX, T
        Sulfamethoxazole   A, D, T, V
        Sulfanilamide   A, D
        Sulfasalazine   A, D, HL, T, V
        Sulfisoxazole   A, D, HL, T, V

7.4.60 TETRACYCLINES
        Chlortetracycline   HL
        Demeclocycline
            (Demethylchlortetracycline)   D, T

Doxycycline	HL, T
Methacycline (Metacycline)	OX
Minocycline	A, D, HL, T, V
Tetracycline	A, D, HL, T, V
Tigecycline	D, V

7.7 ANTI-MYCOBACTERIALS

7.7.1 ANTI-TUBERCULOSIS DRUGS

Cycloserine	D, V
Ethionamide	D, OX
Isoniazid (INH)	A, D, HL, T, V

7.10 ANTI-FUNGAL ANTIBIOTICS

Amphotericin B	D, ED, HL, T, V
Fluconazole	D, V
Flucytosine	A, HL, V
Griseofulvin	A, D, HL, V
Itraconazole	D, HL, T, V
Ketoconazole	D, T
Posaconazole	A, D, EP, HL, T, V, VD
Voriconazole	A, D, EP, HL, N, OE, T, V

7.14 ANTI-PROTOZOALS

Atovaquone/Proguanil	D, T
Eflornithine	D, OX, V
Nitazoxanide	D, EP
Pentamidine	A, D, HL, T, V
Sodium stibogluconate	V
Suramin	OX

7.14.1 AMEBICIDES

Iodoquinol	A, V
Metronidazole	A, D, HL, N, T, V
Tinidazole	A, D, V

7.14.4 ANTI-LEPROSY DRUGS

Dapsone	D, T, V

7.14.8 ANTI-MALARIAL DRUGS

Artemether/Lumefantrine	A, D, N, T, V
Chloroquine	D, HL, OX, T, V
Hydroxychloroquine	A, D, HL, N, T, V
Mefloquine	A, AH, D, EP, HL, HY, LB, T, V, VD
Quinine	A, D, HD, HL, T, V
Sulfadoxine—Pyrimethamine	A, D, T, V

7.17 ANTI-VIRAL DRUGS

Amantadine	A, D
Foscarnet	A, D, EP, HL, N, O, T, V
Hexadimethrine	OX
Ribavirin	D, T
Rimantadine	A, D, T
Vidarabine	A, D

7.17.1 ANTI-RETROVIRALS

7.17.1.1 ANTI-RETROVIRAL PROTEASE INHIBITORS

Cidofovir	A, D, ED, EP, HL, HY, OE, OM, T, V
Darunavir	V
Ganciclovir	A, D, ED, EP, HL, T, V
Indinavir	D, V
Lopinavir	A, D, OM, T
Oseltamivir	D, ED, V
Ritonavir	A, C, D, EP, HL, HY, OM, T, V, VD
Saquinavir	A, D, EP, HL, MP, O, T
Valacyclovir (Acyclovir)	A, AH, D
Valganciclovir	A, D, EP, HL, T

7.17.1.4 ANTI-RETROVIRAL REVERSE TRANSCRIPTASE INHIBITORS

Didanosine	A, D, ED, EP, HL, OE, OM, T
Efavirenz	A, D, EQ, T, V
Etravirine	V
Lamivudine	D, ED, O
Nevirapine	D, V
Stavudine	D, V
Zalcitabine	A, D, EB, EP, EQ, HL, OM, T, V
Zidovudine	A, D, HL, T, V

7.17.1.8 ANTI-RETROVIRAL CC CHEMOKINE RECEPTOR 5 (CCR5) ANTAGONISTS

Maraviroc	AH, D, HL, OM

7.17.1.12 ANTI-RETROVIRAL HIV FUSION INHIBITORS

Enfuvirtide	O, V

7.17.1.16 ANTI-RETROVIRAL INTEGRASE INHIBITORS

Raltegravir	D, L, V

7.17.4 INTERFERONS

Interferon alfa-2a	A, D, EP, HD, HL, T, V
Interferon alfa-2b	A, D, EP, HD, HL, HY, L, N, OM, T, V

Interferon alfacon-1	D, EP, O, T
Interferon alfa-n3	D, T
Interferon beta-1a	A, D, EP, HL, HY, L, ME, N, OE, OM, T, V, VD
Interferon beta-1b	A, D, ED, EP, HL, N, OE, OM, T
Interferon gamma-1b	A, D
Peginterferon alfa-2a	D, EP, HL, OE, T, V
Peginterferon alfa-2b	D, HL, OM, T, V

7.17.8 MONOCLONAL ANTIBODIES

Adalimumab	D, EP, HL, T, V
Alemtuzumab	A, D, HL, OM, V
Bevacizumab	A, D, ED, HL, OM, V
Canakinumab	V
Certolizumab	D, V
Cetuximab	A, D, ED, EP, HL, OE, OM, T, V
Eculizumab	D, T, V
Infliximab	A, C, D, EP, O, OE, OM, V
Muromonab-CD3	AH, D, EB, HL, OM, T, V
Natalizumab	D, V
Omalizumab	D, EP
Palivizumab	ED, OM
Panitumumab	D, V
Ranibizumab	D, EP, EQ, V
Rituximab	D, EP, HL, OE, T, V
Tositumomab	A, D, ED, EP, T, VD
Trastuzumab	A, D, HL, V

7.17.12 NEURAMINIDASE INHIBITORS

Zanamivir	D, O

7.20 URINARY ANTI-INFECTIVES

Fosfomycin	D, ED
Methenamine (Hexamine)	D, OX, T
Nitrofurantoin	A, D, N, V
Trimethoprim	A, D, T, V

10 ANTIHISTAMINES

Dextromethorphan	A, AH, D, N
Levocabastine	D, HL, OE
Methapyrilene	D, N, T
Thonzylamine	A, T, V

Table 14-1

10.1 H₁ RECEPTOR ANTAGONISTS

Azatadine	A, D, L, T, V
Azelastine	D, V
Bromodiphenhydramine	OX, T
Bromopheniramine	D, T
Chlorpheniramine	A, D, L, T, V
Chlorphenoxamine	T
Clemastine	D, T, V
Cyproheptadine	D, L, T, V
Desloratadine	D, OM
Diphenhydramine	A, D, L, T, V
Diphenylhydrazine	OX
Doxylamine	D, T, V
Emedastine	T
Fexofenadine	A, D, EP, OM, T
Loratadine	D, EP, O, T, V
Methdilazine	D, T
Orphenadrine	A, D, N, T, V
Pheniramine	D, T
Promethazine	A, D, T
Pyrilamine	N, T, V
Trimeprazine	D, T
Tripelennamine	A, D, T, V

10.4 H₂ RECEPTOR ANTAGONISTS

Famotidine	D, EP, ET, T, V
Ranitidine	D, V

10.8 PIPERAZINES

Cinnarizine	T
Cyclizine	AH, T, V
Delavirdine	A, D, EP, N, OM, T, V
Flunarizine	D, V
Meclizine	AH, T, V
Piperazine	A, D, V

10.8.1 PIPERAZINE DERIVATIVES

Cetirizine	A, D, EP, HL, OX, T, V
Hydroxyzine	A, D
Levocetirizine	OM

14 ANTI-NEOPLASTICS (ANTI-CANCER DRUGS)

Amonafide (Nafidimide)	D, T
Arsenic trioxide	D, EP, T
Bleomycin	HL, OX, T
Bortezomib	A, D, HL, V
Buserelin	D, ED, EP, HD, T, V
Cytarabine	A, D, HL

Table 14-1

Dactinomycin	OX
Etoposide	V
Gallium nitrate	HL, T
Levamisole	A, D, N, V
Lonidamine	OX
Misonidazole	AD, T
Mitomycin	A, N, V
Nelarabine	A, D, N, VD
Paclitaxel	A, HL, T
Sorafenib	T
Tirapazamine	HL, T

14.1 ALKYLATING DRUGS

Altretamine	A, D, V
Busulfan	D, ED
Carboplatin	D, HL, OX, T
Carmustine (BCNU)	A, D, EQ
Chlorambucil	A
Cisplatin (CDDP)	A, EP, HL, OX, T, V, VD
Cyclophosphamide	D, OX
Ifosfamide	AH, D
Lomustine (CCNU)	A
Mechlorethamine (Nitrogen mustard)	HL, T, V
Oxaliplatin	A, D, HL, OX, V
Temozolomide	A, D, EP, EQ, HL, HY, OM, T, V

14.4 ANTHRACYCLINES

Daunorubicin	
(Liposomal daunorubicin)	A, D, EP, HL, T
Doxorubicin	
(Liposomal doxorubicin)	A, D, N, OM, T, V

14.8 ANTI-METABOLITE DRUGS

Capecitabine	A, D, EB, EP, EQ, HL, OM, V
Dichloromethotrexate	AD, HL, VD
Floxuridine	A, N, V
Fludarabine	AH, HL
Fluorouracil	A, N
Methotrexate	A, D, HL, T
Pentostatin	A, D, EP, HL, L, OM, T, V
Procarbazine	A, D, HD, HL, N

14.12 CYTOKINES

Aldesleukin	A, D

14.16 MITOTIC INHIBITORS

Docetaxel	D, HL

Table 14-1

14.20 NATURAL ANTI-NEOPLASTICS

Irinotecan	D, V
Vinblastine	AD, D, EQ, HL, N, T, V, VD
Vincristine	A, AD, D, EQ, HL, N, V, VD
Vinorelbine	A, AD, D, HL, V, VD

14.24 NON-STEROIDAL AROMATASE INHIBITORS

Aminoglutethimide	A, D, V
Letrozole	D, V

14.28 RETINOIDS

Bexarotene	A, D, EP, OE

14.32 STEROID ANTI-NEOPLASTICS

Cyproterone	A, D, ED

14.36 TUMOR NECROSIS FACTOR MODIFIERS

Abatacept	D, ED, HL, MP, OE, OM, T, V
Etanercept	D, ED, OM, T, V
Lenalidomide	D, V
Thalidomide	A, D, HL, N, T, V

14.40 TYROSINE KINASE INHIBITORS

Dasatinib	D, T, V
Imatinib	D, HL, T, V
Nilotinib	D, EP, HL, V

17 AUTONOMIC NERVOUS SYSTEM DRUGS

17.1 ANTI-CHOLINERGIC DRUGS

Atropine	A, D, OX
Benztropine	A, D
Cyclopentolate	A
Dimenhydrinate	A, D, T, V
Flavoxate	D, V
Homatropine	D, OX, T
Hyoscyamine	A, D
Pinaverium	V
Scopolamine	D, EQ

17.1.1 MUSCARINIC RECEPTOR ANTAGONISTS

Oxybutynin	D, T
Tolterodine	D, V
Trospium	EP

17.4 ERGOT ALKALOIDS

Dihydroergotamine	A, D, EP, T, V
Ergonovine (Ergometrine)	D, T, V

Ergotamine	D, V
Methylergonovine	D, T
Methysergide	A, D, V
Pergolide	A, D, EP, HL, OM, T, V

17.8 INTESTINAL MOTILITY STIMULANTS

Trimebutine	D, HL

17.8.1 SEROTONIN 5-HT$_3$ RECEPTOR ANTAGONISTS

Palonosetron	D, T

17.8.4 SEROTONIN 5-HT$_4$ RECEPTOR PARTIAL AGONISTS

Tegaserod	D, OM, V

17.12 PARASYMPATHOMIMETIC DRUGS

17.12.1 CHOLINERGIC AGONIST DRUGS

Cevimeline	A, EP, HL, OM, T, V
Guanidine	A
Nicotine	D, ED, EP, HD, OM, T, V
Pilocarpine	D, ED, EP, HL, T

17.12.4 CHOLINESTERASE INHIBITORS

Galantamine	A, D, T, V
Pyridostigmine	A, N, V
Rivastigmine	A, D, ED, EP, HL, ME, N, OM, T, V, VD

17.16 SYMPATHOMIMETIC DRUGS

Amezinium	T
Mephentermine	OX, T
Phentermine	D, T
Phenylephrine	D
Phenylpropanolamine	D, L, T, V
Pseudoephedrine	A, D, T

20 CARDIOVASCULAR DRUGS

20.1 ANTI-ANGINALS

Ranolazine	D, T, V
Trimetazadine	D, V

20.4 ANTI-ARRHYTHMICS (HEART RHYTHM REGULATORS)

Adenosine	D, EP
Amiodarone	A, D, N, T, V
Bretylium	D, V
Disopyramide	D, V
Flecainide	A, D, HL, N, T, V
Mexiletine	A, D, N, T

Table 14-1

20.4 ANTI-ARRHYTHMICS (HEART RHYTHM REGULATORS) (CONT'D.)

Moricizine	A, D, N, T, V
Procainamide	D, T
Propafenone	A, D, HL, LB, T, V
Quinidine	A, D, HD, HL, T, V
Tocainide	A, D, EP, HL, N, T, V

20.4.1 CARDIAC GLYCOSIDES

Digoxin	D, OX, V

20.8 ANTI-HYPERTENSIVE DRUGS

Rescinnamine	D, HL

20.8.1 ALPHA ADRENERGIC BLOCKING DRUGS

Alfuzosin	D, V
Bunazosin	OX, T
Doxazosin	A, AH, D, EP, HL, HY, OM, T, V
Prazosin	D, T, V
Tamsulosin	D, V
Terazosin	D, T, V
Thymoxamine	OX, T
Trimazosin	T

20.8.4 ANGIOTENSIN-2-RECEPTOR ANTAGONISTS

Candesartan	D, O, T, V
Eprosartan	A, D, OE, OM, T, V
Irbesartan	D, ED, EP, HD, O, T, V
Losartan	A, D, T, V
Olmesartan	D, V
Telmisartan	D, EP, OM, T, V
Valsartan	D, EP, T, V

20.8.8 ANGIOTENSIN-CONVERTING ENZYME (ACE) INHIBITORS

Benazepril	D, T, V
Captopril	A, D, T
Cilazapril	A, D, EB, T, V
Enalapril (Enalaprilat)	A, D, HL, T, V
Fosinopril	D, EP, T, V
Imidapril	D, T
Lisinopril	A, D, EP, T, V
Moexipril	A, D, EP, HL, OM, T, V
Perindopril	D, EP, O, OM, T, V
Quinapril	A, D, T, V
Ramipril	D, EQ, FF, HL, T, V
Trandolapril	D, LB, T, V

Table 14-1

20.8.12 BETA-ADRENERGIC-BLOCKING DRUGS (BETA-BLOCKERS)

Acebutolol	D, T, V
Atenolol	A, D, HL, T, V
Betaxolol	A, D, EP, HL, L, T, V
Bisoprolol	D, EP, HL, T, V
Carteolol	D, T
Carvedilol	D, HL, T, V
Celiprolol	D, T
Dilevalol	T
Labetalol	D, V
Levobetaxolol	D, EP, OM, T, V
Levobunolol	A, D
Metoprolol	D, EP, FF, HL, T, V
Nadolol	D, T
Nebivolol	D, V
Oxprenolol	D, T, V
Pindolol	D, T, V, VD
Propranolol	A, AH, D, HL, T, V
Sotalol	D, V
Timolol	D, EP, T, V, VD

20.8.16 CALCIUM-CHANNEL-BLOCKING DRUGS (CALCIUM BLOCKERS)

Amlodipine	A, D, EP, T, V
Bepridil	D, T, V
Diltiazem	A, D, EP, OM, T, V
Felodipine	D, V
Isradipine	D, OX
Lacidipine	D, OX
Nicardipine	A, D, ED, T, V
Nifedipine	A, D, HL, LB, T, V
Nilvadipine	D, OX, T
Nimodipine	D, OX, T
Nisoldipine	A, D, EP, OM, T, V
Nitrendipine	OX, T
Verapamil	D, EQ, N, T, V

20.8.16.1 DIHYDROPYRIDINE CALCIUM-CHANNEL BLOCKERS

Lercanidipine	D, LB, V

20.8.20 CENTRALLY ACTING ANTIADRENERGIC DRUGS

Clonidine	AH, D, T, V
Guanabenz	A, D, T
Guanfacine	D, T, V
Methyldopa	D, V

20.8.24 ENDOTHELIN RECEPTOR ANTAGONISTS

Bosentan	T, O, V
Sitaxsentan	A, D, EB, EP, HL, OM, T, V

Table 14-1

20.8.28 Phosphodiesterase type 5 (PDE5) inhibitors

Sildenafil	A, D, ED, EP, HL, T, V
Tadalafil	D, HL, T, V
Vardenafil	D, HL, T, V

20.8.32 Rauwolfia alkaloids

Deserpidine	D, OX
Reserpine	D, HL, V

20.8.36 Renin inhibitors

Aliskiren	V

20.8.40 Vasodilators

Diazoxide	D, HL, T
Minoxidil	D, OE, V
Papaverine	D, V

20.8.40.1 Coronary vasodilators

Isosorbide	D, EP, PE, T, V
Nitroglycerin	D, V

20.12 Anti-lipemics

Dextrothyroxine	D, T
Omega-3-acid ethyl esters	D, V
Probucol	D, T

20.12.1 Bile acid sequestrants

Cholestyramine	D, T, V
Colestipol	D, V

20.12.4 Fibrates

Bezafibrate	D, V
Ciprofibrate	D, V
Fenofibrate	D, EP, OM, T, V
Gemfibrozil	D, V

20.12.8 HMG-CoA reductase inhibitors

Atorvastatin	D, HL, T
Cerivastatin	D, V
Fluvastatin	A, D, V
Lovastatin	D, V
Pravastatin	D, HL, T, V
Rosuvastatin	D, T, V
Simvastatin	D, V

23 Dermatological drugs

23.1 Anti-psoriasis drugs

Etretinate	D, EP, HL, OE, OM

23.4 VITAMIN A ANALOGS

Acitretin	A, C, D, EP, HL, OE, OM, T
Isotretinoin	A, D, HL, T
Tretinoin	A, D, EP, FF, HL, T

26 DIAGNOSTIC DRUGS

26.1 MRI CONTRAST DRUGS

Gadodiamide	A, D, T
Gadopentetate	D, EP, HD, N, T
Gadoteridol	D, T
Gadoversetamide	D, EP, HY, T, V

26.4 RADIOPAQUE DRUGS

Iodixanol	D, EP, HL, T, V
Iohexol	D, HL, N, T, V
Iopromide	D, HL, V
Iotrolan	D, EP, N, T
Ioversol	N, T, V

26.8 ULTRASOUND CONTRAST AGENTS

Perflutren	D, HL, T, V

30 ELECTROLYTIC & WATER BALANCE AGENTS

30.5 DIURETICS

30.5.1 DIURETICS--CARBONIC ANHYDRASE INHIBITORS

Acetazolamide	A, D, HD, HL, T
Dichlorphenamide	A, D, T
Methazolamide	A, D, HD, T, V

30.5.4 DIURETICS—LOOP

Azosemide	OX
Bumetanide	D, EP, HL, T, V
Ethacrynic acid	FF, HL, T, V
Furosemide (Frusemide)	A, D, FF, HL, T, V
Indacrinone	OX
Ozolinone	OX
Piretanide	D, OX
Torsemide (Torasemide)	D, HL, T, V

30.5.8 DIURETICS—POTASSIUM-SPARING

Amiloride	D, T, V
Spironolactone	A, D
Triamterene	D, V

Table 14-1

Table 14-1

30.5.12 DIURETICS—THIAZIDE-RELATED

Bendroflumethiazide	D, HL, T, V
Chlorothiazide	D, V
Chlorthalidone	D, HL, T, V
Hydrochlorothiazide	D, T, V
Hydroflumethiazide	D, V
Indapamide	A, D, ED, EP, O, T, V
Methyclothiazide	D, T, V
Metolazone	D, T, V
Polythiazide	D, V
Quinethazone	V
Trichlormethiazide	D, V

30.10 IRRIGATING SOLUTIONS

30.10.1 HEXITOL IRRIGANTS

Mannitol	D, OX, V
Sorbitol	V

32 ENZYMES & ENZYME INHIBITORS

32.1 ENZYMES

Agalsidase alfa	D, EP, HL, T, V
Agalsidase beta	A, D, HL, T, V
Alglucosidase alfa	D, EP, HL, OH, OM
Galsulfase	EP, OM
Idursulfase	D, ED, V

32.4 ENZYME INHIBITORS

Miglustat	D, V
Nitisinone	O

34 GASTROINTESTINAL DRUGS

34.1 ANTI-EMETICS

Diphenidol	AH, D
Trimethobenzamide	D, V

34.1.1 P/NEUROKININ-1 RECEPTOR ANTAGONISTS

Aprepitant (Fosaprepitant)	D, T

34.1.4 SEROTONIN-RECEPTOR ANTAGONISTS

Alosetron	ED, O
Dolasetron	A, D, T, V
Dronabinol	A, D, EQ, T, V
Granisetron	D, V
Ondansetron	A, D

34.4 ANTIFLATULENTS
   Simethicone   EP

34.8 ANTI-ULCER DRUGS

   34.8.1 GASTRIC MUCOSAL DRUGS
      Misoprostol   D, EP, HL, T, V
      Sucralfate   D, V

   34.8.4 PROTON PUMP INHIBITORS
      Dexlansoprazole   D, EP, T, V
      Esomeprazole   A, D, EP, OM, T, V
      Lansoprazole   D, ED, HL, OM, T, V
      Omeprazole   D, EP, HL, OM, OX, T, V
      Pantoprazole   A, D, EP, HL, OE, T, V
      Rabeprazole   D, ED, EP, HL, OE, OM, T,
                                              V, VD

   34.12 CHLORIDE CHANNEL ACTIVATORS
      Lubiprostone   D, V

   34.16 CHOLELITHOLYTIC AGENTS
      Ursodiol   D, HL, OM, V

   34.20 LIPASE INHIBITORS
      Orlistat   D, O

   34.24 PROKINETIC DRUGS
      Cisapride   D, V
      Metoclopramide   A, D, V

36 HEMATOLOGICAL DRUGS

   36.1 ANTI-CLOTTING DRUGS
      Pentosan   D, N, T
      Ticlopidine   D, T

   36.4 ANTI-FIBRINOLYTIC DRUGS (BLOOD CLOTTING DRUGS)
      Aminocaproic acid   D, HL, T
      Antihemophilic factor   D, OM

   36.8 ANTI-THROMBOTIC DRUGS
      Fondaparinux   D, V

   36.12 BLOOD-FLOW DRUGS
      Pentoxifylline   AH, D, EP

   36.16 COAGULATION DRUGS
      Anistreplase   D, V

Table 14-1

36.20 HEMATOPOIETIC AGENTS
Epoetin alfa	D, EP, O, OM, V
Romiplostim	D, EP, O, OH, T

36.24 PLATELET INHIBITOR DRUGS
Anagrelide	D, ED, T
Cilostazol	D, EP, T, V
Clopidogrel	D, V
Dipyridamole	A, D, EP, T, V

40 HORMONES & HORMONE MODIFIERS

40.1 ADRENAL DRUGS
Mitotane	A, D, HL, V

40.1.1 ADRENOCORTICOTROPHIC HORMONES (ACTH)
Corticotropin	D, T, V
Cosyntropin	D, T, V

40.1.2 CORTICOSTEROIDS
Loteprednol	ED, HD, T

40.1.4 GLUCOCORTICOIDS
Beclomethasone	BS, D, EP, T
Betamethasone	BS, D, V
Budesonide	D, EP, O, OE, OM, V
Ciclesonide	EP
Cortisone	V
Dexamethasone	A, D, HL, N, V
Flunisolide	D, EP, O, V
Fluticasone	D, EP, OM
Hydrocortisone	V
Methylprednisolone	V
Mometasone	EP, OM
Prednisolone	T, V
Prednisone	HL, HY, T, V
Triamcinolone	OM, V

40.1.8 MINERALOCORTICOIDS
Fludrocortisone	V

40.4 ANDROGENS (MALE SEX HORMONES)
Danazol	D, V
Testosterone	D, V

40.8 ANTI-DIABETIC DRUGS (HYPOGLYCEMIC DRUGS)

40.8.1 BIGUANIDE ANTI-DIABETIC DRUGS
Metformin	D, EP

Table 14-1

40.8.4 INSULINS

Insulin aspart	D, V
Insulin detemir	D, ED, EP, VD
Insulin, human	ED, EP, OM

40.8.12 SULFONYLUREAS

Gliclazide	D, HL, OM, T
Glipizide	A, D, V
Glisoxepide	T
Glyburide (Glibenclamide)	D, T
Tolazamide	D, V
Tolbutamide	D, T, V

40.12 CONTRACEPTIVES

Ethinyl estradiol	AD, D, EB, ED, EP, ET, HD, L, OE, OM, T, V
Etonogestrel	D, OM
Norethindrone	AD, D, ED

40.16 ESTROGEN AGONIST—ANTAGONISTS

Clomiphene	D, HL, T, V
Raloxifene	V

40.16.1 ESTROGEN ANTAGONISTS

Fulvestrant	D, V
Tamoxifen	A, D

40.20 ESTROGENS

Estradiol	D, EP, HL, O, OM, T, V
Estradiol-17 beta	D, ED, EP
Estriol	HL

40.24 GONADOTROPINS

Goserelin	D, HY, V
Leuprolide	D, EP, HD, T, V
Menotropins	D, EP, V

40.28 GROWTH FACTOR DRUGS

Mecasermin	D, EP, HL, OM

40.32 PROGESTINS

Levonorgestrel	D, O, V
Medroxyprogesterone	A, D, HL, OX, T, V
Megestrol	D, HL
Norelgestromin	D, ED, EP, HL, OT, T, V, VD
Progesterone	A, D, EP, HL, T, V

Table 14-1

40.36 PROSGLANDINS

       Dinoprostone   D, HL

   40.36.1 PROSTAGLANDIN ANALOGS

       Carboprost   D, T, V

       Travoprost   HL, EP, T, V

40.40 SELECTIVE ESTROGEN RECEPTOR MODIFIERS

       Toremifene   A, D, V

40.42 THYROID DRUGS

   40.42.1 ANTI-THYROID DRUGS

       Methimazole   D, V

       Propylthiouracil   D, HL, V

   40.42.4 PARATHYROID DRUGS

       Calcitonin   D, EP, FF, HL, T, V

       Teriparatide   D, V

40.44 PITUITARY HORMONES

       Histrelin   D, EP, HL

       Nafarelin   D, EP, V

       Somatropin   D, ED, EP, HL, N, O, OM, OR, T, V

       Vasopressin   V

40.48 SOMATOSTATIC DRUGS

       Octreotide   A, D, ED, EP, HL, O, OM, OR, T, V

43 IMMUNOSUPPRESSANT DRUGS

       Cyclosporine   A, D, ED, HL, T, V, VD

       Gusperimus   T

       Mycophenolate   D, ED, EP, HL, T, V

       Pimecrolimus   EP, O, OM

       Sirolimus   D, EP, HL, OM, T

       Tacrolimus   A, D, ED, EP, HL, N, OE, OM, T, V

46 MISCELLANEOUS DRUGS

       Acamprosate   D, HL, T, V

       Cysteamine   A, D, HL

       Gelatin   HL

       Lanthanum   D, V

       Sodium phenylacetate   A

       Sodium phenylbutyrate   HL

Table 14-1

46.1 ANTI-RHEUMATIC DRUGS
Auranofin   OX, T

46.10 XANTHINE OXIDASE INHIBITORS
Allopurinol   A, D, T, V

Febuxostat   A, D, HL, T, V

50 MUSCULOSKELETAL DRUGS
Leflunomide   D, V

50.1 BONE RESORPTION INHIBITORS

50.1.1 BISPHOSPHONATES
Alendronate   D, T, V

Ibandronate   A, D, ED, T, V

Risedronate   D, EP, HL, OM, T, V

Tiludronate   D, EP, T, V

Zoledronic acid   D, V

53 NEUROLOGICAL/NERVOUS SYSTEM DRUGS

53.1 ANTI-CATAPLECTIC DRUGS
Sodium oxybate   A, AH, D, EP, EQ, OE, T, V

53.4 ANTI-ALZHEIMER'S DRUGS

53.4.1 CHOLINESTERASE INHIBITORS
Donepezil   A, D, EP, HL, N, OE, OM, T, V

Tacrine   A, D, EP, HL, L, OM, T, V

53.4.4 NMDA RECEPTOR ANTAGONISTS
Memantine   A, AH, D, ED, EP, HL, OM, T, V

53.8 ANTI-AMYOTROPHIC LATERAL SCLEROSIS (ALS) DRUGS
Riluzole   A, D, EP, HL, HY, V, VD

53.12 ANTI-CONVULSANT DRUGS
Carbamazepine   A, AH, D, EP, HL, HY, N, T, V

Divalproex   A, D, ED, EP, HL, N, OM, T, V

Ethosuximide   A, D

Ethotoin   A, D, N

Felbamate   A, D, HL, N, OM

Fosphenytoin   A, D, EP, HL, HY, N, T, V

Gabapentin   A, D, EP, ET, FF, HL, HY, L, N, OE, OM, PE, T, V, VD

Lacosamide   A, D, EQ, T, V

Lamotrigine   A, D, ED, EP, HL, N, OS, T, V

Levetiracetam   A, D, EP, OM, V

Table 14-1

53.12 ANTI-CONVULSANT DRUGS (CONT'D.)

Methsuximide	A, AH, D
Oxcarbazepine	A, D, EP, N, O, OE, T, V
Phenytoin (Diphenylhydantoin)	A, D, N, OS, V
Pregabalin	A, D, ED, EQ, HL, HY, N, OE, OM, T, V
Primidone	A, D, N, V
Rufinamide	A, D, N, O, V
Tiagabine	A, D, EP, HL, HY, N, OE, OM, T, V
Topiramate	A, D, EP, HL, HY, LB, N, OM, T, V
Valproate	A, D, EP, HL, N, OM, T, V
Valproic acid	A, D, EP, HL, N, OM, T, V
Vigabatrin	A, D, EP, HL, N, T, V
Zonisamide	A, D, HL, N, T, V

53.16 ANTI-PARKINSONIAN DRUGS

Carbidopa	A, D
Entacapone	A, D
Levodopa	A, D
Rotigotine	A, D, T, V
Tolcapone	D, EP, EQ, LB, OM, T, V

53.16.1 DOPAMINE RECEPTOR AGONISTS

Bromocriptine	A, D, HL, V
Cabergoline	D, V
Pramipexole	A, D, ED, EQ, OM, T, V
Ropinirole	A, D, ED, EP, HL, HY, OM, T, V, VD

53.20 ANTI-VERTIGO DRUGS

Nabilone	A, D, EQ, T, V

53.24 DOPAMINE REUPTAKE INHIBITORS

Bupropion	A, AD, D, EP, HL, HY, T, V
Diclofensine	T
Varenicline	D, EQ, HL, ME, N, T, V

53.28 MULTIPLE SCLEROSIS DRUGS

Glatiramer	A, D, EP, HL, N, OE, OM, T, V

53.32 SEROTONIN-RECEPTOR AGONISTS

Almotriptan	A, D, EP, HY, N, OM, T, V
Eletriptan	A, D, ED, EP, OM, T, V
Frovatriptan	A, D, EP, HY, T, V
Naratriptan	D, HL, L, OM, OR, PP, T, V
Rizatriptan	A, D, EP, HL, HY, T, V

Sumatriptan	A, D, EP, FF, HD, HL, HY, ME, N, OE, OM, PP, T, V
Zolmitriptan	A, D, EP, HL, HY, T, V

53.36 SKELETAL MUSCLE RELAXANTS

Baclofen	A, D, N, T, V
Carisoprodol	A, D, N, V
Chlorzoxazone	D, V
Cyclobenzaprine	A, D, T, V
Dantrolene	AH, D
Methocarbamol	D, N, V
Rapacuronium	HL
Tizanidine	D, EP, HL, OM, T, V

53.40 NEUROTOXINS

Abobotulinum Toxin A	D, V
Botulinum Toxin Type A	D, HL, N, T, V
Botulinum Toxin Type B	D, OM, T, V

56 OPTIC/OTIC DRUGS (EYE & EAR DRUGS)

56.1 OPTIC DRUGS

56.1.1 MACULAR DEGENERATION THERAPY ADJUNCT

Pegaptanib	D, HL, T, V
Verteporfin	D, HL, V

56.4 OTIC DRUGS

56.4.1 CERUMENOLYTIC DRUGS (EAR-WAX REMOVERS)

Propylene glycol	A, CH, OX
Triethanolamine (Trolamine)	EP, OE, OX, T

60 PSYCHOTROPIC DRUGS

60.1 ANTI-DEPRESSANT DRUGS

Nefazodone	A, D, EP, HL, HY, OM, T, V, VD

60.1.1 MONOAMINE OXIDASE INHIBITORS (MAO)

Isocarboxazid	A, D
Moclobemide	D, T
Phenelzine	A, D, N, T
Rasagiline	A, D, HL, V, VD
Selegiline	A, D, EP, EQ, HL, LB, OE, OM, T, V
Tranylcypromine	A, D, N, T

Table 14-1

60.1.1.1 MONOAMINE DEPLETER DRUGS
Tetrabenazine   A, D, LB

60.1.4 BICYCLIC ANTI-DEPRESSANTS)
Viloxazine   A, D, V

60.1.8 TRICYCLIC ANTI-DEPRESSANTS
Amitriptyline	A, D, HD, HL, HY, N, T, V
Amoxapine	A, D, T
Clomipramine	A, AH, D, EP, HL, HY, N, OM, T, V, VD
Desipramine	A, D, HY, T
Dothiepin	A, D, T
Doxepin	A, D, T, V
Imipramine	A, D, T
Melitracen	T
Nortriptyline	A, D, T
Protriptyline	A, D, T
Trimipramine	A, D, T, V

60.1.12 TETRACYCLIC ANTI-DEPRESSANTS
Maprotiline	A, D, T, V
Mirtazapine	A, D, EP, HL, HY, N, OM, T, V

60.1.16 HETEROCYCLIC ANTI-DEPRESSANTS
Trazodone   A, D, T, V

60.1.20 SELECTIVE NORADRENALINE REUPTAKE INHIBITORS
Reboxetine   D, V

60.1.24 SELECTIVE NOREPINEPHRINE REUPTAKE INHIBITORS
Atomoxetine   D, O

60.1.28 SELECTIVE SEROTONIN & NOREPINEPHRINE REUPTAKE INHIBITORS
Desvenlafaxine	D, T
Duloxetine	A, D, EP, T, V
Milnacipran	A, D, T, V
Venlafaxine	A, D, EP, HL, HY, L, N, OE, OM, T, V

60.1.32 SELECTIVE SEROTONIN REUPTAKE INHIBITORS (SSRIs)
Citalopram	A, D, EP, OM, T, V
Escitalopram	A, AH, D, ED, EP, HL, ME, N, PE, T, V
Fluoxetine	A, D, EP, HL, HY, N, T, V
Fluvoxamine	A, D, EP, HL, HY, OM, T, V
Paroxetine	A, D, EP, HL, HY, N, OE, OM, T, V

Sertraline	A, D, EP, HL, HY, L, N, OM, T, V
Zimeldine	T

60.1.36 SEROTONIN ANTAGONISTS

Pizotifen	A, D

60.4 ANTI-MANICS

Lithium	A, D, N, T, V

60.8 ANTIPSYCHOTIC DRUGS

Aripiprazole	A, D, EP, HL,OE, OM, T, V
Clozapine	A, AH, D, ED, N, V
Haloperidol	V
Iloperidone	D, T, V
Loxapine	A, D, T
Molindone	D, LB, T
Paliperidone	D, V
Perphenazine	A, D
Pimozide	D, V
Quetiapine	A, D, EP, HL, T, V
Risperidone	A, D, ED, EP, HL, HY, T, V
Thiothixene	A, D
Ziprasidone	A, D, ED, EP, N, OE, OM, T, V
Zotepine	A, D, V

60.8.1 PHENOTHIAZINES

Ethopropazine (Phenopropazine)	A, D
Mesoridazine	A, D
Thiethylperazine	D, T
Thioridazine	D, V
Zuclopenthixol	A, D, HY, T, V

60.12 ANXIOLYTICS, SEDATIVES & HYPNOTICS

Carbromal	A
Chloral hydrate	A, D, MP, V
Methylphenidate	AH, D, ED, EP, OM, V
Zolpidem	A, AH, D, EP, HL, HY, L, LB, OE, OM, T, V

60.12.1 ANXIOLYTICS

Buspirone	A, AD, D, HY, T
Meprobamate	A, D, V

60.12.4 BARBITURATES

Amobarbital	D, V
Butabarbital	D, V
Butalbital	D, EP, T, V

60.12.4 BARBITURATES (CONT'D.)

Mephobarbital	A, D, N
Pentobarbital	A, D, N
Phenobarbital	A, D, N, V
Secobarbital	A, D, V

60.12.8 BENZODIAZEPINES

Alprazolam	A, D, HY, T, V
Brotizolam	A, OX, T
Chlordiazepoxide	A, T, V
Clobazam	A, D, N, V
Clonazepam	A, D, EP, N, O, V
Clorazepate	A, D, T, V
Diazepam	A, D, HL, N, T, V
Estazolam	A, D, EP, HL, N, T
Flunitrazepam	A, V
Flurazepam	A, D, T, V
Loprazolam	A, V
Lorazepam	A, D, HL, T, V
Lormetazepam	A, V
Midazolam	A, D, EB, LB, N, T, V
Nitrazepam	A, D, OX, V
Oxazepam	A, D, N, T, V
Prozepam	T
Quazepam	A, D, T
Temazepam	A, D, N, T, V
Triazolam	A, AH, D, HL, T

60.12.12 PYRAZOLOPYRIMIDINES

Zaleplon	A, D, EP, HL, HY, L, N, T, V

60.16 HYPNOTIC DRUGS

Eszopiclone	A, D, EP, HY, N, OE, OM, T, V, VD
Zopiclone	A, D

60.20 PSYCHOSTIMULANTS

Caffeine	D, T, V
Modafinil	A, AH, D, ED, EP, HL, HY, V
Pemoline	D, N

60.20.1 ANOREXIANTS

Dexfenfluramine	A, D, HL, T, V
Sibutramine	A, D, ED, EP, HL, OE, OM, T, V, VD

63 RESPIRATORY DRUGS

63.1 ANTITUSSIVE DRUGS

Chlophedianol	V

63.4 BRONCHODILATORS—BETA ADRENERGIC AGONISTS

Albuterol (Salbutamol)	A, D, ED, EP, OM, T, V
Bitolterol	D, V
Ephedrine	AH, D, V
Ipratropium	A, D, EQ, T, V
Isoproterenol	D, T
Levalbuterol	D, EP, V
Salmeterol	D, EP, OM, V
Terbutaline	D, T, V
Theophylline	D, T

63.8 RESPIRATORY ANTI-INFLAMMATORY DRUGS

Cromolyn sodium (Sodium cromoglycate)	D, T, V
Montelukast	D, EP, O, OM

66 TOXICOLOGY DRUGS

66.1 ANTIDOTES

66.1.1 ACETAMINOPHEN ANTIDOTES

Acetylcysteine	A, EP

66.1.4 BENZODIAZEPINE ANTAGONISTS

Flumazenil	A, D, HL, HY, T, V

66.4 HEAVY METAL ANTAGONISTS/CHELATING AGENTS

Deferasirox	AD, D, EP, HL, O, V
Deferoxamine (Desferroxamine)	D, HD, HL, T
Penicillamine	T
Succimer	A, D, EB, OM

66.8 SYNTHETIC ALCOHOL DEHYDROGENASE INHIBITORS

Disulfiram	A, V
Fomepizole	D, N, T, V

70 SERUMS, TOXOIDS & VACCINES

70.1 SERUMS

Immune globulin	D, EP, V

70.4 TOXOIDS

Tetanus vaccine	CL, D, EP, OM

Table 14-1

70.8 VACCINES

Haemophilus vaccine	OM
Hepatitis A vaccine	A, D, O, OM, V
Hepatitis B vaccine	D, EP, T, V
Influenza vaccine	D, HL, L, V
Measles vaccine	A, D, HL, OM
Measles, mumps & rubella vaccine	A, D, EP, HL, OM
Measles, rubella vaccine	A, D, HL, OM
Meningococcal serogroup C vaccine	D, OM
Mumps vaccine	A, HL, OM
Pneumococcal vaccine	OM
Rabies vaccine	D, EP, V
Rotavirus vaccine	OM
Rubella & mumps vaccine	D, HL
Rubella vaccine	D, HL, OM
Varicella vaccine	A, D, O

75 SUPPLEMENTS

75.1 AMINO ACIDS

Levocarnitine	D, V

75.4 VITAMINS

Cyanocobalamin (Vitamin B_{12})	A, D
Ergocalciferal (Vitamin D_2)	A, T, V
Niacin (Vitamin B_3)	D, T, V
Paricalcitol	D, V
Pyridoxine (Vitamin B_6)	A

75.8 MINERALS

Iron sucrose	D, EP
Potassium gluconate	HL, T, V
Sodium ferric gluconate	D, ED

Key to Side Effect Abbreviations Used in Table 14-1

A	Ataxia
AD	Auditory disorder, Auditory disturbances
AH	Auditory hallucinations
BS	Burning/stinging in ear canal
C	Ceruminosis, Excessive ear wax
CH	Cholesteatoma
CL	Cochlear lesion, Cochlear damage
D	Dizziness
EB	Ears blocked, Ears feel "plugged"
ED	Ear disorder, Ear disease, unspecified
EP	Ear pain, Earache, Ear discomfort
EQ	Equilibrium disorder, Equilibrium dysfunction
ET	Eustachian tube disorder
FF	Feeling of fullness in ear(s)
HD	Hearing disorder, Hearing disturbances
HL	Hearing loss, Hearing decreased, Hearing impaired, Hypoacusis, Deafness
HY	Hyperacusis
L	Labyrinthitis, Labyrinthine disorder
LB	Loss of balance
ME	Meniere's disease
MP	Middle ear pressure
N	Nystagmus
O	Otitis (not specified)
OE	Otitis externa
OH	Otorrhagia (bleeding from ear)
OM	Otitis media, Fluid in ears, Middle ear disorder
OR	Otorrhea (purulent discharge [puss] from the ear)
OS	Oscillopsia
OT	Otosclerosis
OX	Ototoxicity
PE	Perforated eardrum
PP	Phonophobia
T	Tinnitus
V	Vertigo
VD	Vestibular disorder, Vestibular dysfunction, Vestibular disturbances

Note: See the Appendix for a more complete description of what these terms mean.

Table 14-1

Chapter 15

Ototoxic Herbals

Herbals That Can Damage Our Ears

People have asked me, "We know that some prescription drugs are ototoxic. Are any of the natural remedies made directly from herbs also ototoxic?"

This is a good question. Most herbals, by their very nature, are good for our bodies. If fact, one of the reasons God made them was for us to use in order to stay healthy. Is it any wonder that today, many people take herbs to try to regain the health they once had?

In general, herbs do not have the numerous severe side effects of prescription drugs. In the forward to the *PDR for Herbal Medicines* it states, "Most herbal remedies are notably free of known side effects".[101] (Yes, there are a few exceptions. Some are highly toxic and you need to be aware of them.)

There are two reasons why herbals are generally not ototoxic. First, herbal remedies are not highly concentrated as are pharmaceutical drugs. Therefore, they exert a **mild** action on your body that naturally produces few (and mild) side effects. Second, the active ingredients in herbs do not act alone. Each herb contains a multitude of natural chemical compounds that **work together** to heal your body. Since they are taken in the right proportions to each other, they do good things in your body.

In contrast, pharmaceutical drugs seldom have these two advantages. Generally, the active ingredient has been isolated from the other helpful factors and therefore must **work alone**. As a result, it is not in "harmony" with the rest of your body's bio-chemistry. Furthermore, the active ingredient is highly concentrated. In this form it exerts a much **harsher** action on your body—hence the resulting numerous harmful side effects. You should be aware that the more botanical preparations are refined and concentrated, the more they act like pharmaceuticals in your body and less like natural herbal preparations.

You'll notice that in this section, there are a number of herbals, some of which are listed as causing tinnitus. However, striking by their absence are a number of common herbals that contain salicylates (an ototoxic substance that causes tinnitus), and thus you would think should be listed here, but are not.

A lady wondered about that too. She asked, "I wondered if you knew about the ototoxicity of various foods. I read that tea is high in salicylates, as are also a lot of fruits. Does this mean that drinking/eating these things can make my existing tinnitus worse?"

As attested by the lack of such foods in the following listings, the short answer is typically "no". It is true that salicylates occur naturally in a good number of foods such as fruits, vegetables, dried spices, tea and food flavorings in quite high concentrations, but reports of resulting tinnitus are almost non-existent. Why?

Maybe we should we asking, "Can we ingest sufficient amounts of salicylates in our foods to cause the typical ototoxic side effects of tinnitus, reversible hearing loss, dizziness and vertigo?"

Some people may be allergic to, or particularly sensitive to salicylates. These people may indeed suffer the above side effects. However, the vast majority of people that ingest foods containing salicylates never notice any change in their tinnitus, and thus these foods are not reported to cause tinnitus. Here's why.

People on the average "Western diet" naturally ingest an estimated 10 to 200 mg. a day of salicylates. In comparison, the average dose of (adult) *Aspirin* contains a whopping 650 mg. of Salicylic acid per pill, while a baby *Aspirin* contains 81 mg. of Salicylic acid.

Conventional wisdom says that a person has to take 5 or 6 **adult** *Aspirin* tablets a day before they get tinnitus, or notice a change in their existing tinnitus.

Let's compare a few foods high in salicylates to a person taking a single baby aspirin (81 mg.) a day. Here's how it stacks up.

Curry powder has the highest salicylate content of any food—218 mg. per 100 g.[102] To get 81 mg. of salicylate, you would have to ingest 1.31 oz. of Curry powder at a sitting if you could stand it! If you wanted to consume the equivalent amount of salicylates contained in 6 adult *Aspirin*, you'd have to choke down almost 4 **pounds** of pure curry powder. It's just not going to happen!

Raisins are high in salicylates (6.62 mg. per 100 g.). To even get just one baby's aspirin worth of Salicylic acid, you'd have to eat about three pounds of raisins. And to get the equivalent salicylates contained in 6 adult *Aspirin*, where tinnitus starts to be noticeable, you'd have to gorge yourself with 144 **pounds** of raisins—at one sitting mind you!

Almonds are also considered high in salicylates at 3 mg. per 100 g. To get one baby's aspirin worth of Salicylic acid, you'd have to chomp your way through 6 pounds of almonds at one sitting! I eat a handful of almonds almost every day—but one handful (less than 1 ounce) is a far cry from the 288 **pounds** of almonds I'd have to gobble to begin to have a change in my tinnitus from eating almonds.

Some people are worried about getting tinnitus from eating tomatoes. Tomatoes have 0.13 mg. of salicylates per 100 g. Therefore, to get even one baby's *Aspirin* worth of Salicylic acid, you'd have to stuff yourself with a whopping 134 pounds of tomatoes at one sitting! If you wanted to get the equivalent salicylate content contained in a single adult *Aspirin*, you'd have to devour more than half a ton of tomatoes—again, all at one sitting mind you. In order for you to get tinnitus by eating fresh tomatoes, you'd need to consume 3 TONS of tomatoes at one sitting—and by then tinnitus would be the least of your worries!

Thus, even though you eat natural foods high in salicylates, unless you are particularly sensitive to salicylates, typically you physically could not ingest enough salicylates each day to either cause tinnitus, or affect your existing tinnitus. That is why these natural foods do not appear in these listings.

So feel free to eat your tomatoes, feast on broad beans, lace your food with curry powder and garlic and drink your green tea—all in moderation of course—and you won't have to worry that their ototoxic properties might damage your ears.

There are very few ototoxic herbals. I have combed through hundreds and hundreds of herbal listings to find the few that, under the right conditions, can damage our ears.

As was done in the drug and chemical listings, if dizziness is the only ototoxic side effect reported, I have omitted that herb from the detailed listings since dizziness may or may not be a sign of ototoxicity.

In the detailed herbal listings that follow, notice that generally ototoxicity is not a factor when these herbals are used in **normal** therapeutic dosages. Ototoxic side effects most often only show up when a person begins **overdosing** on these herbals. Even then, many of the resulting ototoxic side effects are often temporary balance issues such as ataxia or vertigo.

Ototoxic Herbal Listings

Abies alba

Common name: White fir

Main active ingredients: alpha-pinene, bornyl acetate, camphene, limonene, santene, tricyclene

Ototoxic effects:
    Vestibular:
        Ataxia: (PDR-H)
        Dizziness: (PDR-H)

Notes:
    Overdosing may cause dizziness and staggering gait (ataxia) (PDR-H).

Aga   (see **Amanita muscaria**)

Allium sativum

Common name: Garlic

Main active ingredients: allylalliin, methylalliin, propenyl alliin

Ototoxic effects:
    Vestibular:
        Vertigo: (PDR-H)

Amanita muscaria

Common name: Aga, Fly agaric

Main active ingredients: ibotenic acid, muscimol

Ototoxic effects:
  Vestibular:
    Ataxia (coordination disorder): (PDR-H)
    Dizziness: (PDR-H)

Notes:

  Highly toxic. Large doses can lead to death (PDR-H).

American hellebore   (see **Veratrum viride**)

American wormseed   (see **Chenopodium ambrosioides**)

Anamirta cocculus

Common name: Fish berry

Main active ingredients: menispermine, paramenispermine, picrotoxin

Ototoxic effects:
  Vestibular:
    Ataxia (coordination disorder): (PDR-H)
    Dizziness: (PDR-H)

Notes:

  Very poisonous (PDR-H).

Aspidosperma quebracho-blanco

Common name: Quebracho

Main active ingredients: aspidospermine, yohimbine

Ototoxic effects:
  Vestibular:
    Vertigo: (PDR-H)

Ayahuasca   (see **Banisteriopsis caapi**)

Banisteriopsis caapi

Common name: Ayahuasca, Yage

Main active ingredients: harmaline, harmalol, harmine, harmol, tetrahydroharmine

Ototoxic effects:
  Cochlear:
    Tinnitus: (PDR-H)

Notes:

  Overdosing may cause tinnitus (PDR-H).

Beans, broad   (see **Vicia faba**)

Bearded darnel   (see **Lolium temulentum**)

Bloodroot   (see **Sanguinaria canadensis**)

Boldo   (see **Peumus boldus**)

Broad beans   (see **Vicia faba**)

Camellia sinensis

Common name: Green tea

Main active ingredients: **Caffeine**

Ototoxic effects:
    Vestibular:
        Vertigo: (PDR-H)

Notes:

> If you drink a lot of Green tea regularly so that you get over 1.5 g of caffeine per day, you may experience vertigo (PDR-H). You can expect that the side effects will be milder forms of the side effects listed in the main drug section under the generic drug **Caffeine**.

> Since there is anywhere from 3 to 75 mg. of caffeine per cup of green tea, you should be able to drink between 20 and 500 cups of green tea a day before you begin to experience any ototoxic side effects.

Cannabis sativa

Common name: Hemp, Marijuana

Main active ingredients: cannabinol

Ototoxic effects:
    Cochlear:
        Auditory hallucinations: (PDR-H)
        Tinnitus: (Ka7, PDR-H)
    Vestibular:
        Ataxia: (NTP)
        Dizziness: (PDR-H)
        Loss of balance: (NTP)

Notes:

> The (illegal) drugs hashish and marijuana ("pot") are derived from this plant.

> Tetrahydrocannabinol, an active ingredient in marijuana, can cause tinnitus (She). (See the generic drug **Dronabinol** in the main drug section for the pharmaceutical version and its specific ototoxic properties.)

Chenopodium ambrosioides

Common name: American wormseed, Wormseed oil

Main active ingredients: ascaridiole

Ototoxic effects:
Cochlear:
Hearing loss: (PDR-H)
Tinnitus: (PDR-H)

Notes:

Damage frequently occurs to the nerves (hair cells) in the cochlea. This damage may cause hearing loss and tinnitus (buzzing in the ears) which can last for years (PDR-H).

Chrysanthemum cinerariifolium

Common name: Pyrethrum

Main active ingredients: pyrethrine

Ototoxic effects:
Cochlear:
Tinnitus: (PDR-H)

Notes:

Overdosing may cause tinnitus (PDR-H).

Cinchona   (see **Cinchona pubescens**)

Cinchona pubescens

Common name: Cinchona, Quinine

Main active ingredients: quinidine, quinine

Ototoxic effects:
Cochlear:
Hearing disorder: (PDR-H)
Hearing loss: (PDR-H)
Tinnitus: (PDR-H)

Notes:

Overdosing may cause tinnitus and hearing loss (ranging up to total deafness) (PDR-H). (See the generic drug **Quinine** in the main drug section for the pharmaceutical version, and for its specific ototoxic properties.)

Crataegus laevigata

Common name: English Hawthorn

Main active ingredients: flavonoides, 6-C and 8-C-glycosyl compounds, oligomeric proan-thocyanidins, biogenic amines and triterpenes

Ototoxic effects:
    Vestibular:
        Dizziness: (PDR-H)
        Vertigo: (PDR-H)

Notes:

    Dizziness and vertigo occur infrequently (PDR-H).

Cyamopsis tetragonoloba

Common name: Guar gum

Main active ingredients: galactomannans

Ototoxic effects:
    Vestibular:
        Vertigo: (PDR-H)

Notes:

    Vertigo occurs rarely (PDR-H).

Darnel, bearded   (see **Lolium temulentum**)

Duck's foot   (see **Podophyllum peltatum**)

English hawthorn   (see **Crataegus laevigata**)

Ephedra sinica

Common name: Ma Huang

Main active ingredients: ephedrine, pseudoephedrine, norephedrine

Ototoxic effects:
    Cochlear:
        Auditory hallucinations: (PDR-H)
    Vestibular:
        Dizziness: (PDR-H)

Fir, white   (see **Abies alba**)

Fish berry   (see **Anamirta cocculus**)

Fly agaric   (see **Amanita muscaria**)

Garlic   (see **Allium sativum**)

Green tea   (see **Camellia sinensis**)

Guar gum   (see **Cyamopsis tetragonoloba**)

Hawthorn, English   (see **Crataegus laevigata**)

Hellebore, American   (see **Veratrum viride**)

Hellebore, white   (see **Veratrum album**)

Hemp   (see **Cannabis sativa**)

Ivy, poison   (see **Rhus toxicodendron**)

Kalmia latifolia

Common name: Mountain laurel

Main active ingredients: andromedotoxin, grayanotoxin I

Ototoxic effects:
    Vestibular:
        Ataxia (coordination disorder): (PDR-H)
        Dizziness: (PDR-H)

Lactuca virosa

Common name: Lactucarium, Prickly lettuce

Main active ingredients: lactucin, lacutcopicrin, taraxasterol

Ototoxic effects:
    Cochlear:
        Tinnitus: (PDR-H)
    Vestibular:
        Dizziness: (PDR-H)

Notes:

    Symptoms may result from an overdose, or eating too many of the fresh leaves in salads (PDR-H).

Lactucarium   (see **Lactuca virosa**)

Laurel, mountain   (see **Kalmia latifolia**)

Lettuce, prickly   (see **Lactuca virosa**)

Lolium temulentum

Common name: Bearded darnel, Taumelloolch

Main active ingredients: temulentic acid, temulentin

Ototoxic effects:
    Vestibular:
        Ataxia: (PDR-H)
        Dizziness: (PDR-H)

Notes:

    Overdosing may cause dizziness and staggering gait (ataxia) (PDR-H).

Lophophora williamsii

Common name: Mescal buttons, Peyote

Main active ingredients: hordenine, mescaline

Ototoxic effects:
    Cochlear:
        Auditory hallucinations: (PDR-H)

Ma Huang   (see **Ephedra sinica**)

Marijuana   (see **Cannabis sativa**)

Mayapple   (see **Podophyllum peltatum**)

Melaleuca alternifolia

Common name: Tea tree

Main active ingredients: terpinenes

Ototoxic effects:
    Vestibular:
        Ataxia (coordination disorder): (PDR-H)

Notes:

    Overdose can result in ataxia (PDR-H).

Mentha x piperita

Common name: Peppermint

Main active ingredients: menthol

Ototoxic effects:
    Cochlear:
        Auditory hallucinations: [1]
    Vestibular:
        Ataxia: [1]
        Dizziness: [1]
        Nystagmus: [1]
        Vertigo: [1]

Notes:

Menthol is made from peppermint oil. Pure menthol is toxic.

[1] Some people are very sensitive to the effects of menthol and can have the above reactions.[103]

Mescal buttons   (see **Lophophora williamsii**)

Mountain laurel   (see **Kalmia latifolia**)

Pausinystalia yohimbe

Common name: Yohimbe bark

Main active ingredients: yohimbine

Ototoxic effects:
Cochlear:
Hearing disorder: (PDR-H)

Notes:

Yohimbe has been associated with a transient impairment in auditory sensory gating (PDR-H).

Peppermint   (see **Mentha x piperita**)

Peumus boldus

Common name: Boldo

Main active ingredients: boldine

Ototoxic effects:
Cochlear:
Auditory hallucinations: (PDR-H)

Notes:

Overdosing may cause auditory hallucinations (PDR-H).

Peyote   (see **Lophophora williamsii**)

Pine, various species   (see **Pinus spp.**)

Pinus spp.

Common name: Pine, various species

Main active ingredients: alpha-pinene, delta3-carene

Ototoxic effects:
    Vestibular:
        Ataxia: (PDR-H)
        Vertigo: (PDR-H)

Notes:

    Overdosing may cause staggering gait (ataxia) and vertigo (PDR-H).

Podophyllum peltatum

Common name: Duck's foot, Mayapple

Main active ingredients: podophyllin

Ototoxic effects:
    Vestibular:
        Ataxia (coordination disorder): (PDR-H)
        Dizziness: (PDR-H)

Notes:

    Overdosing may cause coordination disorders (ataxia) and dizziness (PDR-H).

Poison ivy   (see **Rhus toxicodendron**)

Pontian rhododendron   (see **Rhododendron ponticum**)

Prickly lettuce   (see **Lactuca virosa**)

Pyrethrum   (see **Chrysanthemum cinerariifolium**)

Quebracho   (see **Aspidosperma quebracho-blanco**)

Quillaja   (see **Quillaja saponaria**)

Quillaja saponaria

Common name: Quillaja, Soap tree

Main active ingredients: quillajasaponin

Ototoxic effects:
    Vestibular:
        Vertigo: (PDR-H)

Notes:

    Overdosing may cause vertigo (PDR-H).

Quinine   (see **Cinchona pubescens**)

Rhododendron ferrugineum

Common name: Rust-red rhododendron

Main active ingredients: rhododentrine

Ototoxic effects:
   Vestibular:
      Ataxia (coordination disorder): (PDR-H)

Notes:

   Overdosing may cause coordination disorders (ataxia) (PDR-H).

Rhododendron ponticum

Common name: Pontian rhododendron

Main active ingredients: andromedotoxin, acetylandromedol, rohodotoxin

Ototoxic effects:
   Vestibular:
      Ataxia (coordination disorder): (PDR-H)

Notes:

   Overdosing may cause coordination disorders (ataxia) (PDR-H).

Rhododendron, Pontian   (see **Rhododendron ponticum**)

Rhododendron, rust-red   (see **Rhododendron ferrugineum**)

Rhus toxicodendron

Common name: Poison ivy

Main active ingredients: urushiol

Ototoxic effects:
   Vestibular:
      Vertigo: (PDR-H)

Notes:

   Overdosing may cause vertigo (PDR-H).

Rue   (see **Ruta graveolens**)

Rust-red rhododendron   (see **Rhododendron ferrugineum**)

Ruta graveolens

Common name: Rue

Main active ingredients: gamma-fagarine, rutacultin, skimmianin

Ototoxic effects:
    Vestibular:
        Vertigo: (PDR-H)

Sage   (see **Salvia officinalis**)

Salvia officinalis

Common name: Sage

Main active ingredients: chlorogenic acid, rosmarinic acid, ursolic acid

Ototoxic effects:
    Vestibular:
        Vertigo: (PDR-H)

Notes:

    Overdosing may cause vertigo (PDR-H).

Sanguinaria canadensis

Common name: Bloodroot

Main active ingredients: various isoquinoline alkaloids, chief alkaloid: sanguinarine

Ototoxic effects:
    Vestibular:
        Dizziness: (PDR-H)
        Vertigo: (PDR-H)

Notes:

    The FDA has ruled Bloodroot to be unsafe for use in foods, drugs, herbals and beverages. (PDR-H).

Soap tree   (see **Quillaja saponaria**)

Taumelloolch   (see **Lolium temulentum**)

Taxus baccata

Common name: Yew

Main active ingredients: taxine

Ototoxic effects:
    Vestibular:
        Vertigo: (PDR-H)

Notes:

    Overdosing may cause vertigo (PDR-H).

Tea, green   (see **Camellia sinensis**)

Tea tree   (see **Melaleuca alternifolia**)

Veratrum album

Common name: White hellebore

Main active ingredients: veratrine

Ototoxic effects:
Vestibular:
Vertigo: (PDR-H)

Notes:

Overdosing may cause vertigo (PDR-H).

Veratrum viride

Common name: American hellebore

Main active ingredients: isorubijervine, protoverine

Ototoxic effects:
Vestibular:
Vertigo: (PDR-H)

Notes:

Overdosing may cause vertigo and death. No longer used. (PDR-H).

Vicia faba

Common name: Broad beans

Main active ingredients: convicine, vicine

Ototoxic effects:
Vestibular:
Vertigo: (PDR-H)

Notes:

If you eat large quantities of raw or briefly-cooked broad beans, and depending on your body chemistry, you may experience vertigo (PDR-H).

White fir   (see **Abies alba**)

White hellebore   (see **Veratrum album**)

Wormseed, American   (see **Chenopodium ambrosioides**)

Wormseed oil   (see **Chenopodium ambrosioides**)

Yage   (see **Banisteriopsis caapi**)

Yew   (see **Taxus baccata**)

Yohimbe bark   (see **Pausinystalia yohimbe**)

---

101 *PDR for Herbal Medicines*, 2000. p. v.

102 To learn more about salicylates in foods, read the articles *Salicylates* and *Salicylate Content in Foods*. (See the "Literature Cited" section at back of book for exact references.)

103 *Menthol Toxicology*, 2000. pp. 1-2

Chapter 16

Ototoxic Chemicals

Chemicals Also Can Damage Our Ears

There are many, many chemicals in our world today—more than 1,000,000 in fact. Certainly not all of these chemicals damage our ears. Researchers estimate that maybe between 3,000 and 56,000 may be ototoxic. That's still a lot of ear-damaging chemicals! This book contains information on all the ototoxic "chemicals" I have found to date—a paltry 35 herbals, 148 chemicals and 877 drugs. Obviously, at this point, researchers are only scratching the tip of the iceberg insofar as identifying ototoxic chemicals are concerned.

The two worst classes of ototoxic chemicals are the organic solvents and the heavy metals. Both of these classes of substances are found almost everywhere.

You likely have many ototoxic chemical substances in, or around, your home. Some of these ototoxic chemicals include adhesives, auto emissions, fungicides, glues, grease and spot removers, insecticides, insulation, lacquers, liquid correction fluid (whiteout), organic solvents, paint, paint thinners, resins, room deodorizers, rug cleaners, spray paint, varnishes and wood preservatives to name a few.[101, 102]

In addition, you may be exposed to ototoxic chemicals if you work in one of the many manufacturing plants and factories that use organic solvents or heavy metals. Such processes as electroplating, shoe manufacturing, dry cleaning, cold vulcanization, electronic battery manufacture and polyvinyl chloride manufacturing all use various ototoxic chemicals.[103]

Furthermore, I'll bet you didn't realize that some kinds of air pollution can also hurt your ears. Depending on the type and severity of the air pollution, you could end up with a hearing loss, balance problems or other damage to your ears.[104]

You probably think of air pollution as occurring outside. However, a lot of dangerous air pollution from various organic solvents occurs in your home, in offices and in factories. These organic solvents seem to be everywhere. The problem is that when you breathe in the fumes from many of these solvents, you slowly but surely damage your ears. This damage often does not show up right away. However, if caught in time, the damage is usually reversible.

Early symptoms of organic solvent ototoxicity may include dizziness, vertigo and disequilibrium. Later on, testing may reveal that your brain has problems processing what you hear.[105] For example, a study of workers in one rubber factory revealed that 47% had subclinical abnormalities in the auditory pathways in their brainstems due to the solvents used in manufacturing rubber.[106]

Sometimes, ototoxic damage from organic solvents is clearly obvious such as when it results in massive hearing loss or roaring tinnitus. However, in other cases, like in the above study, the results are more insidious and subtle, showing up as impaired auditory processing in the brain. This means that even though the chemical hasn't caused reduced hearing as such, the person affected can't understand everything they hear.

Ototoxic Chemical Listings

1-Butanol   (see **Butyl alcohol**)

1-Chloronaphthalene   (see **Chloronaphthalene**)

1-Methylhydrazine   (see **Methyl hydrazine**)

1-Naphthyl chloride   (see **Chloronaphthalene**)

1-Pentanol   (see **Pentanol**)

1,1,1-Trichloroethane   (see **Trichloroethane**)

1,1,1,3,3,3-Hexafluoro-2-propanol   (see **Hexafluoro propanol**)

1,1,2,2-Tetrachloroethane   (see **Tetrachloroethane**)

1,2-Dibromo-3-chloropropane   (see **Dibromo-chloropropane**)

1,2-Dichloroethane   (see **Dichloroethane**)

1,2-Diethoxyethane   (see **Ethylene glycol diethyl ether**)

1,2-Epoxypropane   (see **Epoxypropane**)

1,2,3,4-Tetrachloronaphthalene   (see **Tetrachloronaphthalene**)

1,3-Butadiene   (see **Butadiene**)

1,3-Dichloro-2-propanol   (see **Dichloro propanol**)

1,3-Dinitrobenzene   (see **Dinitrobenzene**)

1,4-Dichlorobenzene   (see **Dichlorobenzene**)

1,4-Dioxane   (see **Dioxane**)

1,8-Cineol   (see **Cineol**)

2-Butanone   (see **Methyl ethyl ketone**)

2-Butenone   (see **Methyl vinyl ketone**)

2-Chloro-1,3-butadiene mixture   (see **Chlorobutadiene mixture**)

2-Chloroethanol   (see **Chloroethanol**)

2-Chloronaphthalene   (see **Chloronaphthalene**)

2-Ethoxyethanol   (see **Ethoxyethanol**)

2-Hexanone   (see **Hexanone**)

2-Hydroxybenzamide   (see **Hydroxybenzamide**)

2-Methoxyaniline   (see **Anisidine**)

2-Methoxyethanol   (see **Methoxyethanol**)

2-Nitortoluene   (see **Nitrotoluene**)

2,2-Dichlorovinyl dimethyl phosphate   (see **Vapona**)

2,2'-Dihydroxydiethylamine   (see **Diethanolamine**)

2,3-Dichloro-1-propanol   (see **Dichloro propanol**)

2,4-D   (see **Dichlorophenoxyacetic acid**)

2,4-Dichlorophenoxyacetic acid   (see **Dichlorophenoxyacetic acid**)

2,4-Dinitrophenol   (see **Dinitrophenol**)

2,4-Dinitrotoluene   (see **Dinitrotoluene**)

2,4-DNT   (see **Dinitrotoluene**)

2,4,5-T   (see **Trichlorophenoxyacetic acid**)

2,4,5-Trichlorophenoxyacetic acid   (see **Trichlorophenoxyacetic acid**)

2,5-Dimethylfuran   (see **Dimethylfuran**)

2,5-Dimethylfurane   (see **Dimethylfuran**)

2,6-Dinitrotoluene   (see **Dinitrotoluene**)

2,6-DNT   (see **Dinitrotoluene**)

3-Amino-1,2,4-triazole   (see **Amino triazole**)

3-Cresol   (see **Cresol mixture**)

3-Methoxybenzenamine   (see **Anisidine**)

4-Aminoaniline dihydrochloride   (see **Phenylenediamine dihydrochloride**)

4-Bromoaniline   (see **Bromoaniline**)

4-Cresol   (see **Cresol mixture**)

4-Hydroxyloluene   (see **Cresol mixture**)

4-Methoxybenzenamine   (see **Anisidine**)

4-Methylphenol   (see **Cresol mixture**)

4-Nitroaniline   (see **Nitroaniline**)

4-Nitrobenzenamine   (see **Nitroaniline**)

4-Nitrotoluene   (see **Nitrotoluene**)

4,4'-DDE   (see **DDE**)

6-Amino nicotinamide   (see **Amino nicotinamide**)

6-AN   (see **Amino nicotinamide**)

Aatack   (see **Tetramethylthiuram disulfide**)

Acaraben   (see **Chlorobenzilate**)

Acarin   (see **Dicofol**)

Accelerator thiuram   (see **Tetramethylthiuram disulfide**)

Acetyl ethylene   (see **Methyl vinyl ketone**)

Acetyldimethylamine   (see **Dimethyl acetamide**)

Acetylene tetrachloride   (see **Tetrachloroethane**)

Acetylene trichloride   (see **Trichloroethylene**)

Adipic acid dinitrile   (see **Adiponitrile**)

Adiponitrile

Pronunciation guide: ad-ih-poh-NYE-trel

Other names: Adipic acid dinitrile, Hexanedinitrile

Uses: in the manufacture of nylon; in organic synthesis

Ototoxic effects:
　　Vestibular:
　　　　Vertigo: (NTP)

Aero-cyanamid   (see **Calcium cyanamide**)

Agroceres   (see **Heptachlor**)

Agrocide   (see **Lindane**)

Agrotect   (see **Dichlorophenoxyacetic acid**)

Akar   (see **Chlorobenzilate**)

Aktikon   (see **Atrazine**)

Alcanfor   (see **Camphor**)

Alcohol   (see **Ethanol**)

Aldifen   (see **Dinitrophenol**)

Aldrex   (see **Aldrin**)

Aldrin

Pronunciation guide: OL-drin

Other names: *Aldrex, Aldrosol, Drinox, Octalene, Seedrin*

Uses: insecticide

Ototoxic effects:
　　Vestibular:
　　　　Ataxia: (NTP)
　　　　Dizziness: (NTP)

Aldrosol   (see **Aldrin**)

Algofrene   (see **Dichlorodifluoromethane**)

Algylen   (see **Trichloroethylene**)

Alltox   (see **Toxaphene**)

Alpha-chloronaphthalene   (see **Chloronaphthalene**)

Alpha-dichlorohydrin   (see **Dichloro propanol**)

Alpha-difluromethylornithine   (see **Difluromethylornithine**)

Alpha-hydroquinone   (see **Hydroquinone**)

Alvit   (see **Dieldrin**)

Amerol   (see **Amino triazole**)

Aminobenzene   (see **Aniline**)

Amino nicotinamide

Pronunciation guide: ah-MEEN-oh nih-koe-TIN-ah-mide

Other names: 6-Amino nicotinamide, 6-AN

Uses: in experimental medicine as a modulator in cancer treatments; anti-metabolite

Ototoxic effects:
    Cochlear:
        Hearing loss: [1]
        Tinnitus: [107]

Notes:

    [1] Can cause permanent sensorineural hearing loss. This chemical is both neurotoxic and cochlear toxic.[108]

Amino triazole

Pronunciation guide: ah-MEEN-oh TRY-ah-zole

Other names: 3-Amino-1,2,4-triazole, *Amerol, Amitrol, Cytrol, Diurol, Herbizole, Weedazol*

Uses: herbicide; defoliant; photographic reagent; etc.

Ototoxic effects:
    Vestibular:
        Ataxia: (NTP)

Amitrol   (see **Amino triazole**)

Amyl alcohol   (see **Pentanol**)

Amyl hydride   (see **Pentane**)

Amylol   (see **Pentanol**)

Anesthetic ether   (see **Ethyl ether**)

Anhydrol   (see **Ethanol**)

Aniline

Pronunciation guide: AH-nil-en

Other names: Aminobenzene, Benzenamine, *Blue oil, Cyanol, Kyanol*

Uses: in the manufacture of rubber chemicals, agriculture chemicals and dyestuffs; in dyes and drugs; antioxidants; photographic chemicals; explosives; petroleum refining; herbicides and fungicides; marking inks; in many organic chemicals; etc.

Ototoxic effects:
    Cochlear:
        Tinnitus: (NTP)
    Vestibular:
        Dizziness: (NTP)

Anisidine

Pronunciation guide: ah-NIS-sih-deen

Other names: M-Anisidine, M—3-Aminoanisole, 3-Methoxybenzenamine, O-Anisidine, O—2-Aminoanisole, 2-Methoxyaniline, P-Anisidine, P—4-Aminoanisole, 4-Methoxy-benzenamine

Uses: in azo dyes, triphenylmethane dyes and hair dyes; in preparation of organic compounds; corrosion inhibitor for steel; antioxidant for polymercaptan resins; etc.

Ototoxic effects:
    Vestibular:
        Dizziness: (NTP)
        Vertigo: (NTP)

Antabuse   (see **Tetramethylthiuram disulfide**)

Anti-rust   (see **Sodium nitrite**)

Apavinphos   (see **Mevinphos**)

Aquacat   (see **Cobalt**)

Arasan   (see **Tetramethylthiuram disulfide**)

Armol   (see **Methylaminophenol sulfate**)

Arochlor

Pronunciation guide: ARE-oh-klor

Other names: Arochlor 1254, PCB-1254, Polychlorinated biphenyl 1254

Uses: in electrical capacitors and electrical transformers; vacuum pumps; gas-transmission turbines; high-temperature dielectrics; inks; insecticides; adhesives; etc.

Ototoxic effects:
   Cochlear:
        Hearing loss (hearing difficulties): (NTP)

Arochlor 1254   (see **Arochlor**)

Arsenic

Pronunciation guide: ARE-seh-nik

Other names: Arsenic chloride, Arsenic trioxide

Uses: arsenic compounds; in ceramics, glass manufacturing and enamels; in weed killers, herbicides, rodenticides, insecticides and sheep dips; pharmaceuticals; etc.

Ototoxic effects:
   Cochlear:
        Hearing loss: (Ryb)
        Tinnitus: (Ka7)

Notes:

Hearing losses caused by **Arsenic** are concentrated in the low frequencies—125 Hz to 500 Hz (Ryb).

Arsenic air pollution can cause significant sensorineural hearing loss. (Ryb) Children exposed to airborne **Arsenic** from a power plant had statistically significant hearing losses, especially at the lower frequencies.[109]

Exposure to **Arsenic** and loud noise at the same time can result in greater hearing loss than would normally result from exposure to both **Arsenic** and noise separately (Nia).

See Chapter 8, "The Sinister Partnership Between Ototoxic Agents and Noise" for further information on this chemical.

Arsenic chloride   (see **Arsenic**)

Arsenic trioxide   (see **Arsenic**)

Aspartame

Pronunciation guide: ASS-par-tame

Other names: L-Asparty-L-phenylalanine methyl ester, *NutraSweet*

Uses: artificial sweetener

Ototoxic effects:
 Cochlear:
  Hearing loss: 0.4% [1, 2, 3]
  Tinnitus: [2, 3]
 Vestibular:
  Dizziness: 7.5% [1, 2, 3]
  Equilibrium disorder (balance problems): 7.5% [1, 2, 3]
  Vertigo: [3]

Notes:

[1] An FDA report on **Aspartame** side effects lists these figures as the percent of complaints for this symptom reported to the FDA.[110]

[2] According to Dr. Woodrow Monte, common complaints relative to **Aspartame** include dizziness, tinnitus and loss of equilibrium.[111]

[3] Mark Gold lists dizziness, hearing loss, tinnitus and vertigo as side effects of **Aspartame**.[112] as does Dr. Joseph Mercola.[113]

It is hard to separate the fact from the fiction regarding how **Aspartame** affects our ears. It appears, just like for almost all of the other drugs/chemicals listed in this book, that a given person may consume **Aspartame** without experiencing any obvious side effects. At the same time, it appears just as true that another person taking **Aspartame** may experience one or more adverse side effects. As always—beware. If you think that **Aspartame** is affecting your ears, eliminate it from your diet and see if there are any positive changes. That way you'll know how it affects your own body.

Astrobot (see **Vapona**)

Atgard (see **Vapona**)

Atrazin (see **Atrazine**)

Atrazine

Pronunciation guide: ah-TRA-zeen

Other names: *Aktikon, Atrazin, Candex, Fenatrol, Primatol, Vectal*

Uses: herbicide

Ototoxic effects:
 Vestibular:
  Ataxia: (NTP)

Attac   (see **Toxaphene**)

Azabenzene   (see **Pyridine**)

Azine   (see **Pyridine**)

Azinophos-methyl   (see **Gusathion**)

Azoxybenzene

Pronunciation guide: ah-ZOX-ee-ben-zeen

Other names: Azoxybenzide, Diphenyldiazene oxide, *Fentoxan*

Uses: insecticide; used in organic synthesis; etc.

Ototoxic effects:
    Vestibular:
        Ataxia: (NTP)

Notes:

    During testing, researchers found that **Azoxybenzene** caused ataxia in mice. Ataxia is not yet reported in humans at this point, but be aware of this possibility (NTP).

Azoxybenzide   (see **Azoxybenzene**)

Baycid   (see **Baytex**)

Bayer 21/116   (see **Methyl demeton**)

Bayer 9007   (see **Baytex**)

Bayer 9027   (see **Gusathion**)

Baytex

Pronunciation guide: BAY-tex

Other names: *Baycid, Bayer 9007, Fenthion, Tiguvon*

Uses: insecticide; acaricide

Ototoxic effects:
    Vestibular:
        Ataxia: (NTP)

Belt   (see **Chlordane**)

Benesal   (see **Hydroxybenzamide**)

Benzenamine   (see **Aniline**)

Benzene

Pronunciation guide: BEN-zeen

Other names: *Benzol, Benzolene*, Mineral naphtha, *Pyrobenzol*

Uses: solvent; used in the manufacture of medicines, dyes, linoleum, oil cloth, pesticides, plastics, resins, aviation fuel, detergents, flavors, perfumes, paints, coatings, varnishes, lacquers, explosives; etc.

Ototoxic effects:
Cochlear:
    Hearing loss: (NTP)
    Tinnitus: (NTP)
Vestibular:
    Ataxia: (NTP)
    Dizziness: (ATS, NTP)
    Vertigo: (NTP)

Notes:
See Chapter 8, "The Sinister Partnership Between Ototoxic Agents and Noise" for further information on this chemical.

Benzene hexachloride   (see **Lindane**)

Benzene methanol   (see **Benzyl alcohol**)

Benzenol   (see **Phenol**)

Benzinol   (see **Trichloroethylene**)

Benz-o-chlor   (see **Chlorobenzilate**)

Benzohydroquinone   (see **Hydroquinone**)

Benzol   (see **Benzene**)

Benzolene   (see **Benzene**)

Benzyl alcohol

Pronunciation guide: BEN-zil AL-koe-hall

Other names: Benzene methanol, Hydroxytoluene, Phenyl methanol

Uses: photographic developer; used in perfumes, cosmetics and flavorings; solvent; insect repellant; local anesthetic; etc.

Ototoxic effects:
Vestibular:
    Dizziness: (NTP)
    Vertigo: (NTP)

Beta-chloroethyl alcohol   (see **Chloroethanol**)

Beta-chloronaphthalene   (see **Chloronaphthalene**)

Beta-dichlorohydrin   (see **Dichloro propanol**)

Betadine   (see **Iodine**)

Beta-quinol   (see **Hydroquinone**)

Bichlorendo   (see **Mirex**)

Bichromate of potash   (see **Potassium dichromate**)

Biethylene   (see **Butadiene**)

Binitrobenzene   (see **Dinitrobenzene**)

Bivinyl   (see **Butadiene**)

BL 6623   (see **Photodieldrin**)

Bladan   (see **Tetraethylpyrophosphate**)

Blue oil   (see **Aniline**)

Bonain's solution

Pronunciation guide: Boe-nayns

Other names:

Uses: medicine

Ototoxic effects:
    Unspecified/General Ear Conditions:
        Ototoxicity: [114]

Notes:

Bonain's solution is composed of Cocaine, **Phenol** & Thymol. (See the chemical **Phenol** for its specific ototoxic properties.)

Bonoform   (see **Tetrachloroethane**)

Borer Sol   (see **Dichloroethane**)

Bravo   (see **Chlorothalonil**)

Brevinyl   (see **Vapona**)

Brick oil (see **Creosote**)

Brocide (see **Dichloroethane**)

Brodan (see **Chlorpyrifos**)

Bromic acid potassium salt (see **Potassium bromate**)

Bromide salt of potassium (see **Potassium bromide**)

Bromoaniline

Pronunciation guide: broe-moe-AN-ih-lin

Other names: 4-Bromoaniline, P-Bromoaniline, P-Bromophenylamine

Uses: in preparing azo dyes and dihydroquinazolines

Ototoxic effects:
  Cochlear:
    Tinnitus: (NTP)
  Vestibular:
    Dizziness: (NTP)

Brom-o-Gas (see **Methyl bromide**)

Bromomethane (see **Methyl bromide**)

Brushtox (see **Trichlorophenoxyacetic acid**)

Butadiene

Pronunciation guide: byoo-tah-DIE-een

Other names: 1,3-Butadiene, Biethylene, Bivinyl, Pyrrolyene, Vinylethylene

Uses: in synthetic rubber; synthetic polymeric elastomers; rocket fuels; plastics; resins; latex paint; etc.

Ototoxic effects:
  Vestibular:
    Vertigo: (NTP)

Butanone (see **Methyl ethyl ketone**)

Butoflin (see **Deltamethrin**)

Butoss (see **Deltamethrin**)

Butyl alcohol

Pronunciation guide: BYOO-tul AL-koe-hall

Other names: 1-Butanol, N-Butanol, N-Butyl alcohol, Propylcarbinol

Uses: solvent; in coatings, resins and dyes; etc.

Ototoxic effects:
    Cochlear:
        Hearing loss: (Nia)
    Vestibular:
        Dizziness: [115]
        Vertigo: [116]

Notes:

Exposure to **Butyl alcohol** and loud noise at the same time can result in greater hearing loss than would normally result from exposure to both **Butyl alcohol** and noise separately (Nia).

See Chapter 8, "The Sinister Partnership Between Ototoxic Agents and Noise" for further information on this chemical.

Butyl methyl ketone   (see **Hexanone**)

Butyl nitrite

Pronunciation guide: BYOO-tul NIE-tryte

Other names: Isobutyl nitrite, N-Butyl nitrite

Uses: in room odorizers

Ototoxic effects:
    Cochlear:
        Hearing loss: (Ryb)
    Vestibular:
        Dizziness: (NTP)

Notes:

Studies using rats show that exposure to **Butyl nitrite** causes significant sensorineural hearing loss in the higher frequencies (Ryb).

Exposure to **Butyl nitrite** and loud noise at the same time can result in greater hearing loss than would normally result from exposure to both **Butyl nitrite** and noise separately (Nia).

See Chapter 8, "The Sinister Partnership Between Ototoxic Agents and Noise" for further information on this chemical.

Calcium cyanamide

Pronunciation guide: KAL-see-um sye-AN-ah-mide

Other names: *Aero-cyanamid*, Lime nitrogen, *Nitrolime*

Uses: herbicide and pesticide; refining of iron; etc.

Ototoxic effects:
    Vestibular:
        Dizziness: (NTP)
        Vertigo: (NTP)

Calcium cyanide

Pronunciation guide: KAL-see-um SYE-ah-nyed

Other names: *Calcyanide*, *Cyanogas*

Uses: fumigant; rodenticide; in stainless-steel manufacture; in leaching precious metal ores; etc.

Ototoxic effects:
    Vestibular:
        Dizziness: (NTP)
        Vertigo: (NTP)

Calcyanide   (see **Calcium cyanide**)

Camphechlor   (see **Toxaphene**)

Camphor

Pronunciation guide: KAM-for

Other names: *Alcanfor*, D-Camphor, L-Camphor

Uses: in the manufacture of plastics; insect repellant; in lacquers and varnishes; in explosives; in embalming fluids; etc.

Ototoxic effects:
    Cochlear:
        Tinnitus: (NTP)
    Vestibular:
        Dizziness: (NTP)
        Vertigo: (NTP)

Candex   (see **Atrazine**)

Canogard   (see **Vapona**)

Carbax   (see **Dicofol**)

Carbetox   (see **Malathion**)

Carbinol   (see **Methyl alcohol**)

Carbitol   (see **Diethylene glycol monoethyl ether**)

Carbolic acid   (see **Phenol**)

Carbon bisulfide   (see **Carbon disulfide**)

Carbon dichloride   (see **Tetrachloroethylene**)

Carbon disulfide

Pronunciation guide: KAR-bon die-SUL-fyed

Other names: Carbon bisulfide, Carbon sulfide

Uses: disinfectant; insecticides; solvent; bactericide; wood preservative; used in extracting and processing oils, fats resins and waxes; etc.

Ototoxic effects:
    Cochlear:
            Auditory disorder (auditory disturbances): (NTP)
            Auditory hallucinations: (NTP)
            Hearing loss: (Ryb)
    Vestibular:
            Dizziness: (NTP)
            Vertigo: (NTP)

Notes:

Carbon disulfide causes high-frequency sensorineural hearing loss. **Carbon disulfide** may also cause a conductive loss due to inflammation of the nasal cavity and Eustachian tubes (Ryb).

The longer you are exposed to **Carbon disulfide**, the more likely you will end up with a hearing loss. Also, the longer you are exposed to **Carbon disulfide**, the more severe the resulting hearing loss will likely be (Ryb).

In one study, researchers found that the incidence of hearing loss was higher than expected among workers exposed to both noise and **Carbon disulfide** at the same time. In addition, they also found that the hearing losses were more severe and began sooner than in those workers only exposed to noise and not **Carbon disulfide**. Another study suggested that chronic exposure to **Carbon disulfide** damaged the auditory pathways in the brainstem. In other words, the **Carbon disulfide** didn't damage the cochlea so much as it did the sound processing areas of the brain.[117]

In a study of 259 workers in the viscose industry who were exposed to **Carbon disulfide**, the incidence of sensorineural hearing loss was 60% compared to 46% in the control group who had been exposed to noise alone. In 42% (control group 33%), the hearing damage was not in the cochlea, but in the auditory pathways in the brain (Ryb).

See Chapter 8, "The Sinister Partnership Between Ototoxic Agents and Noise" for further information on this chemical.

Carbon monoxide

Pronunciation guide: KAR-bon mon-OX-eyed

Other names: CO

Uses: Carbon monoxide is a by-product of combustion

Ototoxic effects:
    Cochlear:
        Hearing loss: [118]
        Tinnitus:[119]
    Vestibular:
        Ataxia (gait disturbance): [120]
        Dizziness: [121]
        Vestibular disorder: [122]

Notes:

Hearing might also become distorted.[123]

A 1948 study revealed a whopping 78% incidence of sensorineural hearing loss among 700 cases of **Carbon monoxide** poisoning. **Carbon monoxide** poisoning may result in mild to moderate temporary hearing loss, or it may be severe and permanent (Ryb).

Carbon monoxide can cause abnormal results to auditory brainstem response (ABR) tests indicating damage to the auditory circuits in the brain.[124]

Low levels of **Carbon monoxide** from secondhand smoke and air pollution likely contribute to permanent hearing loss in infants. Damage to hearing was seen with exposure of as little as 25 parts per million in rats.[125]

The ototoxic effects of **Carbon monoxide** are made worse by the presence of noise at the same time (Ryb).

See Chapter 8, "The Sinister Partnership Between Ototoxic Agents and Noise" for further information on this chemical.

Carbon sulfide   (see **Carbon disulfide**)

Carbon tetrachloride

Pronunciation guide: KAR-bon tet-rah-KLOR-eyed

Other names: *Carbona*, *Necatorine*, Perchloromethane, *Tetraform*, *Tetrasol*, *Univerm*

Uses: in fire extinguishers, refrigerants, fumigants; solvent; in dry cleaning; for extracting oils from seeds; etc.

Ototoxic effects:
    Cochlear:
        Hearing loss: (NTP)
    Vestibular:
        Dizziness: (NTP)
        Vertigo: (NTP)

Notes:

> See Chapter 8, "The Sinister Partnership Between Ototoxic Agents and Noise" for further information on this chemical.

Carbona   (see **Carbon tetrachloride**)

Carbophos   (see **Malathion**)

Carfene   (see **Gusathion**)

Cellon   (see **Tetrachloroethane**)

Cellosolve   (see **Ethoxyethanol**)

Ceresan   (see **Ethyl mercury chloride**)

Chemathion   (see **Malathion**)

Chemform   (see **Methoxychlor**)

Chlordan   (see **Chlordane**)

Chlordane

Pronunciation guide: KLOR-dane

Other names: *Belt, Chlordan,* Chlordane technical mixture, *Chlorodane, Dowchlor, Ortho-klor, Toxichlor*

Uses: insecticide; fungicide; wood preservative; etc.

Ototoxic effects:
  Vestibular:
    Ataxia: (NTP)
    Dizziness: (NTP)

Chlordane technical mixture   (see **Chlordane**)

Chlorfenidim   (see **Monuron**)

Chlorilen   (see **Trichloroethylene**)

Chloroalonil   (see **Chlorothalonil**)

Chlorobenzilate

Pronunciation guide: klor-oh-BEN-zih-late

Other names: *Acaraben, Akar, Benz-o-chlor, Folbex, Kop-mite*

Uses: insecticide; miticide; acaricide; etc.

Ototoxic effects:
  Vestibular:
    Ataxia: (NTP)

Chlorobutadiene mixture

Pronunciation guide: klor-oh-byoo-tah-DIE-een

Other names: 2-Chloro-1,3-butadiene mixture, *Chloroprene*, Methyl toluene, *Neoprene*, *Violet 3*

Uses: in manufacture of neoprene rubber; in dyes; cleaning agent; industrial solvent; aviation gasoline; etc.

Ototoxic effects:
  Vestibular:
    Ataxia: (NTP)
    Dizziness: (NTP)

Chlorocamphene   (see **Toxaphene**)

Chlorodane   (see **Chlordane**)

Chloroethanol

Pronunciation guide: klor-oh-ETH-an-all

Other names: 2-Chloroethanol, Beta-chloroethyl alcohol, Ethylene chlorohydrin, Glycol chlorohydrin

Uses: solvent; in manufacture of insecticides; in seed germination; cleaning agent; etc.

Ototoxic effects:
  Vestibular:
    Dizziness: (NTP)
    Vertigo: (NTP)

Chloroethene   (see **Trichloroethane**)

Chloroethylmercury   (see **Ethyl mercury chloride**)

Chloroform

Pronunciation guide: KLO-roe-form

Other names: Methane trichloride, Methyl trichloride, TCM, Trichloromethane

Uses: solvent; used in the manufacture of fluorocarbon plastics, resins, refrigerants and propellants; used as a solvent for fats, oils, plastics, dyes, rubber, alkaloids, waxes resins and dry cleaning; used as a fumigant, insecticide, anesthetic, analgesic, muscle relaxant, carminative, flavoring agent, preservative, bactericide, antispasmodic; used in the manufacture of **Penicillin** and other pharmaceuticals; etc.

Ototoxic effects:
    Cochlear:
        Hearing loss: [1]
    Vestibular:
        Dizziness: (ATS, NTP)

Notes:

    [1] May cause hearing loss.[126]

Chloromethane   (see **Methyl chloride**)

Chloromethylmercury   (see **Methyl mercury chloride**)

Chloronaphthalene

Pronunciation guide: klor-oh-NAP-thah-leen

Other names: 1-Chloronaphthalene, 2-Chloronaphthalene, 1-Naphthyl chloride, Alpha-chloronaphthalene, Beta-chloronaphthalene, *Nalowax*

Uses: solvent; used in manufacture of electrical cable insulation; immersion liquid in microscopy; etc.

Ototoxic effects:
    Vestibular:
        Vertigo: (NTP)

Chlorophos   (see **Trichlorfon**)

Chloropicrin

Pronunciation guide: klor-oh-PIK-rin

Other names: *Dolochlor*, *Larvacide*, Nitrochloroform, *Picride*, Trichloronitromethane

Uses: in dyes; fumigant; fungicides and insecticides; tear gas; disinfectant; etc.

Ototoxic effects:
    Vestibular:
        Vertigo: (NTP)

Chloroprene   (see **Chlorobutadiene mixture**)

Chlorothalonil

Pronunciation guide: klor-roe-thah-LOH-nil

Other names: *Bravo*, Chloroalonil, *Daconil*, *Exotherm*, *Forturf*, *Termil*

Uses: fungicide; preservative in paints and adhesives

Ototoxic effects:
    Vestibular:
        Ataxia: (NTP)

Notes:

    Chlorothalonil caused ataxia in lab animals (NTP). Ataxia is not reported in humans at this point, but be aware of this possibility.

Chloroxone   (see **Dichlorophenoxyacetic acid**)

Chlorpyrifos

Pronunciation guide: klor-PYE-rih-foss

Other names: *Brodan, Durmet, Dursban, Killmaster, Lorsban, Pyrinex, Terial*

Uses: insecticide; acaricide; etc.

Ototoxic effects:
    Vestibular:
        Ataxia: (NTP)
        Dizziness: (NTP)

Cineol

Pronunciation guide:

Other names: 1,8-Cineol, *Cineole, Eucalyptol,* Limonene oxide

Uses: in veterinary medicine, pharmaceuticals, flavoring, and perfumery

Ototoxic effects:
    Vestibular:
        Ataxia: (NTP)
        Vertigo: (NTP)

Cineole   (see **Cineol**)

Cislin   (see **Deltamethrin**)

CO   (see **Carbon monoxide**)

Coal tar   (see **Creosote**)

Coal tar oil   (see **Creosote**)

Cobalt

Pronunciation guide: KOE-balt

Other names: *Aquacat, Super cobalt*

Uses: chemical manufacturing; electroplating; ceramics; lamp filaments; diagnostic aid in medicine; radiation therapy; in metal alloys; etc.

Ototoxic effects:
Cochlear:
Hearing loss: (NTP)

Columbian spirit   (see **Methyl alcohol**)

Combot   (see **Trichlorfon**)

Compound 1080   (see **Fluoroacetic acid sodium salt**)

Crackdown   (see **Deltamethrin**)

Creosote

Pronunciation guide: KREE-oh-sote

Other names: *Brick oil*, Coal tar, Coal tar oil, *Liquid pitch oil*, Naphthalene oil, Wood creosote

Uses: wood preservative; agent for waterproofing; insecticide, fungicide and germicide; in fuel oil; pitch for roofing; animal and bird repellant; antiseptic and disinfectant; etc.

Ototoxic effects:
Vestibular:
Dizziness: (NTP)
Vertigo: (NTP)

Cresol mixture

Pronunciation guide: KREE-sol

Other names: 3-Cresol, 4-Cresol, 4-Hydroxyloluene, 4-Methylphenol, M-,P-Cresol mixture, P-Cresylic acid, P-Oxytoluene

Uses: used in disinfectants, solvents, cleaners, fumigants, photographic developers, explosives, degreasing compounds, paint-brush cleaners; in the manufacture of chemicals, dyes, plastics and antioxidants; etc.

Ototoxic effects:
Cochlear:
Tinnitus: (NTP)
Vestibular:
Dizziness: (NTP)
Vertigo: (NTP)

Cresyl phosphate   (see **Tricresyl phosphate**)

Cristoxo   (see **Toxaphene**)

Crisulfan   (see **Endosulfan**)

Cryptodine   (see **Ethyl mercury chloride**)

Crysthyon   (see **Gusathion**)

Cyanide of sodium   (see **Sodium cyanide**)

Cyanobrik   (see **Sodium cyanide**)

Cyanogas   (see **Calcium cyanide**)

Cyanogran   (see **Sodium cyanide**)

Cyanol   (see **Aniline**)

Cyclodan   (see **Endosulfan**)

Cyclohexane

Pronunciation guide: sye-kloe-HEX-ayne

Other names: Hexahydrobenzene, Hexamethylene, Hexanaphthene

Uses: solvent; in perfume manufacturing; in manufacturing various chemicals; in solid fuels; etc.

Ototoxic effects:
    Cochlear:
        Tinnitus: (Ka8)
    Vestibular:
        Dizziness: (NTP)
        Loss of balance (loss of equilibrium): (NTP)

Cygon

Pronunciation guide: SYE-gon

Other names: *Daphene, De-fend, Dimeton, Ferkethion, Fosfotox, Perfecthion, Rogor, Roxion, Trimetion*

Uses: insecticides, acaricide

Ototoxic effects:
    Vestibular:
        Ataxia: (NTP)
        Dizziness: (NTP)

Cymag   (see **Sodium cyanide**)

Cypona   (see **Vapona**)

Cytrol   (see **Amino triazole**)

Cyuram   (see **Tetramethylthiuram disulfide**)

Dacamine   (see **Trichlorophenoxyacetic acid**)

Daconil   (see **Chlorothalonil**)

Daphene   (see **Cygon**)

D-camphor   (see **Camphor**)

DDE

Pronunciation guide: dee-dee-ee

Other names: 4,4'-DDE, DDT Dehydrochloride, Dichlorodiphenyldichloroethylene, P,P'-DDE

Uses: insecticide; military products

Ototoxic effects:
  Vestibular:
    Ataxia: (NTP)
    Dizziness: (NTP)

DDT Dehydrochloride   (see **DDE**)

DEA   (see **Diethanolamine**)

Decamine   (see **Dichlorophenoxyacetic acid**)

Dechan   (see **Dicyclohexylamine nitrite**)

Dechlorane   (see **Mirex**)

Decis   (see **Deltamethrin**)

De-fend   (see **Cygon**)

Delnatex   (see **Dioxathion**)

Deltamethrin

Pronunciation guide: del-tah-MEE-thrin

Other names: *Butoflin, Butoss, Cislin, Crackdown, Decis, K-Otek, K-Othrin*

Uses: insecticide

Ototoxic effects:
    Cochlear:
        Tinnitus: (NTP)
    Vestibular:
        Ataxia: (NTP)
        Dizziness: (NTP)

Deltan   (see **Dimethyl sulfoxide**)

Demasorb   (see **Dimethyl sulfoxide**)

Demeton methyl   (see **Methyl demeton**)

Developer R   (see **Resorcinol**)

Devisulphan   (see **Endosulfan**)

Devol red GG   (see **Nitroaniline**)

DFMO   (see **Difluromethylornithine**)

Diazoting salts   (see **Sodium nitrite**)

Dibasic sodium arsenate   (see **Sodium arsenate heptahydrate**)

Dibromo-chloropropane

Pronunciation guide: die-BROE-moe klor-oh-PROE-pane

Other names: 1,2-Dibromo-3-chloropropane, *Fumazone, Nemagon, Nemagone, Nematox*

Uses: soil fumigant, nematocide and pesticide; in organic synthesis

Ototoxic effects:
    Vestibular:
        Ataxia: (NTP)

Dichlorobenzene

Pronunciation guide: die-klor-oh-BEN-zeen

Other names: 1,4-Dichlorobenzene, *Globol, Paracide,* Para-dichlorobenzene, *Paramoth, Parazene*

Uses: insecticide, pesticide, fumigant, germicide and miticide; moth balls; air deodorant; chemical intermediate for dyes and organic chemicals; lubricant; disinfectant; etc.

Ototoxic effects:
> Vestibular:
>> Dizziness: (NTP)
>> Vertigo: (NTP)

Dichlorodifluoromethane

Pronunciation guide: die-klor-oh-die-flyoor-oh-meth-ayne

Other names: *Algofrene, Eskimon 12, Fluorocarbon, Freon, Frigen 12*

Uses: refrigerant; aerosol propellant; rocket propellant; foaming agent; etc.

Ototoxic effects:
> Cochlear:
>> Tinnitus: (NTP)

Dichlorodiphenyldichloroethylene   (see **DDE**)

Dichloroethane

Pronunciation guide: die-klor-oh-ETH-ayne

Other names: 1,2-Dichloroethane, *Borer Sol, Brocide, Dutch oil,* Ethane dichloride, Ethylene chloride

Uses: chemical intermediate in manufacturing various chemical compounds; anti-knock additive in leaded fuels; in color films; pesticides; in extraction of oil from seeds; cleaning agent for textiles; solvent; in organic synthesis; fumigant; etc.

Ototoxic effects:
> Vestibular:
>> Dizziness: (NTP)
>> Nystagmus: (NTP)

Dichlorohydrin   (see **Dichloro propanol**)

Dichloromethane   (see **Methylene chloride**)

Dichlorophenoxyacetic acid

Pronunciation guide: die-KLOR-oh-fee-nox-ee-ah-see-tik ASS-id

Other names: 2,4-D, 2,4-Dichlorophenoxyacetic acid, *Agrotect, Chloroxone, Decamine, Evert DT, Monosan, Netagrone, Salvo, Transamine, Trinoxol, Weedone*

Uses: weed-killer; herbicide; defoliant; etc.

Ototoxic effects:
> Vestibular:
>> Vertigo: (NTP)

Dichloro propanol

Pronunciation guide: DIE-klor-oh PROE-pan-all

Other names: 1,3-Dichloro-2-propanol, 2,3-Dichloro-1-propanol, Alpha-dichlorohydrin, Beta-dichlorohydrin, Dichlorohydrin, *Enodrin,* Glycerol-2,3-dichlorohydrin, Propylene dichlorohydrin

Uses: solvent; in organic syntheses; in paints, lacquers and varnishes; in water colors; in manufacture of photographic chemicals; etc.

Ototoxic effects:
Vestibular:
Vertigo: (NTP)

Dichlorophos (see **Vapona**)

Dicofol

Pronunciation guide: DIE-koe-fol

Other names: *Acarin, Carbax, Hifol, Kelthane, Mitigan*

Uses: acaricide

Ototoxic effects:
Vestibular:
Ataxia: (NTP)
Dizziness: (NTP)
Equilibrium disorder: (NTP)

Dicyclohexylamine nitrite

Pronunciation guide: die-SYE-kloe-hex-ee-lah-meen NYE-tryte

Other names: *Dechan,* Dodecahydrophenylamine nitrite

Uses: corrosion inhibitor

Ototoxic effects:
Vestibular:
Vertigo: (NTP)

Dieldrin

Pronunciation guide: die-EL-drin

Other names: *Alvit, Dieldrix, Illoxol, Octalox, Quintox*

Uses: insecticide

Ototoxic effects:
Vestibular:
Dizziness: (NTP)
Nystagmus: (NTP)

Dieldrix   (see **Dieldrin**)

Diethanolamine

Pronunciation guide: die-eth-an-OLE-ah-meen

Other names: 2,2'-Dihydroxydiethylamine, DEA, *Diolamine*, Iminodiethanol

Uses: emulsifying and dispersing agent; a cation in many water soluble salts of drugs; pesticides; industrial basic solvents; in surface active agents; used in textile specialties, herbicides, petroleum demulsifiers, cosmetics and pharmaceuticals; in organic synthesis; in cutting oils, shampoos, cleaners; etc.

Ototoxic effects:
  Vestibular:
    Ataxia: (NTP)

Diethyl cellosolve   (see **Ethylene glycol diethyl ether**)

Diethylene dioxide   (see **Dioxane**)

Diethylene glycol monoethyl ether

Pronunciation guide: die-ETH-il-een GLY-kol MON-oh-eth-il EE-ther

Other names: *Carbitol, Diglycol, Dioxitol, Ethyl Digol, Solvolsol, Transcutol*

Uses: solvent; in brake fluid; in organic synthesis; for setting the twist it yarns and conditioning yarns and cloth; etc.

Ototoxic effects:
  Vestibular:
    Ataxia: (NTP)
    Dizziness: (NTP)

Diethyl ether   (see **Ethyl ether**)

Difluromethylornithine

Pronunciation guide: die-floo-roe-meth-ee-lore-NITH-een

Other names: Alpha-difluromethylornithine, DFMO

Uses: anti-cancer experimental drug

Ototoxic effects:
  Cochlear:
    Hearing disorder: [1]
    Hearing loss: [2]
    Tinnitus: [127]

Notes:

[1] Temporary or permanent dose-related ototoxicity.[128]

[2] Higher doses can cause hearing loss.[129]

Diglycol   (see **Diethylene glycol monoethyl ether**)

Dihydroxybenzene   (see **Hydroquinone**)

Dimethyl acetamide

Pronunciation guide: die-METH-ill ah-SEE-ta-mide

Other names: Acetyldimethylamine, Dimethylamide acetate

Uses: solvent

Ototoxic effects:
   Cochlear:
      Auditory hallucinations: (NTP)

Dimethyl sulfoxide

Pronunciation guide: die-METH-ill sul-FOX-eyed

Other names: *Deltan, Demasorb, Dimexide, Doligur, Dromisol, Durasorb, Dyadur, Somipront, Syntexan*

Uses: in antifreeze, hydraulic fluid, paint and varnish removers; solvent; in the manufacture of industrial cleaners and pesticides; anti-inflammatory agent; analgesic; etc.

Ototoxic effects:
   Vestibular:
      Dizziness: (NTP)
      Vertigo: (NTP)

Dimethylamide acetate   (see **Dimethyl acetamide**)

Dimethylbenzene   (see **Xylene**)

Dimethylfuran

Pronunciation guide: die-meth-il-FYOOR-an

Other names: 2,5-Dimethylfuran, 2,5-Dimethylfurane

Uses: (not available)

Ototoxic effects:
   Vestibular:
      Dizziness: (NTP)
      Vertigo: (NTP)

Dimeton (see **Cygon**)

Dimexide (see **Dimethyl sulfoxide**)

Dinitrobenzene

Pronunciation guide: die-nye-troe-BEN-zeen

Other names: 1,3-Dinitrobenzene, Binitrobenzene, M-Dinitrobenzene

Uses: organic synthesis; intermediates in dye manufacturing

Ototoxic effects:
  Cochlear:
    Hearing loss: (Nia)
  Vestibular:
    Nystagmus: (NTP)
    Vertigo: (NTP)

Notes:

  The ototoxic effects of **Dinitrobenzene** are made worse by the presence of noise at the same time (Nia).

  See Chapter 8, "The Sinister Partnership Between Ototoxic Agents and Noise" for further information on this chemical.

Dinitrophenol

Pronunciation guide: die-nye-troe-FEN-all

Other names: 2,4-Dinitrophenol, *Aldifen, Dinofan, Fenoxyl, Nitorphene, Solfo black*

Uses: in manufacturing dyes, wood preservatives, insecticides, explosives, herbicides, photographic developers; etc.

Ototoxic effects:
  Vestibular:
    Dizziness: (NTP)
    Vertigo: (NTP)

Dinitrophenylmethane (see **Dinitrotoluene**)

Dinitrotoluene

Pronunciation guide: die-nye-troe-TALL-yoo-een

Other names: 2,4-Dinitrotoluene, 2,4-DNT, 2,6-Dinitrotoluene, 2,6-DNT, Dinitrophenyl-methane, Methyldinitrobenzene, TDNT

Uses: organic synthesis; dyes; explosives; urethane polymers; etc.

Ototoxic effects:
> Vestibular:
>> Ataxia: (NTP)
>> Dizziness: (NTP)
>> Vertigo: (NTP)

Dinofan   (see **Dinitrophenol**)

Dinoxol   (see **Trichlorophenoxyacetic acid**)

Diokan   (see **Dioxane**)

Diolamine   (see **Diethanolamine**)

Dioxane

Pronunciation guide: die-OX-ayne

Other names: 1,4-Dioxane, Diethylene dioxide, *Diokan*, Ethylene glycol ethylene ether, P-Dioxane

Uses: solvent; biochemical intermediate; etc.

Ototoxic effects:
> Vestibular:
>> Dizziness: (NTP)
>> Vertigo: (NTP)

Dioxane phosphate   (see **Dioxathion**)

Dioxathion

Pronunciation guide: die-ox-ah-THY-on

Other names: *Delnatex*, Dioxane phosphate, *Dioxation*, *Hercules*, *Kavadel*, *Ruphos*

Uses: insecticide; miticide; acaricide

Ototoxic effects:
> Vestibular:
>> Ataxia: (NTP)
>> Dizziness: (NTP)

Dioxation   (see **Dioxathion**)

Dioxitol   (see **Diethylene glycol monoethyl ether**)

Diphenyldiazene oxide   (see **Azoxybenzene**)

Diphosphoric acid tetraethyl ester   (see **Tetraethylpyrophosphate**)

Dipotassium dichromate   (see **Potassium dichromate**)

Dipropyl   (see **Hexane**)

Dipropylmethane   (see **Heptane**)

Dipterex   (see **Trichlorfon**)

Diurol   (see **Amino triazole**)

Dodecahydrophenylamine nitrite   (see **Dicyclohexylamine nitrite**)

Doligur   (see **Dimethyl sulfoxide**)

Dolochlor   (see **Chloropicrin**)

Dolomide   (see **Hydroxybenzamide**)

Dowchlor   (see **Chlordane**)

Drinox   (see **Aldrin**)

Drinox H-34   (see **Heptachlor**)

Dromisol   (see **Dimethyl sulfoxide**)

Dukeron   (see **Trichloroethylene**)

Durafur black RC   (see **Phenylenediamine dihydrochloride**)

Duraphos   (see **Mevinphos**)

Durasorb   (see **Dimethyl sulfoxide**)

Duratox   (see **Methyl demeton**)

Durmet   (see **Chlorpyrifos**)

Dursban   (see **Chlorpyrifos**)

Dutch oil   (see **Dichloroethane**)

Dyadur   (see **Dimethyl sulfoxide**)

Dylox   (see **Trichlorfon**)

Econazole nitrate

Pronunciation guide: ee-KON-ah-zole NYE-trate

Other names: *Ecostatin, Ifenec, Micofugal, Palavale, Pargin, Spectazole*

Uses: anti-fungal agent

Ototoxic effects:
    Cochlear:
        Auditory hallucinations: (NTP)
    Vestibular:
        Dizziness: (NTP)

Notes:

    Auditory hallucinations are mild and temporary (NTP).

Ecostatin   (see **Econazole nitrate**)

Elon   (see **Methylaminophenol sulfate**)

Emulsion 212   (see **Tris dichloro propyl phosphate**)

Endocel   (see **Endosulfan**)

Endosulfan

Pronunciation guide: end-oh-SUL-fan

Other names: *Crisulfan, Cyclodan, Devisulphan, Endocel, Malix, Thifor, Thiodan*

Uses: insecticide, pesticide

Ototoxic effects:
    Vestibular:
        Ataxia: (NTP)

Endrex   (see **Endrin**)

Endrin

Pronunciation guide: EN-drin

Other names: *Endrex, Hexadrin, Mendrin, Nendrin*

Uses: insecticide; avicide; rodenticide; pesticide

Ototoxic effects:
    Cochlear:
        Hearing loss: (NTP)
    Vestibular:
        Ataxia: (NTP)
        Dizziness: (NTP)

Notes:

Hearing loss is temporary (NTP).

Enodrin   (see **Dichloro propanol**)

Epoxypropane

Pronunciation guide: ee-POX-ee-proe-pane

Other names: 1,2-Epoxypropane, Methyl ethylene oxide, Methyloxirane, Propene oxide, Propylene epoxide, Propylene oxide

Uses: fumigant; solvent; used in polyols for urethane foams, propylene glycols, surfactants, detergents, synthetic lubricants, elastomers; etc.

Ototoxic effects:
    Vestibular:
        Ataxia: (NTP)
        Dizziness: (NTP)

Erinitrit   (see **Sodium nitrite**)

Eskimon 12   (see **Dichlorodifluoromethane**)

Essence of mirbane   (see **Nitrobenzene**)

Esteron   (see **Trichlorophenoxyacetic acid**)

Ethane dichloride   (see **Dichloroethane**)

Ethanol

Pronunciation guide: ETH-ah-nol

Other names: Alcohol, Anhydrol, Ethyl alcohol, Ethyl hydrate, Grain alcohol, Molasses alcohol, Potato alcohol, Spirits of wine

Uses: solvent; antiseptic; sedative; alcoholic beverages; in the manufacture of perfumes, pharmaceuticals and various chemical compounds; etc.

Ototoxic effects:
    Cochlear:
        Tinnitus: (Ka7)
    Vestibular:
        Ataxia: (NTP)
        Dizziness: (NTP)

Ethenylbenzene   (see **Styrene**)

Ether   (see **Ethyl ether**)

Ethoxyethane   (see **Ethyl ether**)

Ethoxyethanol

Pronunciation guide: eth-ox-ee-ETH-ah-nol

Other names: 2-Ethoxyethanol, *Cellosolve*, Ethylene glycol ethyl ether, Glycol ethyl ether, Hydroxy ether, *Oxitol*

Uses: solvent; anti-icing additive for aviation fuels; in varnish removers, cleaning solutions, dyes; etc.

Ototoxic effects:
    Vestibular:
        Vertigo: (NTP)

Ethyl alcohol   (see **Ethanol**)

Ethyl benzene   (see **Xylene**)

Ethyl Digol   (see **Diethylene glycol monoethyl ether**)

Ethyl ether

Pronunciation guide: ETH-il EE-ther

Other names: Anesthetic ether, Diethyl ether, Ether, Ethoxyethane, Ethyl oxide

Uses: solvent; reagent in organic synthesis; primer for gasoline engines; refrigerant; used in diesel fuels, in dry cleaning, inhalation anesthetic; etc.

Ototoxic effects:
    Vestibular:
        Ataxia: (NTP)
        Dizziness: (NTP)
        Vertigo: (NTP)

Ethyl glyme   (see **Ethylene glycol diethyl ether**)

Ethyl hydrate   (see **Ethanol**)

Ethyl mercury chloride

Pronunciation guide: ETH-il MER-kyoo-ree

Other names: *Ceresan*, Chloroethylmercury, *Cryptodine*, *Granosan*

Uses: Polymerization catalyst; seed and bulb fungicide

Ototoxic effects:
    Vestibular:
        Ataxia: (NTP)

Ethyl methyl ketone   (see **Methyl ethyl ketone**)

Ethyl oxide   (see **Ethyl ether**)

Ethylene alcohol   (see **Ethylene glycol**)

Ethylene chloride   (see **Dichloroethane**)

Ethylene chlorohydrin   (see **Chloroethanol**)

Ethylene dihydrate   (see **Ethylene glycol**)

Ethylene glycol

Pronunciation guide: ETH-il-een GLY-call

Other names: Ethylene alcohol, Ethylene dihydrate, Glycol, Monoethylene glycol, *Tescol*

Uses: solvent; used in antifreeze, in hydraulic brake fluid, in the formulation of inks; softening agent; used in the synthesis of explosives and other chemical compounds; etc.

Ototoxic effects:
Vestibular:
Dizziness: (NTP)
Nystagmus: (NTP)

Ethylene glycol diethyl ether

Pronunciation guide: ETH-il-een GLY-call die-ETH-ill EE-ther

Other names: 1,2-Diethoxyethane, *Diethyl cellosolve, Ethyl glyme*

Uses: solvent

Ototoxic effects:
Vestibular:
Ataxia: (NTP)
Nystagmus: (NTP)
Vertigo: (NTP)

Ethylene glycol ethyl ether   (see **Ethoxyethanol**)

Ethylene glycol ethylene ether   (see **Dioxane**)

Ethylene glycol methyl ether   (see **Methoxyethanol**)

Ethylene tetrachloride   (see **Tetrachloroethylene**)

Ethylene trichloride   (see **Trichloroethylene**)

Eucalyptol   (see **Cineol**)

Evert DT   (see **Dichlorophenoxyacetic acid**)

Exotherm   (see **Chlorothalonil**)

Fast red base GG   (see **Nitroaniline**)

Fenatrol   (see **Atrazine**)

Fenoxyl   (see **Dinitrophenol**)

Fenthion   (see **Baytex**)

Fentoxan   (see **Azoxybenzene**)

Ferkethion   (see **Cygon**)

Fermide   (see **Tetramethylthiuram disulfide**)

Fernasan   (see **Tetramethylthiuram disulfide**)

Ferriamicide   (see **Mirex**)

Filmerine   (see **Sodium nitrite**)

Fluoroacetic acid sodium salt

Pronunciation guide: flure-oh-ah-SEE-tik ASS-id

Other names: *Compound 1080, Ratbane 1080,* Sodium fluoacetate, Sodium monofluoroacetate

Uses: rodenticide; insecticide

Ototoxic effects:
  Vestibular:
    Nystagmus: (NTP)

Fluorocarbon   (see **Dichlorodifluoromethane**)

Folbex   (see **Chlorobenzilate**)

Formaldehyde

Pronunciation guide: for-MAL-deh-hyde

Other names: *Formalin,* Formic aldehyde, *Formol, Karsan, Lysoform,* Methyl aldehyde, Methylene glycol, Oxomethane, *Paraform*

Uses: preservative; disinfectant; antiseptic; germicide; fungicide; in organic chemicals; in the manufacture of phenolic resins; in ceiling and wall insulation; etc.

Ototoxic effects:
    Vestibular:
        Dizziness: (NTP)
        Vertigo: (NTP)

Formalin   (see **Formaldehyde**)

Formic aldehyde   (see **Formaldehyde**)

Formol   (see **Formaldehyde**)

Forron   (see **Trichlorophenoxyacetic acid**)

Forturf   (see **Chlorothalonil**)

Foschlor   (see **Trichlorfon**)

Fosdrin   (see **Mevinphos**)

Fosfothion   (see **Malathion**)

Fosfotox   (see **Cygon**)

Fosvex   (see **Tetraethylpyrophosphate**)

Fourrine   (see **Phenylenediamine dihydrochloride**)

Fourrine EW   (see **Resorcinol**)

Freon   (see **Dichlorodifluoromethane**)

Frigen 12   (see **Dichlorodifluoromethane**)

Fumazone   (see **Dibromo-chloropropane**)

Fyrol FR 2   (see **Tris dichloro propyl phosphate**)

Geniphene   (see **Toxaphene**)

Genol   (see **Methylaminophenol sulfate**)

Germalgene   (see **Trichloroethylene**)

Gestid   (see **Mevinphos**)

Globol   (see **Dichlorobenzene**)

Glycerin   (see **Glycerol**)

Glycerol

Pronunciation guide: GLISS-er-ol

Other names: Glycerin

Uses: solvent; emulsifying agent; food additive; sweetening agent; used in plasticizer manufacturing; in nitroglycerine, antifreeze, antibiotics, cosmetics, liquid soap and printing inks; laxative; etc.

Ototoxic effects:
    Cochlear:
        Hearing loss: (NTP)
    Vestibular:
        Dizziness: (NTP)

Notes:

    Hearing loss is temporary (NTP).

Glycerol-2,3-dichlorohydrin   (see **Dichloro propanol**)

Glycol   (see **Ethylene glycol**)

Glycol chlorohydrin   (see **Chloroethanol**)

Glycol ethyl ether   (see **Ethoxyethanol**)

Grain alcohol   (see **Ethanol**)

Granosan   (see **Ethyl mercury chloride**)

Graphol   (see **Methylaminophenol sulfate**)

Grisol   (see **Tetraethylpyrophosphate**)

Gusathion

Pronunciation guide: GUS-ah-thy-on

Other names: Azinophos-methyl, *Bayer 9027*, *Carfene*, *Crysthyon*, Methyl guthion, Methylazinphos

Uses: insecticide; acaricide

Ototoxic effects:
    Vestibular:
        Ataxia: (NTP)
        Dizziness: (NTP)
        Vertigo: (NTP)

Halon 1001   (see **Methyl bromide**)

Heptachlor

Pronunciation guide: HEP-tah-klor

Other names: *Agroceres, Drinox H-34,* Heptachlorane, *Heptagran, Heptamul, Heptox, Rhodiachlor*

Uses: insecticide; fumigant

Ototoxic effects:
Vestibular:
Ataxia: (NTP)

Heptachlorane   (see **Heptachlor**)

Heptagran   (see **Heptachlor**)

Heptamul   (see **Heptachlor**)

Heptane

Pronunciation guide: HEP-tane

Other names: Dipropylmethane, Heptylhydride, N-Heptane, Normal heptane

Uses: solvent; in rubber tire manufacture; in chemical synthesis; etc.

Ototoxic effects:
Cochlear:
Hearing loss: [1]
Vestibular:
Dizziness: [130]
Ataxia: [131, 132]
Vertigo: [133]

Notes:

[1] Exposure to **Heptane** and loud noise at the same time can result in greater hearing loss than would normally result from exposure to both **Heptane** and noise separately (Nia).

See Chapter 8, "The Sinister Partnership Between Ototoxic Agents and Noise" for further information on this chemical.

Heptox   (see **Heptachlor**)

Heptylhydride   (see **Heptane**)

Herbizole   (see **Amino triazole**)

Hercules   (see **Dioxathion**)

Herkal   (see **Vapona**)

Hermal   (see **Tetramethylthiuram disulfide**)

Hexadrin   (see **Endrin**)

Hexafluoroisopropanol   (see **Hexafluoro propanol**)

Hexafluoro propanol

Pronunciation guide: HEX-ah-flyoo-oh PROE-pan-all

Other names: 1,1,1,3,3,3-Hexafluoro-2-propanol, Hexafluoroisopropanol, HFIP

Uses: esterification agent

Ototoxic effects:
    Vestibular:
        Dizziness: (NTP)
        Vertigo: (NTP)

Hexahydrobenzene   (see **Cyclohexane**)

Hexamethylene   (see **Cyclohexane**)

Hexamite   (see **Tetraethylpyrophosphate**)

Hexanaphthene   (see **Cyclohexane**)

Hexane

Pronunciation guide: HEX-ayne

Other names: Dipropyl, Hexyl hydride, N-Hexane, *Skellysolve B*

Uses: solvent; used in low-temperature thermometers; paint diluent; laboratory reagent; etc.

Ototoxic effects:
    Cochlear:
        Hearing loss: (Nia)
        Tinnitus: (Ka8)
    Vestibular:
        Dizziness: (NTP)
        Vertigo: (NTP)

Notes:

    Hexane appears to damage the auditory pathways in the brain (Ryb).

    Exposure to **Hexane** and loud noise at the same time can result in greater hearing loss than would normally result from exposure to both **Hexane** and noise separately (Nia).

    See Chapter 8, "The Sinister Partnership Between Ototoxic Agents and Noise" for further information on this chemical.

Hexanedinitrile   (see **Adiponitrile**)

Hexanone

Pronunciation guide: HEX-ah-noan

Other names: 2-Hexanone, Butyl methyl ketone, Methyl N-butyl keytone

Uses: solvent for fats, ink thinners, lacquers, nitrocellulose, oils, resins and waxes; used in printing plasticized fabrics

Ototoxic effects:
  Cochlear:
      Tinnitus: (Ka8)

Hexit   (see **Lindane**)

Hexyl hydride   (see **Hexane**)

HFIP   (see **Hexafluoro propanol**)

Hifol   (see **Dicofol**)

Hydrazomethane   (see **Methyl hydrazine**)

Hydrocyanic acid sodium salt   (see **Sodium cyanide**)

Hydroquinone

Pronunciation guide: hye-droe-KWIN-ohn

Other names: Alpha-hydroquinone, Benzohydroquinone, Beta-quinol, Dihydroxybenzene, P-Benzenediol, *Quinol, Tecquinol*

Uses: photographic reducer and developer; stabilizer in paints, varnishes, motor fuels and oils; antioxidant for fats and oils; etc.

Ototoxic effects:
  Cochlear:
      Tinnitus: (NTP)
  Vestibular:
      Dizziness: (NTP)

Hydroxybenzamide

Pronunciation guide: hye-drox-ee-BEN-zah-mide

Other names: 2-Hydroxybenzamide, *Benesal, Dolomide, Salicylamide, Salymid, Urtosal*

Uses: used in medicine as an analgesic, antipyretic and anti-inflammatory agent; in C.I. 43815 mordant dye

Ototoxic effects:
    Cochlear:
        Hearing loss: (NTP)
    Vestibular:
        Dizziness: (NTP)

Hydroxybenzene   (see **Phenol**)

Hydroxy ether   (see **Ethoxyethanol**)

Hydroxymethylmercury   (see **Methyl mercury hydroxide**)

Hydroxytoluene   (see **Benzyl alcohol**)

Ifenec   (see **Econazole nitrate**)

Illoxol   (see **Dieldrin**)

Iminodiethanol   (see **Diethanolamine**)

Inhibisol   (see **Trichloroethane**)

Iodine (Iodophor, Povidone iodine)

Pronunciation guide: EYE-eh-dine (eye-OH-deh-for, POH-vih-done EYE-eh-dine)

Other names: *Betadine*, Polyvinylpyrrolidone, *Proviodine*

Uses: antimicrobial; antiseptic; bactericide; contact sanitizer; disinfectant; fungicide; virucide

Ototoxic effects:
    Unspecified/General Ear Conditions:
        Ototoxicity: (Str) [134]

Iodophor (see **Iodine**)

Iopezite   (see **Potassium dichromate**)

Isobutyl nitrite   (see **Butyl nitrite**)

Kamfochlor   (see **Toxaphene**)

Karbofos   (see **Malathion**)

Karmex   (see **Monuron**)

Karsan   (see **Formaldehyde**)

Kavadel   (see **Dioxathion**)

Kelthane   (see **Dicofol**)

Killax   (see **Tetraethylpyrophosphate**)

Killmaster   (see **Chlorpyrifos**)

Kop-mite   (see **Chlorobenzilate**)

K-Otek   (see **Deltamethrin**)

K-Othrin   (see **Deltamethrin**)

Kronitex   (see **Tricresyl phosphate**)

Kwell   (see **Lindane**)

Kyanol   (see **Aniline**)

Larvacide   (see **Chloropicrin**)

L-Asparty-L-phenylalanine methyl ester   (see **Aspartame**)

L-Camphor   (see **Camphor**)

Lead

Pronunciation guide: LED

Other names:

Uses: in lead paints, leaded gasoline and lead crystal glassware; in imported or old pottery; lead chromates used in colored plastics

Ototoxic effects:
    Cochlear:
        Hearing loss: (ATS, Ryb)
        Tinnitus: (ATS)
    Vestibular:
        Vertigo: (Ryb)

Notes:

Most of the **Lead** pollution in our environment today comes from all the **Lead** once used in leaded gasoline. This **Lead** is leached from the soil by acid pH. Thus acid rain may increase our exposure to **Lead** in food and drinking water (Ryb).

Children under 6 years of age are particularly susceptible to the effects of **Lead**. Note that **Lead** exposure is especially dangerous to unborn children. **Lead** affects the nervous system. Adverse effects from **Lead** can happen at levels once thought to be safe. Childhood **Lead** toxicity can have permanent effects.[135]

Sensorineural hearing loss increases with increasing blood **Lead** levels. The longer you are exposed to **Lead**, the greater the hearing loss. Hearing loss is greater at the higher frequencies (Ryb).

It seems that there is no safe threshold below which **Lead** does not affect hearing.[136]

Hearing loss may contribute to the apparent learning disabilities or poor classroom behavior exhibited by children with **Lead** toxicity. Hearing loss is not uncommon in children exposed to **Lead**.[137]

In addition to hearing loss, **Lead** slows down the normal auditory activity along the auditory pathways in our brains (Ryb). It also damages the myelin sheath that surrounds and insulates the auditory nerve.[138]

Tinnitus (ringing in the ears) can be associated with severe anemia caused by **Lead** toxicity.[139]

Note that iron and calcium deficiencies enhance the body's absorption of **Lead**.[140, 141]

The ototoxic effects of **Lead** are made worse by the presence of noise at the same time (Nia).

See Chapter 8, "The Sinister Partnership Between Ototoxic Agents and Noise" for further information on this chemical.

Lead dimethyldithiocarbamate

Pronunciation guide: LED die-METH-ill-die-THY-oh-KAR-bah-mate

Other names: *Ledate*, Methyl ledate

Uses: vulcanization accelerator

Ototoxic effects:
    Vestibular:
        Ataxia: (NTP)
        Dizziness: (NTP)

Ledate   (see **Lead dimethyldithiocarbamate**)

Lime nitrogen   (see **Calcium cyanamide**)

Limonene oxide   (see **Cineol**)

Lindan   (see **Vapona**)

Lindane

Pronunciation guide: LYNN-dane

Other names: *Agrocide*, Benzene hexachloride, *Hexit*, *Kwell*

Uses: ectoparasiticide; insecticide; pesticide; scabicide

Ototoxic effects:
    Cochlear:
        Tinnitus: (Ka8)
    Vestibular:
        Ataxia: (AHF, NTP)
        Dizziness: (NDH, NTP)
        Loss of balance: (NTP)

Lindol   (see **Tricresyl phosphate**)

Liquid pitch oil   (see **Creosote**)

Lirobetarex   (see **Monuron**)

Lirohex   (see **Tetraethylpyrophosphate**)

Liromat   (see **Malaoxon**)

Lorsban   (see **Chlorpyrifos**)

Lunar caustic   (see **Silver nitrate**)

Lyddite   (see **Picric acid**)

Lysoform   (see **Formaldehyde**)

M—3-Aminoanisole   (see **Anisidine**)

Malacide   (see **Malathion**)

Malaoxon

Pronunciation guide: mah-lah-OX-on

Other names: *Liromat*, Malaoxone, Oxycarbophos

Uses: pesticide

Ototoxic effects:
    Vestibular:
        Ataxia: (NTP)
        Dizziness: (NTP)
        Nystagmus: (NTP)

Malaoxone   (see **Malaoxon**)

Malathion

Pronunciation guide: mal-ah-THY-on

Other names: *Carbetox, Carbophos, Chemathion, Fosfothion, Karbofos, Malacide, Mercaptothion*

Uses: insecticide; acaricide; etc.

Ototoxic effects:
  Vestibular:
      Ataxia: (NTP)
      Dizziness: (NTP)

Malix   (see **Endosulfan**)

Manganese

Pronunciation guide: MANG-gah-neese

Other names:

Uses: in metallurgy of ferrous metals; electroplating; etc.

Ototoxic effects:
  Cochlear:
      Hearing loss: (Ryb)
  Vestibular:
      Vestibular disorder: (Ryb)

Notes:

> Sensorineural hearing loss from exposure to **Manganese** is in both the low and high frequencies, leaving the mid-frequencies with better hearing (Ryb). An audiogram typically would show an inverted "cookie bite" loss.

> **Manganese** can cause abnormal results to auditory brainstem response (ABR) tests indicating damage to the auditory circuits in the brain.[142]

> The ototoxic effects of **Manganese** are made worse by the presence of noise at the same time (Nia).

> See Chapter 8, "The Sinister Partnership Between Ototoxic Agents and Noise" for further information on this chemical.

Manganese sulfate monohydrate (see also Manganese)

Pronunciation guide: MANG-gah-neese SUL-fate mon-oh-HYE-drate

Other names: Manganese (II) sulfate monohydrate, Manganous sulfate monohydrate

Uses: porcelain glaze; fertilizer additive; used in fungicides, paints, varnishes, textile dyes, medicines and ceramics; dietary supplement; etc.

Ototoxic effects:
  Cochlear:
    Hearing loss: (NTP)
  Vestibular:
    Ataxia: (NTP)
    Loss of balance: (NTP)

Manganese (II) sulfate monohydrate   (see **Manganese sulfate monohydrate**)

Manganous sulfate monohydrate   (see **Manganese sulfate monohydrate**)

M-Anisidine   (see **Anisidine**)

Maralate   (see **Methoxychlor**)

Masoten   (see **Trichlorfon**)

M-Dihydroxybenzene   (see **Resorcinol**)

M-Dinitrobenzene   (see **Dinitrobenzene**)

Meetco   (see **Methyl ethyl ketone**)

Melinite   (see **Picric acid**)

Mendrin   (see **Endrin**)

Menite   (see **Mevinphos**)

Mercaptothion   (see **Malathion**)

Mercury (see also Methyl mercury)

Pronunciation guide: MER-kyoo-ree

Other names:

Uses: in producing chlorine gas and caustic soda; in thermometers, dental fillings, batteries

Ototoxic effects:
  Cochlear:
    Hearing loss: (ATS, Ryb)
    Tinnitus: (Ka7)
  Vestibular:
    Ataxia: (Ryb)

Notes:

  Exposure to **Mercury** (and **Methyl mercury**) can cause sensorineural hearing loss.[143]

Mercury combines with other elements to form inorganic mercury compounds. **Mercury** also combines with carbon to form organic mercury compounds. The most common one, **Methyl mercury**, is produced mainly by small organisms (bacteria) in the water or soil. We can ingest **Mercury** in the food we eat, the water we drink and the air we breathe.[144]

Minamata disease (**Mercury** poisoning) is named after the place in Japan where it was described back in 1953. Many people became sick from eating seafood contaminated with **Mercury**-containing effluent that was discharged from a nearby chemical factory. Minamata disease begins with various symptoms followed by ataxia and hearing loss. In fact, up to 80% of people with Minamata disease have hearing loss (Ryb).

Hearing loss from **Mercury** poisoning is usually permanent although in some cases it is temporary. In one follow-up study between 14 and 24 years after being exposed to Mercury, 28% of those exposed to **Mercury** still had hearing loss while 7% showed improvement (Ryb).

In 1965 a **Methyl mercury** poisoning from eating contaminated seafood (also in Japan) had the symptoms of Minamata disease. Of 149 people with neurologic disturbances, 35% had mild hearing losses, 16% had moderate hearing losses while 46% had normal hearing (Ryb).

Of 49 Iraqi children poisoned with **Methyl mercury**, 24 (49%) had hearing losses ranging from mild to total deafness (Ryb).

It appears that the early and middle stages of **Mercury** toxicity damage the cochlea, whereas the final stage affects the auditory pathways in the brain. Mercury also damages the myelin sheath that surrounds and insulates the auditory nerve.[145] Hearing loss develops quite early in **Methyl mercury** poisoning. The hearing loss covers the whole hearing spectrum from low to high frequency (Ryb).

Exposure to **Mercury** and loud noise at the same time can result in greater hearing loss than would normally result from exposure to both **Mercury** and noise separately (Nia).

See Chapter 8, "The Sinister Partnership Between Ototoxic Agents and Noise" for further information on this chemical.

Metasystox   (see **Methyl demeton**)

Methacide   (see **Toluene**)

Methane dichloride   (see **Methylene chloride**)

Methane trichloride   (see **Chloroform**)

Methanol   (see **Methyl alcohol**)

Methoxcide   (see **Methoxychlor**)

Methoxychlor

Pronunciation guide: meth-OX-ee-klor

Other names: *Chemform, Maralate, Methoxcide, Metox*

Uses: insecticide; ectoparasiticide

Ototoxic effects:
Vestibular:
Ataxia: (NTP)

Methoxyethanol

Pronunciation guide: meth-ox-ee-ETH-an-ol

Other names: 2-Methoxyethanol, Ethylene glycol methyl ether, Methyl glycol

Uses: solvent; jet fuel deicing additive; used in nail polish, quick-drying varnishes and enamels; etc.

Ototoxic effects:
Cochlear:
Hearing disorder: (NTP)
Vestibular:
Ataxia: (NTP)
Dizziness: (NTP)

Methyl acetone   (see **Methyl ethyl ketone**)

Methyl alcohol

Pronunciation guide: METH-il AL-koe-hall

Other names: *Carbinol, Columbian spirit*, Methanol, Methyl hydroxide, Wood alcohol, Wood naphtha

Uses: solvent; used in organic synthesis; antifreeze; food additive; used in paint, varnish removers, cleaning and dewaxing preparations, embalming fluids, dyes; etc.

Ototoxic effects:
Vestibular:
Dizziness: (NTP)
Vertigo: (NTP)

Methyl aldehyde   (see **Formaldehyde**)

Methylaminophenol sulfate

Pronunciation guide: METH-il-ah-meen-oh-fee-nall SUL-fate

Other names: *Armol, Elon, Genol, Graphol, Metol, Photol, Pictol*, P-Methylaminophenol sulfate, *Rhodol, Verol*

Uses: photographic developer; hair and fur dyes

Ototoxic effects:
  Vestibular:
    Vertigo: (NTP)

Methylazinphos   (see **Gusathion**)

Methylbenzene   (see **Toluene**)

Methylbenzol   (see **Toluene**)

Methyl bromide

Pronunciation guide: METH-il BROE-mide

Other names: *Brom-o-Gas*, Bromomethane, *Halon 1001*, *Pestmaster*, *Zytox*

Uses: used in ionization chambers; refrigerant; fire extinguishing agent; soil fumigant; industrial solvent; herbicide; insecticide; used in degreasing wool, nuts and seeds; in manufacturing many drugs; etc.

Ototoxic effects:
  Cochlear:
    Hearing loss: (NTP)
  Vestibular:
    Ataxia: (NTP)
    Dizziness: (NTP)
    Nystagmus: (NTP)
    Vertigo: (NTP)

Methyl chloride

Pronunciation guide: METH-il KLOR-eyed

Other names: Chloromethane, Monochloromethane

Uses: in organic chemistry; extractant for greases, oils and resins; solvent; refrigerant; local anesthetic; fumigant; food additive; herbicide; in the manufacture of various chemical substances; etc.

Ototoxic effects:
  Cochlear:
    Tinnitus: (Ka8)
  Vestibular:
    Ataxia: (NTP)
    Dizziness: (NTP)
    Nystagmus: (NTP)
    Vertigo: (NTP)

Methyl chloroform   (see **Trichloroethane**)

Methyl chlorophos   (see **Trichlorfon**)

Methyl demeton

Pronunciation guide: METH-il DEM-eh-ton

Other names: *Bayer 21/116*, Demeton methyl, *Duratox*, *Metasystox*

Uses: insecticide; acaricide

Ototoxic effects:
 Cochlear:
  Auditory disorder (inner ear irritation): (NTP)
 Vestibular:
  Ataxia: (NTP)
  Dizziness: (NTP)

Methyldinitrobenzene   (see **Dinitrotoluene**)

Methylene acetone   (see **Methyl vinyl ketone**)

Methylene chloride

Pronunciation guide: METH-ih-leen KLOR-eyed

Other names: Dichloromethane, Methane dichloride, *Narkotil*, *Solaesthin*

Uses: in rubber adhesives; in pharmaceuticals; paint and varnish remover; solvent; refrigerant; fumigant; in organic synthesis; etc.

Ototoxic effects:
 Cochlear:
  Auditory hallucinations: (NTP)
  Hearing loss: (ATS)
  Tinnitus: (Ka8)
 Vestibular:
  Dizziness: (NTP)
  Vertigo: (NTP)

Notes:

 Exposure to lower levels of **Methylene chloride** in air can lead to slight hearing loss.[146]

Methylene glycol   (see **Formaldehyde**)

Methyl ethyl ketone

Pronunciation guide: METH-il ETH-il KEE-tone

Other names: 2-Butanone, Butanone, Ethyl methyl ketone, *Meetco*, Methyl acetone

Uses: solvent; used in manufacture of synthetic resins; intermediate in drug manufacture; intermediate in manufacture of ketones and amines; etc.

Ototoxic effects:
>   Vestibular:
>> Dizziness: (NTP)
>> Vertigo: (NTP)

Notes:

>   Vertigo is mild (NTP).

Methyl ethylene oxide   (see **Epoxypropane**)

Methyl glycol   (see **Methoxyethanol**)

Methyl guthion   (see **Gusathion**)

Methyl hydrazine

Pronunciation guide: METH-il HYE-drah-zeen

Other names: 1-Methylhydrazine, Hydrazomethane, Monomethylhydrazine

Uses: solvent; intermediate in chemical synthesis; rocket fuel

Ototoxic effects:
>   Vestibular:
>> Ataxia: (NTP)

Methyl hydroxide   (see **Methyl alcohol**)

Methylhydroxymercury   (see **Methyl mercury hydroxide**)

Methyl ledate   (see **Lead dimethyldithiocarbamate**)

Methyl mercury chloride (see also Mercury)

Pronunciation guide: METH-il MER-kyoo-ree KLOR-eyed

Other names: Chloromethylmercury, Methyl mercury (II) chloride

Uses: fungicide

Ototoxic effects:
>   Cochlear:
>> Hearing loss: (NTP)
>   Vestibular:
>> Ataxia: (NTP)

Methyl mercury (II) chloride   (see **Methyl mercury chloride**)

Methyl mercury hydroxide (see also Mercury)

Pronunciation guide: METH-il MER-kyoo-ree hye-DROX-eyed

Other names: Hydroxymethylmercury, Methylhydroxymercury, *Panogen soil drench*

Uses: defoliant; fungicide; epoxidation catalyst

Ototoxic effects:
Cochlear:
Hearing loss: (NTP)
Vestibular:
Ataxia: (NTP)
Dizziness: (NTP)
Nystagmus: (NTP)

Notes:

Symptoms may not appear until weeks or months after acute exposure to toxic concentrations. Damage tends to be permanent (NTP).

Methyl N-butyl keytone   (see **Hexanone**)

Methyl N-Valerate   (see **Methyl valerate**)

Methyloxirane   (see **Epoxypropane**)

Methyl pentanoate   (see **Methyl valerate**)

Methyl thiram   (see **Tetramethylthiuram disulfide**)

Methyl toluene   (see **Chlorobutadiene mixture**)

Methyl trichloride   (see **Chloroform**)

Methyl valerate

Pronunciation guide: METH-il VAL-er-ate

Other names: Methyl N-Valerate, Methyl pentanoate

Uses: (not available)

Ototoxic effects:
Vestibular:
Dizziness: (NTP)
Vertigo: (NTP)

Methyl vinyl ketone

Pronunciation guide: METH-il VIE-nil KEE-tone

Other names: 2-Butenone, Acetyl ethylene, Methylene acetone, Vinyl methyl ketone

Uses: monomer for vinyl resins; alkylating agent; intermediate for plastics; in cigarette smoke; etc.

Ototoxic effects:
    Vestibular:
        Dizziness: (NTP)
        Vertigo: (NTP)

Metol   (see **Methylaminophenol sulfate**)

Metox   (see **Methoxychlor**)

Mevinphos

Pronunciation guide: meh-VIN-fos

Other names: *Apavinphos, Duraphos, Fosdrin, Gestid, Menite,* Phosdrin, Phosfene

Uses: insecticide; acaricide

Ototoxic effects:
    Vestibular:
        Ataxia: (NTP)
        Dizziness: (NTP)

M-Hydroquinone   (see **Resorcinol**)

Micofugal   (see **Econazole nitrate**)

Mineral naphtha   (see **Benzene**)

Mirbane oil   (see **Nitrobenzene**)

Mirex

Pronunciation guide: MY-rex

Other names: *Bichlorendo,* Dechlorane, *Ferriamicide,* Perchloropentacyclodecane

Uses: insecticide; pesticide; flame retardant; used in paper, paint, rubber, electrical, adhesive and textile applications; etc.

Ototoxic effects:
    Vestibular:
        Ataxia: (NTP)

Mitigan   (see **Dicofol**)

Molasses alcohol   (see **Ethanol**)

Monochloromethane   (see **Methyl chloride**)

Monoethylene glycol   (see **Ethylene glycol**)

Monomethylhydrazine   (see **Methyl hydrazine**)

Monosan   (see **Dichlorophenoxyacetic acid**)

Monurex   (see **Monuron**)

Monuron

Pronunciation guide: moh-NYOOR-on

Other names: *Chlorfenidim, Karmex, Lirobetarex, Monurex, Monuruon, Telvar*

Uses: herbicide; plant growth regulator; etc.

Ototoxic effects:
    Vestibular:
        Ataxia: (NTP)

Monuruon   (see **Monuron**)

M-,P-Cresol mixture   (see **Cresol mixture**)

Nalowax   (see **Chloronaphthalene**)

Naphthalene oil   (see **Creosote**)

Narcogen   (see **Trichloroethylene**)

Narkotil   (see **Methylene chloride**)

N-Butanol   (see **Butyl alcohol**)

N-Butyl alcohol   (see **Butyl alcohol**)

N-Butyl nitrite   (see **Butyl nitrite**)

NCI-C00599   (see **Photodieldrin**)

Necatorine   (see **Carbon tetrachloride**)

Neguvon   (see **Trichlorfon**)

Nemagon   (see **Dibromo-chloropropane**)

Nemagone   (see **Dibromo-chloropropane**)

Nematox   (see **Dibromo-chloropropane**)

Nendrin   (see **Endrin**)

Neoprene   (see **Chlorobutadiene mixture**)

Nerkol   (see **Vapona**)

Netagrone   (see **Dichlorophenoxyacetic acid**)

N-Heptane   (see **Heptane**)

N-Hexane   (see **Hexane**)

Nifos   (see **Tetraethylpyrophosphate**)

Nitorphene   (see **Dinitrophenol**)

Nitric acid silver salt   (see **Silver nitrate**)

Nitroaniline

Pronunciation guide: NYE-troe-an-ih-lin

Other names: 4-Nitroaniline, 4-Nitrobenzenamine, *Devol red GG, Fast red base GG,* Paranitroaniline, P-Nitroaniline

Uses: intermediate for dyes, antioxidants and gasoline; corrosion inhibitor; in pesticides; in pharmaceutical synthesis; etc.

Ototoxic effects:
    Vestibular:
        Ataxia: (NTP)
        Dizziness: (NTP)

Nitrobenzene

Pronunciation guide: nye-troe-BEN-zeen

Other names: Essence of mirbane, Mirbane oil, Nitrobenzol

Uses: solvent; in chemical manufacture; in refining lubricating oils; etc.

Ototoxic effects:
    Vestibular:
        Vertigo: (NTP)

Nitrobenzol   (see **Nitrobenzene**)

Nitrochloroform   (see **Chloropicrin**)

Nitrolime   (see **Calcium cyanamide**)

Nitrotoluene

Pronunciation guide: nye-troe-TALL-yoo-een

Other names: 2-Nitrotoluene, 4-Nitrotoluene, O-Nitrophenylmethane, O-Nitrotoluene, P-Methylnitrobenzene, P-Nitrotoluene

Uses: manufacture of dyes; toluidines; nitrobenzoic acids; etc.

Ototoxic effects:
  Vestibular:
    Ataxia: (NTP)
    Dizziness: (NTP)

Nitrous acid sodium salt   (see **Sodium nitrite**)

Nitroxanthic acid   (see **Picric acid**)

Nogos   (see **Vapona**)

Normal heptane   (see **Heptane**)

N-Pentane   (see **Pentane**)

N-Pentanol   (see **Pentanol**)

NutraSweet   (see **Aspartame**)

O—2-Aminoanisole   (see **Anisidine**)

O-Anisidine   (see **Anisidine**)

Octafluoropropane   (see **Perfluoropropane**)

Octalene   (see **Aldrin**)

Octalox   (see **Dieldrin**)

O-Nitrophenylmethane   (see **Nitrotoluene**)

O-Nitrotoluene   (see **Nitrotoluene**)

Ortho-klor   (see **Chlordane**)

Oxitol   (see **Ethoxyethanol**)

Oxomethane   (see **Formaldehyde**)

Oxybenzene   (see **Phenol**)

Oxycarbophos   (see **Malaoxon**)

P—4-Aminoanisole   (see **Anisidine**)

Palavale   (see **Econazole nitrate**)

P-Anisidine   (see **Anisidine**)

Panogen soil drench   (see **Methyl mercury hydroxide**)

Paracide   (see **Dichlorobenzene**)

Para-dichlorobenzene   (see **Dichlorobenzene**)

Paraform   (see **Formaldehyde**)

Paramoth   (see **Dichlorobenzene**)

Paranitroaniline   (see **Nitroaniline**)

Parazene   (see **Dichlorobenzene**)

Pargin   (see **Econazole nitrate**)

P-Benzenediamine dihydrochloride   (see **Phenylenediamine dihydrochloride**)

P-Benzenediol   (see **Hydroquinone**)

P-Bromoaniline   (see **Bromoaniline**)

P-Bromophenylamine   (see **Bromoaniline**)

PCB-1254   (see **Arochlor**)

P-Cresylic acid   (see **Cresol mixture**)

P-Dioxane   (see **Dioxane**)

Pelagol CD   (see **Phenylenediamine dihydrochloride**)

Pelagol RS   (see **Resorcinol**)

Pentane

Pronunciation guide: PEN-tane

Other names: Amyl hydride, N-Pentane

Uses: solvent extraction; fuel; chemical synthesis; natural gas processing plants; tube oil additives; hydraulic fluids; in pesticides, paint removers, insecticides; etc.

Ototoxic effects:
Vestibular:
Vertigo: (NTP)

Pentanol

Pronunciation guide: PEN-tah-nall

Other names: 1-Pentanol, Amyl alcohol, *Amylol*, N-Pentanol, *Pentasol*, Pentyl alcohol

Uses: solvent; in organic synthesis; in manufacture of petroleum additives; in urea-formaldehyde plastics processing; in pharmaceuticals

Ototoxic effects:
Cochlear:
Hearing loss: (NTP)
Vestibular:
Dizziness: (NTP)
Vertigo: (NTP)

Notes:

Hearing loss may be partial or total (NTP).

Pentasol   (see **Pentanol**)

Pentyl alcohol   (see **Pentanol**)

Perchlor   (see **Tetrachloroethylene**)

Perchloroethylene   (see **Tetrachloroethylene**)

Perchloromethane   (see **Carbon tetrachloride**)

Perchloropentacyclodecane   (see **Mirex**)

Perclene   (see **Tetrachloroethylene**)

Perfecthion   (see **Cygon**)

Perfluoropropane

Pronunciation guide: PER-fluoo-roe-proe-pane

Other names: Octafluoropropane

Uses: medical uses include liquid ventilation, contrast agents, blood extenders, surgical applications, etc.

Ototoxic effects:
  Cochlear:
    Tinnitus: (She)

Perklone   (see **Tetrachloroethylene**)

Pertite   (see **Picric acid**)

Pestmaster   (see **Methyl bromide**)

Petzinol   (see **Trichloroethylene**)

Phenacide   (see **Toxaphene**)

Phenol

Pronunciation guide: FEE-nall

Other names: Benzenol, Carbolic acid, Hydroxybenzene, Oxybenzene, Phenyl hydroxide, Phenylic acid

Uses: disinfectant; solvent; in manufacture of artificial resins; in many medical and industrial organic compounds and dyes; in gericides, antioxidants, preservatives, explosives, fertilizers, paints, paint removers; used as an anesthetic and antiseptic; etc.

Ototoxic effects:
  Cochlear:
    Tinnitus: (NTP)
  Vestibular:
    Dizziness: (NTP)
    Vertigo: (NTP)

Phenylenediamine dihydrochloride

Pronunciation guide: FEE-nih-len-ee-die-aye-meen die-HIE-droe-klor-eyed

Other names: 4-Aminoaniline dihydrochloride, *Durafur black RC*, *Fourrine*, P-Benzene-diamine dihydrochloride, *Pelagol CD*, P-Phenylenediamine dihydrochloride

Uses: in dyeing furs; analytical reagent; etc.

Ototoxic effects:
  Vestibular:
    Vertigo: (NTP)

Phenylethylene   (see **Styrene**)

Phenyl hydroxide   (see **Phenol**)

Phenylic acid   (see **Phenol**)

Phenylmethane   (see **Toluene**)

Phenyl methanol   (see **Benzyl alcohol**)

Phortox   (see **Trichlorophenoxyacetic acid**)

Phosdrin   (see **Mevinphos**)

Phosfene   (see **Mevinphos**)

Phosphoric acid tritolyl ester   (see **Tricresyl phosphate**)

Phosvit   (see **Vapona**)

Photodieldrin

Pronunciation guide: FOE-toe-die-el-drin

Other names: *BL 6623, NCI-C00599*

Uses: (not available)

Ototoxic effects:
　　Vestibular:
　　　　Ataxia: (NTP)
　　　　Dizziness: (NTP)
　　　　Nystagmus: (NTP)

Photol   (see **Methylaminophenol sulfate**)

Picric acid

Pronunciation guide: PIK-rik ASS-id

Other names: *Lyddite, Melinite*, Nitroxanthic acid, *Pertite, Shimose*

Uses: used in explosives, matches and batteries; reagent; antiseptic; astringent; etching copper; etc.

Ototoxic effects:
　　Vestibular:
　　　　Vertigo: (NTP)

Picride   (see **Chloropicrin**)

Pictol   (see **Methylaminophenol sulfate**)

P-Methylaminophenol sulfate   (see **Methylaminophenol sulfate**)

P-Methylnitrobenzene   (see **Nitrotoluene**)

P-Nitroaniline   (see **Nitroaniline**)

P-Nitrotoluene   (see **Nitrotoluene**)

Polychlorinated biphenyl 1254   (see **Arochlor**)

Polyvinylpyrrolidone   (see **Iodine**)

Pomarsol   (see **Tetramethylthiuram disulfide**)

Potassium bichromate   (see **Potassium dichromate**)

Potassium bromate

Pronunciation guide: poe-TASS-see-um BROE-mate

Other names: Bromic acid potassium salt

Uses: laboratory reagent; oxidizing agent; food additive; analytical chemistry; etc.

Ototoxic effects:
Cochlear:
    Hearing loss: (NTP)

Potassium bromide

Pronunciation guide: poe-TASS-see-um BROE-mide

Other names: Bromide salt of potassium, Tripotassium tribromide

Uses: in photography manufacture; in process engraving and lithography; in special soaps; as lab reagent; formerly used as a sedative and anticonvulsant

Ototoxic effects:
Vestibular:
    Ataxia: (NTP)
    Dizziness: (NTP)
    Vertigo: (NTP)

Potassium dichromate

Pronunciation guide: poe-TASS-see-um die-KROE-mate

Other names: Bichromate of potash, Dipotassium dichromate, *Iopezite*, Potassium bichromate

Uses: tanning leather; in dyeing, painting, photolithography, staining wood, pyrotechnics and safety matches; oxidizer; corrosion inhibitor; etc.

Ototoxic effects:
Vestibular:
    Vertigo: (NTP)

Potato alcohol   (see **Ethanol**)

Povidone iodine (see **Iodine**)

P-Oxytoluene   (see **Cresol mixture**)

P,P'-DDE   (see **DDE**)

P-Phenylenediamine dihydrochloride   (see **Phenylenediamine dihydrochloride**)

Primatol   (see **Atrazine**)

Propene oxide   (see **Epoxypropane**)

Propylcarbinol   (see **Butyl alcohol**)

Propylene dichlorohydrin   (see **Dichloro propanol**)

Propylene epoxide   (see **Epoxypropane**)

Propylene oxide   (see **Epoxypropane**)

Proviodine   (see **Iodine**)

Pyridine

Pronunciation guide: PYRE-rid-een

Other names: Azabenzene, *Azine*

Uses: solvent; in analytical chemistry; intermediate in pesticide production; in pharmaceuticals; in waterproofing; in the manufacture of paints; in explosives, dyestuffs, rubber, vitamins and disinfectants; as a dyeing assistant; etc.

Ototoxic effects:
Vestibular:
Dizziness: (NTP)
Vertigo: (NTP)
Notes:
Vertigo is temporary (NTP).

Pyrinex   (see **Chlorpyrifos**)

Pyrobenzol   (see **Benzene**)

Pyrrolyene   (see **Butadiene**)

Quinol   (see **Hydroquinone**)

Quintox (see **Dieldrin**)

Ratbane 1080 (see **Fluoroacetic acid sodium salt**)

Reddon (see **Trichlorophenoxyacetic acid**)

Resorcine (see **Resorcinol**)

Resorcinol

Pronunciation guide: ree-ZORSE-in-all

Other names: *Developer R, Fourrine EW*, M-Dihydroxybenzene, M-Hydroquinone, *Pelagol RS, Resorcine*

Uses: tanning; manufacture of resins; resin adhesives; explosives; dyes; cosmetics; dyeing and printing textiles; antiseptic; etc.

Ototoxic effects:
    Vestibular:
        Vertigo: (NTP)

Rhodiachlor (see **Heptachlor**)

Rhodol (see **Methylaminophenol sulfate**)

Rogor (see **Cygon**)

Roxion (see **Cygon**)

Ruphos (see **Dioxathion**)

Salicylamide (see **Hydroxybenzamide**)

Salvo (see **Dichlorophenoxyacetic acid**)

Salymid (see **Hydroxybenzamide**)

Seedrin (see **Aldrin**)

Shimose (see **Picric acid**)

Silver nitrate

Pronunciation guide: SIL-ver NYE-trate

Other names: Lunar caustic, Nitric acid silver salt

Uses: photography; manufacture of mirrors; silver plating; indelible inks; hair dyes; reagent in analytical chemistry; topical anti-infective; etc.

Ototoxic effects:
    Vestibular:
        Vertigo: (NTP)

Skellysolve B   (see **Hexane**)

Sodium arsenate   (see **Sodium arsenate heptahydrate**)

Sodium arsenate heptahydrate

Pronunciation guide: SOE-dee-um AR-seh-nate hep-tah-HYE-drate

Other names: Dibasic sodium arsenate, Sodium arsenate

Uses: dyeing; germicides; printing fabrics; in treating parasitism in animals; formerly used as an anthelmintic and dermatological agent; etc.

Ototoxic effects:
    Vestibular:
        Dizziness: (NTP)
        Vertigo: (NTP)

Sodium cyanide

Pronunciation guide: SOE-dee-um SYE-ah-nide

Other names: Cyanide of sodium, *Cyanobrik*, *Cyanogran*, *Cymag*, Hydrocyanic acid sodium salt

Uses: extracting gold and silver from ores; in electroplating baths; fumigant; in case-hardening steel; insecticides; cleaning metals; in manufacturing dyes and pigments; in rodenticides; in metal polishes; in metallurgical and photographic processes; etc.

Ototoxic effects:
    Vestibular:
        Dizziness: (NTP)
        Vertigo: (ATS, NTP)

Sodium fluoacetate   (see **Fluoroacetic acid sodium salt**)

Sodium monofluoroacetate   (see **Fluoroacetic acid sodium salt**)

Sodium nitrite

Pronunciation guide: SOE-dee-um NYE-tryte

Other names: *Anti-rust*, Diazoting salts, *Erinitrit*, *Filmerine*, Nitrous acid sodium salt

Uses: rubber accelerator; color fixative and preservative in cured meats, meat products and fish; in pharmaceuticals; photographic and analytic reagent; dye manufacture; antidote for cyanide poisoning

Ototoxic effects:
    Vestibular:
        Vertigo: (NTP)

Solaesthin   (see **Methylene chloride**)

Solfo black   (see **Dinitrophenol**)

Solvolsol   (see **Diethylene glycol monoethyl ether**)

Somipront   (see **Dimethyl sulfoxide**)

Spectazole   (see **Econazole nitrate**)

Spirits of wine   (see **Ethanol**)

Spontox   (see **Trichlorophenoxyacetic acid**)

Strobane   (see **Trichloroethane**)

Strobane-T   (see **Toxaphene**)

Strychnine

Pronunciation guide: STRIK-nine

Other names:

Uses: rodenticide

Ototoxic effects:
    Cochlear:
        Hyperacusis:[147]
    Unspecified/General Ear Conditions:
        Ototoxicity: [148]

Styrene

Pronunciation guide: sty-REEN

Other names: Ethenylbenzene, Phenylethylene, Styrol

Uses: organic solvent; used in making plastics, synthetic rubber and resins; insulator

Ototoxic effects:
    Cochlear:
        Hearing loss: (Ryb)
        Tinnitus: (Ka8)

Notes:

In studies using rats, **Styrene** has caused marked hearing loss. This is also true for humans. For example, in one study there was significant high-frequency sensorineural hearing loss in workers exposed to varying amounts of **Styrene**. Also, **Styrene** messes up the auditory circuits in the brain that process speech and other complex sound (Ryb). In a plastic boat plant, 7 of the 18 workers exposed to **Styrene** displayed abnormal central auditory system results.[149]

People working in factories for 5 or more years where the concentration of **Styrene** fumes in the air they were breathing was well below the occupational exposure limit of 50 ppm still had hearing losses. Although their conventional hearing tests were normal, high-frequency testing revealed hearing loss at the highest frequency they could hear. Researchers concluded that this upper limit of hearing is a sensitive indicator for early detection of ototoxicity in workers exposed to **Styrene**.[150]

The ototoxic effects of **Styrene** are made worse by the presence of noise at the same time (Nia).

See Chapter 6, "The Shocking Truth about Hearing Testing and Ototoxic Drugs" and Chapter 8, "The Sinister Partnership Between Ototoxic Agents and Noise" for further information on this chemical.

Styrol   (see **Styrene**)

Super cobalt   (see **Cobalt**)

Syntexan   (see **Dimethyl sulfoxide**)

Task   (see **Vapona**)

TCM   (see **Chloroform**)

TCPP   (see **Tris dichloro propyl phosphate**)

TDNT   (see **Dinitrotoluene**)

Tecquinol   (see **Hydroquinone**)

Teg   (see **Triethylene glycol**)

Telvar   (see **Monuron**)

Terial   (see **Chlorpyrifos**)

Termil   (see **Chlorothalonil**)

Tersan   (see **Tetramethylthiuram disulfide**)

Tescol   (see **Ethylene glycol**)

Tetracap   (see **Tetrachloroethylene**)

Tetrachloroethane

Pronunciation guide: TET-rah-klor-oh-eth-ayne

Other names: 1,1,2,2-Tetrachloroethane, Acetylene tetrachloride, *Bonoform, Cellon, Westron*

Uses: solvent; in manufacturing paints, varnish and rust removers; in soil sterilants, weed killers and insecticides; in cleaning and degreasing metals; fumigant; dry cleaning agent; herbicide; etc.

Ototoxic effects:
Cochlear:
Tinnitus: (Ka8)
Vestibular:
Dizziness: (NTP)
Vertigo: (NTP)

Tetrachloroethylene

Pronunciation guide: tet-rah-klor-oh-ETH-il-een

Other names: Carbon dichloride, Ethylene tetrachloride, *Perchlor*, Perchloroethylene, *Perclene, Perklone, Tetracap, Tetroguer*

Uses: solvent; in dry cleaning; in degreasing metals; anthelmintic; fumigant; drying agent; in printing inks; etc.

Ototoxic effects:
Cochlear:
Tinnitus: (NTP)
Vestibular:
Dizziness: (NTP)
Vertigo: (NTP)

Tetrachloronaphthalene

Pronunciation guide: tet-rah-klor-oh-NAP-thah-leen

Other names: 1,2,3,4-Tetrachloronaphthalene

Uses: synthetic waxes; dielectrics in capacitors; wire insulation

Ototoxic effects:
Vestibular:
Vertigo: (NTP)

Tetraethyl diphosphate   (see **Tetraethylpyrophosphate**)

Tetraethylpyrophosphate

Pronunciation guide: tet-rah-eth-il-PYRE-roe-fos-fate

Other names: *Bladan*, Diphosphoric acid tetraethyl ester, *Fosvex, Grisol, Hexamite, Killax, Lirohex, Nifos*, Tetraethyl diphosphate, *Tetron, Vapotone*

Uses: insecticide; rodenticide

Ototoxic effects:
Vestibular:
Ataxia: (NTP)

Tetraform   (see **Carbon tetrachloride**)

Tetramethylthiuram disulfide

Pronunciation guide: tet-rah-meth-il-THY-yoor-am die-SUL-fyed

Other names: *Aatack, Accelerator thiuram, Antabuse, Arasan, Cyuram, Fermide, Fernasan, Hermal*, Methyl thiram, *Pomarsol, Tersan*, Tetrathiuram disulfide, *Thiram, Thiuram, Vulkacit*

Uses: fungicide, bacteriostat, insecticide and pesticide; disinfectant; animal repellant; antiseptic; vulcanization accelerator; antioxidant; the drug *Antabuse* used in the treatment of alcoholism; etc.

Ototoxic effects:
Vestibular:
Ataxia: (NTP)
Dizziness: (NTP)

Tetrasol   (see **Carbon tetrachloride**)

Tetrathiuram disulfide   (see **Tetramethylthiuram disulfide**)

Tetroguer   (see **Tetrachloroethylene**)

Tetron   (see **Tetraethylpyrophosphate**)

Thifor   (see **Endosulfan**)

Thiodan   (see **Endosulfan**)

Thiram   (see **Tetramethylthiuram disulfide**)

Thiuram   (see **Tetramethylthiuram disulfide**)

Threthylene   (see **Trichloroethylene**)

Tiguvon   (see **Baytex**)

Tin (see **Trimethyltin**)

TMT   (see **Trimethyltin**)

Toluene

Pronunciation guide: TALL-yoo-een

Other names: *Methacide*, Methylbenzene, Methylbenzol, Phenylmethane, *Toluol*

Uses: chemical manufacture; in artificial leather, fabric and paper coatings; in explosives, dyes and other organic compounds; solvent for paints, lacquers, gums, oils, rubber, vinyls and resins; gasoline additive; adhesive solvent; in saccharin; in perfumes; in the cleaning industry; insecticide; constituent of asphalt and naphtha; etc.

Ototoxic effects:
    Cochlear:
        Hearing loss: [151] (ATS, Ryb)
        Tinnitus:[152]
    Vestibular:
        Ataxia: (NTP)
        Equilibrium disorder: (ATS)
        Dizziness: (ATS, NTP)
        Nystagmus: (NTP)
        Vertigo: (NTP)

Notes:

Toluene is commonly found in many consumer products. It is also found in motor vehicle emissions. You likely are exposed to **Toluene** in your own home without realizing it (Ryb).

I have an anecdotal report in my files of a woman who ended up with a hearing loss from the cumulative effects (over several years) of using a spray varnish containing **Toluene** in an enclosed garage.

Of six workers accidentally exposed to **Toluene** fumes, three had resulting hearing losses. After 6 months, one had recovered her hearing, but the other two were left with "notch" hearing losses at between 3 and 6 kHz (Ryb).

Low to moderate repeated occupational exposure to **Toluene** can cause sensorineural hearing loss. In some cases, the hearing loss occurs months after the exposure to **Toluene**.[153] Also, combinations of **Toluene** and some common medicines like **Aspirin** and **Acetaminophen** may increase the hearing loss caused by exposure to **Toluene**.[154]

Toluene, like other organic solvents, disturbs our balance system. But that is not all, in studies where people inhaled **Toluene** fumes, the results revealed dramatic hearing losses originating in the brain's auditory pathways. Other studies show high-frequency hearing losses due to cochlear damage (Ryb). Incidentally, **Toluene** can damage hearing whether inhaled, or absorbed by contact with the liquid form.[155]

In one study using rats, **Toluene** alone and noise alone caused considerable hearing loss, particularly in the high frequencies. However, the hearing loss of rats exposed to

Toluene followed by noise was greater than the sum of the effects of **Toluene** and noise alone (Ryb).

In another study, workers were grouped into one of four groups—those exposed to both noise and **Toluene**, those exposed to **Toluene** alone, those exposed to noise alone, and those not exposed to either **Toluene** or noise (the control group). The results were dramatic. The risk of hearing loss of those exposed to noise alone was 4 times greater than the control group; the risk of hearing loss of those exposed to **Toluene** alone was 5 times greater; and the risk of hearing loss of those exposed to both noise and **Toluene** was 11 times greater![156]

In yet another study those exposed to both noise and **Toluene** had a 53% incidence of high-frequency sensorineural hearing loss, those exposed to noise alone, 26% and the control group 8%. When these results are adjusted for age, they show that noise exposure increases the risk of hearing loss by 4.6 times. When the noise is combined with exposure to **Toluene**, the risk jumps a whopping 27.5 times (Ryb).

See Chapter 8, "The Sinister Partnership Between Ototoxic Agents and Noise" for further information on this chemical.

Toluol   (see **Toluene**)

Toxadust   (see **Toxaphene**)

Toxaphene

Pronunciation guide: TOX-ah-feen

Other names: *Alltox, Attac,* Camphechlor, Chlorocamphene, *Cristoxo, Geniphene, Kamfochlor, Phenacide, Strobane-T, Toxadust, Toxyphen, Vertac*

Uses: in insecticides and pesticides

Ototoxic effects:
    Cochlear:
        Hyperacusis (Auditory reflex excitability): (NTP)
    Vestibular:
        Vertigo: (NTP)

Toxichlor   (see **Chlordane**)

Toxyphen   (see **Toxaphene**)

Transamine   (see **Dichlorophenoxyacetic acid**)

Transcutol   (see **Diethylene glycol monoethyl ether**)

Tri-2-propenylamine   (see **Triallyamine**)

Triallyamine

Pronunciation guide: try-AL-lee-aye-meen

Other names: Tri-2-propenylamine

Uses: intermediate in chemical processes

Ototoxic effects:
Vestibular:
Vertigo: (NTP)

Tributon　(see **Trichlorophenoxyacetic acid**)

Trichloran　(see **Trichloroethylene**)

Trichlorfon

Pronunciation guide: try-KLOR-oh-fon

Other names: *Chlorophos, Combot, Dipterex, Dylox, Foschlor, Masoten,* Methyl chlorophos, *Neguvon, Trinex, Tugon, Votexit*

Uses: insecticide; used to treat certain human parasitic infections

Ototoxic effects:
Vestibular:
Ataxia: (NTP)
Nystagmus: (NTP)
Vertigo: (NTP)

Trichloroethane

Pronunciation guide: try-klor-oh-ETH-ayne

Other names: 1,1,1-Trichloroethane, Chloroethene, *Inhibisol,* Methyl chloroform, *Strobane*

Uses: used in cold-type metal cleaning; in plastic cleaning; in vapor degreasing; as a chemical intermediate; in adhesives; as a coolant and lubricant; stain repellant for upholstery; in wig cleaning; solvent; etc.

Ototoxic effects:
Vestibular:
Ataxia: (NTP)
Dizziness: (NTP)
Loss of balance: (NTP)

Trichloroethylene

Pronunciation guide: try-klor-oh-ETH-il-een

Other names: Acetylene trichloride, *Algylen, Benzinol, Chlorilen, Dukeron,* Ethylene trichloride, *Germalgene, Narcogen, Petzinol,* Threthylene, *Trichloran, Trilene, Vestrol*

Uses: in dry cleaning; in metal degreasing; solvent; refrigerant; heat exchange liquid; in organic synthesis; fumigant; diluent in paints and adhesives; in textile processing; disinfectant; chemical intermediate in production of pesticides, gums, resins, tars, paints, varnishes; etc.

Ototoxic effects:
 Cochlear:
  Hearing loss: (ATS, Ryb)
  Tinnitus: (ATS, NTP)
 Vestibular:
  Ataxia: (NTP)
  Dizziness: (ATS, NTP)
  Vertigo: (ATS, NTP)

Notes:

Exposure to **Trichloroethylene** (TCE) can result in sensorineural hearing loss in both ears. In one study of 40 workers exposed to **Trichloroethylene**, 26 (65%) had bilateral sensorineural hearing loss.[157] They also had lesions of their balance systems that could result in such things as ataxia and vertigo.[158] The characteristics of the hearing loss were sensorineural, the same loss in both ears and high-frequency loss with a dip beginning at 2,000 to 3,000 Hz. The longer workers were exposed, the more likely they were to have abnormal audiograms (Ryb).

Trichloroethylene can cause abnormal results to auditory brainstem response (ABR) tests indicating damage to the auditory circuits in the brain.[159]

The ototoxic effects of **Trichloroethylene** are made worse by the presence of noise at the same time (Nia). One study showed that the longer you are exposed to **Trichloroethylene**, the worse your hearing gets.[160]

See Chapter 8, "The Sinister Partnership Between Ototoxic Agents and Noise" for further information on this chemical.

Trichloromethane   (see **Chloroform**)

Trichloronitromethane   (see **Chloropicrin**)

Trichlorophenoxyacetic acid

Pronunciation guide: try-klor-oh-fee-nox-ee-ah-SEE-tik ASS-id

Other names: 2,4,5-T, 2,4,5-Trichlorophenoxyacetic acid, *Brushtox, Dacamine, Dinoxol, Esteron, Forron, Phortox, Reddon, Spontox, Tributon, Veon, Weedone*

Uses: herbicide

Ototoxic effects:
 Cochlear:
  Hearing loss: (NTP)

Tricresyl phosphate

Pronunciation guide: try-KRES-il FOS-fate

Other names: Cresyl phosphate, *Kronitex, Lindol,* Phosphoric acid tritolyl ester, Tritolyl phosphate

Uses: plasticizer; flame-retardant; solvent; additive to high-pressure lubricants; sterilizer; in linseed oil; in china wood oil; etc.

Ototoxic effects:
Vestibular:
Vertigo: (NTP)

Triethylene glycol

Pronunciation guide: try-ETH-il-een GLY-kol

Other names: *Teg, Trigen, Triglycol, Trigol*

Uses: in plastics; in air disinfectants; solvent; in dehydration of natural gas; in printing inks; fungicide; etc.

Ototoxic effects:
Vestibular:
Nystagmus: (NTP)

Trigen　(see **Triethylene glycol**)

Triglycol　(see **Triethylene glycol**)

Trigol　(see **Triethylene glycol**)

Trilene　(see **Trichloroethylene**)

Trimethyltin

Pronunciation guide: try-METH-il-tin

Other names: TMT

Uses: in polyvinyl chloride piping, siding and window casings; catalyst for polyurethane foam; vulcanization of silicone rubber; anti-fouling marine paints; wood preservatives; fungicides; acaricides; etc.

Ototoxic effects:
Cochlear:
Hearing loss: (Ryb)

Notes:

Studies with rats show that exposure to **Trimethyltin** damages the auditory circuits in the brain and can produce a flat hearing loss. This sensorineural hearing loss is generally reversible except in the very high frequencies (Ryb).

Damage to the outer hair cells of rats is evident as early as 48 hours after exposure to **Trimethyltin**. By 9 days, inner hair cell damage can be detected. The outer hair cell damage is directly related to the amount of exposure to **Trimethyltin** (Ryb).

Trimethyltin can damage the central auditory system as well as damage the myelin sheath (the "insulation" that coats the nerve cells). It also causes swelling of the white matter of the brain.[161]

Exposure to **Trimethyltin** and loud noise at the same time can result in greater hearing loss than would normally result from exposure to both **Trimethyltin** and noise separately (Nia).

Researchers are trying to find ways to block the ototoxic effects of the heavy metals. The exciting news is that the glutamate receptor antagonist MK-801 appears to block the ototoxic effects of **Trimethyltin**.[162]

See Chapter 8, "The Sinister Partnership Between Ototoxic Agents and Noise" for further information on this chemical.

Trimetion   (see **Cygon**)

Trinex   (see **Trichlorfon**)

Trinoxol   (see **Dichlorophenoxyacetic acid**)

Tripotassium tribromide   (see **Potassium bromide**)

Tris (1,3-dichloro-2-propyl) phosphate   (see **Tris dichloro propyl phosphate**)

Tris dichloro propyl phosphate

Pronunciation guide: TRIS die-KLOR-oh PROE-pul FOS-fate

Other names: *Emulsion 212, Fyrol FR 2, TCPP,* Tris (1,3-dichloro-2-propyl) phosphate

Uses: flame retardant

Ototoxic effects:
Vestibular:
Ataxia: (NTP)

Tritolyl phosphate   (see **Tricresyl phosphate**)

Tugon   (see **Trichlorfon**)

Univerm   (see **Carbon tetrachloride**)

Urtosal   (see **Hydroxybenzamide**)

Vapona

Pronunciation guide: vay-POE-nah

Other names: 2,2-Dichlorovinyl dimethyl phosphate, *Astrobot, Atgard, Brevinyl, Canogard, Cypona, Dichlorophos, Herkal, Lindan, Nerkol, Nogos, Phosvit, Task, Vaponite*

Uses: insecticide; fumigant; veterinary anthelmintic; etc.

Ototoxic effects:
    Vestibular:
        Ataxia: (NTP)
        Dizziness: (NTP)

Vaponite   (see **Vapona**)

Vapotone   (see **Tetraethylpyrophosphate**)

Vectal   (see **Atrazine**)

Veon   (see **Trichlorophenoxyacetic acid**)

Verol   (see **Methylaminophenol sulfate**)

Vertac   (see **Toxaphene**)

Vestrol   (see **Trichloroethylene**)

Vinylethylene   (see **Butadiene**)

Vinyl methyl ketone   (see **Methyl vinyl ketone**)

Violet 3   (see **Chlorobutadiene mixture**)

Votexit   (see **Trichlorfon**)

Vulkacit   (see **Tetramethylthiuram disulfide**)

Weedazol   (see **Amino triazole**)

Weedone   (see **Dichlorophenoxyacetic acid**)

Weedone   (see **Trichlorophenoxyacetic acid**)

Westron   (see **Tetrachloroethane**)

Wood alcohol   (see **Methyl alcohol**)

Wood creosote   (see **Creosote**)

Wood naphtha   (see **Methyl alcohol**)

Xylene

Pronunciation guide: ZYE-leen

Other names: Dimethylbenzene, Ethyl benzene, *Xylol*

Uses: aviation gasoline; solvent; synthesis of organic chemicals; in dye manufacture; etc.

Ototoxic effects:
> Cochlear:
>> Hearing loss: (ATS, Ryb)
> Vestibular:
>> Ataxia: (NTP)
>> Equilibrium disorder: (ATS)
>> Dizziness: (ATS, NTP)

Notes:

> Sensorineural hearing loss has been observed in animals exposed to moderate to high levels (1,300 to 2,000 ppm) of **Xylene**.[163] Hearing loss was greater with greater concentrations of **Xylene**. Also, the higher frequencies were affected with lower concentrations, but all frequencies were affected at high concentrations (Ryb).

> **Xylene** can cause abnormal results to auditory brainstem response (ABR) tests indicating damage to the auditory circuits in the brain.[164]

> The ototoxic effects of **Xylene** are made worse by the presence of noise at the same time (Nia).

> See Chapter 8, "The Sinister Partnership Between Ototoxic Agents and Noise" for further information on this chemical.

Xylol (see **Xylene**)

Zytox (see **Methyl bromide**)

---

101 Haybach, 1998. p. 7.

102 Haybach, 1999. pp. 22-23.

103 Haybach, 1999. pp. 22-23.

104 Bisesi, 1994. p. 1.

105 Odkvist, 1992. pp. 687-690.

106 Kumar, 1997. p. 469.

107 *Statement of Principles concerning Tinnitus*, 1986. p. 3.

108 Troost, 1998d. p. 1.

109 Bisesi, 1994. p. 4.

110 *Symptoms Attributed to Aspartame in Complaints Submitted to the FDA*, 1995. pp. 2-3.

111 Monte, 1984. p. 2.

112 Gold, 1995. pp. 2-5.

113 Mercola, 2004, p. 1.

114 Haybach, 1999. p. 23.

115 *MSDS n-Butanol*, 1998. p. 3.

116 *Chemical Sampling Information—n-Butyl Alcohol*, 2000, p. 2.

117 Morata, 1994. pp. 359-366.

118 Shochat, 2001. p. 5

119 Matheson Tri-gas, Inc., 2001. p. 2.

120 Shochat, 2001. p. 5

121 Shochat, 2001. p. 4

122 Shochat, 2001. p. 5

123 Adams, 1999. p. 2.

124 Bisesi, 1994. p. 7.

125 Reinberg, 2003. pp. 1-2.

126 Carmen, 1977. p. 161.

127 *Statement of Principles concerning Tinnitus*, 1986. p. 3.

128 Troost, 1998d. p. 1.

129 Doyle, 2001. pp. 553-558.

130 *MSDS Heptane*, 1998. p. 2.

131 *MSDS Heptane*, 1998. p. 2.

132 *Occupational Safety & Health Guideline for Heptane*, 1999. p. 4.

133 *Occupational Safety & Health Guideline for Heptane*, 1999. p. 4.

134 Haybach, 1999. p. 23.

135 *Lead*, 1990. p. 2.

136 *Public Health Assessment: Dupage County Landfill (Blackwell Forest Preserve) Warrenville, Dupage County, Illinois.* 1997.

137 *Case Studies in Environmental Medicine: Lead Toxicity*, 1995. p. 9.

138 Bisesi, 1994. p. 8.

139 *Public Health Assessment: Hipps Road Landfill, Jacksonville, Duval County, Florida.* 1995.

140 *Case Studies in Environmental Medicine: Lead Toxicity*, 1995. pp. 8-12.

141 *Lead*, 1990. p. 2.

142 Bisesi, 1994. p. 7.

143 *Public Health Assessment: Nyanza Chemical Waste Dump, Ashland, Middlesex County, Massachusetts*, 1994.

144 *Mercury*, 1999. pp. 1-2.

145 Bisesi, 1994. p. 8.

146 *Methylene chloride*, 1993. p. 2.

147 Braund, 2001. p. 1.

148 Haybach, 1998. p. 7.

149 Morata, 1994. pp. 359-366.

150 Morioka, 1999. pp. 1-5.

151 *Toluene*, 1995. p. 2.

152 Morata, 1994. pp. 359-366.

153 Hendrix, 2001. p. 3.

154 *Public Health Assessment: Miami County Incinerator, Troy, Miami County, Ohio*, 1997.

155 Hendrix, 2001. p. 3.

156 Morata, 1994. pp. 359-366.

157 Gist, 1995. p.18.

158 Morata, 1994. pp. 359-366.

159 Bisesi, 1994. p. 7.

160 Vernick, 1993. p. 157.

161 Hendrix, 2001. p. 4.

162 *Environmental Impact on Hearing: Is Anyone Listening*, 1994. p. 4.

163 *Xylene*, 1990. p. 3.

164 Bisesi, 1994. p. 7.

Appendix

Glossary of Terms

Adverse side effect: A harmful result of a drug as opposed to the desired therapeutic effect. Often just referred to as a "side effect". For example, tinnitus and dizziness are common side effects of many drugs.

Agonist: A drug that can combine with receptors in the nervous system that **cause** a particular action to take place. The opposite of agonist is antagonist. (See antagonist.)

Aminoglycoside: A class of antibiotics used to treat serious bacterial infections. This class of drugs is generally very ototoxic. Five of the more common AMINOGLYCOSIDES are **Amikacin**, **Gentamicin**, **Neomycin**, **Streptomycin** and **Tobramycin**.

Analgesic: A class of pain-relieving drugs.

Anesthetic: A class of drugs that temporarily causes loss of ability to feel pain.

Antagonist: A drug that blocks or works against the action of another drug, or prevents a particular body action from taking place. An antagonist is the opposite of an agonist. (See agonist.)

Anti-arrhythmics: A class of drugs used to treat irregular heartbeats.

Antibacterial: A class of drugs that kills or slows the growth of bacteria.

Antibiotics: Drugs used to treat infections.

Antidepressants: A class of drugs used to treat mental depression.

Antihistamines: A class of drugs used to prevent or relieve allergy symptoms.

Anti-hypertensives: A class of drugs used to help lower high blood pressure.

Anti-infectives: A class of drugs used to treat infections.

Anti-inflammatory drugs, non-steroidal: Commonly referred to as NSAIDs (Non-steroidal anti-inflammatory drugs). This class of anti-inflammatory drugs is not steroid-like. As well as their anti-inflammatory effects, they also commonly help to reduce pain and fever. Common drugs in this class include **Aspirin**, **Acetaminophen** and **Ibuprofen**.

Anti-inflammatory drugs, steroidal: A class of anti-inflammatory drugs that are Cortisone-like. Common drugs in this class include **Cortisone**, **Dexamethasone** and **Prednisone**.

Anti-inflammatory: A class of drugs used to relieve pain, swelling and other symptoms of inflammation.

Anti-neoplastics: A class of drugs used to treat cancer.

Anti-protozoals: A class of drugs used to treat infections caused by protozoa.

Anti-psychotics: A class of drugs used to treat some mental and emotional conditions.

Antipyretics: A class of drugs used to reduce fever.

Antiseptics: Drugs that prevent infections by inhibiting the growth of infectious agents. Normally used on the skin to prevent infections in cuts, scrapes and wounds.

Antivirals: A class of drugs used to treat infections caused by viruses.

Ataxia: ("A" in Table 14-1) Impaired coordination that typically reveals itself in a staggering gait. Gait ataxia is one of the results of a damaged vestibular (balance) system.

Audiogram: A graph of your hearing loss showing your hearing loss measured in decibels for each of the test frequencies. (See also "Conventional audiogram".)

Auditory disorder: ("AD" in Table 14-1) In this book, I have lumped together under the heading of "Auditory disorder" the following vague conditions—auditory damage, auditory defects, auditory disorders, auditory disturbances, auditory ototoxicity and inner ear abnormalities. Researchers used these various terms for apparently similar conditions during the drug studies that are reported in sources like the PDR and CPS. Unfortunately, the researchers did not define exactly what they meant by these terms. (See somewhat similar terms under "Hearing disorder" and "Hearing loss".)

Auditory hallucinations: ("AH" in Table 14-1) "Hearing" voices and other sounds that are not there (phantom sounds). This can be a manifestation of mental illness such as schizophrenia, one of the side effects of taking certain drugs, or something not working quite right in the auditory circuits in the brain. (See "Musical Ear Syndrome" for more information on this latter point.)

Auditory reflex: Any reflex occurring in response to a sound. If the ear is essentially deaf, there will not be any auditory reflex. For example, a deaf baby won't startle when you clap your hands near its head.

Auditory reflex excitability: (See under "Hyperacusis".)

Bacteremia: Live bacteria present in your bloodstream. This is often due to an infection somewhere in your body.

Blind trials: Drug trials where the people in the study don't know if they are taking the drug being tested or the placebo. (See also "Double-blind trials".)

Burning/stinging: ("BS" in Table 14-1) This side effect may occur when the drug is used in the external ear canal, resulting in a burning or stinging sensation.

Central Nervous System: Commonly abbreviated to CNS. That part of the nervous system composed of the brain and spinal cord. Technically, the hair cells in the cochlea and the auditory nerves are also part of the CNS. Problems in the auditory parts of the CNS can distort hearing and "mess up" the way your brain processes what you hear so you may not understand what you hear.

Ceruminosis: ("C" in Table 14-1) Variously listed by researchers as increased ear wax, ear wax, ear wax build-up, excessive ear wax formation and increased cerumen. Cerumen is the medical term for ear wax. When ear wax builds up, it can block the ear canal and cause some degree of temporary hearing loss.

Chelator: A molecule that binds a metal ion to itself. This can be used to remove an ion from participation in biological processes. For example, chelators can bind heavy metals such as lead and mercury and prevent them from damaging the body.

Cholesteatoma: ("CH" in Table 14-1) A non-cancerous tumor in the middle ear largely composed of skin cells. This condition usually is the result of chronic otitis media.

Clinical hearing loss: A hearing loss that can be detected by "normal" audiological testing using the conventional test frequencies between 125 Hz and 8,000 Hz.

CNS: (See Central nervous system.)

Cochlear lesions: ("CL" in Table 14-1) A lesion is the site of some sort of damage. Thus cochlear lesions are damage to the cochlea. They have been variously listed by researchers as cochlear damage, cochlear infarctions and cochlear lesions. Cochlear lesions are generally otosclerotic lesions from trauma or vaccinations, or adverse effects from other things. The active lesions are crumbly and bleed. Inactive lesions are hard. These lesions end up deforming the turns in the cochlea. Also, cochlear lesions can cause partial nerve atrophy in the cochlea.

Cochlear nerve: Sometimes called the auditory nerve or the acoustic nerve. One of the two branches of the eighth cranial nerve. It conducts the hearing signals from the inner ear to the brain. (See also "Eighth cranial nerve".)

Cochlear system: The hearing system of your inner ear consisting of the cochlea and the auditory nerve.

Conductive hearing loss: (See "Hearing loss, conductive".)

Conventional audiogram: An audiogram that covers the frequencies from 125 hertz to 8,000 hertz. (See also "Audiogram".)

Cookie-bite hearing loss: Named for the shape of this kind of hearing loss on an audiogram. Both the high and low frequencies are normal or near-normal, but there is a broad dip in the mid frequencies that looks like someone took a bite out of the top of the audiogram. (See also "Audiogram".)

CPS: *Compendium of Pharmaceuticals and Specialties*. The main drug reference book used by doctors, pharmacists and hospitals in Canada.

Deafness: The PDR and CPS sometimes use the term "deafness" to describe some degree of hearing loss, not just total deafness. Instead of using this term, I use the term "hearing loss". (See under "Hearing loss".)

Discrimination: The ability to tell apart similar-sounding words such as "fun" and "sun". People with normal hearing have close to 100% discrimination. If your discrimination scores drop below 50%, you can't understand much of what you hear. Speech then sounds more like gibberish or a foreign language. Some drugs don't cause hearing loss as such, but cause discrimination problems so you can't understand what you are hearing.

Diuretics: A class of drugs used to increase urine production. This helps the kidneys get rid of excess water and salt. *LOOP DIURETICS* such as **Furosemide** and **Ethacrynic acid** can be quite ototoxic, especially when taken with other ototoxic drugs.

Dizziness: ("D" in Table 14-1) This is a general term that people describe variously as feeling faint, giddy, light-headed, unsteady or woozy. Others feel a sense of imbalance or disequilibrium. Very often dizziness is one of the first signs that a drug is beginning to affect the balance system.

Double-blind trials: Drug trials where neither the people in the study nor the doctors doing the study know who is taking the new drug and who is taking the placebo. This information only comes out after the study is over and the results have been compiled.

Ear disorder: ("ED" in Table 14-1) In this book, I have lumped together under the heading of "Ear disorder" the following vague conditions—ear abnormality, ear disease (unspecified) and ear disorder. Researchers used these various terms for apparently similar conditions during the drug studies that are reported in sources like the PDR and CPS. Unfortunately, the researchers did not define exactly what they meant by these terms.

Ear pain: ("EP" in Table 14-1) In this book, I have lumped together under the heading of "Ear pain" the following conditions—earache, ear discomfort, ear pain and otalgia. Researchers used these various terms during the drug studies that are reported in sources like the PDR and CPS. (See also "Otalgia".)

Ears blocked: ("EB" in Table 14-1) In this book, I have lumped together under the heading of "Ears blocked" the following vague conditions—clogged ears, congestion in ears, ears blocked, ears feel "plugged up," ears plugged, ear stuffiness and plugged ears. Researchers used these various terms for apparently similar conditions during the drug studies that are reported in sources like the PDR and CPS. (See also "Feeling of fullness in ears".)

Eighth cranial nerve: Sometimes called the vestibulocochlear nerve. It divides into two parts—the cochlear (auditory) nerve responsible for hearing, and the vestibular nerve responsible for balance. This nerve carries hearing and balance information from the inner ear to the brain. If it is damaged or diseased, you could experience things such as hearing loss, tinnitus, hyperacusis, dizziness, loss of balance, vertigo, nausea and vomiting.

Equilibrium disorder: ("EQ" in Table 14-1) In this book, I have lumped together under the heading of "Equilibrium disorder" the following vague conditions—balance difficulties, balance disorder, balance problems, equilibrium disorders, equilibrium disturbances, equilibrium dysfunction and loss of equilibrium. Researchers used these various terms for apparently similar conditions during the drug studies that are reported in sources like the PDR and CPS. Unfortunately, the researchers did not define exactly what they meant by these terms. (See also "Loss of balance".)

Eustachian tube disorder: ("ET" in Table 14-1) This is a condition relating to the Eustachian tubes that go from the back of the throat to the middle ears. It is variously called Eustachian tube disorder and Eustachian tube dysfunction. These terms probably refer to the Eustachian tubes becoming clogged as a result of a middle ear infection.

FDA: The United States Food and Drug Administration. This is the government agency that is responsible for approving and regulating drug use in the USA. One of its purposes is to help protect your health by keeping unproven and unsafe drugs off the market.

Feeling of fullness in ears: ("FF" in Table 14-1) This is likely the same condition as the various terms described under "Ears blocked". However, when you rapidly lose your hearing, often it seems like your ears feel full or stuffed or blocked. This is a psychological feeling, not a physical reality. This term may also refer to this feeling.

Fluid in ear: Fluid typically builds up in the middle ear when you have an ear infection. (See also "Otitis media".)

Free radicals: An atom or molecule having at least one unpaired electron. Free radicals are usually unstable and highly reactive. Your body produces some free radicals. Many come from outside your body—from smoking, breathing polluted air or being exposed to ultraviolet radiation. Free radicals often damage nearby cells. The hair cells in your inner ears are particularly susceptible to damage by free radicals. Some drugs produce free radicals that can damage your ears. Antioxidants neutralize free radicals so they can't do any further damage.

Hearing disorder: ("HD" in Table 14-1) In this book, I have lumped together under the heading of "Hearing disorder" the following vague conditions—disturbed hearing, ear/hearing disorder, hearing abnormality, hearing alterations, hearing disturbance, hearing dysfunction and hearing problems. Researchers used these various terms for apparently similar conditions during the drug studies that are reported in sources like the PDR and CPS. Unfortunately, the researchers did not define exactly what they meant by these terms, but I think they used these terms to mean some degree of hearing loss. (See somewhat similar terms under "Auditory disorder" and "Hearing loss".)

Hearing loss, conductive: A hearing loss that originates in the outer or middle ear. It involves the ear canal, the eardrum or the three tiny bones in the middle ear. Conductive hearing losses are "mechanical" losses.

Hearing loss, sensorineural: Sometimes abbreviated as SNHL. A hearing loss involving the cochlea, auditory nerves and/or the central auditory pathways in the brain. Formerly commonly called "nerve deafness". Ninety percent of adults with hearing losses have this kind of hearing loss.

Hearing loss: ("HL" in Table 14-1) In this book, I have lumped together under the heading of "Hearing loss" the following similar terms—auditory acuity decrease, change in the ability to perceive tones, deafness, decreased hearing, diminished hearing, hearing difficulty, hearing impaired, hearing loss, hearing toxicity, hypoacusis, nerve deafness, partial transitory deafness and reversible hearing loss. Researchers used these various terms for apparently similar conditions during the drug studies that are reported in sources like the PDR and CPS. Unfortunately, the researchers did not define how these terms differ from each other. (See also "Auditory disorder" and "Hearing disorder".)

Hyperacusis: ("HY" in Table 14-1) Abnormal hearing sensitivity. Sometimes described as "noise intolerance" and "auditory reflex excitability". If you have hyperacusis, you now perceive normal-volume sounds as much too loud. In fact, you may perceive normal sounds as being painfully loud. Hyperacusis can be caused by exposure to loud noise and/or certain ototoxic drugs.

Hypoacusis (Hypoacousia): (listed under "HL" in Table 14-1) Low sensitivity to sound—in other words, hearing loss.

Intravenous: Commonly abbreviated as I.V. This term is used when drugs are injected directly into a vein. Taking ototoxic drugs intravenously can result in a higher risk of ototoxic damage since the drugs can be given fairly rapidly and in high doses.

I.V.: (See "Intravenous".)

Labyrinthitis: ("L" in Table 14-1) Labyrinthitis is an inflammation of the labyrinth. It can result in hearing loss and/or balance problems. It can cause abnormal (not necessarily decreased) function of the sensors in the labyrinth. In this book, I have lumped together under the heading of "Labyrinthitis" the following vague conditions—acute labyrinthitis, labyrinth disorder, labyrinthine disorder and labyrinthitis. Researchers used these various terms for apparently similar conditions during the drug studies that are reported in sources like the PDR and CPS. Unfortunately, the researchers did not define exactly what they meant by these terms.

Loss of balance: ("LB" in Table 14-1) This is one of the signs of vestibular damage. (See also "Equilibrium disorder".)

Meniere's disease: ("ME" in Table 14-1) A syndrome consisting of progressive fluctuating hearing loss, vertigo, tinnitus, dizziness, nausea and a feeling of fullness in the ear (the ear feels stuffed up or blocked). The nausea from severe vertigo is often its most debilitating aspect.

Middle ear pressure: ("MP" in Table 14-1) In this book, I have lumped together under the heading of "Middle ear pressure" the following similar, but vague, conditions—ear pressure, middle ear pressure and pressure/throbbing in ears. Researchers used these various terms for apparently similar conditions during the drug studies that are reported in sources like the PDR and CPS. Unfortunately, the researchers did not define exactly what they meant by these terms.

Middle ear: That portion of the ear lying immediately behind the ear drum and containing the three tiny bones—malleus (hammer), incus (anvil) and stapes (stirrup)—that conduct sound from the eardrum to the inner ear.

Musical Ear Syndrome (MES): Hearing complex phantom sounds such as voices and music. These sounds may be clear, or vague, and are often heard by hard of hearing people. People hearing MES sounds are not mentally ill. These sounds are somewhat akin to tinnitus sounds, and are sometimes called musical tinnitus. For further information on Musical Ear Syndrome, check out my book *Phantom Voices, Ethereal Music and Other Spooky Sounds*—see the back of this book for further information. (See also "Auditory hallucinations" and "Tinnitus".)

Myelin sheath: The "insulation" surrounding nerve bundles. Some metals like **Lead**, **Mercury** and **Tin** can damage the myelin sheath that surrounds and insulates the auditory nerve. This causes various problems related to hearing.

Nephrotoxic: Drugs that are toxic (poisonous) to cells in the kidneys.

Nerve deafness: The old term for sensorineural hearing loss. (See "Sensorineural hearing loss".)

Non-steroidal inflammatory drugs: (See "Anti-inflammatory drugs, non-steroidal".)

NSAIDs: Non-steroidal inflammatory drugs. (See "Anti-inflammatory drugs, non-steroidal".)

Nystagmus: ("N" in Table 14-1) Abnormal, rapid, rhythmic, involuntary, alternating movements of the eyeball. Your eyes may jerk from side to side or up and down. Ototoxic drugs can cause horizontal nystagmus. Nystagmus results from damage to the vestibular system or to the central nervous system.

Oscillopsia: ("OS" in Table 14-1) Oscillating or bouncing vision caused by excessive motion of an image on the retina. Oscillopsia results when the vestibular system is destroyed or severely damaged.

Otalgia: Earache or ear pain (ear discomfort). A common cause is middle ear infections. About 25% of ototoxic drugs can cause this symptom. (See also "Ear pain".)

OTC: Abbreviation for "over-the-counter". These are drugs that are available without a prescription.

Otic: Relating to the ear.

Otitis: ("O" in Table 14-1) An inflammation (infection) of the ear without specifying exactly where it occurs. I have included the general term "ear infection" under this heading. (See also "Otitis externa" and "Otitis media".)

Otitis externa: ("OE" in Table 14-1) Inflammation of the external ear canal usually caused by an infection. Includes the term "swimmer's ear".

Otitis media: ("OM" in Table 14-1) Inflammation of the middle ear or eardrum. This is the fancy way of referring to a middle ear infection. In this book, I have lumped together under the heading of "Otitis media" the following vague conditions—fluid in ears, middle ear disorder, middle ear disturbance and otitis media. Researchers used these various terms for apparently similar conditions during the drug studies that are reported in sources like the PDR and CPS. Unfortunately, the researchers did not define exactly what they meant by these terms. (See also "Fluid in ears".)

Otorrhea: ("OR" in Table 14-1) A purulent discharge (pus) from the ear; ear drainage.

Otorrhagia: ("OH" in Table 14-1) Bleeding from the ear canal; ear hemorrhage.

Otosclerosis: ("OT" in Table 14-1)) (OH-toe-sklair-ROW-sis) An inherited dominant genetic condition that causes abnormal spongy bone growth on the tiny bones in the middle ear and surrounding bone. Often this results in the stirrup (stapes) becoming fixed to the oval window of the cochlea. Because the stapes no longer vibrates freely, this causes a progressive conductive hearing loss. If the otosclerosis eventually invades the cochlea (cochlear otosclerosis), the result is additional (sensorineural) hearing loss.

Ototoxic: ("OX" in Table 14-1) Drugs that are injurious or harmful to the ear, sometimes limited to damage to the organs or nerves of the ear concerned with hearing and balance (cochlear and vestibular organs and associated nerves). In this book, I use the term "ototoxic" in its fullest sense.

PDR: *Physicians' Desk Reference*. The main drug reference book used by doctors, pharmacists and hospitals in the USA.

Perforated eardrum: ("PE" in Table 14-1) An eardrum that has ruptured or has a hole in it. The fancy term is tympanic membrane perforation. This is commonly a result of a middle ear infection.

Phonophobia: ("PP" in Table 14-1) Technically, phonophobia is a fear of sound. Phonophobia could result from having severe hyperacusis such that louder sounds hurt. When you know a sound will hurt, you may become afraid of such sounds, or afraid of being around louder sounds.

Placebo: A "medicine" (sometimes called a "sugar pill") that—unknown to the patient—has no active medicinal ingredients. It is used in drug studies to compare the efficacy of a new drug to no treatment at all without the patient being aware of which "treatment" they are getting.

Potentiation: The interaction between two drugs such that the pharmacologic response is greater than the sum of the individual responses to each drug. For example, taking two ototoxic drugs at the same time may cause the side effects to be much more severe to your ears than would be the case if you had taken the same drugs, but at different times. A synergistic effect. (See synergistic.)

Prodrug: A drug that exerts its pharmacological action as it is converted by metabolic processes into another closely-related drug by the body. For example, **Acemetacin** is a prodrug of **Indomethacin**. Likewise **Alatrofloxacin** is a prodrug of **Trovafloxacin**. It is rapidly and completely converted in your body to **Trovafloxacin.**

Proprioceptive system: (proh-pree-oh-SEP-tiv) One of the three separate balance systems in your body. It consists of nerve sensors in the muscles, tendons and joints, especially in your legs, that help you keep your balance. The other two systems are your visual system and the vestibular system in your inner ears. When your vestibular system is damaged, your proprioceptive system works with your visual system to give you some semblance of balance.

Pure-tone audiogram: An audiogram based on listening to pure tones (the normal situation) as opposed to listening to speech.

Radiopaque agents: A class of drugs that makes it easier to see an area of the body with x-rays. This makes it easier to diagnose certain medical conditions.

Recruitment: An abnormally greater increase in loudness in response to increased sound intensity as compared with a normal ear. In practical terms, if you have recruitment, you perceive louder sounds as much louder than normal and they often hurt. Recruitment is one result of the greatly reduced dynamic range found in people with sensorineural hearing loss.

Salicylism: Poisoning by salicylic acid or any of its compounds such as **Acetylsalicylic acid** (*Aspirin*) and **Bismuth subsalicylate** (*Pepto-Bismol*). Symptoms of salicylism include nausea, vomiting, headaches, tinnitus, hearing loss, mental dullness, confusion, quickened pulse and increased respirations.

Sensorineural hearing loss: (See "Hearing loss, sensorineural".)

Side effect: (See "Adverse side effect".)

Sign: An abnormality indicative of disease that your doctor can see or feel upon examination. An objective indication of disease. For example, bleeding from your ear canal would be a sign of ear damage. (See also "Symptom".)

Ski-slope hearing loss: The shape of your hearing loss as displayed on your audiogram. If you have a ski-slope hearing loss, your low frequency hearing is normal or near normal and your hearing loss quickly drops to profound by the mid to high frequencies. It looks like a ski hill sloping down from the left side of your audiogram.

Sub-clinical hearing loss: A hearing loss above 8,000 Hz. It can only be detected using a special audiometer calibrated to test hearing in the frequencies between 8,000 and 20,000 Hz. Conventional hearing testing only tests those frequencies between 125 Hz and 8,000 Hz. Many ototoxic drugs cause sub-clinical hearing loss, at least in the beginning.

Symptom: Any deviation from normal that is experienced by a patient and is indicative of disease. A symptom is a subjective indication of disease and something your doctor can't see or feel. For example, tinnitus would be a symptom of ear damage. (See also "sign".)

Synergistic: A reaction where the total is more than the sum of the individual parts. For example, noise and certain drugs have a synergistic effect on hearing loss. Assume that a given amount of noise normally causes 1 unit of hearing loss. Also, assume that a given drug normally causes 2 units of hearing loss. Therefore, if you were exposed to both the noise and the drug, you would expect to have 3 units of hearing loss. However, in this hypothetical example, when tested, you find you have 7 units of hearing loss. The extra 4 units above what you would have expected by adding up the two figures, is caused by the synergistic action of noise and ototoxic drugs working together.

Tinnitus: ("T" in Table 14-1) Tinnitus sounds are simple phantom sounds. Tinnitus is the sensation of hearing sounds in your ears when these sounds are not present. Tinnitus is sometimes described as your ears ringing or buzzing. It may be a ringing, swishing, buzzing whooshing, clanging, shrieking or other type of noise that seems to originate in your ears or head. It is not a disease, but a symptom of various abnormal underlying conditions in the auditory system. (Compare with "Musical Ear Syndrome" which comprises more complex phantom sounds.)

Turner syndrome: A rare chromosomal (genetic) disorder of females characterized by short stature and the lack of sexual development at puberty. Among a host of other physical defects/abnormalities are hearing disorders.

Vertigo: ("V" in Table 14-1) Vertigo is the illusion of movement—the sensation of motion when none is present. It may feel like you are spinning around, or that the room is spinning around you. Frequently vertigo is accompanied by feelings of imbalance and/or nausea. Vertigo is a common result of damage to the balance system of the inner ear (vestibular system). Less often, it is caused by abnormal conditions in the brain (central nervous system). Many ototoxic drugs can cause vertigo.

Vestibular disorder: ("VD" in Table 14-1) Vestibular disorders are disorders that affect your balance. In this book, I have lumped together under the heading of "Vestibular disorder" the following vague conditions—vestibular damage, vestibular defects, vestibular disorder, vestibular disturbances, vestibular dysfunction, vestibular ototoxicity, vestibular stimulation and vestibular toxicity. Researchers used these various terms for apparently similar conditions during the drug studies that are reported in sources like the PDR and CPS. Unfortunately, the researchers did not define exactly what they meant by these terms.

Vestibular system: That portion of the inner ear and the central nervous system involved with the sense of balance. This system controls your equilibrium (balance) and stabilizes your eyes in space. It works together with your brain to sense, maintain and regain your balance and a sense of where your body and its parts are positioned. It regulates movement (walking, running, etc.) and keeps objects in visual focus as the body moves. Many ototoxic drugs can damage your vestibular system. This gives rise to a whole host of balance-related problems.

Vestibulocochlear nerve: (See "Eighth cranial nerve".)

Literature Cited

10 Best and Worst Foods for You. In: Bottom Line Secrets "Daily Health News" newsletter. April 22, 2010.

AARP Bulletin. October, 2009.

Abdulla, Sara. 1996. *Action call to halt antibiotic-induced hearing loss*. British Medical Journal. 313(7058).

About Benzodiazepines. 2005. TRANX—Tranquillizer Recovery and New Existence. http://www.tranx.org.au/benzodiaz.html.

Adams, John. 1999. *Fact sheet 4—Health risks of carbon monoxide*. Iowa State University Extension, Polk County. http://www.exnet.iastate.edu/polk/health/carbon/fact4.html.

Agency for Toxic Substances and Disease Registry (ATSDR). 2001. *ToxFAQs*. U.S. Department of Health and Human Services, Public Health Service. http://www.atsdr.cdc.gov/toxfaq.html.

AHFS Drug Information, 2002. American Hospital Formulary Service. American Society of Health-System Pharmacists. 7272 Wisconsin Avenue, Bethesda, MD 20814.

AHFS Drug Information, 2009. American Hospital Formulary Service. American Society of Health-System Pharmacists. 7272 Wisconsin Avenue, Bethesda, MD 20814.

"Amazing Grace"…Pentoxifylline-induced musical hallucinations. 1993. In: Neurology 1993; 43:1621. CSM West Midlands re: Action August 1994, No. 5. http://www.csmwm.org/reaction/No5.htm.

American Heritage Dictionary of the English Language. 2000. 4th Edition. Boston & New York: Houghton Mifflin Company.

Amonafide. 2000. Lexi-Comp Inc. http://www.library.duq.edu/clinref/datasets/cancer_f/html/chapter/mono/mm006375.htm.

Anipryl. 1999. Animal Health, a division of Pfizer, Inc. Exton, PA.

Antibiotics index. 2001. http://is.icc.u-tokai.ac.jp/~arai/drugs.html.

Are you dizzy? 2001. Audiologic Consultants, Inc. Queen Street Professional Center, 1776 South Queen Street, York, PA 17403. e-mail: audcon@netrax.net.

Are You Taking Too Many Medications? April 27, 2007. Bottom Line Secrets.

Articaine. 2003. Drug Information. Genesis Health System. http://www.genesishealth.com/micromedex/quickdrug/dnx1059.aspx.

Asaju, Tunde. 2001. *Once Scared, Twice Adamant.* Abuja Bureau. Africa News Service. April 10, 2001. Lagos, Nigeria.

Ashton, Heather. 2002. *Benzodiazepines: How They Work and How to Withdraw.* http://www.benzo.org.uk/manual/contents.htm.

Aspirin component prevents antibiotic-induced deafness. 1999. Journal Laboratory Investigation (July). University of Michigan. Ann Arbor, MI. http://www.umich.edu/~newsinfo/Releases/1999/Jul99/r071399a.html.

Audiological aspects of ototoxicity. 1996. Boys Town National Research Hospital. Omaha, Nebraska 68131. http://wvww.boystown.org/btnrh/chlc/ototox.htm.

Avandia—How Dangerous Is It Really? 2010.

Azapropazone (NSAID). 1994. Electronic Doctor. http://www.edoc.co.za/medilink/actives/91.html.

Barry, Patricia. 2002. *What's fueling drug costs?* AARP Bulletin. 43(3):3-18. Washington, D.C.

Bauman, Neil G. 2016. *Take Control of Your Tinnitus—Here's How.* Integrity First Publications, 1013 Ridgeway Dr., Lynden, WA 98264. http://hearinglosshelp.com/shop/category/books/.

Bauman, Neil. 2005. *Loud Music and Hearing Loss.* http://hearinglosshelp.com/blog/loud-music-and-hearing-loss/.

Bauman, Neil. 2009. *Will Taking Sodium Thiosulfate Prevent Ototoxicity?* http://hearinglosshelp.com/blog/will-taking-sodium-thiosulfate-prevent-ototoxicity/.

Be an active member of your health care team. 2001. U.S. Food and Drug Administration. Center for Drug Evaluation and Research. http://www.fda.gov/cder/consumerinfo/active_member.htm.

Be careful when mixing grapefruit juice with your Rx. 1999. American Association of Pharmaceutical Scientists (AAPS). http://www.newswise.com/articles/1999/4/GRAPFRUT.APS.html.

Benjamin, Mark. 2004. *Drug Causing GIs Permanent Brain Damage.* United Press International. 5/26/2004.

Benzodiazepine Addiction, Withdrawal & Recovery. 2006. http://www.benzo.org.uk.

Berner, Mark, and Gerald Rotenberg. 1996. *New guide to prescription and over-the-counter drugs.* Canadian Medical Association/Reader's Digest.

Bisesi, Michael, and Allan Rubin. 1994. *Chemical air pollutants and otorhinolaryngeal toxicity.* Journal of Environmental Health. 56(7):24.

Boniva (Ibandronic Acid)—Adverse Event Reports—Other Serious Reactions—Arthralgia. Page 1. 2009. DrugLib.com—Drug Information Portal. http://www.druglib.com/adverse-reactions_side-effects/boniva/seriousness_other/reaction_arthralgia/.

Boniva (Ibandronic Acid)—Adverse Event Reports—Other Serious Reactions—Pain in Jaw. 2009. DrugLib.com—Drug Information Portal. http://www.druglib.com/adverse-reactions_side-effects/boniva/seriousness_other/reaction_pain_in_jaw/.

Bowen, James. 1998. *Dizziness: A diagnostic puzzle.* In: Hospital medicine. Medscape, Inc. http://www.medscape.com.

Braund, K. G. 2001. *Neurotoxic disorders.* In: Clinical neurology in small animals—Localization, diagnosis and treatment. Ithaca: International Veterinary Information Service. http://www.ivis.org/special_books/Braund/braund22/chapter_frm.asp.

British National Formulary (BNF 44). September 2002. Published by the British Medical Association and the Royal Pharmaceutical Society of Great Britain. Pharmaceutical Press, PO Box 151, Wallingford, Oxon, OX10 8QU, UK. http://www.pharmpress.com.

British National Formulary (BNF 58). September 2009. Published by the British Medical Association (BMJ) and the Royal Pharmaceutical Society of Great Britain. Pharmaceutical Press (RPS Publishing), London, UK. http://www.bnf.org.

Brotizolam. 1997. Electronic Doctor. Zambia. http://www.edoc.co.za/medilink/actives/142.html.

Busto, Usoa, et. al. 1988. *Protracted Tinnitus after Discontinuation of Long-Term Therapeutic use of Benzodiazepines.* New England Journal of Medicine 315:854-859. http://www.benzo.org.uk/busto.htm.

Carmen, Richard. 1977. *Our endangered hearing—Understanding & coping with hearing loss.* Rodale Press. Emmaus, PA.

Carmen, Richard. 1999. *Chemicals & hearing—Danger ahead*. Hearing Health Magazine (March/April).

Cary, R., S. Clarke, and J. Delic. 1997. *Effects of combined exposure to noise and toxic substances—Critical review of the literature*. Ann. Occup. Hyg. 41(4):455-465.

Case studies in environmental medicine: Lead toxicity. 1995. Agency for Toxic Substances and Disease Registry. Atlanta, GA. http://www.atsdr.cdc.gov/HEC/caselead.html.

Celiprolol. 2001. Our-Doctor Ltd. http://www.our-doctor.co.uk/Generic/Drugs/celiprolol.html.

Chemical sampling information-n-Butyl alcohol. 2000. Occupational Safety & Health Administration. http://osha-slc.gov/dts/chemicalsampling/data/CH_222900.html.

Chockley, Nancy. 2001. *Drug ads "A tool to sell a product"*. AARP Bulletin. 42(8). Washington, D.C.

Climara forte. 2000. Patient Information Leaflet. H. E. Clissmann, Schering AG, Ireland.

Clinical pharmacology 2000. 2001. Gold Standard Multimedia. http://cp.gsm.com.

Clinical trials of tirapazamine enter final phase. 2001. http://www-radonc.stanford.edu/tirapaz.html.

Cohen, Sharon. 2000. Personal communication. Jan. 2000 and November 2001.

Compendium of Pharmaceuticals and Specialties. 1998. 33rd Edition. Canadian Pharmacists Association, 1785 Alta Vista Drive, Ottawa, Ontario, Canada K1G 3Y6.

Compendium of Pharmaceuticals and Specialties. 2000. 35th Edition. Canadian Pharmacists Association, 1785 Alta Vista Drive, Ottawa, Ontario, Canada K1G 3Y6.

Compendium of Pharmaceuticals and Specialties. 2003. 38th Edition. Canadian Pharmacists Association, 1785 Alta Vista Drive, Ottawa, Ontario, Canada K1G 3Y6.

Compendium of Pharmaceuticals and Specialties. CPS 2010. Canadian Pharmacists Association, 1785 Alta Vista Drive, Ottawa, Ontario, Canada K1G 3Y6.

Consumer Warning: Medical Study Indicates Commonly Prescribed Pain Killer Abuse Can Cause Rapid, Profound Hearing Loss. April 26, 1999. PRNewswire.

Cosyntropin–Injectable. 2009. http://www.medicinenet.com/conyntropin-injectable/article.htm.

Curhan, Sharon G., et. al. 2010. *Analgesic Use and the Risk of Hearing Loss in Men*. The American Journal of Medicine. Mar. 123(3):231-237.

Dancer, Jess. Sep. 14, 2007. *Advance for Audiologists*.

Davison, Steven P., and Mitchell S. Marion. 1998. *Sensorineural hearing loss caused by NSAID-induced aseptic meningitis*. ENT: Ear, Nose & Throat Journal. 77(10):820-825.

de la Cruz, M. 1999. *Carbamazepine-induced sensorineural hearing loss*. Arch Otolaryngol Head Neck Surg. Feb; 125(2):225-7.

Desyrel (Trazodone hydrochloride). In: MedWatch—2004 Safety Alerts for Drugs, Biologics, Medical Devices and Dietary Supplements. http://www.fda.gov/medwatch/SAFETY/2004/safety04.htm.

Dextromethorphan. ~2000. Drugs and Human Performance Fact Sheets. National Highway Traffic Safety Administration. http://www.nhtsa.dot.gov/people/injury/research/job185drugs/dextromethorphan.htm.

Diabetes Health Warning. In: October 8, 2010 personal email.

DiSogra, Robert. 2001. *Adverse drug reactions and audiology practice*. Audiology Today. Special Issue.

Disorders of the inner ear. 2000. Chapter 8. In: Hearing and balance; the inner ear. Department of Neurophysiology. University of Wisconsin-Madison. http://www.neurophys.wisc.edu/~ychen/textbook/chap-8.html.

Don't be a silent victim of a drug's side effects. Mon. June 2, 2008. In: "Healthier News", The W. C. Douglass newsletter.

Dothiepin. 2002. Medizine. http://www.cix.co.uk/~cyberville/medizine/dothiepi.htm.

Dothiepin (tricyclic). 1994. Electronic Doctor. Zambia. http://www.edoc.co.za/medilink/actives/354.html.

Doyle, Karen, et al. 2001. *Effects of difluoromethylornithine chemoprevention on audiometry thresholds and otoacoustic emissions*. Arch. Otolaryngol. Head & Neck Surgery. 127:553-558. http://archotol.ama-assn.org/issues/v127n5/abs/ooa00061.html.

Drug Facts and Comparisons. 2009. Wolters Kluwer Health. St. Louis, MO. http://www.factsandcomparisons.com.

Drug Information Online. 2010. http://www.drugs.com.

Drug Prevents Chemotherapy-induced Hearing Loss, Study Finds. August 10, 2004. Advance for Audiologists.

eHealth Treats—Medicine & Cure—Adalimumab. 2009. http://www.ehealthtreats.com/medicine.asp?Medicine=Adalimumab.

Elbe, Dean. 1999a. *GJDIs with benzodiazepines*. http://www.powernetdesign.com/grapefruit/benzos.htm.

Elbe, Dean. 1999b. *GJDIs with calcium-channel blockers (CCBs)*. http://www. powernetdesign.com/grapefruit/ccbs.htm.

Elbe, Dean. 1999c. *Cholesterol-lowering drugs*. http://www.powernetdesign.com/grapefruit/ cholesterol.htm.

Elbe, Dean. 1999d. *GJDIs with immunosuppressants*. http://www.powernetdesign.com/ grapefruit/immunosuppressants.htm.

Elbe, Dean. 1999e. *Miscellaneous GJDIs*. http://www.powernetdesign.com/grapefruit/ misc.htm.

Elbe, Dean. 1999f. *Studies showing lack of GJDI*. http://www.powernetdesign.com/ grapefruit/nogjdi.htm.

Elbe, Dean. 1999g. *Unconfirmed potential GJDIs*. http://www.powernetdesign.com/ grapefruit/potential.htm.

Environmental impact on hearing: is anyone listening? 1994. In: Focus. Environmental health perspectives. 102(11). http://ehpnet1.niehs.nih.gov/docs/1994/102-11/ focus2.html.

Epstein, Steven, M.D., 1995. *What you should know about ototoxic medications*. SHHH Journal (October). http://trfn.clpgh.org/shhh/epstein.html.

Epstein, Steven, M.D., 2002. *Drugs That Can Cause Hearing Loss/Drugs That Can Cause Tinnitus*. Notes distributed at meeting, May 2002. Washington, DC.

Estrada, Benjamin. 1997. *Infectious causes of hearing loss beyond otitis media*. Infect Med. 14(3):239-244. http://www.medscape.com/SCP/IIM/1997/v14.no3/m2076.estrada/ m2076.estrada.html.

Evenson, Brad. 2002. *Ear Drops May Be Hazardous: Health Canada*. National Post.

Fausti, S. A., et al. 1992. *High-frequency audiometric monitoring for early detection of aminoglycoside ototoxicity*. Journal of Infectious Diseases. 165(6):1026-32.

Fausti, S. A., et al. 1993a. *High-frequency monitoring for early detection of cisplatin ototoxicity*. Arch Otolaryngol Head Neck Surg. 119 (6):661-6.

Fausti, S. A., et al. 1993b. *High-frequency testing techniques and instrumentation for early detection of ototoxicity*. J. Rehabil. Res. Dev. 30(3):333-41.

Fausti, S. A., et al. 1994. *High-frequency audiometric monitoring strategies for early detection of ototoxicity*. Ear Hear. 15(3):232-9.

Fausti, S. A., et al. 1999. *An individualized sensitive frequency range for early detection of ototoxicity*. Ear Hear. 20(6):497-505.

FDA Announces Revisions to Labels for Cialis, Levitra and Viagra. October 18, 2007. http://www.fda.gov/bbs/topics/NEWS/2007/NEW01730.html.

FDA MedWatch – Benicar (Olmesartan) Ongoing Safety Review. June 11, 2010.

FDA MedWatch – Meridia (Sibutramine): Market Withdrawal Due to Risk of Serious Cardiovascular Events. October 8, 2010.

Femtran. 2000. Health Answers Australia: Drug finder. http://healthanswers.telstra.com/drugdata/appco/00098847.asp.

Food and medication interactions can be very harmful. Fact sheet 32. 1999. http://www.aidsnutrition.org/fact32.shtml.

Flieger, Ken. 1995. *Testing drugs in people.* FDA Consumer Special Report. U.S. Food and Drug Administration. http://www.fda.gov/fdac/special/newdrug/testing.html.

Forge, Andrew. 1999. *Industrial chemicals are hazardous to hearing.* Lancet. 353(9160):1250.

Fortimicin for injection. 1998. Kyowa Hakko Kogyo Co., Ltd. Japan. http://www.jpma.or.jp/jpr/PDF/KYOWA03.PDF.

Freundlich, Naomi. 1998. *When the cure may make you sicker.* Review of *Prescription for disaster—The hidden dangers in your medicine cabinet,* by Thomas J. Moore. http://www.businessweek.com/1998/11/b3569025.htm.

Fruchtengarten, Ligia. 1998. *Nitrazepam.* International Programme on Chemical Safety. Poison Control Centre of Sao Paulo, Brazil. http://www.inchem.org/documents/pims/pharm/pim675.htm.

Fusetti, M, et. al. 1999. *Mefloquine and Ototoxicity: A Report of 3 Cases.* Clin. Ter. 1999 Sep-Oct;150(5):379-82. (Abstract in PubMed.)

Gist, Ginger L., and JeAnne R. Burg. 1995. *Trichloroethylene—A review of the literature in view of the results of the trichloroethylene subregistry results.* Agency for Toxic Substances and Disease Registry. Atlanta, GA. http://www.atsdr.cdc.gov/NER/TCE/a6rev.html.

Gold, Mark D. *The bitter truth about artificial sweeteners.* 1995. http://www.nexusmagazine.com//Aspartame.html.

Goodman, Robert. 2002. *Can drug ads lead to unnecessary spending?* AARP Bulletin. 43(3):17. Washington, D.C.

Grapefruit and serious drug interactions. 2000. From: Clinical Pharmacology and Therapeutics. 61(4). http://paganism.com/ag/herbs/druginter.html.

Grapefruit interferes with select medications. January, 2000. http://www.bayfront.org/information/side.html.

Grapefruit juice and drugs. January, 2000. http://www.emphysemafoundation.org/Grapejuice.html.

Grapefruit juice and medications. 1997. Ask the Pharmacist. The University of Mississippi Medical Center. http://umcnews.com/askthepharmacist/grapefruitjuice.html.

Grapefruit juice can interact with medications. 1999. Harvard Heart Letter. Harvard Medical School. http://www.mylifepath.com/article/iac/100059316.

Grapefruit juice effect. 1997. http://pharminfo.com/pubs/msb/gfj_effect.html.

Griffiths, Slade. 1999. *Digitalis (digoxin, lanoxin).* In: Cowley College's Emergency Medicine Formulary. http://www.kcmetro.cc.mo.us/pennvalley/emt/digox.htm.

Guidelines for the audiologic management of individuals receiving cochleotoxic drug therapy. 1994. American Speech-Language-Hearing Association. 36(3), Supplement No. 12.

Hain, Timothy. 1999. *Bilateral vestibulopathy and ototoxicity.* Northwestern University Medical School. http://www.cscd.nwu.edu/public/balance/bilateral.html.

Hain, Timothy. 2001a. *Gentamicin toxicity.* http://www.tchain.com/otoneurology/disorders/bilat/gentamicin%20toxicity.htm.

Hain, Timothy. 2001b. *Ototoxic medications.* http://www.tchain.com/otoneurology/disorders/bilat/ototoxicns.html.

Halmagyi, C. M., et al. *Gentamicin vestibulotoxicity.* 1994. Otolaryngology and Head and Neck Surgery. 111(5):571-4.

Halmagyi, C. M., et al. 1995. *Ototoxicity.* http://www.bme.jhu.edu/labs/chb/disorders/abototox.html.

Haybach, Patty J. 1999. *Balance and hearing: At risk from drugs.* Course #170. http://nurse.cyberchalk.com/nurse/COURSES/NURSEWEEK/NW170/menu.html.

Haybach, Patty J. 1998. *Ototoxicity for nurses.* http://www.geocities.com/otolithic/ototox.htm.

Haybach, Patty J. 1996. *Ototoxicity.* http://www.vestibular.org/ototox.html.

Helal, Amal. 1997. *Aminoglycoside ear drops and ototoxicity.* Canadian Medical Association Journal. 156(7).

Hendrix, Robert A. & Grant A. Berry. 2001. *The effects of pollution on hearing and balance.* http://members.aol.com/tiermensch/pollutionhearing.html.

Homatropine hydrobromide. 2000. InteliHealth. http://www.intelihealth.com/IH/ihtIH/WSIHW000/19689/11509/213982.html.

Hormone-replacement Therapy Causes Hearing Loss, Study Finds. Sept. 9, 2006. http://www.medicalnewstoday.com/articles/51301.php.

House, Dr. John. 2008. *House vs. House: Vicodin Addiction and Hearing Loss*. Sept. 20, 2008. ABC News. http://a.abcnews.com/Health/PainNews/story?id=5841784&page=1.

Hull, Jeffrey W, Dr. 2000. *Nystagmus*. http://www.drhull.com/EncyMaster/N/nystagmus.html.

Inner Ear. 2001. Section 7, Chapter 85, Merck Manual. http://www.merck.com/pubs/mmanual/section7/chapter85/85j.htm.

InteliHealth. 2001. Harvard Medical School's Consumer Health Information. http://www.intelihealth.com.

International retail prices for prescription drugs. 2001. http://e-pharmacy.md/generics_Q-Z.html.

Iqbal, S. M., et. al. 1999. *Metronidazole ototoxicity—report of two cases*. Journal of Laryngology & Otology. 113 (4): pp. 355-357. http://journals.cambridge.org/action/displayAbstract?fromPage=online&aid=1047676

It's not pulp fiction: Taking medications with grapefruit juice may increase their potency. January 22, 1996. http://www.med.umich.edu/opm/newspage/grapefru.htm.

Jaeger, Christina. 2001. *Hearing loss turned into deafness*. Los Angeles Times. 10 September.

Janes, Malisa, Rh.D. 2000. Personal communication.

Kafetzis, D. A., et al. 1999. *Isepamicin versus amikacin for the treatment of acute pyelonephritis in children*. International Journal of Antimicrobial Agents. 14 (2000).

Kalinec, Federico, Ph.D. 2010. Personal communication. House Ear Institute. Los Angeles, CA.

Kalkanis, James. 2001. *Inner ear—Ototoxicity*. eMedicine. 2(7). http://www.emedicine.com/ent/topic699.htm.

Kanda, Yukihiko, and Kohichiro Shigeno. 1994. *Sudden hearing loss associated with interferon*. Lancet. 343(8906):1134-5.

Kaufman, Orin, D.O. 1997. *Ototoxic medications: Drugs that can cause hearing loss and tinnitus*. Hearing Rehabilitation Quarterly. 22(2). http://www.lhh.org/hrq/22-2/ototoxic.htm.

Kaufman, Orin, D.O. 1998 *Ototoxic drugs*. NYSA of SHHH, Inc. http://www.netprocorp.com/shhhh/nys/fall98/art4.htm.

Keeley, Paul, et. al. Dec. 23, 2000. *Hear My Song: Auditory Hallucinations with Tramadol Hydrochloride*. British Medical Journal. http://articles.findarticles.com/p/articles/mi_m0999/is_7276_321/ai_69057220.

Ketek. 2004. Aventis Pharmaceuticals. http://www.aventis-us.com/PIs/ketek_TXT.html.

Kilpatrick, Jefferson, et al. 2000. *Low-dose oral methotrexate management of patients with bilateral Meniere's disease*. ENT: Ear, Nose & Throat Journal. 79(2):82-88.

Kumar, Dinesh. 1998. *Drugs that can cause deafness*. UNI. 12 November. http://www.tribuneindia.com/98nov12/punjab.htm.

Kumar, V. and O. Tandon. 1997. *Neurotoxic effects of rubber factory environment. An auditory evoked potential study*. Department of Physiology, University of Medical Sciences, Delhi, India. Electromyogr. Clin. Neurophysiol. 37(8):469-73.

Lacidipine. 1994. Electronic Doctor. Zambia. http://www.edoc.co.za/medilink/actives/557.html.

Lariam (Mefloquine) Info. 2005. http://www.indiana.edu/~primate/lariam.html.

Lawford, R. & Sorrell, T. C. 1994. *Amebic abscess of the spleen complicated by Metronidazole-induced neurotoxicity: case report*. Clin. Infect. Dis. 19 (2) pp. 346-348. http://www.ncbi.nlm.nih.gov/pubmed/7986915.

Lead. 1990. Agency for Toxic Substances and Disease Registry. Atlanta, GA. http://www.atsdr.cdc.gov/ToxProfiles/phs8817.html.

Lederfen Tablets. 1994. Lederle Laboratories, Cyanamid House, Gosport, Hampshire, England. http://www.itri.bton.ac.uk/projects/pills/corpus/Wyeth:Lederfen_Tablets.

Lercanidipine Hydrochloride. 2004. Tiscali. http://www.tiscali.co.uk/lifestyle/healthfitness/health_advice/netdoctor/archive/100003985_2.html.

Lidocaine helps relieve ringing in the ears. 2000. Reuters Health. 19 May.

Lotemax. 2007. Bausch & Lomb GmbH. Electronic Medicines Compendium. http://emc.medicines.org.uk/emc/assets/c/html/DisplayDoc.asp?DocumentID=20686.

Lyos, Andrew. 1992. *Ototoxicity*. The Bobby R. Alford Department of Otorhinolaryngology and Communicative Sciences. Grand Round Archives. http://www.bcm.tmc.edu/oto/grand/82092.html.

Mannitol. 2001. Delmar, a division of Thompson Learning. http://www.nursespdr.com/members/database/ndrhtml/mannitol.html.

Matheson Tri-Gas, Inc. 2001. *Material Safety Data Sheet for product 00202883*. Parsippany, N. J. http://www.mathesongas.com/msds/CarbonMonoxideCarbonDioxideLessthan3000ppmPropane.htm.

McIntyre, P. B. 1997. *Dexamethasone reduces hearing loss in childhood Hib meningitis and in pneumococcal meningitis when given early*. JAMA. 278:925-31.

McPheeters, Harold, M.D. 1999-2001. Personal communication.

Medications That Can Cause Tinnitus, 2007. Yahoo Health. http://health.yahoo.com/ency/ healthwise/aa147614.

Medizine: *Benorylate*. 2001. http://www.cix.co.uk/~cyberville/medizine/benoryla.htm.

Medline Plus Health Information. 2001. Micromedex, Inc. http://www.nlm.nih.gov/ medlineplus/druginfo/drug_Aa.html.

Medroxyprogesterone acetate. 2001. The CancerBACUP Factsheet. http://www.cancerbacup. org.uk/info/medroxyprogesterone.htm.

Medscape. 1998-2010. Medscape from WebMD. http://www.medscape.com.

Menthol Toxicology. 2000. http://goodhealth.freeservers.com/MentholToxicology.htm.

Mercola, Joseph. 2004. *Aspartame: What You Don't Know Can Hurt You*. http://www. mercola.com/article/aspartame/dangers.htm.

Mercury. 1999. ToxFAQ. Agency for Toxic Substances and Disease Registry. Atlanta, GA. http://www.atsdr.cdc.gov/tfacts46.html.

Methylene chloride. 1993. ToxFAQ. Agency for Toxic Substances and Disease Registry. Atlanta, GA. http://www.atsdr.cdc.gov/tfacts14.html.

Minocha, Anil, MD. June 9, 2010. *Don't Let Heartburn Turn Deadly*. In: Bottom Line Secrets.

Mintz, Morton. 1979. *Upjohn's Shuck and Jive Routine*. http://www.motherjones.com/ mother_jones/N79/mintz.html.

Monte, Woodrow C. 1984. *Aspartame: Methanol and the public health*. Journal of Applied Nutrition. 36(1). http://www.dorway.com/monte84.txt.

Morata, Thais C., and Derek E. Dunn. 1994. *Occupational exposure to noise and ototoxic organic solvents*. Archives of Environmental Health. 49(5):359.

Morioka, Ikuharu and Mototsugu Kuroda. 1999. *Evaluation of organic solvent ototoxicity by the upper limit of hearing*. Archives of Environmental Health. 54(5):341.

MSDS n-Butanol. 1998. Union Carbide Chemicals and Plastics Tech. Corp. http://arpltd. com/n-butano.htm.

MSDS Heptane. 1998. Mallinckrodt Baker, Inc. http://www.jtbaker.com/msds/h0584.htm.

Namenda Tablets. 2003. Forest Pharmaceuticals, Inc. St. Louis, MO 63045. www.namenda.com.

National Toxicology Program. 2001. Chemical Health and Safety Data. National Institutes of Health's National Institute of Environmental Health Sciences (NIEHS) located in Research Triangle Park, NC. http://ntp-server.niehs.nih.gov/Main_Pages/Chem-HS.html.

New Grapefruit Juice—Drug Interactions Found. 1998. Clinical Pharmacology and Therapeutics. 64:286-288. http://www.nutritionfarm.com/health_news/1998/grapefruit.htm.

Niall, Paul. 1998. *The effects of industrial ototoxic agents and noise on hearing*. University College, London, England. http://www.racp.edu.au/afom/nlii9907.htm.

Nitrazepam. 2000. C Health Drug Database. http://www.mediresource.net/canoe/health/DrugInfo.asp?BrandNameID=341.

Nivadil. 2001. Fujisawa Pharmaceutical Co., Ltd. 4-7, Doshomachi 3-chome, Chuo-ku, Osaka, Japan.

Noise and Hearing Loss. 1990. National Institutes of Health Consensus Development Conference Statement. January 22-24. http://isis.nlm.nih.gov:80/nih/cdc/www/76txt.html.

Nursing 2010 Drug Handbook. 30th Anniversary Edition. 2010. Wolters Kluwer—Lippincott Williams & Wilkins. Ambler, PA 19002.

Occupational Safety and Health Guideline for Heptane. 1999. Occupational Safety and Health Administration, U.S. Department of Labor. http://www.osha-slc.gov/SLTC/healthguidelines/heptane/recognition.html.

Odkvist, Lars, Claes Moller, and Karl-Ake Thuomas. 1992. *Otoneurologic disturbances caused by solvent pollution*. Otolaryngology-Head and Neck Surgery. 106(5).

Oghalai, John. 1996. *Ototoxicity*. The Bobby R. Alford Department of Otorhinolaryngology and Communicative Sciences. Grand Round Archives. Baylor College of Medicine. Houston, Texas. http://www.bcm.tmc.edu/oto/grand/42596.html.

O'Hara, Jane. 1998. *Whistle-blower*. Maclean's. (November 16):64-68.

Omeprazole (Prilosec) OPDA Post-marketing Safety Review. 2000. Department of Health and Human Services, Public Health Service, Food and Drug Administration. NDA #19-810. http://www.fda.gov/ohrms/dockets/ac/00/backgrd/3650b1b_tab_05.pdf.

Oransky, Ivan & Jeanne Lenzer. 2002. *Ties to drug manufacturers deform medical reviews*. In: USA Today. August 1. p. 11A.

Otology. 1991. Chapter 8: Otorhinolaryngology: Section I. In: United States Naval Flight Surgeon's Manual. Third Edition. Clinical ENT. http://www.vnh.org/FSManual/08/02Otology.html.

Panimycin injection. 1998. Meiji Seika Kaisha, Ltd. 2-4-16, Kyobashi, Chuo-ku, Tokyo 104-8002, Japan. http://www.jpma.or.jp/jpr/PDF/MEIJIS08.PDF.

Parikh, Rajesh. January, 2000. *Newer Drugs in Cardiology*. In: Bombay Hospital Journal Special Issue on Family Medicine. Vol. 42, No. 1. http://www.bhj.org/journal/2000_4201_jan00/SP_75.HTM.

Paromomycin-oral. 2001. First DataBank, Inc. San Bruno, CA. http://personalmd.com/drgdb/9254.htm.

PDR for Nonprescription Drugs, Dietary Supplements, and Herbs. 29th Edition. 2008. Thompson Healthcare, Inc. Montvale, NJ 07645-1725.

PDR for Nonprescription Drugs, Dietary Supplements, and Herbs. 30th Edition. 2009. Thompson Reuters. Montvale, NJ 07645-1725.

Phenylpropanolamine (PPA) information page. 2001. Center for Drug Evaluation and Research. U.S. Food and Drug Administration. http://www.fda.gov/cder/drug/infopage/ppa/default.htm.

Physicians' Desk Reference. 51st Edition. 1997. Medical Economics Company, Inc. Montvale, NJ 07645-1742.

Physicians' Desk Reference. 54th Edition. 2000. Medical Economics Company, Inc. Montvale, NJ 07645-1742.

Physicians' Desk Reference. 54th Edition. Supplement A. 2000. Medical Economics Company, Inc. Montvale, NJ 07645-1742.

Physicians' Desk Reference. 56th Edition. 2002. Medical Economics Company, Inc. Montvale, NJ 07645-1742.

Physicians' Desk Reference. 57th Edition. 2003. Thompson PDR. Montvale, NJ 07645-1742.

Physicians' Desk Reference. 61st Edition. 2007. Thompson PDR. Montvale, NJ 07645-1725.

Physicians' Desk Reference. 62nd Edition. 2008. Thompson Healthcare, Inc. Montvale, NJ 07645-1725.

Physicians' Desk Reference. 63rd Edition. 2009. Physicians' Desk Reference, Inc. Montvale, NJ 07645-1725.

Physicians' Desk Reference. 64th Edition. 2010. PDR Network, LLC. Montvale, NJ 07645-1725.

Physicians' Desk Reference. 2001. On-line version. Medical Economics Company, Inc. Montvale, NJ 07645-1742. http://physician.pdr.net/physician/index.htm.

Physicians' Desk Reference for Herbal Medicines. 2nd Edition. 2000. Medical Economics Company, Inc. Montvale, NJ 07645-1742.

Physicians' Desk Reference for Herbal Medicines. 4th Edition. 2007. Thompson Healthcare, Inc. Montvale, NJ 07645-1725.

Physicians' Desk Reference. for Nonprescription Drugs and Dietary Supplements. 23rd Edition. 2002. Thompson Medical Economics. Montvale, NJ 07645-1742.

Physicians' Desk Reference for Ophthalmic Medicines. 30th Edition. 2002. Medical Economics Company, Inc. Montvale, NJ 07645-1742.

Piretanide (potassium depletion). 1994. Electronic Doctor. Zambia. http://www.edoc.co.za/medilink/actives/826.html.

Popular medication also causes hearing loss. 1991. Nutrition Health Review. (Winter).

Potassium gluconate. Generic Online Pharmacy. 2004-2009. http://tarnow.oaza.pl/laskowa/images/avatars/bug/Potassium-Gluconate.html.

Preservex. 1995. Bristol-Myers Squibb Pharmaceuticals Limited. England. http://www.itri.bton.ac.uk/projects/pills/corpus/Bristol-Myers-Squibb::Preservex_Tablets.

Priest, Lisa. 2009. *Chemotherapy's link to hearing loss found.* The Globe and Mail. Canada. November 8, 2009. http://www.theglobeandmail.com/news/national/chemotherapys-link-to-hearing-loss-found/article1355986/.

Priuska, Eric, and Jochen Schacht. 1997. *Mechanism and prevention of aminoglycoside ototoxicity: Outer hair cells as targets and tools.* ENT: Ear, Nose & Throat Journal. 76(3):164.

Procain. 2001. Sopharma Bulgaria. http://www.bpg.bg/sopharma/categories/418/41812procaine.html.

Procardia (Nifedipine) Capsules. 2002. MedWatch-February 2002 Safety-Related Drug Labeling Changes. http://www.fda.gov/medwatch/SAFETY/2002/Feb02.htm.

Product Information—Stilnox. 2002. Sanofi-Synthelabo Australia Pty Limited. New South Wales, Australia. http://www.sanofi-synthelabo.com.au/pdf/Stilnox PI 1002.pdf.

Prograf. 2002. Fujisawa. http://www.fujisawa.com/medinfo/pi/pi_page_pg.htm.

Public health assessment: Dupage County Landfill (Blackwell Forest Preserve) Warrenville, Dupage County, Illinois. 1997. Agency for Toxic Substances and Disease Registry. Atlanta, GA. http://www.atsdr.cdc.gov/HAC/pha/dupage/dup_p2.html.

Public health assessment: Hipps Road Landfill, Jacksonville, Duval County, Florida. 1995. Agency for Toxic Substances and Disease Registry. Atlanta, GA. http://www.atsdr.cdc.gov/HAC/pha/hipps/hip_p2c.html.

Public health assessment: Miami County Incinerator, Troy, Miami County, Ohio. 1997. Agency for Toxic Substances and Disease Registry. Atlanta, GA. http://www.atsdr. cdc.gov/HAC/pha/miami/mia_p2.html.

Public health assessment: Nyanza Chemical Waste Dump, Ashland, Middlesex County, Massachusetts. 1994. Agency for Toxic Substances and Disease Registry. Atlanta, GA. http://www.atsdr.cdc.gov/HAC/pha/nyanza/ncw_p2.html.

Questions about CDER. 2001. U.S. Food and Drug Administration. Center for Drug Evaluation and Research. http://fda.gov/cder/about/faq/default.htm.

Quinacrine hydrochloride. 2001. http://sparc.airtime.co.uk/bse/quinacrine.html.

Rantudil Retard. 2002. Bayer Turk Kimya San. Ltd. Istanbul. http://www.bayer.com.tr/ pharma/english/rantudilretard.html.

Recent Questions and Answers about Lotemax. 2007. Patientsville.com. http://www. patientsville.com/medication/lotemax_side_effects.htm.

Reinberg, Steven. October 17, 2003. *Secondhand Smoke May Damage Infants' Hearing— Mild levels of carbon monoxide impair hearing in young rats.* Health Day News. http://www.hon.ch/News/HSN/515578.html.

Rickey, Tom. 2004. *Scientists raise caution about effects of HRT on hearing.* University of Rochester Medical Center. http://www.eurekalert.org/pub_releases/2004-02/uorm-src022004.php.

Rimadyl carprofen. 2000. Animal Health, Exton, PA, a division of Pfizer Inc., NY, NY.

Roberts, Daniel, et al. 2001. *Musical Hallucinations Associated With Seizures Originating From an Intracranial Aneurysm.* Mayo Clin Proc. 2001;76:423-426. Mayo Clinic. Scottsdale, AZ.

Rofecoxib. 2010. Wikipedia. http://en.wikipedia.org/wiki/Rofecoxib.

Rosen, Elizabeth. 2001. *Noise Inducted Hearing Loss.* Grand Rounds Presentation, UTMB, Dept. of Otolaryngology. January 10, 2001. http://www2.utmb.edu/otoref/Grnds/ Hear-Loss-Noise-000110/Hear-Loss-Noise.htm.

Roxithromycin Consumer Information. 2008. http://www.rx-market.net/med/Roxithromycin. html.

RxList Monographs. 1997-2010. Neil Sandow owner. www.rxlist.com.

Rybacki, James, and James Long. 1998. *The Essential Guide to Prescription Drugs.* Harper Perennial. A Division of HarperCollins Publishers.

Rybacki, James, and James Long. 2001. *The Essential Guide to Prescription Drugs.* Harper Resource. An Imprint of Harper-Collins Publishers.

Rybacki, James. 2006. *The Essential Guide to Prescription Drugs*. Collins. An Imprint of Harper-Collins Publishers.

Rybak, Leonard. 1992. *Hearing: The effects of chemicals*. Otolaryngology-Head and Neck Surgery. 106(6):677-686.

Salicylate Content of Foods. 2007. http://www.plantpoisonsandrottenstuff.info/print/salicylates.aspx.

Salicylates. Food Intolerance Network Factsheet. Updated, June, 2010. http://www.fedupwithfoodadditives.info/factsheets/Factsalicylates2.htm#avoid.

Sagamicin injection 60. 1998. Kyowa Hakko Kogyo Co., Ltd. Japan. http://www.jpma.or.jp/jpr/PDF/KYOWA07.PDF.

Sanders, Melodie. 1997. *Drugs which can cause ototoxicity and/or tinnitus*. Extracted from the database "Micromedex Computerized Clinical Information System/DRUGDEX System" of Drug Evaluation Monographs/Adverse Drug Reactions Index. Baylor Health Sciences Library. Dallas, TX.

Schacht, Jochen. 1997. *Common drugs may prevent antibiotic-induced deafness*. Ann Arbor, MI. http://pslgroup.com/dg/3c296.htm.

Shachtman, Noah. December 19, 2003. *Pop a Pill, Save Your Hearing?* Wired News. http://www.wired.com/news/medtech/0,1286,61646,00.html.

Shea, John J., Jr. 1994. *Streptomycin perfusion of the labyrinth through the round window plus intravenous streptomycin*. Otolaryngologic Clinics of North America. 27(2):317-324.

Shearer, Catherine. 1991. *Living with a hearing loss, Level III*. Student notes.

Shearer, Catherine. 1994. *Ototoxic (harmful to the ear) drugs*. Mimeographed class notes.

Shemesh, Zecharya. 2001. *List of drugs which may cause tinnitus*. Hadassah Department of Laryngology. Israel. http://www.hadassah.org.il/hmo/tinnitus/tinnitus_14_1_faq_drugs.htm.

Shlafer, Marshal. 2000. *Ototoxic drugs*. University of Michigan Medical School. http://www-personal.umich.edu/~mshlafer/ototox.html.

Shochat, Guy, MD. 2001. *Toxicity, carbon monoxide*. eMedicine Journal. 2(5). http://www.emedicine.com/EMERG/topic817.htm.

Side effects caused by Roxithromycin. 2008. http://www.roxithromycin.com/roxithromycin_sideeffects.

Silverman, Harold M. 2000. *The Pill Book*. 9th Edition. Bantam Books. New York, NY.

Snow, James B. and Philip A. Wackym. 2008. *Ballenger's Otorhinolaryngology Head and Neck Surgery*, 17th edition. Pmph. USA.

Soh, K. 1999. *Noise is a public health and social problem in Singapore*. Singapore Med. J. 40(9). http://www.sma.org.sg/smj/4009/articles/4009e2.html.

Staab, Dr. Wayne J. 1991. *The Rexton guide to better hearing*. 512 East Canterbury Lane, Phoenix, Arizona 85022.

Stanten, Michele. 1996. *150 secrets to erase the signs of aging*. Rodale Press. Emmaus, PA.

Statement of principles concerning tinnitus. 1986. Department of Veterans' Affairs. Australia. http://www.dva.gov.au/pensions/statemnt/f034bp.htm.

Stedman's Medical Dictionary. 2000. 27th Edition. Lippincott Williams & Wilkins. Baltimore, Maryland.

Strain, George M. 1996. *Aetiologies of deafness*. School of Veterinary Medicine. Louisiana State University. http://www.lsu.edu/deafness/aetiologies.htm.

Sumatriptan. 2009. Daily Med. http://dailymed.nlm.nih.gov/dailymed/drugInfo. cfm?id=9285.

Suss, Elaine. 1993. *When the hearing gets hard*. Insight Books. Plenum Press. New York.

Suter, Alice. 1991. *Noise and its effects*. Administrative Conference of the United States. November. http://www.nonoise.org/library/suter/suter.htm.

Symptoms attributed to aspartame in complaints submitted to the FDA. 1995. http://aspartametruth.com/92symptoms.html.

Synapause-E3. 2003. South African Electronic Package Inserts. http://home.intekom.com/pharm/donmed/synap-e3.html.

Tange, R. A., W. A. Dreschler, and R. J. van der Hulst. 1985. *The Importance of high-tone audiometry in monitoring for ototoxicity*. Arch. Otorhinolaryngol. 242(1).

Teicoplanin (antibiotic). 1997. Electronic Doctor. http://www.edoc.co.za/medilink/actives/978.html.

Teicoplanin sodium. 1997. JBC Handbook. 4th edition. http://members.ozemail.com.au/~jamesbc/pages/drugs/227.htm.

Toluene. 1995. ToxFAQ. Agency for Toxic Substances and Disease Registry. Atlanta, GA. http://www.atsdr.cdc.gov/tfacts56.html.

Top 200 Prescriptions. 2001. RxList. The Internet Drug Index. http://www.rxlist.com/top200.htm.

Top 200 Prescriptions. 2008. RxList. http://www.rxlist.com/script/main/hp.asp.

Trivedon-20 Tablets. 2004. Cipla. http://www.cipla.com/ourproducts/04/trivedon.htm.

Troost, B. Todd, and Melissa A. Walker. 1998a. *Drug induced vestibulocochlear toxicity.* In: Iatrogenic Neurology. Butterworth-Heinman. Boston. http://ivertigo.net/ototoxicity/otcochlear.html.

Troost, B. Todd, and Melissa A. Walker. 1998b. *Drug induced vestibulocochlear toxicity.* In: Iatrogenic Neurology. Butterworth-Heinman. Boston. http://ivertigo.net/ototoxicity/otvestibular.html.

Troost, B. Todd, and Melissa A. Walker. 1998c. *Drug induced vestibulocochlear toxicity.* In: Iatrogenic Neurology. Butterworth-Heinman. Boston. http://ivertigo.net/ototoxicity/otgentamicin.html.

Troost, B. Todd, and Melissa A. Walker. 1998d. *Drug induced vestibulocochlear toxicity.* In: Iatrogenic Neurology. Butterworth-Heinman. Boston. http://ivertigo.net/ototoxicity/otother.html.

Trudexa, Annex 1, Summary of Product Characteristics. 2009. EMEA (European Medicines Agency). http://www.emea.europa.eu/humandocs/PDFs/EPAR/trudexa/H-482-PI-en.pdf.

UAB Study Examines Hearing Loss, Viagra Use. May 17, 2010. University of Alabama at Birmingham. (Reported from findings published in the May 18, 2010 issue of the Archives of Otolaryngology-Head and Neck Surgery).

United States Pharmacopeia. 1998 Edition. 1997. *Complete Drug Reference.* Consumer Reports. A Division of Consumers Union. Yonkers, New York.

United States Pharmacopeia. 2001 Edition. 2001. *Complete Drug Reference.* Micromedex Thompson Healthcare & U.S. Pharmacopeia. Consumer Reports. A Division of Consumers Union. Yonkers, New York.

Use of CellCept (Mycophenolate mofetil) associated with increased pregnancy loss and congenital malformations, Oct. 29, 2007. FDA bulletin. CDER MedWatch Listserv.

Venapulse tablets. 1993. South African Electronic Package Inserts. http://home.intekom.com/pharm/lennon/venapuls.html.

Vernick, David M., and Constance Grzelka. 1993. *The hearing loss handbook.* Consumer Reports Books. Yonkers, N.Y.

Vestibular Apparatus. 2000. Chapter 8. In: Hearing and balance; the inner ear. Department of Neurophysiology. University of Wisconsin-Madison. http://www.neurophys.wisc.edu/~ychen/textbook/chap-7.html.

Vestibular frequently asked questions. 1995. The Johns Hopkins School of Medicine. http://www.bme.jhu.edu/labs/chb/faq/faq.html

Vetbase: List of drugs. 2000. Dutch Veterinary Information Systems. Graafschap 7, Utrecht, The Netherlands. http://www.vetinfo.demon.nl/drugs.htm.

Veterinary Formulary. 2001. Research Animal Resources. University of Minnesota. http://www.ahc.umn.edu/rar/umnuser/formulary.html.

Waltermire, Richard, R. Ph., MS. 1998. *Direct-to-customer advertising of RX drugs can be harmful to your health.* From Drug benefit trends. http://www.medscape.com/SCP/DBT/1998/v10.n10/ d5637.watt/d5637.watt.html. p. 1.

WebMDHealth. 2001. *Genetics of hearing loss.* DNA Sciences Article. http://my.webmd.com/content/article/3204.675.

What is a serious adverse event? 2001. MedWatch. The FDA Medical Products Reporting Program. http://www.fda.gov/medwatch/report/DESK/ADVEVNT.HTM.

White, Linda, MD and Steven Foster. 2000. *The Herbal Drugstore.* Rodale Inc.

Wikipedia. 2010. http://en.wikipedia.org.

Wingert, Pat and Barbara Kantrowitz. 2006. *Listen Up, Women—It's true that women hear better than men. But new research suggests that one female hormone may actually hurt their hearing.* Newsweek, 9/12/2006. http://msnbc.msn.com/id/14789510/site/newsweek.

Wolfe, Sidney, M.D. 2010. *Frequently Asked Questions.* Public Citizen—Worst Pills, Best Pills. http://www.worstpills.org/public/page.cfm?op_id=49#five.

WorkPro. 1999. Southeastern Ohio Regional Medical Center. http://www.seormc.org/workpro/newsletters/august_99.htm.

Worst Pills Best Pills News. September, 2007.

Xylene. 1990. Public Health Statement. Agency for Toxic Substances and Disease Registry. Atlanta, GA. http://www.atsdr.cdc.gov/ToxProfiles/phs9030.html.

Yagi, M. et al. 1999. *Rescue of hair cells from aminoglycoside ototoxicity by adenoviral-mediated over-expression of GDNF.* Kresge Hearing Research Institute. Abstract #243. http://www.aro.org/archives/1999/243.html.

Yorgason, Joshua, et al. 2010. *Acetaminophen ototoxicity after acetaminophen/Hydrocodone abuse: Evidence from two parallel in vitro mouse models.* Otolaryngology—Head and Neck Surgery, 2010 Jun, 142 (6): 814-819.

Zanidip Product Information. 2005. Solvay Pharmaceuticals. http://www.pbs.gov.au/pi/smpzanid31205.pdf.

Zolpidem (Oral Route, Oromucosal Route), 2009. MayoClinic.com. http://www.mayoclinic.com/health/drug-information/DR601839/DSECTION-side-effects.

Zuger, Abigail. 1997. *How grapefruit juice makes some pills more powerful*. The New York Times on the Web. October 7. wysiwyg://105/http://www.geocities.com/CollegePark/Quad/5442/grapefruit.htm.

Good Books on Hearing Loss

Integrity First Books in the series:

Everything You Wanted to Know About Your Hearing Loss But Were Afraid to Ask

(Because You Knew You Wouldn't Hear the Answers Anyway!)

by Neil G. Bauman, Ph.D.

If you enjoyed this book and would like to learn more about hearing loss and how you can successfully live with it, you may be interested in the other helpful books in this series by Dr. Neil. Each book is packed with the things you need to know in order to thrive in spite of your various hearing loss issues. The direct link for ordering the following books is http://hearinglosshelp.com/shop/category/books/.

Ototoxic Drugs Exposed—The Shocking Truth About Prescription Drugs, Medications, Chemicals and Herbals That Can (and Do) Damage Our Ears ($52.45; eBook $39.95)

This book, now in its third edition, reveals the shocking truth that many prescription drugs can damage your ears. Some drugs slowly and insidiously rob you of your hearing, cause your ears to ring or destroy your balance. Other drugs can smash your ears in one fell swoop, leaving you with profound, permanent hearing loss and bringing traumatic change into your life. Learn how to protect your ears from the ravages of ototoxic drugs and chemicals. Describes the specific ototoxic effects of 877 drugs, 35 herbals and 148 chemicals (798 pages).

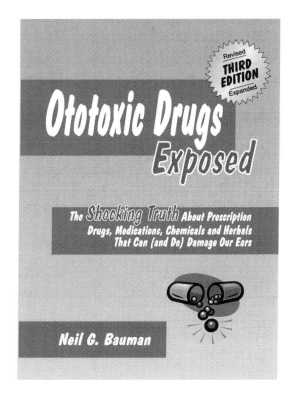

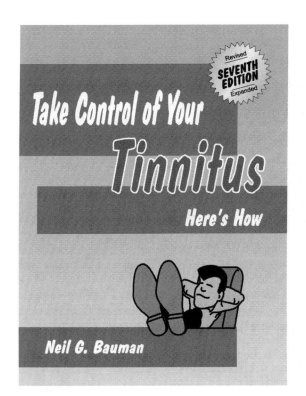

Take Control of Your Tinnitus—Here's How
($29.95; eBook $22.99)

If your ears ring, buzz, chirp, hiss, click or roar, you know just how annoying tinnitus can be. The good news is that you do not have to put up with this racket for the rest of your life. You can take control of your tinnitus. Recent studies show that a lot of what we thought we knew about tinnitus is not true at all. Exciting new research reveals a number of things that you can do to eliminate or greatly reduce the severity of your tinnitus so that it no longer bothers you. This totally-revised, up-to-date and expanded 7th edition contains the very latest in tinnitus research and treatment. In this book you will learn what tinnitus is, what causes tinnitus and things you can do to take control of your tinnitus (356 pages).

Phantom Voices, Ethereal Music & Other Spooky Sounds ($22.49; eBook $16.99)

When you realize you are hearing phantom sounds, you immediately think that something has gone dreadfully wrong "upstairs"—that you are going crazy. Because of this, few people openly talk about the strange phantom voices, music, singing and other spooky sounds they hear. This book, the first of its kind in the world, lifts the veil on "Musical Ear syndrome" and reveals numerous first-hand accounts of the many strange phantom sounds people experience. Not only that, it explains what causes these phantom sounds, and more importantly, what you can do to eliminate them, or at least, bring them under control (178 pages).

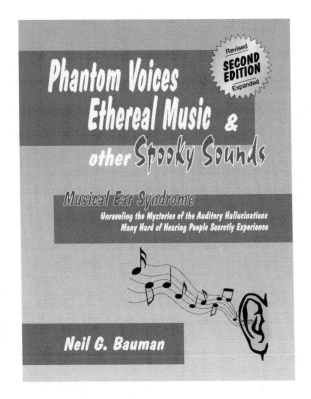

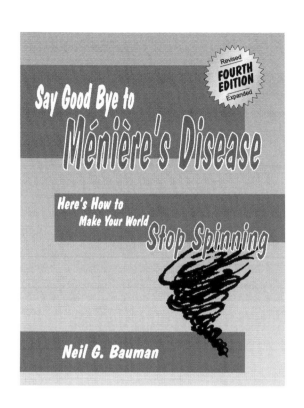

Say Good Bye to Ménière's Disease—Here's How to Make Your World Stop Spinning ($21.95; eBook $16.49)

Ménière's disease is one of the more baffling and incapacitating conditions a person can experience. If you suffer from your world spinning, have a fluctuating hearing loss, tinnitus and a feeling of fullness in your ears, this book is for you. It details what Ménière's disease is like; explains the recent breakthrough into the underlying cause of Ménière's; and shows you how, at last, you can be free from the ravages of this debilitating condition. Each page is packed with practical information to help you successfully conquer your Meniere's disease. Join the hundreds and hundreds of people whose worlds have now stopped spinning (128 pages).

Keys to Successfully Living with Your Hearing Loss ($19.97; eBook $15.49)

Do you know: a) the critical missing element to successfully living with your hearing loss? b) that the No. 1 coping strategy hard of hearing people instinctively use is wrong, wrong, wrong? c) what the single most effective hearing loss coping strategy is? d) how you can turn your hearing aids into awesome hearing devices? This book addresses the surprising answers to these and other critical questions. Applying them to your life will put you well on the road to successfully living with your hearing loss (84 pages).

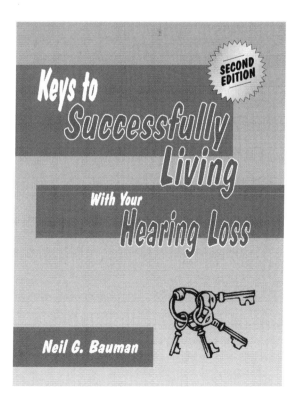

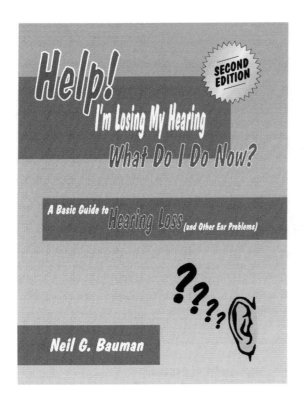

Help! I'm Losing My Hearing—What Do I Do Now? ($18.95; eBook $14.49)

Losing your hearing can flip your world upside down and leave your mind in a turmoil. You may be full of fears, wondering how you will be able to live the rest of your life as a hard of hearing person. You don't know where to turn. You lament, "What do I do now?" Set your mind at rest. This easy to read book, written by a fellow hard of hearing person, is packed with the information and resources you need to successfully deal with your hearing loss and other ear conditions (116 pages).

Grieving for Your Hearing Loss—The Rocky Road from Denial to Acceptance ($12.95; eBook $9.95)

When you lose your hearing you need to grieve. This is not optional—but critical to your continued mental and physical health. This book leads you through the process of dealing with the grief and pain you experience as a result of your hearing loss. It explains what you are going through each step of the way. It gives you hope when you are in the depths of despair and depression. It shows you how you can lead a happy vibrant life again in spite of your hearing loss. This book has helped many (56 pages).

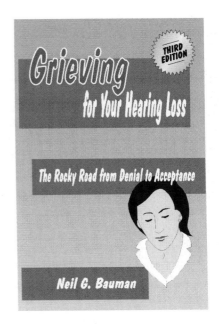

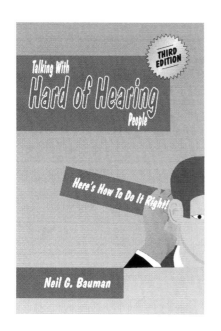

Talking with Hard of Hearing People—Here's How to Do It Right! ($9.95; eBook $7.95)

Talking is important to all of us. When communication breaks down, we all suffer. For hard of hearing people this happens all the time. This book is for you—whether you are hearing or hard of hearing! It explains how to communicate with hard of hearing people in one-to-one situations, in groups and meetings, in emergency situations, and in hospitals and nursing homes. When you use the principles given in this book, good things will happen and you will finally be able to have a comfortable chat with a hard of hearing person (38 pages).

When Hearing Loss Ambushes Your Ears— Here's What Happens When Your Hearing Goes on the Fritz ($14.95; eBook $11.95)

Hearing loss often blind-sides you. As a result, your first step should be to learn as much as you can about your hearing loss; then you will be able to cope better. This most interesting book explains how your ears work, the causes of hearing loss, what you can expect to hear with different levels of hearing loss and why you often can't understand what you hear. Lots of audiograms and charts help make things clear. You will also discover a lot of fascinating things about how loud noises damage your ears (88 pages).

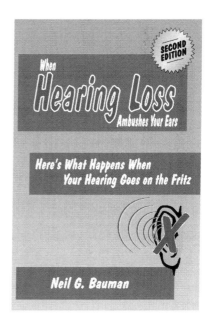

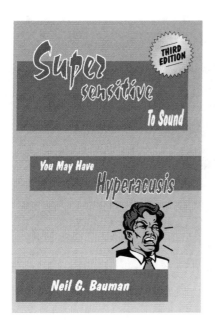

Supersensitive to Sound? You May Have *Hyperacusis* ($9.95; eBook $7.95)

If some (or all) normal sounds seem so loud they blow your socks off, this is the book you want to read! You don't have to avoid noise or lock yourself away in a soundproof room. Exciting new research on this previously baffling problem reveals what you can do to help bring your hyperacusis under control (42 pages).

Here! Here! You and Your Hearing Loss/ You and Your Hearing Aids ($12.95; eBook $10.95)

Part I of this book contains a series of my newspaper articles on hearing loss such as, "Hear Today. Gone Tomorrow?" "Hearing Loss Is Sneaky!" "The Wages of Din Is Deaf!" "When Your Ears Ring..." "Get In My Face Before You Speak!" "How's That Again?" "Being Hard of Hearing Is Hard" "I'm Deaf, Not Daft!" Part II contains articles on hearing aids such as, "You Better Watch Out..." "Before Buying Your First Hearing Aid..." "Please Don't Lock Me Away in Your Drawer" "Good-bye World of Silence!" "Becoming Friends with Your Hearing Aids" "Two's Better Than One!" (56 pages).

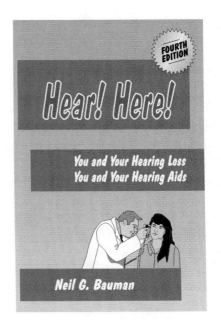

You can order any of the foregoing books/eBooks (plus you can read more than 1,000 helpful articles about hearing loss and related issues) from the
Center for Hearing Loss Help
web site at
http://hearinglosshelp.com
or order them from the address below

Center for Hearing Loss Help

1013 Ridgeway Drive,
Lynden, WA 98264-1057
Phone: (360) 778-1266
FAX: (360) 389-5226
E-mail: info@hearinglosshelp.com
Web site: http://hearinglosshelp.com

Made in the USA
Columbia, SC
29 September 2019